LABORATORY PROCEDURES FOR VETERINARY TECHNICIANS

LABORATORY PROCEDURES FOR VETERINARY TECHNICIANS

THIRD EDITION

Edited by

Paul W. Pratt, VMD

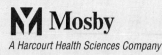

Mosby

A Harcourt Health Sciences Company

St. Louis   London   Philadelphia   Sydney   Toronto

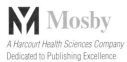

A Harcourt Health Sciences Company
Dedicated to Publishing Excellence

Vice President and Publisher: Don Ladig
Executive Editor: Linda L. Duncan
Developmental Editors: Jo Salway and Melba Steube
Project Manager: John Rogers
Senior Production Editor: Helen Hudlin
Book Designer: Yael Kats
Manufacturing Manager: Linda Ierardi

THIRD EDITION
Copyright © 1997 by Mosby, Inc.

Previous editions copyrighted 1985 and 1992 by American Veterinary Publications, Inc.

Printed in the United States of America

Mosby, Inc.
11830 Westline Industrial Drive
St. Louis, Missouri 63146

Library of Congress Cataloging-in-Publication Data

Laboratory procedures for veterinary technicans / edited by Paul W.
   Pratt.—3rd ed.
      p.   cm.
   Includes bibliographical references and index.
   ISBN 0-8151-7326-1
   1. Veterinary clinical pathology—Laboratory manuals.
   2. Veterinary medicine—Laboratory manuals.   I. Pratt, Paul W.
SF772.6.L36
636.089'60756—dc20   96-43451

00   01   /   9   8   7   6   5   4

Contributors

Joann L. Colville, DVM
Associate Professor
Department of Veterinary and
  Microbiological Sciences
North Dakota State University
Fargo, North Dakota

**Rick L. Cowell, DVM, MS, Dipl
ACVP**
Professor of Veterinary Clinical
  Pathology
Department of Veterinary Pathology
Oklahoma State University
College of Veterinary Medicine
Stillwater, Oklahoma

Bernard F. Feldman, DVM, PhD
Professor of Clinical Hematology
  and Biochemistry
Department of Biomedical Sciences
  and Pathobiology
Virginia-Maryland Regional College
  of Veterinary Medicine
Virginia Polytechnic Institute and
  State University
Blacksburg, Virginia

Rafael Ruiz de Gopegui, DVM, PhD
Assistant Professor
Department of Pathology and
  Animal Production
Veterinary Faculty of Barcelona
Autonomous University of Barcelona
Bellaterra (Barcelona), Spain

Charles M. Hendrix, DVM, PhD
Associate Professor
Department of Pathobiology
Auburn University
College of Veterinary Medicine
Auburn University, Alabama

Eloyes Hill, MT (ASCP)
Research Specialist II
Department of Veterinary and
  Microbiological Sciences
North Dakota State University
Fargo, North Dakota

PETER J. IHRKE, VMD, DIPL ACVD
Professor of Dermatology
Department of Medicine and
    Epidemiology
University of California
School of Veterinary Medicine
Davis, California

MUHAMMED IKRAM, DVM, MSc, PhD
Coordinator
Department of Animal Health
    Technology
Fairview College
Fairview, Alberta, Canada

BRUCE W. PARRY, BVSc, PhD, DIPL ACVP
Senior Lecturer
Department of Veterinary Science
University of Melbourne
Director of Veterinary Clinic and
    Hospital
University of Melbourne
Werribee, Victoria, Australia

ALBERT C. STRAFUSS, DVM, PhD
Professor Emeritus
Kansas State University
College of Veterinary Medicine
Manhattan, Kansas

MARY ANNA THRALL, BA, DVM, MS, DIPL ACVP
Professor
Department of Pathology
Colorado State University
College of Veterinary Medicine and
    Biomedical Sciences
Fort Collins, Colorado

M. GLADE WEISER, DVM, DIPL ACVP
Professor
Department of Pathology
Colorado State University
College of Veterinary Medicine and
    Biomedical Sciences
Fort Collins, Colorado

JOSEPH G. ZINKL, DVM, PhD, DIPL ACVP
Professor of Clinical Pathology
Department of Pathology,
    Microbiology, and Immunology
University of California
School of Veterinary Medicine
Davis, California

PREFACE

Veterinary practice has changed markedly in the 12 years since publication of the first edition of this text, especially with regard to the practice laboratory. The laboratory of many veterinary practices at that time consisted of a piecemeal collection of instruments for the most basic laboratory examinations. Technicians, and many veterinarians, were often not well trained to use and maintain those few laboratory instruments.

Today, technologically advanced and modularized instruments, inexpensive and rapid test kits, state-of-the-art assays, and a higher level of technician education have made laboratory procedures an important part of most veterinary practices, both diagnostically and financially.

NEW TO THIS EDITION

With each new edition we have strived to improve this book. Changes in this third edition include:

- All sections have been updated according to recent advances in laboratory technology and clinical practice.
- Color illustrations have been added to the chapter on Hematology to aid in identification of blood cells.
- Illustrations have been upgraded and enlarged.
- The graphic presentation has been improved for ease of reading.
- The protocols for many laboratory procedures have been highlighted in boxed summaries for rapid review.
- Information on Cytologic Examination now appears as a separate chapter.
- The chapters on Function Tests and Serology and Immunology include information on sophisticated assays now available from referral laboratories and new in-office test kits.
- The index has been expanded for more easy location of topics.

ACKNOWLEDGMENTS

I am grateful to our group of highly respected contributors, who have diligently revised their sections to reflect the most current standards of excellence in clinical pathology and laboratory medicine. I am also indebted to my colleagues at Mosby–Year Book, Linda Duncan, Jo Salway, and Melba Steube, whose careful planning and oversight minimized the gray hairs I might have otherwise sprouted during production of this book. Finally, I thank the veterinary technicians, technician educators, and veterinary clinicians whose thoughtful suggestions have helped us improve this book with each new edition.

PAUL W. PRATT, VMD

CONTENTS

LABORATORY PROCEDURES FOR VETERINARY TECHNICIANS

THE VETERINARY PRACTICE LABORATORY

one

J. Colville

Our understanding of the information we can gain from laboratory tests has increased greatly over the last few decades. Veterinarians depend on laboratory results to help establish diagnoses, track the course of diseases, and offer prognoses to clients. Many veterinarians routinely request presurgical laboratory screening tests to help identify "at risk" patients before general anesthesia.

Even with the availability of large commercial veterinary reference laboratories, some practices must still wait 2 or 3 days for results. At times, especially when dealing with a critically ill animal, the veterinarian needs laboratory test results much more rapidly. At other times, only one value is sought, and it is not practical to send the sample to a reference laboratory for a single test. Reference laboratories offer panels or batteries of tests that are most useful as screening tests, but these typically are not readily available for immediate or emergency analyses. Such tests as CBCs, fecal examinations, skin scrapings and urinalyses are more economically performed in-house than sending them to a reference laboratory. For these reasons, many veterinarians have purchased or leased analytic instruments for routine in-house testing.

Veterinary practice laboratories are more common and sophisticated today than they were 15 years ago. The availability of educated veterinary technicians to set up and operate the laboratories has played a major role in development of in-house diagnostic systems. Increased availability of affordable analytic instruments has made the purchase of these instruments economically feasible for veterinary practitioners. As practice laboratories become more sophisticated, the list of assays performed by veterinary technicians becomes longer and veterinary technicians become more indispensable in the practice.

ROLE OF THE VETERINARY TECHNICIAN

The veterinary technician/veterinarian team approach works very efficiently in a laboratory situation. A veterinarian is trained to interpret test results, while a veterinary technician is trained to generate these results. It takes an educated veterinary technician to consistently generate reliable laboratory results. A veterinary technician must understand the value of quality control in the laboratory. It is easy for a person without the educational background to follow "cookbook" instructions, but a veterinary technician must be prepared to make educated decisions if something goes wrong or to recognize a test result that is out of the ordinary.

GENERAL CONSIDERATIONS

Although each veterinary practice is unique, every practice laboratory must meet four criteria.

DEDICATED AREA

A specific area should be designated as the laboratory. This area can range from a dedicated space on a counter, to an entire room, depending on the physical facility. The area should be out of the main flow of traffic in the practice but easily accessible when needed. Room temperature controls should provide a constant environment, which in turn provides for optimal quality control. A draft-free area is preferable to one with open windows or with air conditioning or heating ducts blowing air on the area. Drafts can carry dust, which can contaminate specimens and interfere with test results.

SINK

The laboratory area needs a sink and a source of running water. This provides a place to rinse, drain, or stain specimens and reagents and to discard fluids.

STORAGE SPACE

Adequate storage space must be available for reagents and supplies. This keeps them from cluttering the laboratory counter space. Some reagents and specimens must be kept refrigerated or frozen. A refrigerator/freezer should be readily available. A compact countertop refrigerator is sufficient for most practice laboratories. *Note:* Frost-free freezers remove fluid from frozen samples, making them more concentrated if they are left in the freezer too long. For long-term storage of fluid samples (serum, plasma, etc.), use a chest freezer or freezer that is not self-defrosting.

ELECTRICAL OUTLETS

Consider placement of electrical equipment. Take extreme care to ensure that sufficient electrical outlets and circuit breakers are available. Do not overload circuits with ungrounded 3-prong adaptors or extension cords. Avoid working with fluids around electric wires or instruments.

EQUIPMENT AND INSTRUMENTATION

The size of the veterinary practice and the tests routinely performed in the laboratory determine the equipment and instrumentation needed. Minimal equipment includes a microscope, refractometer, microhematocrit centrifuge, and tabletop centrifuge. Additional instrumentation, including blood chemistry analyzers, cell counters, incubators, and microbiology and parasitology equipment, depends on the type and size of the practice, geographic locale of the practice, and the special interests of practice personnel.

MICROSCOPE

A good compound light microscope is essential, even in the smallest laboratory. It can be used to evaluate blood, urine, semen, exudates, and transudates; other body fluids; feces; and other miscellaneous specimens. It also can be used to detect internal and external parasites and to initially characterize bacteria.

By definition, a compound light microscope consists of two separate lens systems: the ocular system and the objective system.

The *ocular lens system* is located in the eyepiece(s) and most often has a magnification of 10X. This means that the ocular lens magnifies an object 10 times. A monocular microscope has one eyepiece, while a binocular microscope, the most commonly used type today, has two eyepieces.

Most compound light microscopes have three or four *objective lenses,* each with a different magnification power. The most common objective lenses are 4X (scanning), 10X (low power), 40X (high dry) and 100X (oil immersion). The scanning lens is not found on all microscopes. An optional fifth lens, a 50X (low oil immersion), is found on some microscopes.

Total magnification of the object being viewed is calculated as the ocular power times objective power. For example, an object viewed under the 40X objective is 400 times larger in diameter than the unmagnified object (10X ocular lens times 40X objective lens equals 400X total magnification).

When viewed through a compound light microscope, an object appears upside down and reversed. The actual right side of an image is seen as its left side, and the actual left side is seen as its right side. Movement of the slide by the mechanical stage is also reversed. When you move the stage to the left, the object appears to move to the right.

Figures 1-1 and 1-2 show the parts of a compound light microscope. The *ocular lens system* and the *objective lens system* have already been discussed. The *optical tube length* is the distance between the objective lens and the eyepiece. In most microscopes this distance is 160 mm. The mechanical *stage* holds the slide being evaluated. It contains an assembly to move the slide smoothly so one can evaluate numerous sections of the slide. *Coarse and fine focus knobs* are used to focus the image of the object being viewed.

The substage *condenser* consists of two lenses that focus light from the light source on the object being viewed. Light is focused by raising or lowering the condenser. Without a substage condenser, haloes and fuzzy rings appear around the object. The *iris (aperture) diaphragm* consists of a number of leaves that are opened or closed to control the amount of light illuminating the object.

In modern microscopes, the *light source* is contained within the microscope itself (Figure 1-3). A transformer controlled by a rheostat controls the intensity of the light entering the condenser. If a *field diaphragm* is contained in the light source, it can be used to focus the light entering the condenser. Older microscopes used an external light source and a mirror to project rays of light from the light source to the condenser system. For instructions in the use of a microscope see Procedure 1-1.

The financial investment in a good-quality compound light microscope is offset by the potential income-generating analyses the practice can perform with the instrument. The initial price of the microscope is important but so also is the quality of the microscope.

A poor-quality microscope may sit unused on the laboratory bench because of inferior performance and frequent down time for repairs. Durability and the

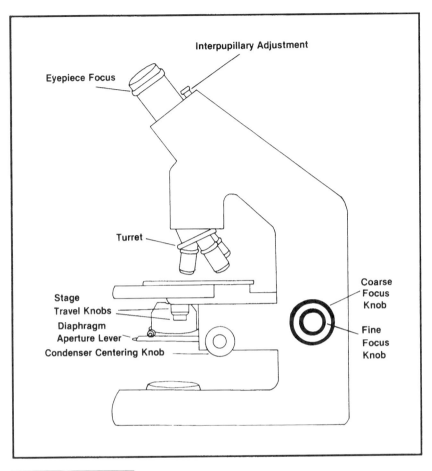

FIGURE 1-1. Components of a compound microscope.

availability of repair service with replacement or loaner microscopes must be considered. A microscope that must be sent away for repair is of no value to the practice.

Microscope prices vary, depending on quality and accessories included. The best microscope for an average practice is most often neither the most expensive nor the least expensive one. The quality of the microscope purchased depends partly on the special interests of practice personnel. For example, if a veterinarian has a special interest in cytology, the practice should purchase a better-quality microscope than a practice that sends all of its hematologic and cytologic samples to a reference laboratory. Such accessories as phase-contrast or darkfield capabilities, cameras, and lighted pointers add to the price but also

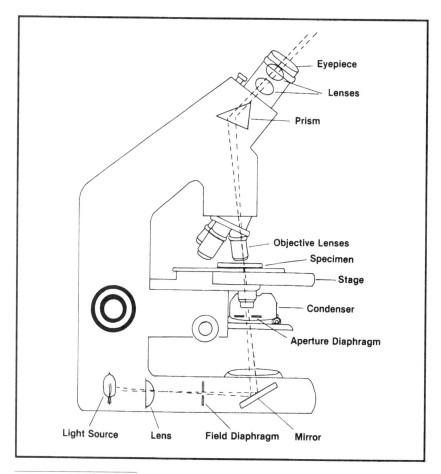

FIGURE 1-2. Light path through a compound microscope.

increase the versatility of the microscope. Reconditioned microscopes are sometimes available through medical or optical equipment suppliers.

CARE AND MAINTENANCE

Only lens paper or a soft brush should be used to clean the lenses and eyepieces. Lens paper is designed for this purpose and will not scratch the lenses.

Remove dust, smudges, marks or fingerprints with gauze, lens paper, or a soft brush.

Remove oil from the oil-immersion objective with lens paper each time the objective is used. Any oil left on the objective will seep into the inside of the lens.

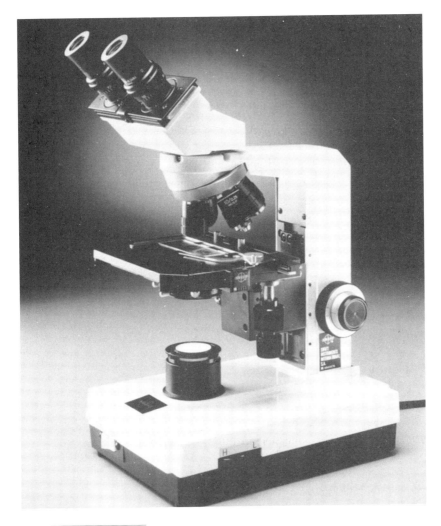

Figure 1-3. Modern binocular microscope. (Courtesy Swift Instruments.)

Use xylene, methanol, ethanol, or commercial lens cleaner sparingly. Because of the solvent qualities of the solutions, with time they may loosen the adhesive that holds the lens in place. Xylene is carcinogenic and ethanol is a controlled substance. Also, methanol, ethanol, and xylene are flammable and toxic.

Keep extra light bulbs on hand. To change a light bulb, turn off the power and unplug the microscope. When the defective bulb has cooled, remove it, and replace it with a new bulb, following the manufacturer's instructions. Use only identical replacement bulbs.

PROCEDURE 1-1. Microscope operating procedures

1. Lower the stage to its lowest point.
2. Turn on the light.
3. Inspect the eyepieces, objectives, and condenser lens and clean as necessary. (Consult the manufacturer's operating manual for any special cleaning instructions.)
4. Place the slide or counting chamber on the stage, appropriate side up.
5. Move the 10X objective into position by turning the turret, not the objective lens.
6. Looking through the eyepieces, adjust the distance between them so that each field appears nearly identical, and the two fields can be viewed as one.
7. Using the coarse and fine focus knobs, bring the image into focus.
8. Adjust the condenser and diaphragms according to the manufacturer's instructions. This allows you to take full advantage of the microscope's resolving power.
9. When using the **40X (high-dry) objective:**
   • Look for a suitable examination area using the 10X (low-power) objective.
   • Swing the high-dry objective into place.
   • Do not use oil on the slide when using the high-dry objective.
10. When using the **100X (oil-immersion) objective:**
    • Locate a suitable examination area using the 10X (low-power) objective.
    • Place a drop of oil on the slide.
    • Swing the oil-immersion objective into place.
11. When finished:
    • Turn the light off.
    • Lower the stage completely.
    • Swing the 4X or 10X objective into place.
    • Remove the slide or counting chamber.
    • Clean the oil-immersion lens, if necessary.

If the field of study appears dirty, the cause may be debris on the eyepiece. Rotate the eyepieces one at a time while looking through them. If the debris also rotates, it is located on the eyepiece. Clean the eyepiece with lens paper or a soft brush.

Locate the microscope in an area where it will not have to be moved frequently and where it will not be jarred by vibrations from centrifuges or slamming doors or be splashed with liquids. Keep it out of sunlight and drafts. Cover it when not in use to prevent dust from accumulating on the lenses.

Carry the microscope with both hands, one under the base and the other holding the supporting arm.

If the microscope is frequently used throughout the day, some people recommend leaving the microscope light on all day. This saves the wear and tear that occur when the light is constantly turned on and off and may extend the life of the bulb.

CENTRIFUGE

Another vital instrument in the veterinary practice laboratory is the centrifuge. It is used to separate cells and particulate matter from the fluids in which they are suspended. The centrifuged fluid (supernatant), such as plasma or serum from a blood sample, can be decanted from the particulate matter (sediment) and stored, shipped, or analyzed. Centrifuges also concentrate cells or other sediment material for analysis, as in preparation of urine or fecal sediment for analysis.

Most centrifuges encountered in veterinary laboratories are one of two types, depending on the style of the centrifuge head. A *horizontal centrifuge head,* also known as the swinging-arm type, has specimen cups that hang vertically when the centrifuge is at rest (Figure 1-4). During centrifugation, the cups swing out to the horizontal position. As the specimen is centrifuged, centrifugal force drives the particles through the liquid to the bottom of the tube. When the centrifuge stops, the specimen cups fall back to the vertical position.

This type of centrifuge has two disadvantages. At excessive speeds (>300 revolutions/min), air friction causes heat buildup. Also, there may be some remixing of the sediment with the supernatant (fluid) when the specimen cups fall back to the vertical position.

The second type of centrifuge head available is the *angled centrifuge head* (Figure 1-5). The specimen tubes are inserted through drilled holes that hold the tubes at a fixed angle, usually at about 52 degrees. This type rotates at

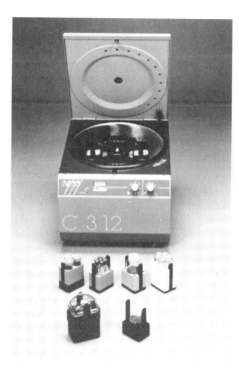

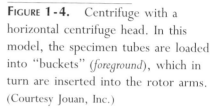

FIGURE 1-4. Centrifuge with a horizontal centrifuge head. In this model, the specimen tubes are loaded into "buckets" (*foreground*), which in turn are inserted into the rotor arms. (Courtesy Jouan, Inc.)

higher speeds than the horizontal-head centrifuge, without excessive heat buildup.

In addition to a standard *on/off switch,* most centrifuges have a *timer* that automatically turns the centrifuge off after a preset time and a *tachometer* or dial to set the speed of the centrifuge. Some centrifuges do not have a tachometer and always run at maximum speed. A centrifuge may also have a *braking device* to rapidly stop it.

Specimens must be centrifuged for a specific time at a specific speed for maximum accuracy. A centrifuge that is run too fast or for too long may rupture cells and destroy the morphology of cells in the sediment. A centrifuge that is run too slowly or for less than the proper time may not completely separate the specimen or concentrate the sediment. Information regarding speed and time of centrifugation should be developed for all laboratory procedures and should be followed for maximum accuracy.

When using a centrifuge, it must be exactly balanced. Similar tubes containing equal weights of sample should be placed in specimen cups opposite each other. Water-filled tubes may be used to balance the centrifuge.

Never operate the centrifuge with the lid unlatched.

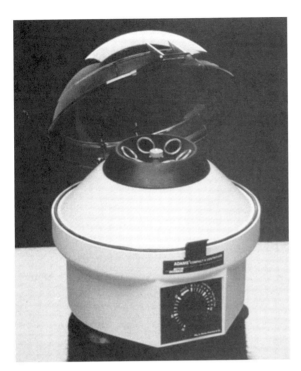

FIGURE 1-5.   Centrifuge with an angled centrifuge head. (Courtesy Becton-Dickinson.)

The centrifuge should be cleaned immediately if anything is spilled inside it. Tubes sometimes crack or break during centrifugation. Pieces of broken tubes must be removed when the centrifuge stops. If these are not removed, they could permanently damage the centrifuge.

Check the operator's manual for maintenance schedules of the different components of the centrifuge. Some centrifuges require periodic lubrication of the bearings. Others may need the brushes checked or replaced regularly. A regular maintenance schedule prevents costly breakdowns and keeps the centrifuge running at maximum efficiency.

A *microhematocrit centrifuge* (Figure 1-6) is used to separate blood cells of different densities from the plasma in which the cells are suspended. With a small blood sample collected in a microhematocrit tube, the microhematocrit centrifuge rapidly provides the packed cell volume (PCV) and a visual assessment of lipemia, hemolysis, jaundice, and leukocytosis. Plasma from the hematocrit tube may be placed in a refractometer to determine total plasma protein concentration. Using a microscope to examine the microhematocrit tube, microfilariae present can be seen in a spun hematocrit sample near the interface of the plasma and cells.

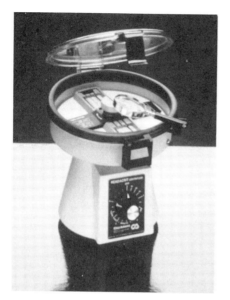

FIGURE 1-6. Microhematocrit centrifuge used to determine the packed cell volume. (Courtesy Becton-Dickinson.)

REFRACTOMETER

A refractometer, or total solids meter, is used to measure fluid specific gravity or protein concentration. The most common uses of the refractometer are determination of the specific gravity of urine or other fluids and the protein concentration of plasma or other fluids.

A refractometer is a cylindric instrument with a built-in prism and calibration scale (Figure 1-7). Refraction is bending of light rays as they pass from one medium (e.g., air) into another medium (e.g., urine) with a different optical density.

Refractometers are calibrated to a zero reading (zero refractive index) with distilled water at a temperature between 60° and 100° F.

Although refractometers measure the refractive index of a solution, scale readings in the instrument have been calibrated in terms of specific gravity and protein concentrations (g/dl). The specific gravity or protein concentration of a solution is directly proportional to its concentration of dissolved substances. Because no solution can be more dilute or have a lower concentration of dissolved substances than distilled water, the scale calibration and readings (either specific gravity or protein concentration) are always greater than zero. The refractometer is read on the scale at the distinct light-dark interface.

Various refractometer models are available. Some are temperature compensated between 60° and 100° F. As long as the temperature remains between

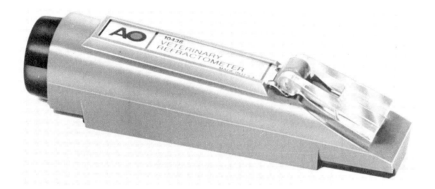

FIGURE **1-7.**   Refractometer or total solids meter. (Courtesy A.O. Reichert Scientific Instruments.)

these two extremes, even as the refractometer is held in the hands, the temperature fluctuation will not affect the accuracy of the reading.

The advantages of a refractometer over other instruments used for similar purposes are precision, accuracy, durability, simplicity of operation, moderate expense, and small required sample volume.

The specific gravity of a urine sample can be determined with just a drop of urine. This becomes significant in some renal diseases if only very small amounts of urine are available and specific gravity measurement is essential for diagnosis, prognosis, and treatment.

Similarly, the plasma protein concentration can be determined from the small amount of plasma in a spun microhematocrit tube. The tube is broken above the cell-fluid interface after reading the hematocrit, and the plasma is placed on the refractometer prism (Procedure 1-2).

PROCEDURE **1-2.**   Refractometer use

1. Inspect and clean the prism cover glass and cover plate.
2. Place a drop of sample fluid on the prism cover glass.
3. Point the refractometer toward bright artificial light or sunlight.
4. Bring the light-dark boundary line into focus by turning the eyepiece.
5. Read and record the result using the appropriate scale (specific gravity, protein).
6. Clean the refractometer following the manufacturer's recommendations.

CARE AND MAINTENANCE

The refractometer should be cleaned after each use. Wipe the prism cover glass and cover plate dry. Some manufacturers suggest cleaning the cover glass and plate with alcohol. Check the manufacturer's cleaning instructions.

The refractometer should be calibrated regularly (weekly or daily, depending on use). Distilled water at room temperature placed on the refractometer should have a zero refractive index and therefore read zero on all scales. If the light-dark boundary deviates from the zero mark by more than one-half division, adjust the refractometer by turning the adjusting screw as directed by the manufacturer's instruction manual. Do not use the refractometer if you are unable to zero it with distilled water.

CHEMISTRY ANALYZERS

Many veterinarians are purchasing their own chemistry analyzers as they become increasingly dependent on clinical chemistry data to diagnose disease and monitor therapy. Manufacturers of chemistry analyzers have become aware of the veterinary market, and a number of them now have veterinary models available, accompanied by an increasing number of analytical tests.

Although most chemistry analyzers are accurate, other factors determine their appropriateness for a veterinary practice laboratory. Ease of operation, availability of applicable tests, shelf life of reagents, technician time and skill needed or available, and degree of calibration and quality control needed should be considered before an instrument is purchased. Talking with someone who operates the same instrument in another veterinary facility is one way of evaluating a chemistry analyzer. Most sales representatives have a list of people who have purchased the instrument and can vouch for its quality. Many manufacturers offer lease programs for chemistry analyzers.

TYPES OF CHEMISTRY ANALYZERS

Photometric colorimetry (also called direct colorimetry) is based on a solution's color increasing as its concentration increases. This type of analyzer is more often used in veterinary practice laboratories than visual colorimetry analyzers.

Colorimetric instruments differ from spectrophotometers in that colorimeters use filters to separate light into wavelengths, while spectrophotometers use prisms or gratings to separate light into wavelengths. Both types of analyzers are "wet" chemistry instruments that generate light of specific wavelengths, pass the light through a liquid sample, measure the intensity of the emergent light, convert the light intensity into electrical energy, and display the electrical energy digitally or on a meter (Figure 1-8).

Several manufacturers have developed "dry" chemistry analyzers (Figure 1-9). Reagents are provided on impregnated premeasured reagent strips or pads. The sample (serum, plasma, whole blood) is placed on the reagent pad or strip and inserted into the analyzer. The analyzer reads a bar code (like a UPC symbol) to identify the assay being performed and automatically adjusts the analyzer to the proper light wavelength and temperature. The entire reaction takes place on the reagent pad or strip and usually involves a color change. These analyzers use *reflective photometric* principles to measure the concentrations of solutions being analyzed. The reagent pads or strips are solid and light cannot pass through them. The degree of color change is proportional to the solution's concentration. The analyzer measures the solution's concentration by the intensity of the light reflected from the reagent pad or strip and generates a digital reading or computer printout.

Advantages of these "dry" chemistry analyzers over "wet" chemistry analyzers are ease of operation, elimination of the necessity to handle and measure liquid reagents (a common source of error), and elimination of test tube or cuvette costs. One disadvantage may be initial purchase cost of the analyzer.

Manufacturers of wet chemistry analyzers are continuing to improve the simplicity and accuracy of their analyzers to compete with the increasingly popular dry chemistry analyzers (Figure 1-10).

Dedicated-use analyzers are available for certain tests. These analyzers sample for only one substance, such as blood glucose. They are generally found

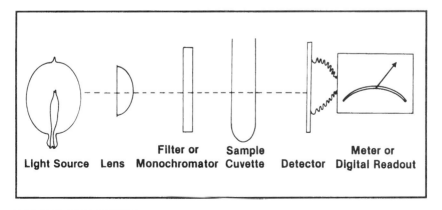

FIGURE 1-8.   Components of a spectrophotometer.

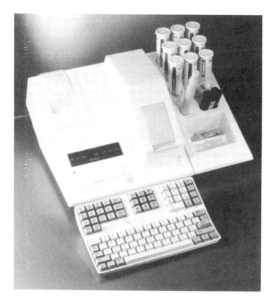

FIGURE 1-9. Reflotron System Blood Chemistry Analyzer can test samples as small as 30 µl and provide results for up to 14 assays in a few minutes. (Courtesy Boehringer Mannheim Diagnostics.)

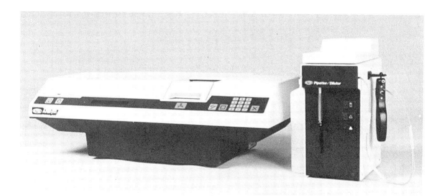

FIGURE 1-10. DuPont Analyst Blood Chemistry Analyzer provides results for up to 15 different assays in a few minutes. (Courtesy DuPont Co.)

in larger laboratories, where larger analyzers are used to run panels or batteries of tests. Dedicated analyzers can be used if only a single test is requested or in emergency situations.

INSTRUMENT USE AND CARE

Chemistry analyzers are sensitive instruments that must be carefully maintained. Follow the manufacturer's operating instructions. Instruments generally have a warmup period to allow the light source, photodetector, and incubator, if present, to reach equilibrium before they are used. It is best to turn on the instrument in the morning and leave it on all day. In this way, the instrument is ready to use at any time during the day, especially in emergency situations.

To prolong the life of the chemistry analyzer, follow the manufacturer's maintenance schedule. Set up a schedule sheet for each instrument in the laboratory (Figure 1-11). At a glance you can review the maintenance history of an instrument.

Most manufacturers have a toll-free number to call if trouble arises.

Electronic cell counters

Just as chemistry analyzers have become more affordable and available in veterinary laboratories, so also have electronic cell counters used in veterinary hematology. A number of electronic cell counters used in human medical laboratories have been adapted to veterinary use. This adaptation was necessary because of the variation in blood cell size among different animal species. Some companies have developed dedicated veterinary multispecies hematology systems that not only count cells but also determine the hematocrit, hemogloblin concentration, MCHC, a partial WBC, and platelet count.

Types of electronic cell counters

An *impedance counter* counts cells by measuring the cells' ability to alter electric resistance as they pass through a small aperture. Two electrodes are placed in an electrically conductive diluent. A bridge with a small aperture is placed between the two electrodes. Cells to be counted are suspended in the diluent and drawn through the aperture. The concentration of cells and the size of the aperture ensure that most cells pass through the aperture singly. Horse, goat, and sheep blood must be diluted more than the blood of other species because of their characteristically high red blood cell counts.

When a cell passes through the aperture, it decreases, or impedes, the electrical flow between the two electrodes. The instrument electronically counts the impedances and reports them as counted cells. The degree of impedance (measured as a voltage pulse) is proportional to the cell volume, so the counter can distinguish cell types based on the varying cell volumes. Most impedance counters have threshold cell size settings that allow the instrument to exclude cells or particles below the threshold setting in the cell count. It is important in a veterinary practice to have a cell counter with an adjustable

(1997) Day	Tech	Clean printhead (weekly)	Check light source (monthly)	Clean and inspect thermocuvette (monthly)	Check linearity (monthly)	Clean syringe (monthly)	Change purge valve tubing (every 2 mos)	Change O rings (annually)	Other
January									
January									
January									
January									
February									
February									
February									
February									
March									
March									

FIGURE 1-11.   Maintenance schedule can be prepared for each instrument so that maintenance procedures are not overlooked.

threshold that can accommodate varying red and white blood cell sizes among different animal species.

Impedance counters provide red blood cell, white blood cell, and platelet counts, along with mean corpuscular volume. They use the number of red blood cells per unit volume to calculate the hematocrit.

Darkfield illumination counters measure cell numbers by detecting light diffraction as a cell passes through a light beam. These counters produce a microscopic focal point of light. The cells are uniformly suspended in solution and drawn singly through the focal point of light. When the light hits a cell, it is measurably diffracted. This diffraction sets up an impulse that is used to electronically count the cells. Darkfield counters are not discriminating enough to measure mean cell volumes.

Some newer electronic cell counters use a laser light beam. They use the same principles as the darkfield counters, but also can determine mean cell volumes.

Multifunctional instruments combine either impedance or darkfield illumination counters with photometric capability to measure hemoglobin concentration. Additionally, they may be programmed to calculate the mean corpuscular hemoglobin and mean corpuscular hemoglobin concentration.

When white blood cell or platelet counts are performed, a lysing solution is added to the blood sample to destroy red blood cells so they do not interfere with the counts. When red blood cell counts are performed, white blood cells and platelets also are counted, but their numbers are so few as compared with red blood cells that they normally are not a significant source of error. Error due to presence of white blood cells is usually less than 1%. An elevated white blood cell count may elevate the reported red blood cell count using an electronic cell counter.

ADVANTAGES, SOURCES OF ERROR

Electronic cell counters offer a fast, reliable method for determining cell counts. They minimize technician error and require decreased technician time to provide results. Several manufacturers offer cell counters with variable threshold settings needed for veterinary hematology. Some of these instruments have preset thresholds for different species (QBC VetAutoread System, Idexx Laboratories; Cell-Dyn 3500, Abbott Diagnostics; Mascot Multispecies Hematology Systems, CDC Technologies). Depending on the degree of sophistication desired, the initial cost of an electronic cell counter can range from less than a thousand dollars to thousands of dollars.

Electronic cell counters do have problems. Voltage fluctuations may cause undetectable errors. Pumps, tubing and valves must be maintained. Diluting fluid and dusty glassware may be contaminated with particles large enough to be counted. The aperture may become partially or totally obstructed. The threshold setting may be improperly set on a counter with a variable threshold control.

Cold agglutinins may cause a decreased red blood cell count because of cell clumping. Before processing, make sure refrigerated blood samples are warmed to room temperature. Fragile lymphocytes, as seen with some lymphocytic leukemias, may rupture in the lysing solution used to lyse red blood cells. This can result in a decreased white blood cell count. The presence of spherocytes may alter the mean corpuscular volume, thus reducing the calculated hematocrit. Elevated serum viscosity may interfere with cell counts.

MAINTENANCE

Electronic cell counters, like chemistry analyzers, are sophisticated instruments that require careful maintenance. Follow the manufacturer's recommendations for routine maintenance. Daily maintenance for many electronic cell counters requires flushing the entire system with bleach and fresh diluting solution to keep the aperture open. Background counts are done periodically to make sure the diluting solution is not contaminated or the glassware and tubing are not dirty. The vacuum pump must be checked at regular intervals to make sure the proper amount of blood and diluting fluid is being drawn into the counter.

QUALITY CONTROL

One of your responsibilities as a veterinary technician in a clinical laboratory is to provide accurate results of your analyses. The various steps performed to ensure this accuracy are collectively known as *quality control* or *quality assurance*.

INSTRUMENT QUALITY CONTROL

A well-planned and carefully executed quality-control program entails evaluation of equipment performance, the technician's analytic skills, and variation of results obtained by different technicians performing the same test.

Depending on the chemistry analyzer or electronic cell counter in your laboratory, you will use a number of solutions in your quality-control program. *Control serum* consists of pooled freeze-dried serum from many patients (usually human) that must be rehydrated before use. Be careful to rehydrate these accurately. "Assayed" control serum has been analyzed repeatedly for each of the many constituents present in serum (glucose, urea nitrogen, calcium, etc.) Data are statistically analyzed and a range of acceptable values for each constituent is established. The manufacturer of the control serum provides a chart listing the *range* (lowest acceptable value to highest acceptable value obtained during the many assays) and the *mean* (average value) for each constituent.

Control serum is used for technician and instrument assessment. It is handled exactly as are patient test samples and should be regularly assayed (with each test batch, daily or weekly) at the same time patient serum samples are assayed. After the assay is completed, check to make sure the control value falls within the manufacturer's reported range. If it does not, repeat the assays of both the patient and control samples.

Control serum can be produced in your own laboratory. Serum obtained from at least 20 clinically healthy animals of one species can be pooled and analyzed numerous times in the laboratory. Data collected from these tests can be statistically analyzed to establish appropriate ranges and mean values. This procedure is very time consuming, especially for smaller laboratories. For this reason, it is much more convenient to purchase commercial control sera.

Aliquots of control serum are placed in small tubes, covered tightly, and frozen, to be used one at a time. At regular intervals (with each test batch, daily or weekly), assay one of the aliquots of control serum at the same time patient serum is assayed. Record the results of the control serum on a chart or log for each assay (Figure 1-12). The values for tests performed on control serum should not significantly vary from one time to another.

Some analytic instruments require a *blank* to prepare them for assays. A blank contains all the reagents used in the assay except the patient specimen. The instrument is adjusted to read 100% transmittance (or zero absorbance) using the blank. By "blanking" the instrument, you are in effect telling it to ignore chemicals or colors contained in the reagents that might interfere with the assay.

A *standard* is a solution containing an exact known amount of a constituent. It is used to calibrate some instruments. Many newer instruments no longer require a blank or standard for use, but control samples are required for any quality-control program.

ACCURACY, PRECISION, RELIABILITY

Accuracy, precision, and reliability are terms frequently used to describe quality control and are the premises of any quality-control program. *Accuracy*

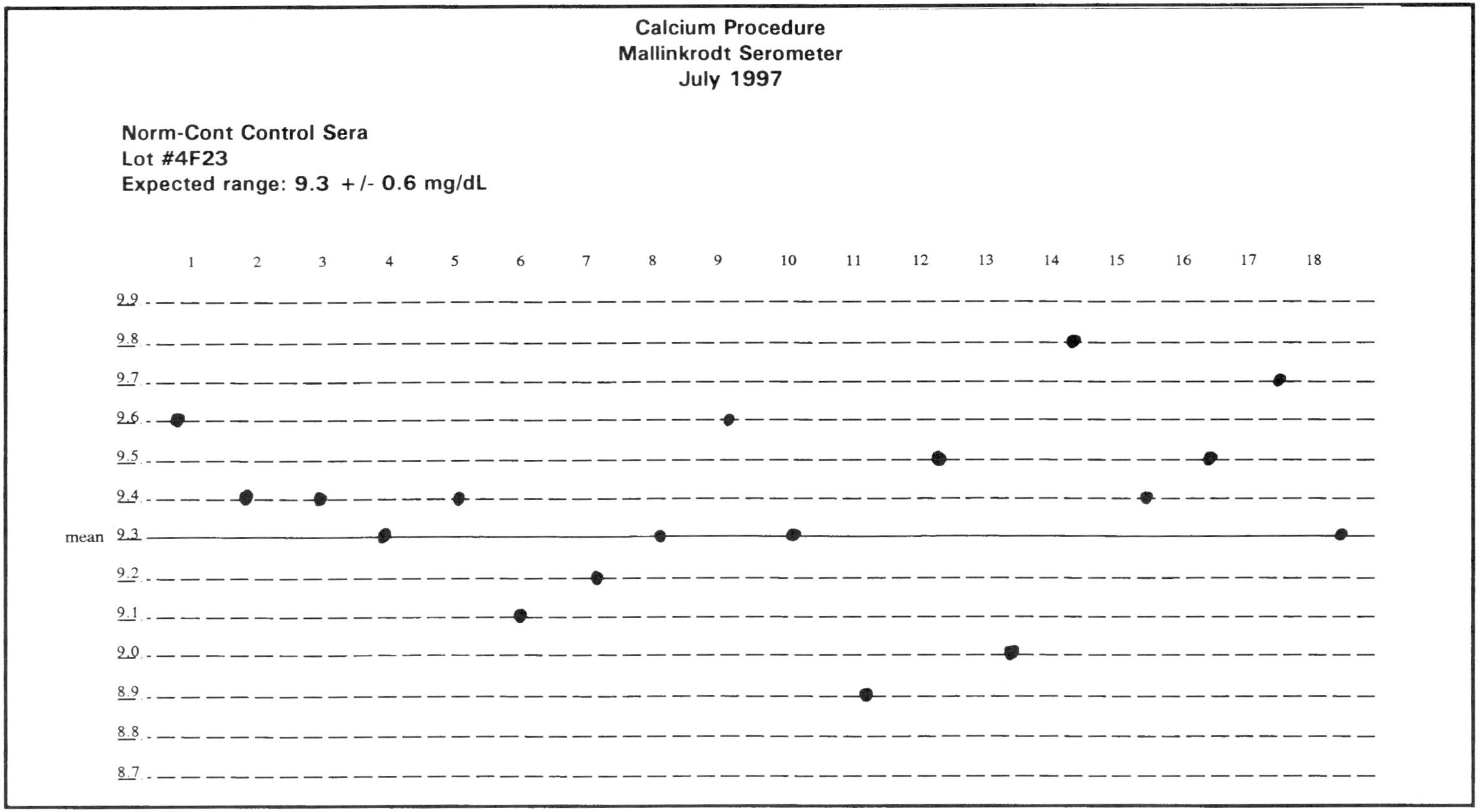
Calcium Procedure
Mallinkrodt Serometer
July 1997
Norm-Cont Control Sera
Lot #4F23
Expected range: 9.3 +/- 0.6 mg/dL
1 2 3 4 5 6 7 8 9 10 11 12 13 14 15 16 17 18
9.9
9.8
9.7
9.6
9.5
9.4
mean 9.3
9.2
9.1
9.0
8.9
8.8
8.7

FIGURE 1-12. Results of periodic quality-control tests on control samples can be charted so as to detect any deterioration in accuracy.

refers to how closely your results agree with the true quantitative value of the constituent. *Precision* is the magnitude of random errors and the reproducibility of measurements. *Reliability* is the ability of a method to be both accurate and precise.

Errors

Three types of errors are common to all systems: clerical, random, and systematic.

Clerical errors are avoidable and include incorrect labeling, delays in transporting samples, incorrect calculations, transcription errors, and sampling the wrong patient. A well-trained and conscientious staff produces very few clerical errors. Some of the most common problems related to sample handling are mislabeling and incomplete or incorrect requisition forms. All tubes, slides, and sample containers should be labeled with the patient's name (with the owner's last name), species, identification number (if available), and date.

Systematic errors cause shifts or trends in results obtained with a specific assay method. They often result in gradual changes, causing the mean value of results to shift in one direction (elevated or decreased). Some factors causing systematic errors are using inaccurate standard sera, reagent instability, and method nonspecificity (using a test method unsuitable for the constituent being assayed).

Random errors, such as variation found in glassware and pipettes, electronic and optic variations of instruments, and temperature controls and timing, occur in all parts of a system. These random errors increase the variability of results.

Applied quality control

Instrument maintenance is a must, both to prolong the life of the instrument and to prevent expensive "down time." All instruments come with an owner's manual. If the manual has been misplaced, contact the manufacturer for a replacement. The manual lists the instrument components that must be inspected and attended to regularly. A notebook listing a schedule with the types of maintenance required for each instrument facilitates instrument maintenance. Prepare a page for each instrument and include the following: instrument name, serial number, model number, purchase date, points to be checked, frequency of checks, record of test readings, changes made to restore accuracy and precision of readings, cost and time associated with necessary repairs and restoration, and the name or initials of the person performing the maintenance (Figure 1-11).

Control serum is analyzed to check the accuracy of an assay method. Some manufacturers provide a quality-control service in which "test" samples are sent to many laboratories for assay each month. The results from all the laboratories are collected and compared. From these results the manufacturer can identify laboratories with accuracy problems.

Ideally, control serum should be tested with each batch of tests run. Controls with normal and/or abnormal concentrations of constituents are run because an assay method may not perform the same at all concentrations tested by a particular method. *Normal control serum* has constituent concentrations that approximate levels normal for that constituent. *Abnormal control serum* has constituent concentrations that are either higher or lower than normal. These abnormal concentrations represent concentrations seen clinically in disease conditions. If there is an abnormal concentration of a constituent in a patient sample, the results can be trusted if the abnormal control serum concentration was assayed as "in range."

For example, a dog with uncontrolled diabetes mellitus could have serum glucose levels many times higher than the normal 91 mg/dl $\pm$ 12 mg/dl. By using an abnormal control serum that has an abnormally high glucose concentration, you can feel confident that the elevated patient glucose reading is accurate if the abnormal control serum assays are in range.

Results obtained using control serum are recorded and kept in a permanent record. It is helpful to graph results so changes or trends can be visually detected (Figure 1-12).

Data can be analyzed in two ways. You can detect shifts or trends and tell if results for control samples are within the range established by the manufacturer. If a control serum result does not fall within the range, it should be retested. If it still fails to come into range, the reagents, instrument, and your technique must be checked. When control values are successively distributed on one or the other side of the mean, there has been a shift of the mean itself and a systematic error is involved.

The frequency of control testing depends on the laboratory's goals. To ensure reliability, control samples *must* be tested when a new assay is set up, a new technician runs the test, a new lot number of reagents is used, or when an instrument is known to perform erratically. Ideally, a control sample is tested with each batch of patient samples. If you are having a problem with a particular assay, it may be wise to increase the frequency of control testing.

If attention is paid to detail and as many sources of all three types of error can be eliminated, your laboratory can provide reliable results. Sloppy, inattentive work habits can lead to diagnostic and therapeutic disasters that may result in the death of an animal. Careful attention ensures the veterinarian has all the correct information needed to make a proper diagnosis, prescribe appropriate treatment, and offer an educated prognosis.

LABORATORY RECORDS

Laboratory records are divided into internal and external record systems. Complete, up-to-date records are necessary for both systems.

INTERNAL RECORDS

Internal records are those by which the laboratory logs assay results and the methods by which they are obtained. They consist of a procedures book and quality-control data and graphs. The procedures book contains the instructions on how to perform all analyses run in the laboratory. Each procedure is described on a separate page. The easiest way to maintain the book is to insert the instruction sheets accompanying each commercial test kit in a three-ring binder, along with typewritten pages of any other procedures performed in the laboratory. Each procedure not performed with commercial kits is described on a separate typewritten page, including the name of the test, synonyms (if any) for the test, the rationale, reagent list, and step-by-step instructions for a single analysis. Individual pages can be inserted into plastic overlays for protection. The procedures book is reviewed from time to time and updated as needed.

Quality-control records are essential, as they document the reliability of assay results and identify results that may be inaccurate. In addition to logs, daily quality-control data can be depicted graphically. This allows early identification of subtle performance changes by instruments, reagents, or operators (Figure 1-12).

EXTERNAL RECORDS

External records are those by which laboratory personnel communicate with people throughout the veterinary clinic or hospital and in other laboratories.

They consist of request forms that accompany the sample to the laboratory, report forms for assay results, laboratory log books with individual test results, and a book containing pertinent information on samples sent to reference laboratories.

Information provided on the accompanying request form includes: the patient's full identification (including identification number, if available) and presenting signs; date and method used to obtain the sample; pertinent history; tests desired; any special notes regarding sample handling; and to whom and by what method results are to be reported (telephone, FAX, written report).

The report form should include complete patient identification and presenting signs, test results (appropriate units), and notation of any extraordinary observations or explanatory comments, if applicable.

For additional backup, the laboratory should keep a log book with all test results recorded in it. If the original laboratory report form is lost in transit, the results are retrievable.

SUPPLIES AND REAGENTS

PREPACKAGED SUPPLIES AND REAGENTS

When possible, buy reagents and supplies in ready-to-use form. Although the initial purchase price may be higher, ready-to-use reagents or test kits offer several advantages over reagents prepared in the laboratory. Labor costs and investments in supplies and special equipment necessary for bulk-reagent preparation are eliminated. Test kits often have reagents premeasured and packaged individually for each test, so there are fewer chances for inaccurate measurements, spoilage after opening, and contamination. Test kit reagents are often packaged to aid proper mixing of reagents and samples. Instructions included with kits are often clear and easy to follow. Finally, many kits and ready-to-use reagents are packaged in small amounts and in a manner that maximizes shelf life, so even laboratories with a small workload use the reagents before their expiration date.

PURCHASING REAGENTS AND SUPPLIES

Purchasing reagents and supplies is easy for most practices. Most veterinary pharmaceutical companies and supply houses have sales representatives who regularly visit practices in their sales territories. Many other companies have catalogs from which to order pharmaceuticals and supplies. Orders can be mailed, telephoned (usually toll-free), or FAXed to the companies, and the merchandise is shipped in a short time if items are in stock. Important points to remember when ordering are: identify your practice by name, address and account number; if applicable, state the date by which you must receive the order; specify any handling or shipping specifications; and identify each item ordered by description and catalog number, followed by the quantity desired. Write the complete order on paper before placing a telephone order. Use an up-to-date catalog provided by the supplier. The few minutes spent in preparation save telephone time and help avoid confusion that could otherwise result in an incomplete or incorrect order.

Any supplier may be temporarily out of stock or discontinue an item; therefore, it is wise to maintain active accounts with at least two veterinary supply houses.

REAGENT HANDLING AND STORAGE

It is impossible to generate consistently reliable test results with improper, inferior, outdated, or contaminated reagents. Most common problems can be avoided by observing some general guidelines. Never use outdated reagents. Do not leave containers uncapped and subject to evaporation and contamination. Store all reagents at the proper temperature. Do not expose reagents to prolonged sunlight or artificial light, which may inactivate the reagent. Avoid contamination and incorrect measurements when you prepare your own reagents.

STAINS

Clinical microscopy is a very important part of a veterinary laboratory. Because so much of microscopy depends on proper staining technique, stain quality must be maintained. Table 1-1 provides a list of stains commonly used in veterinary laboratories. Nearly all of these stains are available in ready-to-use form or in a form that requires very little preparation.

The two most common problems related to stain integrity are dye depletion in solutions and excessive precipitate accumulation in the stain solutions. Solutions should be replaced at least once a month, more often if

TABLE 1-1. Common stains and their use

STAIN	USE
Romanowsky stains (Wright's, Diff-Quik, DipStat)	General cytology and demonstration of bacteria
Gram	Demonstration of bacteria and Gram reaction
New methylene blue	General cytology, reticulocyte count, demonstration of Heinz bodies
India ink	Demonstration of *Cryptococcus neoformans*
Lactophenol cotton blue	Demonstration of fungal elements
Sudan III and IV oil-red-O	Demonstration of lipid
Iodine	Demonstration of parasites

they are heavily used. Do not add new stain to old stain; completely change the stain solution. Keep bottles tightly capped when they are not in use so as to prevent concentration changes due to evaporation. Filter the stain every few weeks. If a dip staining method is being used, the precipitate settles at the bottom of the stain container and not on the slide. Keeping the containers tightly capped when not in use also prevents contamination, colonization by microbes, and pH changes.

ITEMS REQUIRED FOR SPECIFIC TESTS

Tables 1-2 to 1-7 list, on a test-by-test basis, equipment, supplies, and reagents necessary for various laboratory procedures. Details pertaining to methodology and specific supply and reagent use are discussed throughout the remainder of this book. References listed at the end of each chapter, as well as textbooks of clinical pathology and laboratory technology, provide additional information.

TABLE 1-2. Equipment, supplies, and reagents required for hematologic tests

TEST	ITEMS NEEDED FOR PROCEDURE
WBC count	WBC/platelet Unopette (Becton-Dickinson) or diluting pipette; acetic acid; hemacytometer with coverslip; microscope; cell counter
Platelet count	WBC/platelet Unopette or diluting pipette; hemacytometer with coverslip; microscope; cell counter
Reticulocyte count	Test tube (12 × 75 mm); Pasteur pipette; pipette bulb; new methylene blue; glass slide and coverslip; microscope; cell counter
Hemoglobin concentration	Cyanide reagents; spectrophotometer; test tube (12 × 75 mm); pipette (20 ml)
Hematocrit	Microhematocrit reader; microhematocrit centrifuge; microhematocrit tubes; sealing clay
Protein (total solids)	Refractometer; microhematocrit centrifuge; microhematocrit tubes; single-edge razor blade
Plasma fibrinogen	56° C heating block or water bath; microhematocrit tubes; single-edge razor blade; microhematocrit centrifuge; refractometer; test tube
Differential cell count	Glass slide; hematologic stain; phosphate buffer; distilled water; microscope; cell counter
Crossmatch	Centrifuge; saline; test tubes (12 × 75 mm); Parafilm; wooden applicator stick; 37° C heating block; refrigerator; glass slide with coverslip; microscope
Erythrocyte sedimentation rate	Sedimentation stand; Wintrobe tubes; 9¾" Pasteur pipettes; clock
Bone marrow evaluation	Microscope; glass slide with coverslip; stain
Bleeding time	Lancet or scalpel; stopwatch; filter paper; clippers; gauze sponge
Lee-White clotting time	Syringe (5 ml); needle (20 ga); 3 test tubes (12 × 75 mm); 37° C water bath
Fibrin degradation products	Thrombo-Wellco test kit (Wellcome); test tubes (12 × 75 mm)

TABLE 1-3. Equipment, supplies, and reagents required for urinalysis

TEST	ITEMS NEEDED FOR PROCEDURE
Rapid test strip (dipstick) analyses	Reagent test strips; test tube
Protein concentration	Test tube (12 × 75 mm); 3% sulfosalicylic acid; Pasteur pipette with bulb
Occult blood detection	Reagent test strip; blood tablet test kit
Bile detection	Bile tablet test kit; Pasteur pipette
Urobilinogen detection	Reagent test strip
Sediment examination	Test tube (12 × 75 mm); centrifuge; Pasteur pipette with bulb; glass slide with coverslip; stain
Glucose concentration (reducing method)	Reagent tablet; test tube (12 × 75 mm)

TABLE 1-4. Equipment, supplies, and reagents required for parasitologic tests

TEST	ITEMS NEEDED FOR PROCEDURE
Fecal flotation	Magnesium sulfate; zinc sulfate; test tube (16 × 100 mm); strainer; paper cup; distilled water; centrifuge; glass slide with coverslip; wooden applicator stick; microscope; micrometer; cell counter
Ectoparasite evaluation	Potassium hydroxide; glass slide with coverslip
Microfilariae detection by modified Knott's method	Distilled water; 37% formaldehyde; Parafilm; new methylene blue; conical tube; 1-ml pipette; graduated cylinder; centrifuge; glass slide with coverslip; microscope; micrometer
Microfilariae detection by microhematocrit method	Microhematocrit tube; microhematocrit centrifuge; microscope
Microfilariae detection by glass slide examination	Glass slide with coverslip; microscope
Microfilariae detection by filtration method	Filtration test kit; glass slide with coverslip; microscope

TABLE 1-5. Equipment, supplies, and reagents required for fecal analysis

TEST	ITEMS NEEDED FOR PROCEDURE
Parasite detection	See Table 1-4
Occult blood detection	Blood table test kit; distilled water; Pasteur pipette with bulb; glass slide
Fiber content	Applicator stick; Pasteur pipette with bulb; glass slide with coverslip; microscope
Qualitative fat content	Applicator stick; Pasteur pipette with bulb; glass slide with coverslip; Sudan or oil-red-O stain; distilled water; acetone; glacial acetic acid; 70% ethanol; Bunsen burner or alcohol lamp; microscope
Trypsin activity	Radiographic film or gelatin; test tube (16 × 100 mm); pipette (9 ml); 37° C heating block or water bath; distilled water; sodium bicarbonate; refrigerator

TABLE 1-6. Equipment, supplies, and reagents required for serologic and immunologic tests

TEST	ITEMS NEEDED FOR PROCEDURE
Coombs' test	37° C heating block or water bath; refrigerator; test tubes (12 × 75 mm); species-specific Coombs' reagent (Miles Labs); 0.9% saline; glass slide with coverslip; microscope; centrifuge
LE cell detection	Strainer; beaker (100 ml); test tube (16 × 100 mm); 37° C heating block or water bath; Wintrobe tube; 9¾" Pasteur pipette with bulb; glass slide with coverslip; hematologic stain; microscope
Rheumatoid factor detection	Test kit; slide agglutination plate
Canine brucellosis test	Test kit; slide agglutination plate
Feline leukemia virus test	Test kit; Pasteur pipette with bulb
Canine heartworm antigen test	Test kit

TABLE 1-7. Equipment, supplies, and reagents required for bacteriologic and myco-logic tests

TEST	ITEMS NEEDED FOR PROCEDURE
Gram-stained slide examination	Glass slide with coverslip; Gram's stain; distilled water; fixative or Bunsen burner; microscope
Dermatophyte detection	Wood's lamp
Microscopic detection of dermatophytes	Glass slide with coverslip; 15% potassium hydroxide; alcohol lamp or Bunsen burner; microscope
Microscopic detention of systemic fungi	Glass slide with coverslip; 15% potassium hydroxide; lactophenol cotton blue stain; microscope
Aerobic culture	Bunsen burner or alcohol lamp; inoculation loop; agar plates; 37° C incubator
Fungal culture	Sabouraud's agar or Dermatophyte Test Medium (Pitman-Moore)

REFERENCES

1. Tietz: *Fundamentals of clinical chemistry,* ed 2, Philadelphia, 1982, WB Saunders.

2. Henry: *Clinical diagnosis and management by laboratory methods,* ed 17, Philadelphia, 1984, WB Saunders.

3. Bologna: *Understanding laboratory medicine,* St Louis, 1971, Mosby.

4. Jain: *Schalm's veterinary hematology,* ed 4, Philadelphia, 1986, Lea & Febiger.

5. Wintrobe: *Clinical hematology,* ed 8, Philadelphia, 1981, Lea & Febiger.

6. *Operator's manual for the Reflotron system.* Indianapolis, 1985, Boehringer Mannheim Diagnotics.

7. *Operator's manual for the DuPont analyst,* Wilmington, DE, 1993, DuPont Company.

HEMATOLOGY

M.A. Thrall and M.G. Weiser

Accurate hematologic data are essential for diagnosis of many disorders. Blood to be used for hematologic tests should be taken from a large vein and immediately placed in the anticoagulant, potassium ethylenediaminotetraacetate (EDTA). Vacuum tubes containing potassium EDTA are commercially available and should be filled with the specified amount of blood. Blood films should be prepared at once and kept dry at room temperature. If hematologic tests will not be performed within 2 hours of collection, the blood tube should be refrigerated.

Blood samples must be adequately mixed before performing any tests; inadequate mixing results in erroneous data. For example, red blood cells in horses start to settle within seconds, and a packed cell volume performed on an unmixed sample may be erroneous. Tubes of blood can be mixed by gently inverting for several seconds by hand or by placing the tube on a commercially available tilting rack or rotator.

THE COMPLETE BLOOD COUNT

A complete blood count (CBC) provides a minimum set of values that can be determined reliably and cost effectively in the hospital setting. Various techniques are used to determine hematologic values for the CBC. These may be done manually or with automated systems designed for use in veterinary hospitals. The basic components of the CBC may be accurately performed with manual procedures by persons exercising attention to detail.

The CBC should consist of at least the following basic information:

- Packed cell volume (PCV)
- Plasma protein concentration
- Total white blood cell (WBC) count

- Blood film examination: differential WBC count; erythrocyte morphology; estimation of platelet concentration
- Reticulocyte count when patient is anemic

When using hematology instruments designed for the veterinary hospital, the following determinations may be added to the CBC:

- Hemoglobin concentration
- Mean corpuscular volume (MCV) and other erythrocytic indices
- Platelet count

It is no longer viewed as appropriate to perform hemoglobin concentration and erythrocyte counts using manual procedures. These were done historically for purposes of calculating erythrocytic indices detailed in traditional textbooks of hematology. Some of the erythrocytic indices are now regarded as useful when measured on more precise and controlled automated hematology analyzers.

When the CBC is performed by a commercial laboratory, additional values may be reported because automated instruments are used. These may include the erythrocyte concentration, hemoglobin concentration, erythrocytic indices, and erythrocyte size distribution histograms. These additional values vary in their interpretive usefulness. They are packaged together, partly out of necessity, by virtue of the way automated hematology analyzers function. As these automated systems are improved and their cost decreases, they will become more available for use in veterinary hospitals.

INSTRUMENTATION

Instrumentation designed for veterinary hospital use is available to facilitate generation of hematologic data for the CBC. Options are cost effective and convenient in situations where five or more CBCs are performed per day. Benefits of instrumentation include reduced labor investment, more complete information, and improvement of data reliability. The discussion presented here is a brief overview and is not intended to provide an in depth understanding of instrument system options. It is the responsibility of individual users to become thoroughly familiar with detailed documentation that accompanies the specific instrument being used.

Instrumentation for the veterinary hospital falls into two general categories: electronic cell analysis systems and the quantitative buffy coat analysis system.

ELECTRONIC CELL COUNTERS

Electronic cell counters are based on passage of electric current across two electrodes separated by a glass tube containing a small opening or aperture. Electrolyte fluid on either side of the aperture conducts the current. Cells are moved through the aperture for counting by use of vaccuum or positive pressure. Because cells are relatively poor conductors of electricity compared with the electrolyte fluid, they impede flow of current while within the aperture. These transient changes in current may be counted to determine the blood cell concentration. In addition, the volume or size of the cell is proportional to the change in current, allowing the system to catalogue cell sizes. Size information may be displayed in a distribution histogram of the cell population (Figure 2-1). Leukocytes, erythrocytes, and platelets may be analyzed by these systems.

These instruments are calibrated to count cells only above a certain size, known as a *threshold*. This is done to prevent erroneous interpretation of small debris and electronic noise as cells. Because cell populations vary in size between species, the threshold settings must either be set by the operator or are predetermined by an instrument setting for a given species. These settings

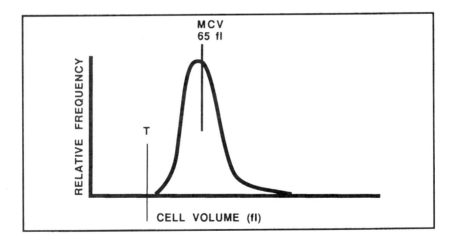

FIGURE **2-1.**   Representative histogram curve showing the distribution of canine erythrocyte volume. From the data in the curve, the mean corpuscular volume (MCV) can be determined. In this example, the MCV is indicated by the vertical line marked *MCV 65 fl.* The position of a counting threshold relative to the cell population is indicated by the vertical line *T.*

should be provided by the manufacturer. Comprehensive hematology systems designed specifically for veterinary applications are now available. By inherent engineering designs, these instruments greatly simplify what the operator needs to know about threshold settings. Species-specific threshold configurations may be part of the on-board software (e.g., Mascot and Hemavet Multispecies Hematology Analyzers, CDC Technologies, Oxford, CT). These systems incorporate the advantages of individual cell analysis that provide sophisticated information about blood cell populations.

The blood sample must be diluted to count cells. For WBC, a dilution is treated with a lytic agent that destroys cell membranes, leaving only nuclei for counting. Erythrocytes (red blood cells, RBCs) may be analyzed on systems that count the RBCs and also provide cell size information. This is done using a much greater blood dilution to which no lytic agent is added. Erythrocyte analysis on automated systems provides diagnostic information about cell volume and an alternative method for determining the hematocrit. The *mean corpuscular volume (MCV)* may be directly measured from analysis of the erythrocyte volume distribution. The hematocrit is then calculated by multiplying the MCV by the erythrocyte concentration. On more sophistocated systems, the volume distribution curve of the erythrocyte population is displayed (Figure 2-1). A relatively new value, termed the *red cell distribution width (RDW)*, is determined by mathematical analysis of the distribution. This value is an index of erythrocyte volume heterogeneity. Abnormally high values indicate increased volume heterogeneity and an underlying disturbance of the erythron. When used in conjunction with the MCV value, the RDW may alert the veterinarian to diseases of erythrocytes that alter RBC size. The same counting and sizing functions exist for counting platelets on more advanced systems.

QUANTITATIVE BUFFY COAT SYSTEM

The quantitative buffy coat system (QBC: Becton Dickinson, Franklin Lakes, NJ) uses differential centrifugation and quantitation of cellular elements by measurements on an expanded buffy coat layer in a specialized microhematocrit tube. It provides a hematocrit value and estimates of leukocyte concentration and platelet concentration. Partial differential count information is provided in the form of total granulocytes and lymphocyte/monocytes categories. One limitation of these leukocyte groupings is that such abnormalities as left shift and eosinophilia may be undetected unless the blood film is examined as defined for the minimum CBC.

Disadvantages of automated systems are related to deviation from the manufacturers' guidelines for operation in a way that compromises the reliability of the results. For example, failure to monitor instrument performance with control samples may lead to erroneous results. A common problem is that CBCs are performed without microscopic examination of the blood film.

MANUAL PROCEDURES

PACKED CELL VOLUME

The packed cell volume (PCV; also called *hematocrit*) is that percentage of whole blood composed of erythrocytes or red blood cells (RBCs). Whole blood is collected in an anticoagulant, such as EDTA or heparin, and placed in a capillary tube (75 × 1 mm). Microhematocrit tubes should be filled about three fourths full, with one end plugged with clay sealant, placed in a centrifuge with the plugged end facing outward, then centrifuged in a microhematocrit centrifuge for 5 minutes (see Figure 1-6, Chapter 1). Of the blood cells, RBCs have the highest specific gravity and gravitate to the bottom of the tube, appearing as a dark red layer. The PCV is then measured by using a hematocrit tube reader, many of which have a linear scale, so that the amount of blood in the tube need not be exact. The bottom of the RBC layer should be at the zero line and the top of the plasma on the top line. The percentage can then be read as the line level with the top of the RBC layer.

A white to gray layer just above the RBC layer is termed the *buffy coat* and consists of WBCs and platelets. The *plasma* is the clear to yellow fluid at the top. Plasma obtained by this method can be used to determine the plasma protein concentration by refractometry. Plasma color and transparency may be helpful in determining a diagnosis and should be recorded.

WHITE BLOOD CELL COUNT

The manual Unopette hemacytometer method (Becton-Dickinson, Rutherford, NJ) of counting WBCs is appropriate for most veterinary hospital laboratories. Unopette WBC test kits contain diluting reservoirs and capillary pipettes for making a 1:100 dilution of blood in ammonium oxalate or acetic acid, both of which lyse erythrocytes. Cells are counted using a hemacytometer and cover glass. An instruction sheet accompanies the kit.

Briefly, the appropriate amount of blood is added to the diluent (lysing solution). After about 10 minutes, the reservoir is shaken to evenly mix the cells and is converted to a dropper assembly. The iris diaphragm of the microscope must be closed to a point where the cells are most visible. The hemacytometer and coverslip must be free of dust and grease. The hemacytometer, with coverslip applied, is loaded with the solution and placed on the microscope, and the counting grid is found, using the 4X objective. Cells are counted in the nine primary squares, using the 10X objective (Figure 2-2).

The number of cells counted is multiplied by dilution and volume factors (total cells counted plus 10% of those counted, multiplied by a dilution factor of 100). Counts are expressed as cells per microliter (µl) of blood. For example, if 80 cells are counted, 80 + 8 = 88 × 100 = 8800/µl.

EVALUATION OF BLOOD FILMS

Blood films are prepared by placing a small drop of blood on a clean glass microscope slide. The end of a second slide is placed against the surface of the first slide at a 30-degree angle and drawn back into the drop of blood (Figure 2-3). When the blood has spread along most of the width of the spreader slide, it is then pushed forward with a steady, even, rapid motion. A properly prepared blood film is thin, with even distribution of cells. After air drying, the films should be stained with Wright's or Wright's-Giemsa stain. A particularly good method of Wright's staining has been described.[1] A quick stain that gives acceptable results is Diff-Quik (Harleco).

The blood film is used to perform the differential WBC count, estimate platelet numbers, and evaluate morphology of WBCs, RBCs, and platelets. The blood film should be inspected under low-power magnification (10X) to note cell numbers and to scan the *feathered edge* (Figure 2-4) for platelet clumps,

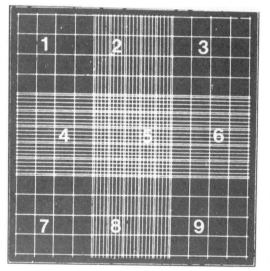

FIGURE 2-2. Nine primary squares of the hemacytometer are used for a Unopette total WBC count.

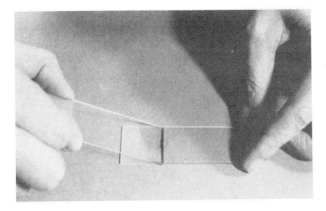

FIGURE 2-3. Blood film preparation. The spreader slide has been drawn back into the drop of blood and the blood has spread along most of its width. It will then be pushed rapidly to the right.

large abnormal cells, and microfilariae. The observer should then select a portion of the film near the thin end, referred as the *counting area,* and switch to the oil-immersion objective (100X) to complete the evaluation.

RED BLOOD CELLS

CLASSIFICATION OF ANEMIA

The function of red blood cells (RBCs; also called *erythrocytes*) is to transport and protect hemoglobin, the oxygen-carrying pigment. Daily production of erythrocytes equals the daily loss (from destruction of aged cells) in a healthy animal. If RBC production is decreased or destruction and/or loss is increased, anemia results. *Anemia* is defined as a condition in which there is a reduced number of circulating RBCs, reduced PCV, or a reduced concentration of hemoglobin.

Anemia may be classified according to bone marrow response (regenerative or nonregenerative) or RBC size and hemoglobin concentration (mean corpuscular volume, mean corpuscular hemoglobin concentration).

CLASSIFICATION BY BONE MARROW RESPONSE. This classification is most clinically applicable because it distinguishes between regenerative and nonregenerative anemias.

In *regenerative anemia,* the bone marrow responds to anemia by increasing erythrocyte production and releasing immature erythrocytes. These immature RBCs (polychromatophilic RBCs or *reticulocytes)* can be observed on the blood film and indicate that the marrow is responsive. The ability of bone marrow to

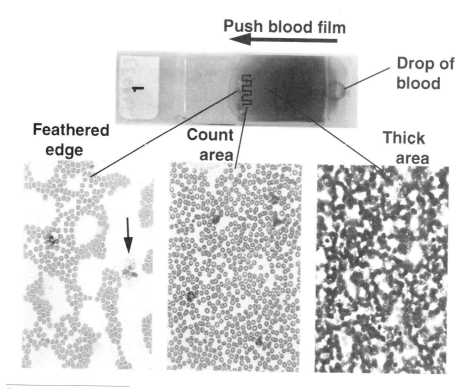

Push blood film

Drop of blood

Feathered edge

Count area

Thick area

FIGURE 2-4.　Gross and microscopic views of different areas on a blood film. The blood film on the glass slide at the top was made by pushing the blood from the drop (indicated *drop of blood*) at the right to the left (*large arrow*). The three major areas of the blood film (*feathered edge, count area, thick area*) are indicated by the lines connected to the respective microscopic views. The rectangular pattern on the glass slide indicates a recommended movement pattern for examining the slide under high magnification. The feathered edge (*left lower*) should be avoided because of artifacts. Note that erythrocyte central pallor is artifactually absent. Leukocytes may be broken (*arrow*). In the count area (*middle lower*), erythrocytes are present in a monolayer and have central pallor. Leukocytes are flattened so that intracellular detail is best. This is the optimal area for evaluating erythrocyte abnormalities and identifying leukocytes. In the thick area (*right lower*), it is not possible to evaluate erythrocyte morphology because the cells are extensively superimposed. Leukocytes are rounded and appear as dark spots, making identification very difficult.

respond indicates that the cause of the anemia is probably either blood loss (hemorrhage) or blood destruction (hemolysis).

In *nonregenerative anemia,* the bone marrow is unable to respond to the anemic state, and reticulocytes are absent on blood films, suggesting bone marrow dysfunction. A bone marrow aspiration biopsy is then indicated (see Bone Marrow Collection), once common endocrine and metabolic causes of nonregenerative anemia are excluded.

CLASSIFICATION BY RBC SIZE AND HEMOGLOBIN CONCENTRATION. Anemias may be classified as *normocytic* (RBCs of normal size), *macrocytic* (RBCs larger than normal), or *microcytic* (RBCs smaller than normal), depending on RBC size. In domestic animals, the most common cause of macrocytic anemia is the transitory increase in RBC size seen with regenerative anemia (*reticulocytosis*). In people, macrocytic anemia is frequently associated with vitamin B_{12} and folic acid deficiencies. These conditions are rarely, if ever, seen in domestic animals.

Microcytic anemia is almost always the result of iron deficiency. Division of immature erythrocytes stops when a critical concentration of hemoglobin is reached. With inadequate iron for hemoglobin synthesis, extra division may occur, resulting in smaller erythrocytes. While chronic blood loss is the most common cause of iron deficiency in adult animals, inadequate dietary iron results in iron-deficiency anemia in very young nursing animals, such as kittens and baby pigs.

Normocytic anemia is characterized by RBCs of normal size and is secondary to a variety of chronic disorders.

Anemias may be *hypochromic* (reduced hemoglobin concentration) or *normochromic* (normal hemoglobin concentration). A hyperchromic state is not possible. Newly released polychromatophilic erythrocytes (*reticulocytes*) are hypochromic because the full concentration of hemoglobin is not yet attained. *Macrocytic hypochromic anemia* suggests regeneration. Iron deficiency also results in hypochromic anemia but is also characterized by microcytosis. Most other types of anemia are *normochromic.*

ERYTHROCYTE INDICES

Determination of erythrocyte indices is helpful in classification of certain anemias.

MEAN CORPUSCULAR VOLUME. The mean corpuscular volume (MCV) is the mean volume for a group of erythrocytes. For many years, the MCV was calculated by dividing PCV by the RBC concentration and multiplying by 10. The unit of volume is the femtoliter (fl), which is 1×10^{-15} liters.

$$\text{MCV (in femtoliters)} = \frac{\text{PCV (\%)} \times 10}{\text{RBC (millions/}\mu\text{l)}}$$

For example, if a dog has a PCV of 42% and a RBC count of 6.0 million/μl, the MCV is 70 fl. Normal ranges for MCV vary among species (Table 2-1).

The size of the erythrocytes can now be determined electronically by automated systems (see Electronic Cell Counters). The PCV can then be calculated by multiplying the MCV by the erythrocyte concentration, eliminating the need to determine the PCV by microcentrifugation.

Anemias may be normocytic, macrocytic, or microcytic. In domestic animals, the most common cause of macrocytic anemia is the transitory increase in MCV seen with reticulocytosis (i.e., large, immature cells being released at the beginning of regenerative anemia). Iron-deficiency anemia is the most common cause of microcytic anemia.

MEAN CORPUSCULAR HEMOGLOBIN.   Mean corpuscular hemoglobin (MCH) is the mean weight of hemoglobin (Hb) contained in the average RBC. It is calculated by dividing the hemoglobin concentration by the RBC concentration and multiplying by 10.

$$\text{MCH (in picograms)} = \frac{\text{Hb (g/dl)} \times 10}{\text{RBC (millions/}\mu\text{l)}}$$

The MCH is the least accurate of the indices, simply because Hb determinations and RBC counts are less accurate than the PCV. Normal MCH values vary with the species (Table 2-1).

MEAN CORPUSCULAR HEMOGLOBIN CONCENTRATION.   The mean corpuscular hemoglobin concentration (MCHC) is the concentration of hemoglobin in the average erythrocyte (or the ratio of weight of hemoglobin to the volume in which it is contained). The MCHC is calculated by dividing the hemoglobin concentration by the PCV and multiplying by 100.

$$\text{MCHC (g/dl)} = \frac{\text{Hb (g/dl)} \times 100}{\text{PCV (\%)}}$$

For example, if a dog has a hemoglobin concentration of 14 g/dl and a PCV of 42%, the MCHC is 33.3 g/dl. The normal range for MCHC is 30 to 36 g/dl for all mammals, with the exception of some sheep and all members of the family Camellidae (camels), which have MCHC values of 40 to 45 g/dl.

TABLE 2-1. Red blood cell characteristics in normal domestic animals

SPECIES	DIAMETER	ROULEAUX	CENTRAL PALLOR	ANISOCYTOSIS	BASOPHILIC STIPPLING IN REGENERATIVE RESPONSE	RETICULOCYTES (NORMAL PCV)	POIKILOCYTES	MCV (FL)	MCHC (G/DL)
Dogs	7.0	+	++++	—	—	±1.0%	—	60-77	32-36
Pigs	6.0	++	±	±	—	±1.0%	++++	50-68	30-34
Cats	5.8	++	+	±	±	±0.5%	—	39-55	30-36
Horses	5.7	++++	±	—	—	0% (will not increase in response to anemia)	—	34-58	31-37
Cattle	5.5	—	+	++	+++	0% (will increase in response to anemia)	—	40-60	30-36
Sheep	4.5	±	+	+	+++	0% (will increase)	—	23-48	31-38
Goats	3.2	—	—	—	++	0% (will increase)	++ (in young)	15-30	35-42

RETICULOCYTE COUNT

A *reticulocyte* is an immature erythrocyte that contains organelles (ribosomes) that are lost as the cell matures (Plate 1). These organelles account for the diffuse blue-gray or polychromatophilic staining of immature cells with Wright's stain. When these immature cells are stained with new methylene blue or brilliant cresyl blue, the organelles clump into visible granules referred to as *reticulum.* This reticulum is present as aggregates or chains of blue granules. White blood cells do not stain well with this type of stain.

Cats, unlike other species, have two morphologic forms of reticulocytes. The aggregate form contains large clumps of reticulum, is similar to reticulocytes in other species, and is the same cell that stains polychromatophilic with Wright's stain. The punctuate form, unique to cats, contains 2 to 8 small, singular, basophilic granules. These cells do not stain polychromatophilic with Wright's stain. In normal nonanemic cats, about 0.4% of the RBCs are aggregate reticulocytes, whereas 1.5% to 10% of the RBCs are punctate reticulocytes. For a meaningful reticulocyte count in cats, only the aggregate form of reticulocyte should be counted.

A *reticulocyte count* is an expression of the percentage of RBCs that are reticulocytes. A reticulocyte count should be performed on the blood of all anemic domestic animals except horses, which do not release reticulocytes from the bone marrow, even in the face of regenerative anemia. Reticulocyte concentration is very useful in assessing the bone marrow's response to anemia.

Blood is stained by placing a few drops of blood and an equal number of drops of new methylene blue or brilliant cresyl blue stain in a small test tube and allowing the mixture to stand for about 10 minutes. Tubes containing premeasured brilliant cresyl blue are commercially available (Curtin Matheson Scientific, Houston, TX). A drop of the mixture is then used to prepare a conventional air-dried blood film, which can then be examined or counterstained with Wright's stain. The percentage of reticulocytes per 1000 erythrocytes is determined.

Reticulocyte counts should be interpreted according to the degree of anemia because fewer mature erythrocytes are present in anemic animals, and reticulocytes are released earlier and persist longer than in normal animals. Higher percentages may be seen in hemolytic than in hemorrhagic types of anemia. Although reticulocytes are often reported as a percentage, a more useful method is to multiply the percentage by the erythrocyte count, to give reticulocytes/μl. Guidelines for reticulocyte interpretation are listed in Table 2-2.

TABLE 2-2.   Interpretation of absolute reticulocyte counts in dogs, cats, and ruminants

	NORMAL	NONREGENERATIVE ANEMIA	MODERATE REGENERATION	MAXIMUM REGENERATION
Dogs, cats	>60,000/μl	<60,000/μl	100,000-200,000/μl	up to 500,000/μl
Ruminants	0	0	±100,000/μl	±300,000/μl

If an erythrocyte count has not been performed, reticulocyte counts may be reported as a percentage. Reticulocyte counts can be corrected for the degree of anemia as follows:

$$\frac{\text{Corrected}}{\text{reticulocyte \%}} = \text{Observed reticulocyte \%} \times \frac{\text{Patient's PCV}}{\text{Normal mean PCV}}$$

For example, if a dog has a PCV of 15% and an observed reticulocyte count of 15%, the corrected reticulocyte count equals:

$$15\% \times \frac{15\%}{45\%} = 5\%$$

Typical reticulocyte responses for dogs (given as percentage) are as follows:

NORMAL	MILD REGENERATIVE RESPONSE	MODERATE REGENERATIVE RESPONSE	MARKED REGENERATIVE RESPONSE
<1%	1% to 8%	9% to 15%	>15%

ERYTHROCYTE MORPHOLOGY

Normal erythrocyte morphology (Plate 2) varies among different species of domestic animals (Table 2-1). Morphology of erythrocytes can be categorized according to cell arrangement on the blood film, size, color, shape, and presence of structures in or on erythrocytes.

CELL ARRANGEMENT.   *Rouleaux formation* is grouping of erythrocytes in stacks (Figure 2-5 and Plate 3). Increased rouleaux formation is seen with increased fibrinogen or globulin concentrations. Marked rouleaux formation is seen in healthy horses.

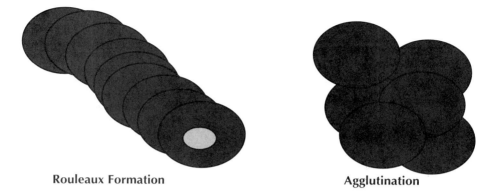

Rouleaux Formation   **Agglutination**

FIGURE 2-5.   Drawing depicting rouleaux formation and agglutination.

Agglutination of erythrocytes should be distinguished from rouleaux formation (Figure 2-5 and Plate 4). Agglutination occurs in immune-mediated disorders, in which antibody coats the erythrocyte, resulting in bridging and clumping of RBCs. It is sometimes observed macroscopically as well as microscopically.

SIZE.   *Anisocytosis* is variation in the size of RBCs (Plates 5 and 6) and may be due to the presence of macrocytes (large cells) or microcytes (small cells) or both.

Macrocytes are RBCs that are larger than normal, with an increased MCV. Macrocytes are usually young, polychromatophilic erythrocytes (reticulocytes) (Plate 6).

Microcytes are RBCs with a diameter less than that of normal erythrocytes, with a decreased MCV. Microcytic cells may be seen with iron deficiency (Plate 7).

COLOR.   *Polychromasia* or polychromatophilic erythrocytes are RBCs exhibiting a bluish tint when stained with Romanowsky (Wright's-type) stain (Plates 6 and 7). The blue tint is due to organelles remaining within the cytoplasm; thus, these are young cells. This is the same cell that, when stained with new methylene blue, or brilliant cresyl blue, appears as a reticulocyte.

Hypochromia is decreased staining intensity caused by insufficient hemoglobin within the cell (Plate 7). Iron deficiency is the most common cause, although macrocytic erythrocytes often appear hypochromic due to their large diameter. Hypochromic cells should be distinguished from bowl-shaped or "punched-out" cells, which are insignificant. Animals with true hypochromia almost always have microcytosis as well, as determined by a decreased MCV.

Normochromia is a normal staining intensity.

SHAPE. Abnormally shaped erythrocytes are called *poikilocytes*. This terminology is not very helpful because it does not suggest a specific diagnosis. Shape and color changes (Figure 2-6) are considered important when they are frequently associated with specific disorders.

Spiculated cells are erythrocytes with one or more surface spicules. This general term includes schistocytes, keratocytes, acanthocytes, and echinocytes. It is better to be as specific as possible when describing shape changes, as certain types of spiculated cells have been associated with certain diseases.

Schistocytes (Plates 1 and 8), a term for RBC fragments, are usually formed as a result of shearing of the red cell by intravascular trauma. Schistocytes may be observed with disseminated intravascular coagulopathy (DIC) (when erythrocytes are broken by fibrin strands), with vascular neoplasms (e.g., hemangiosarcoma), and with iron deficiency. In animals with DIC, there is usually a

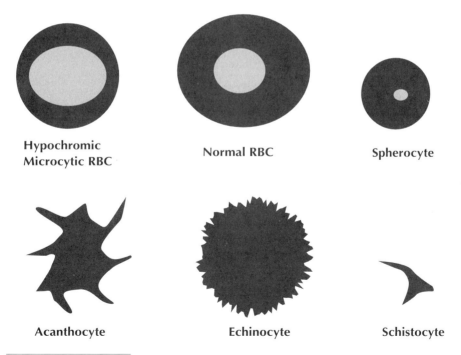

Hypochromic Microcytic RBC   Normal RBC   Spherocyte

Acanthocyte   Echinocyte   Schistocyte

FIGURE 2-6. Erythrocyte shape and color abnormalities that may be helpful in diagnosis.

concurrent thrombocytopenia. In dogs with hemangiosarcoma, there are usually acanthocytes present as well as fragments (Figures 2-6 and Plate 9). In iron-deficiency anemia, the fragmentation is apparently the result of oxidative injury, leading to membrane lesions or increased susceptibility to intravascular trauma. Initially the RBC develops what appears to be a blister or vacuole (Plates 7 and 10), which is thought to represent an oxidative injury occurring when inner membrane surfaces are cross linked across the cell. Exclusion of hemoglobin may account for the colorless area. These lesions subsequently enlarge and break open to form *"apple-stem cells"* (Plates 7 and 10) and *keratocytes* (Plate 10), spiculated red cells with two or more pointed projections. The projections from the keratocytes probably then fragment from the cell (Plates 8 and 10). This process is depicted in Figure 2-7.

Acanthocytes or *spur cells* are irregular, spiculated red cells with a few, unevenly distributed surface projections of variable length and diameter (Plates 6 and 11). They are thought to result from changes in cholesterol concentration at the red cell membrane. They are seen in patients with altered lipid metabolism, such as may occur in cats with hepatic lipidosis and, occasionally, in dogs with liver disease. They are seen quite consistently in dogs with hemangiosarcoma of the liver. The presence of acanthocytes in middle-aged to old large-breed dogs with concurrent regenerative anemia is very suggestive of hemangiosarcoma.

Echinocytes (*burr cells*) are spiculated cells with numerous short, evenly spaced, blunt to sharp surface projections of uniform size and shape. Echinocyte formation can be an artifactual, *in vitro* process associated with pH change from slow drying of blood films; it is then termed *crenation*. Echinocytes have also been associated with renal disease and lymphosarcoma in dogs, following exercise in horses, and with rattlesnake envenomation in dogs (Plate 12).

Spherocytes are small, darkly staining red cells with reduced or no central pallor (Plates 5 and 13). Spherocytes with a small amount of central pallor are referred to as "imperfect spheres." Spherocytes are not easily detected in species other than dogs. They have a reduced amount of membrane as a result of partial phagocytosis by macrophages, which occurs because of antibody and/or complement on the surface of the RBC. They are very significant in that they suggest immune-mediated destruction of red blood cells, resulting in hemolytic anemia. They may also be seen following transfusion with mismatched blood. Immune-mediated hemolytic anemia (IMHA) is usually a very regenerative anemia, with marked polychromasia and high reticulocyte count. However, in some instances, the anemia is non-regenerative as a result of antibodies against RBC precursors within the bone marrow. In these cases,

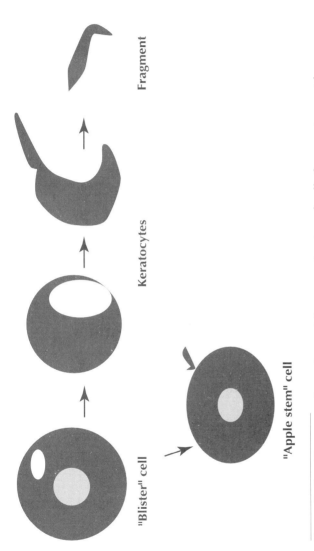

FIGURE 2-7. Keratocyte formation and fragmentation in red cells from patients with iron-deficiency anemia.

spherocytes are often difficult to detect because the presence of large polychromatophilic cells facilitates recognition of the small spherocytes. Although spherocytes appear small or microcytic, their volume is normal, and dogs with IMHA do not have decreased MCV.

Other abnormally shaped erythrocytes, such as *leptocytes* and *bowl-shaped cells,* are less important because they are not associated with specific disorders. Other abnormalities, such as *stomatocytes,* are seen in dogs with very rare inherited disorders (Plate 14).

Leptocytes are thin erythrocytes with increased membrane or decreased volume. Because of this, the cell membrane can fold or become distorted. Leptocytes have a tendency to accumulate in the lower portion of the buffy coat at centrifugation. The most common forms of leptocytes are *target cells* and *folded cells* (Figure 2-8 and Plate 11). *Target cells* are RBCs with a central, rounded area of hemoglobin, surrounded by a clear zone, with a dense ring of hemoglobin around the periphery. *Folded cells* have a transverse, raised fold extending across the center of the cell. Leptocytes are common in patients with nonregenerative anemia.

Inclusions. *Basophilic stippling,* the presence of very small, dark-blue bodies within the erythrocyte, is observed in Wright's-stained cells containing residual RNA. It is common in immature RBCs of ruminants and occasionally in cats during a response to anemia. It is usually characteristic of lead poisoning when seen in dogs (Plate 15).

Howell-Jolly bodies are basophilic nuclear remnants seen in young erythrocytes during the response to anemia (Plate 13). As cells containing nuclear remnants pass through the spleen, phagocytic cells remove the remnants.

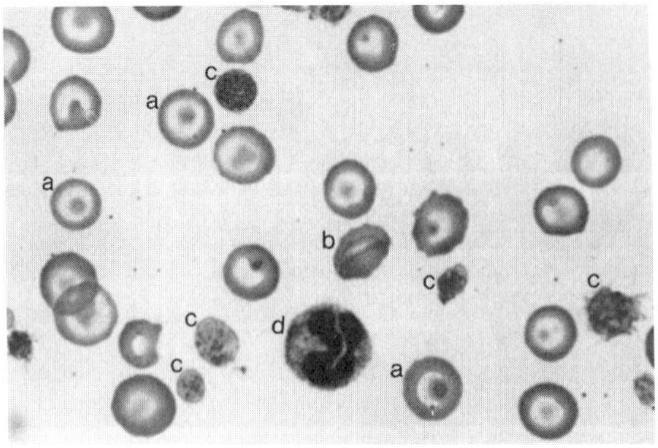

Figure 2-8. Numerous target cells (*a*) and a folded cell (*b*) on a blood film from a dog. *c*, platelets; *d*, neutrophil.

Consequently, increased numbers may be seen after removal of the spleen or with splenic disorders.

Nucleated erythrocytes represent early release of immature cells during anemia but may also be observed in nonanemic animals (Plate 13). An increase in nucleated RBCs out of proportion to the degree of anemia is sometimes caused by lead poisoning. All red blood cells of non-mammalians, such as birds and reptiles, contain nuclei (Plate 16).

Heinz bodies are round structures representing denatured hemoglobin, caused by certain oxidant drugs or chemicals. The denatured hemoglobin becomes attached to the cell membrane and appears as a pale area with Wright's stain (Plate 17). When stained with new methylene blue (same technique used for reticulocytes), the Heinz bodies appear blue (Plate 18). In dogs, they are 1 to 2 µ in diameter. Unlike other domestic animals, normal cats have Heinz bodies in as many as 5% of their RBCs, and Heinz bodies are often increased in concentration with such diseases as lymphosarcoma, hyperthyroidism, and diabetes mellitus in cats.

BLOOD PARASITES

Parasites may be present in or on erythrocytes. Stain precipitate and drying artifacts are sometimes confused with red cell parasites. Drying artifact usually appears refractile (Plate 19).

HEMOBARTONELLA FELIS. This is a fairly common parasite of feline erythrocytes. The disease is referred to as hemobartonellosis (feline infectious anemia). The organisms appear as small (0.2 to 0.5 µ) coccoid, rod-shaped, or ring-line structures that stain dark purple with Wright's stain (Plate 20). They most frequently appear as short rods on the periphery of RBCs. The parasitemia is cyclic; if hemobartonellosis is suspected, the blood should be examined several times before the infection is ruled out. Once antibiotics are given, the parasite disappears rapidly.

HEMOBARTONELLA CANIS. Hemobartonellosis is rare in dogs and usually is only observed in splenectomized or immunosuppressed dogs. The organism most commonly appears as a chain of small cocci or rods that stretch across the surface of the erythrocyte (Plate 21). The chains may appear to branch.

Eperythrozoonosis in swine, cattle, and llamas is quite similar to hemobartonellosis; the organisms are closely related. *Eperythrozoon* appear as small (0.8

to 1.0 μ) cocci, rods, or rings on the RBC surface or free in the plasma. The ring form is most common (Plate 22).

ANAPLASMA MARGINALE.   This intracellular blood parasite causes anaplasmosis in cattle as well as wild ruminants. It appears as small, dark-staining cocci at the margin of RBCs (Figure 2-9) and must be differentiated from Howell-Jolly bodies, as their sizes are similar. Early in the course of the disease as many as 50% of RBCs may contain parasites. By the time the anemia is severe, usually less than 5% of RBCs are affected.

CYTAUXZOON FELIS.   This is a very rare cause of hemolytic anemia in cats. The organism appears as small (1.0 to 2.0 μ), irregular ring forms within erythrocytes, lymphocytes, and macrophages (Figure 2-10).

BABESIA.   Babesiosis of cattle is caused by *Babesia bigemina* and *B. bovis*. The disease is also called Texas fever, redwater fever, and cattle tick fever. *Babesia* appears as a large (3 to 4 μ), pleomorphic, teardrop-shaped intracellular organism, frequently seen in pairs. Babesiosis in horses (piroplasmosis) is caused by *Babesia equi* and *B. caballi*, which are similar to *B. bigemina*. Babesiosis is rare in horses, and the few cases reported in the United States have been seen in the south, especially Florida. Babesiosis in dogs is caused by *Babesia canis* and *B. gibsoni*. They are also similar to *B. bigemina*, but *B. gibsoni* is slightly smaller and appears as rings. Only a small percentage of erythrocytes may be affected. The organisms are more commonly observed in RBCs at the feathered edge.

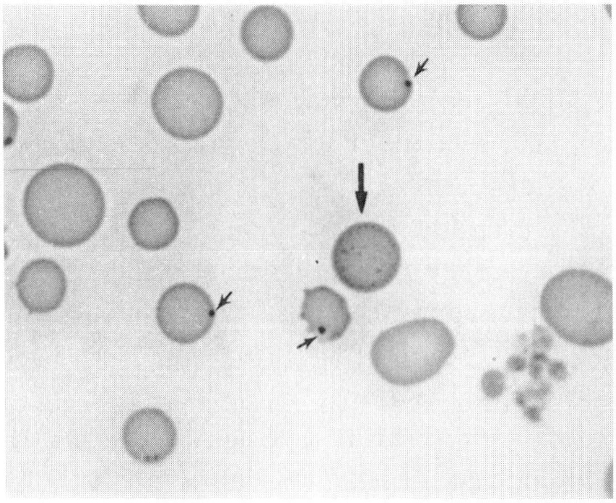

FIGURE 2-9.   *Anaplasma marginale* (*small arrows*) in blood from a cow. Note the anisocytosis and basophilic stippling (*large arrow*). (1400X)

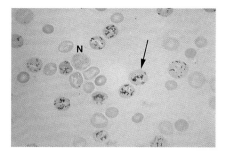

Plate 1. Numerous reticulocytes in blood from a dog with regenerative anemia. Representative reticulocyte *(arrow)*. N, neutrophil. (Brilliant cresyl blue stain.)

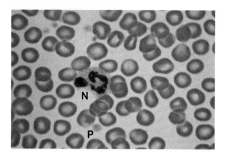

Plate 2. Blood film from a normal dog. Central pallor is evident in the erythrocytes. N, neutrophil. P, platelet. (Wright's stain.)

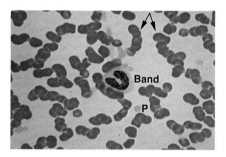

Plate 3. Blood film from a horse. Rouleaux formations are indicated *(arrows)* and a band neutrophil. P, platelet. (Wright's stain.)

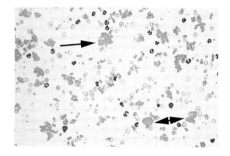

Plate 4. Low-power magnification of blood film from a dog with erythrocyte agglutination *(arrows)*. (Wright's stain.)

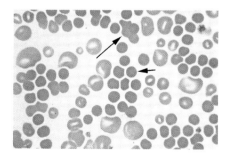

Plate 5. Anisocytosis on a blood film from a dog with immune-mediated hemolytic anemia. The small cells are spherocytes *(short arrow)*. Agglutination is indicated *(long arrow)*. (Wright's stain.)

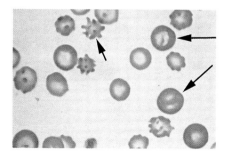

Plate 6. Large (macrocytic) polychromatophilic erythrocytes *(long arrows)* on a blood film from a dog with regenerative anemia resulting from a bleeding intraabdominal hemangiosarcoma. An acanthocyte is indicated *(short arrow)*. (Wright's stain.)

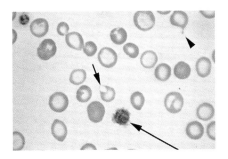

Plate 7. Microcytic hypochromic erythrocytes on a blood film from a dog with iron-deficiency anemia from blood loss. Blister formation *(short arrow)* and "apple stem" formation *(arrowhead)* are common. A large platelet *(long arrow)* is indicated. (Wright's stain.)

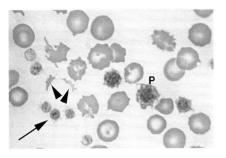

Plate 8. Blood film from a dog with iron-deficiency anemia. Red cell fragments (schistocytes) *(arrowheads)* and normal platelets *(arrow)* are indicated. P, giant platelet. (Wright's stain.)

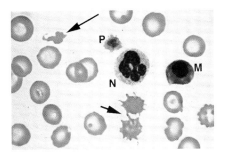

Plate 9. Red cell fragment *(long arrow)* and acanthocytes *(short arrow)* on a blood film from a dog with hemangiosarcoma of the liver and spleen. P, platelet; M, metarubricyte; N, neutrophil. (Wright's stain.)

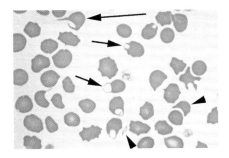

Plate 10. Blood film from a cat with iron-deficiency anemia resulting from chronic gastrointestinal blood loss. Numerous blister cells *(short arrows)*, a keratocyte *(long arrow)*, and fragments *(arrowheads)* are typical membrane changes. (Wright's stain.)

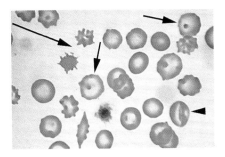

Plate 11. Acanthocytes *(long arrow)*, target cells *(short arrows)*, and folded cells *(arrowhead)* in a blood film from a dog with hemangiosarcoma. (Wright's stain.)

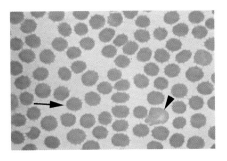

Plate 12. Many echinocytes *(arrow)* on a blood film from a dog bitten by a rattlesnake. Polychromatophilic erythrocytes *(arrowhead)* do not become echinocytic. (Wright's stain.)

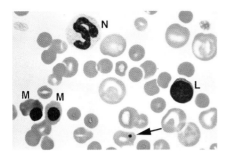

Plate 13. Numerous spherocytes on a blood film from a dog with immune-mediated hemolytic anemia. Several large polychromatophilic red cells are present, indicating the anemia is regenerative. *Arrow,* Howell-Jolly body; *M,* metarubricytes; *N,* neutrophil; *L,* lymphocyte. (Wright's stain.)

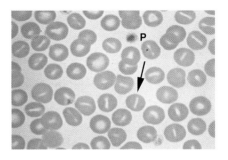

Plate 14. Stomatocytes *(arrow)* on a blood film from a Schnauzer with inherited stomatocytosis. *P,* platelet. (Wright's stain.)

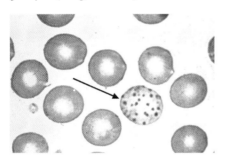

Plate 15. Basophilic stippling *(arrow)* on a blood film from a dog with lead poisoning. (Wright's stain.)

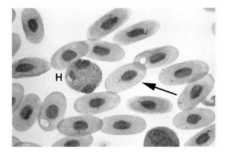

Plate 16. Nucleated erythrocytes *(arrow)* on a blood film from a reptile. Reptiles, like birds, have heterophils *(H)* with eosinophilic granules, rather than neutrophils. (Wright's stain.)

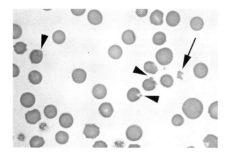

Plate 17. Heinz bodies *(arrowheads)* and fragment *(arrow)* on a blood film from a cat with diabetes mellitus. (Wright's stain.)

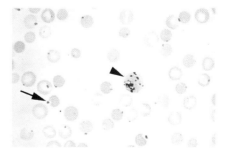

Plate 18. Many Heinz bodies *(arrow)* on a blood film from the cat mentioned in Plate 17. Heinz bodies are more easily seen with this new methylene blue stain. *Arrowhead,* reticulocyte.

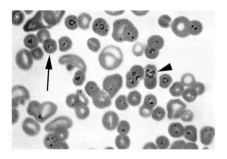

Plate 19. Drying artifacts appear as dots *(arrow)* and ring forms *(arrowhead)*. These artifacts can be distinguished from red cell parasites by their refractile, amorphous appearance. (Wright's stain.)

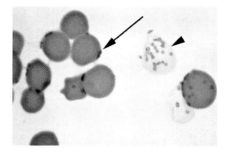

Plate 20. *Hemobartonella felis* organisms *(arrow)* on the periphery of red cells. Ring forms *(arrowhead)* can be easily visualized because the erythrocyte is lysed. (Wright's stain.)

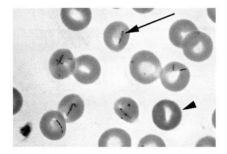

Plate 21. *Hemobartonella canis* organisms *(arrow)* appear as chains of cocci across the surface of red blood cells. *Arrowhead,* polychromatophilic erythrocyte. (Wright's stain.)

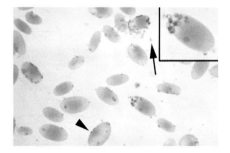

Plate 22. *Eperythrozoon* in a blood film from a llama. Numerous organisms *(arrowhead)* are present on the surface of all red cells (very high magnification, *inset* in upper right corner) and are also free in the plasma, as indicated by their presence between erythrocytes *(arrow)*. (Wright's stain.)

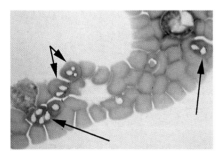

Plate 23. *Babesia canis* organisms *(arrows)* in erythrocytes on the feathered edge of a blood film from a dog. (Wright's stain.)

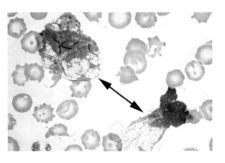

Plate 24. Broken nuclei, often termed "smudge cells" *(arrows)*, should be ignored when performing differential white cell counts. (Wright's stain.)

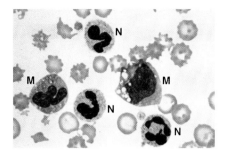

Plate 25. Blood film from a dog with normal neutrophils *(N)* and monocytes *(M)*. Many of the red blood cells are acanthocytic and fragmented. (Wright's stain.)

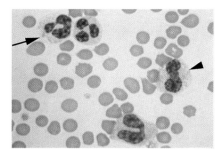

Plate 26. Blood film from an ill cat with numerous toxic neutrophils and bands, as evidenced by Döhle bodies *(arrow)*, "foamy" cytoplasm *(arrowhead)*, and basophilic cytoplasm. (Wright's stain.)

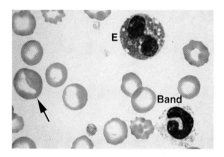

Plate 27. Normal band neutrophil and eosinophil *(E)* from a dog with regenerative anemia, as evidenced by polychromatophilic erythrocytes *(arrow)*. (Wright's stain.)

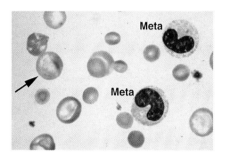

Plate 28. Metamyelocytes on a blood film from a dog with regenerative anemia, as evidenced by polychromatophilic erythrocytes *(arrow)*. Numerous imperfect spherocytes are also present, suggesting immune-mediated hemolytic anemia. (Wright's stain.)

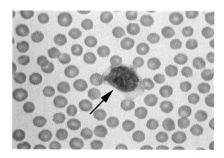

Plate 29. Normal bovine blood film. Large lymphocyte with nucleolar rings *(arrow)*. (Wright's stain.)

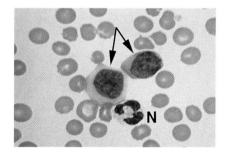

Plate 30. Lymphoblasts *(arrows)* with pale-staining nucleoli within the nuclei. This blood film is from a dog with lymphoblastic leukemia. *N*, neutrophil. (Wright's stain.)

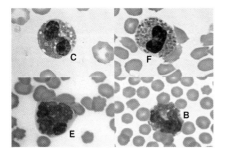

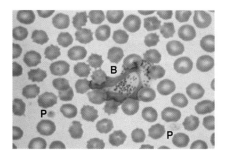

Plate 31. Canine *(C)*, feline *(F)*, equine *(E)*, and bovine *(B)* eosinophils showing varied color and shape of the granules. (Wright's stain.)

Plate 32. Normal basophil *(B)* and platelets *(P)* on a blood film from a dog. Many of the erythrocytes are echinocytes. (Wright's stain.)

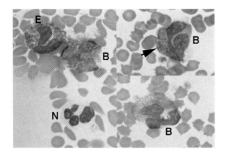

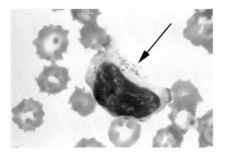

Plate 33. Normal feline basophils *(B)*. One basophil *(arrow)* contains darkly staining granules, which are not commonly observed in cats. *E*, eosinophil; *N*, neutrophil. (Wright's stain.)

Plate 34. Large granular lymphocyte *(arrow)* on a blood film from a dog with chronic ehrlichiosis. (Wright's stain.)

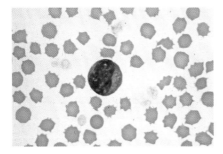

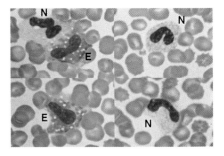

Plate 35. Reactive lymphocyte from a cat with hepatic lipidosis. Numerous acanthocytes are present. (Wright's stain.)

Plate 36. Nuclear hyposegmentation in neutrophils *(N)* and eosinophils *(E)* from a dog with Pelger-Huet anomaly. (Wright's stain.)

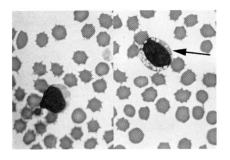

Plate 37. One normal and one vacuolated *(arrow)* lymphocyte from a cat with type A Niemann-Pick disease, an inherited lysosomal storage disorder. (Wright's stain.)

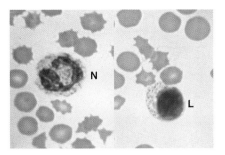

Plate 38. Neutrophil *(N)* and lymphocyte *(L)* that contain granules on a blood film from a cat with GM$_2$ gangliosidosis, a lysosomal storage disease. Numerous erythrocytes are acanthocytic, likely related to the associated liver disease. (Wright's stain.)

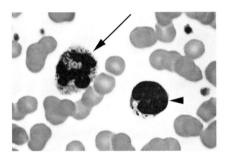

Plate 39. Blood film from a cat with mucopolysaccharidosis VI, a lysosomal storage disease. Lymphocytes contain vacuoles and granules *(arrowhead)*. Neutrophils *(arrow)* contain granules (Alder-Reilly bodies). (Wright's stain.)

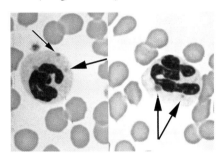

Plate 40. Blood film from a cat with Chediak-Higashi syndrome. Fused lysosomes appear as pink granules *(large arrows)* in the cytoplasm of neutrophils. Döhle body *(small arrow)* is indicated. (Wright's stain.)

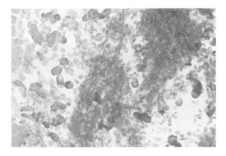

Plate 41. Large masses or clumps of platelets on a blood film from a horse. (Wright's stain.)

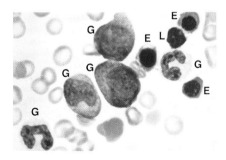

Plate 42. Bone marrow aspirate from a normal dog. Granulocytic cells *(G)* can be differentiated from erythroid cells *(E)* based on nuclear and cytoplasmic characteristics. *L*, lymphocyte. (Wright's stain.)

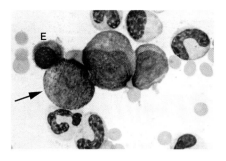

Plate 43. Bone marrow aspirate from a cat. Primary granules within granulocytic precursors are evident *(arrow)*. All cells are granulocytic except one rubricyte *(E)*. (Wright's stain.)

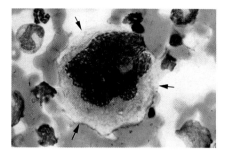

Plate 44. Bone marrow aspirate from a normal dog. A megakaryocyte *(arrows)* is indicated. (Wright's stain.)

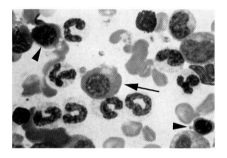

Plate 45. Bone marrow aspirate from a normal dog. A plasma cell *(arrow)* is indicated. Rubricytes *(arrowheads)* have nuclei similar to those of plasma cells but have less cytoplasm. The remaining cells are granulocytic precursors. (Wright's stain.)

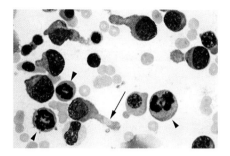

Plate 46. Bone marrow aspirate from a cat with erythremic myelosis. Un-differentiated cells have cytoplasmic projections *(arrow)*. Numerous cells are in mitosis *(arrowheads)*. (Wright's stain.)

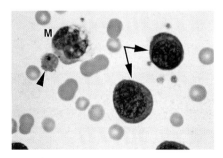

Plate 47. Blood film from a cat with erythremic myelosis (bone marrow is shown in Plate 46). Two rubriblasts *(arrows)* and a cytoplasmic fragment *(arrowhead)* are indicated. *M*, megakaryocyte. (Wright's stain.)

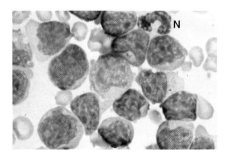

Plate 48. Bone marrow aspirate from a dog with late-stage lymphoblastic leukemia. Note the almost complete absence of granulocytic and erythroid precursors. Numerous lymphoid cells contain cytoplasmic granules. *N*, neutrophil. (Wright's stain.)

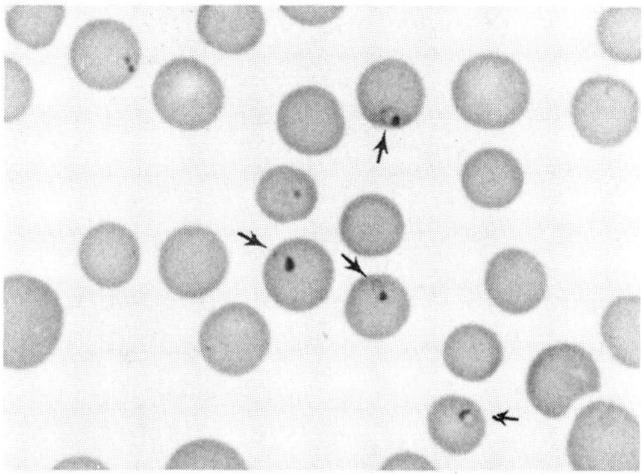

FIGURE **2-10.**   *Cytauxzoon felis*
(*arrows*) in blood from an
experimentally infected cat.
(1400X)

EHRLICHIA.   Ehrlichiosis of dogs (tropical pancytopenia) is caused by *Ehrlichia canis,* an intracellular parasite of monocytes and neutrophils (Plate 23). It is transmitted by the brown dog tick. The organism appears as small clusters, called morulae (3 to 6 μ), in the cytoplasm (Figure 2-11). The disease may result in neutropenia, thrombocytopenia, and anemia. Chronically affected animals may be severely anemic, with marked leukopenia and thrombocytopenia, but sometimes the only hematologic abnormality is lymphocytosis. The total plasma protein level is usually increased. The organisms are best demonstrated during the acute phase but are usually present in very small numbers. Films made from the buffy coat (where monocytes are concentrated)

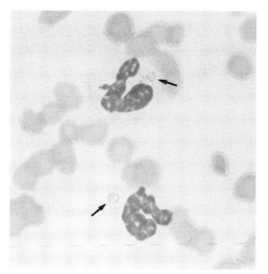

FIGURE **2-11.**   *Ehrlichia (arrows)* in
the neutrophils of a horse. (1400X)

may aid diagnosis. However, in most cases organisms are not seen and the diagnosis is made by serologic testing.

WHITE BLOOD CELLS

Mature and immature neutrophils, lymphocytes, monocytes, eosinophils, and basophils make up the leukocytes (white blood cells, WBCs) found in blood. Each type of cell plays an important role in the body's defense system, and their total concentration is extremely valuable in the diagnosis of various diseases.

DEFINITIONS

The following are some definitions of hematologic terms used in this section:

-penia: Decreased number of cells in the blood. For example, *neutropenia* refers to decreased numbers of neutrophils in the blood. *Lymphopenia* describes decreased numbers of lymphocytes in the blood.

-philia or *cytosis:* Increased number of cells in the blood. For example, *neutrophilia* refers to increased numbers of neutrophils in the blood. *Leukocytosis* refers to increased numbers of leukocytes in the blood.

Left shift: Increased numbers of immature neutrophils in the blood.

Leukemia: Neoplastic cells in the blood or bone marrow. Leukemias are often described as leukemic, subleukemic, or aleukemic, indicating the variation in the tendency for neoplastic cells to be released in the blood.

Leukemoid response: Condition that can be mistaken for leukemia. It is characterized by marked leukocytosis (>50,000/µl) and is usually the result of inflammatory disease.

Lymphoproliferative disorders: Conditions in which lymphocytes or plasma cells proliferate abnormally.

Myeloproliferative disorders: A group of bone marrow disorders, usually neoplastic, characterized by proliferation of one, several, or all of the bone marrow cell lines.

DIFFERENTIAL WHITE BLOOD CELL COUNTS

After examination of the blood film with the 10X objective (see Evaluation of Blood Films), the 100X (oil-immersion) objective is used to count and classify at least 100 nucleated WBCs in the counting area, using a commercially available differential cell counter to keep a running tally of cell types (Figure 2-12). The cells should be counted in the area near, but not on, the feathered edge, where the erythrocytes do not overlap. Broken "smudged" cells (Plate 24) should be ignored. The quantities of all cell types are then expressed as percentages of the total 100-cell count. The absolute number of each type of cell counted is then obtained by multiplying the percentile fraction by the total WBC count.

Differential WBC counts should *always* be expressed in absolute numbers to be diagnostically useful. Percentages are not useful for interpretive purposes. For example, a cat has a total leukocyte count of 3000/µl, with 300 (10%) neutrophils and 2700 (90%) lymphocytes. A second cat has a total count of 40,000/µl, with 4000 (10%) neutrophils and 36,000 (90%) lymphocytes. Although the percentages of cells are the same in both cats, the absolute numbers of cells are vastly different. The first cat has neutropenia, with a normal lymphocyte count. The second cat has extreme lymphocytosis, suggesting lymphoid leukemia, with a normal neutrophil count.

Nucleated RBCs (NRBCs) are included in the total WBC count performed on hemacytometers and electronic cell counters. When performing a differential cell count, NRBCs may be counted separately and reported as NRBCs/100 WBCs. The number of NRBCs encountered while counting 100 WBCs is incorporated into the following equation to calculate a corrected leukocyte count.[3]

$$\text{Corrected WBC count} = \frac{\text{Observed WBC count} \times 100}{100 + \% \text{ nucleated RBCs}}$$

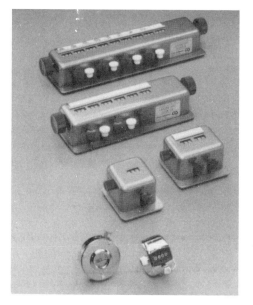

FIGURE 2-12. Various types of counters used for manual cell counts. (Courtesy Becton-Dickinson.)

An alternative and much more practical method is to include the NRBCs within the 100-cell differential count.[1] For example, an animal has a total WBC count of 10,000/µl, with 5000 (50%) neutrophils, 3000 (30%) lymphocytes, 1000 (10%) monocytes, and 1000 (10%) NRBCs. The corrected WBC count can then be calculated by subtracting the absolute number of NRBCs (1000/µl) from the total WBC count (10,000/µl), giving a corrected total WBC count of 9000/µl (10,000 − 1000 = 9000).

APPEARANCE OF LEUKOCYTES IN PERIPHERAL BLOOD

NEUTROPHIL. The nucleus of neutrophils is irregular and elongated; true filaments between nuclear lobes are rare (Plates 2, 8, 13, and 25). The nucleus of equine neutrophils has heavily clumped, coarse chromatin. The cytoplasm stains pale pink, with fine, diffuse granules. Bovine neutrophils have darker-pink cytoplasm. Toxic neutrophils have blue cytoplasm and may contain *Döhle bodies,* which are small (0.5 to 2 µ), angular, blue-gray granules (Plate 26 and Figure 2-13). Other changes with toxicity include vacuoles in the cytoplasm and increased size. The toxic appearance of neutrophils should be recorded, as it may signify bacterial infection.

BAND NEUTROPHIL. The nucleus of band neutrophils is horseshoe shaped, with large round ends (Plate 27). Although slight indentations may be present in the nucleus, if the constriction is greater than one third the width of the nucleus,

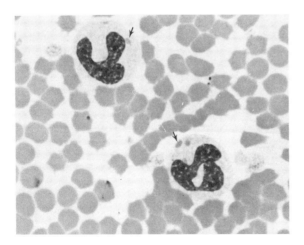

FIGURE 2-13. Döhle bodies (*arrows*) in toxic neutrophils in blood from a cat with pyothorax.

the cell is usually classified as a *segmented neutrophil*. More immature neutrophils (myelocytes, metamyelocytes) are rare in peripheral blood (Plate 28).

LYMPHOCYTE. Small lymphocytes are about 7 to 9 μ in diameter and have a slightly indented nucleus (Plate 13). The chromatin is coarsely clumped, and the cytoplasm is light blue and quite scanty. *Chromocenters,* areas of condensed chromatin, should not be confused with nucleoli; they appear as dark clumps within the nucleus. Medium-sized to large lymphocytes are 9 to 11 μ in diameter, with more abundant cytoplasm. The cytoplasm may contain pink-purple granules. Normal bovine lymphocytes may contain nucleolar rings and may be quite large and difficult to distinguish from neoplastic lymphoid cells (Plate 29).

LYMPHOBLAST. Lymphoblasts are immature lymphoid cells that contain a nucleolus within the nucleus (Plate 30). The nucleolus is a light-blue structure, often surrounded by a ring of chromatin. Lymphoblasts may be observed rarely in the blood of normal animals. Their presence should be recorded, as increased numbers suggest a lymphoproliferative disorder.

MONOCYTE. Monocytes are large cells that contain variably shaped nuclei (Plate 25). The nucleus is occasionally kidney bean shaped but is often elongated and lobulated. The nuclear chromatin is more diffuse in monocytes than in neutrophils, where it is coarsely clumped. The cytoplasm of monocytes is blue-gray and may contain vacuoles and/or small, fine, pink granules. Monocytes may be difficult to distinguish from band neutrophils or metamy-elocytes that are toxic. If a left shift is not present, the cells in question are probably monocytes.

EOSINOPHIL. Eosinophils contain a nucleus similar to that of neutrophils, but the chromatin is usually not as coarsely clumped. The shape of the eosinophilic granules varies considerably among species (Plate 31). The granules in canine eosinophils often vary, with small and large granules within the same cell, and stain less intensely than those of other species; they usually are hemoglobin colored (Plates 27 and 31). Feline eosinophils contain granules that are small, rod shaped, and numerous. The rod shape of the granules is more easily observed in broken than in intact eosinophils. Equine eosinophil granules are very large and round to oval, staining an intense orange-red. Eosinophil granules in cattle, sheep, and pigs are round and much smaller than those in horses. They are uniform in size and stain an intense pink.

Basophil.   The nucleus of basophils is similar to that of monocytes. Basophil granules in dogs are few in number and stain purple to blue-black (Plate 32). Equine and bovine basophil granules are usually more numerous and may completely pack the cytoplasm. Feline basophil granules are round and light lavender (Plate 33) and rarely contain dark granules.

While morphologic abnormalities of leukocytes are sometimes diagnostically useful, quantitative data obtained from the CBC are usually more helpful. A brief description of some acquired and inherited leukocyte morphologic abnormalities follows.

ACQUIRED MORPHOLOGIC ABNORMALITIES

Nuclear hyposegmentation.   Such hyposegmentation usually simply reflects early release of band neutrophils. *Pseudo-Pelger-Huet anomaly* has been reported and is either a variant on a normal inflammatory response or may be due to an idiosyncratic drug reaction. In general, in pseudo-Pelger-Huet anomaly, fewer neutrophils are hyposegmented than in the congenital anomaly.

Nuclear hypersegmentation.   Canine and feline neutrophils with five or more lobes are considered hypersegmented. This is usually due to aging of neutrophils, either *in vivo,* as would be seen with endogenous or exogenous glucocorticoids, which prolong the half-life of circulating neutrophils, or *in vitro,* as a result of prolonged storage of blood before making blood films. Hypersegmented neutrophils are also seen in blood films from Poodles with Poodle macrocytosis.

Toxic change.   The most common disease-induced cytoplasmic changes in neutrophils are referred to as *toxic changes* and are associated with inflammation, infection, drug toxicity, etc. These changes are more significant when they occur in dogs; if severe they often suggest bacterial infection. However, toxic changes are seen quite commonly in cats that are not severely ill. Types of toxic change include cytoplasmic basophilia, Döhle bodies, vacuoles, or "foaminess" (Plate 26), and, very rarely, intensely stained primary granules (toxic granulation). These "toxic" changes are thought to be due to decreased time of neutrophil maturation within the marrow.

Intracytoplasmic neutrophil inclusions in infectious diseases.   Canine distemper inclusions may appear in RBCs and are pale blue to magenta. Rickettsial inclusions (*Ehrlichia* species) are rarely seen within the cytoplasm of neutrophils (Figure 2-11), as are the gametocytes of *Hepatozoon canis.*

"ATYPICAL" LYMPHOCYTES.   Azurophilic granules in the cytoplasm of lymphocytes (Plate 34) are often associated with chronic antigenic stimulation, especially in canine ehrlichiosis. "Reactive" lymphocytes (Plate 35) have increased basophilia in the cytoplasm, may have more abundant cytoplasm, and sometimes contain a larger, more convoluted nucleus. These changes are usually due to antigenic stimulation secondary to vaccination or infection.

INHERITED MORPHOLOGIC ABNORMALITIES

PELGER-HUET ANOMALY.   Most of the neutrophils and eosinophils in heterozygotes for Pelger-Huet anomaly have hyposegmented nuclei. Cells have an immature-shaped nucleus (band or myelocyte form) but a coarse, mature chromatin pattern (Plate 36). Neutrophils function normally and affected animals are healthy.

LYSOSOMAL STORAGE DISORDERS.   These are a group of rare inherited diseases in which a substance is abnormally stored within cells, usually due to an intracellular enzyme deficiency. Numerous types have been reported in animals and clinical signs vary, depending on the specific enzyme deficiency. Most types have either skeletal abnormalities or progressive neurologic disease. Because most cells of the body are affected, the stored substance can often be seen in leukocytes, usually monocytes, lymphocytes, or neutrophils. The appearance of the leukocytes varies, depending on the type of lysosomal storage disease. Lymphocytes may be vacuolated (Plate 37) or contain granules (Plate 38) and/or neutrophils may contain granules (Plates 38 and 39). Examples of these disorders and the accompanying leukocyte abnormality are provided in Table 2-3.

BIRMAN CAT NEUTROPHIL GRANULATION ANOMALY.   Neutrophils from affected cats contain fine eosinophilic to magenta granules. This anomaly is inherited as an autosomal recessive trait. Neutrophil function is normal and affected cats are healthy. This granulation must be distinguished from toxic granulation and the granulation seen in neutrophils of cats with mucopolysaccharidosis and GM_2 gangliosidosis, two of the lysosomal storage disorders.

TABLE 2-3.   Lysosomal storage disorders and associated changes

DISORDER	SPECIES	VACUOLATED LYMPHOCYTES	GRANULATED NEUTROPHILS
Mucopolysaccharidosis I	Dog, cat	+	±
Mucopolysaccharidosis VI	Dog, cat	+	+++
Mucopolysaccharidosis VII	Dog, cat	+	+++
Niemann-Pick, type A	Cat	+++	−
Niemann-Pick, type C	Cat	+	−
GM$_1$ gangliosidosis	Cat	++	−
GM$_2$ gangliosidosis	Dog, cat, pig	+	+++
Fucosidosis	Dog	+	−
α-Mannosidosis	Cat	++	−
Acid lipase deficiency	Cat	++	−

CHEDIAK-HIGASHI SYNDROME.   Neutrophils in cats with Chediak-Higashi syndrome have large, fused 0.5 to 2 μ lysosomes within the cytoplasm and stain lightly pink or eosinophilic (Plate 40). Approximately one in three or four neutrophils contains fused lysosomes. Granules of eosinophils appear slightly plump and large. These cats have a slight tendency to bleed, as platelet function is abnormal. Although neutrophil function is also abnormal, affected cats are generally healthy.

PLATELETS

PLATELET COUNT

Platelets (*thrombocytes*) are a very important component of hemostasis. The best procedure for platelet evaluation is examination of the blood film. When platelet numbers appear decreased, it is appropriate to determine platelet concentration by a more quantitative procedure. This measurement should be done in a commercial laboratory because the expertise required to manually count platelets is difficult to develop and maintain. Both hemacytometer and electronic methods are used to count platelets.

Most domestic animals have increased bleeding if the platelet count drops below 50,000/μl. Platelet numbers should be evaluated in the counting area of the blood film (Figure 2-4). The size of the oil-immersion field depends on the type of microscope used. When using older microscopes, an average of three to five or more platelets per oil-immersion field is considered adequate. When using newer models, you should see eight to ten platelets per oil-immersion field.

If platelet numbers appear decreased, the 10X objective should be used to scan the feathered edge for clumps of platelets (Plate 41). Platelet clumping is common in cats. If clumps are observed, platelets are probably adequate in number. The presence of unusually large platelets (Plate 9) should be noted, as it may suggest early release of platelets from the bone marrow. Platelets, especially in cats, may be larger than erythrocytes. If decreased platelet numbers are suspected on the basis of the blood film examination, a platelet count is indicated.

PLASMA PROTEINS

PLASMA PROTEIN CONCENTRATION

Plasma protein level estimation by refractometry is an important component of the CBC in all species. The plasma with which the PCV was determined is used by breaking the hematocrit tube just above the buffy coat–plasma interface. The plasma is allowed to flow onto the refractometer prism (see Figure 5-3, Chapter 5). The refractometer is then held to a bright light and the reading is made at the dividing line between the bright and dark field. The protein value (in g/dl) is read directly from a scale inside the refractometer. Lipemia results in a false increase in the total protein reading.

PLASMA FIBRINOGEN CONCENTRATION

Fibrinogen is a plasma protein that is important in coagulation and inflammation. Elevated plasma fibrinogen concentrations are common in inflammatory conditions, particularly in cattle. Fibrinogen determination is thus an important component of the CBC in cattle.

Two microhematocrit capillary tubes are filled, as for a PCV, and centrifuged in a hematocrit centrifuge for 5 minutes. The plasma protein level is determined by refractometry (see above) with 1 tube. The other tube is suspended in a 56°-C (133°-F) water bath for 5 minutes, then centrifuged again to spin down the precipitated fibrinogen. (Heating plasma to 56° C precipitates fibrinogen but not albumin or globulin.) The protein concentration is then measured by refractometry in the fibrinogen-free plasma. The difference between the two plasma protein readings is the fibrinogen concentration, in mg/dl. For example, if the total plasma protein level in the unheated tube is 8.3 g/dl and the plasma protein level in the heated tube is 7.5 g/dl, the fibrinogen concentration is 800 mg/dl (0.8 g/dl). The normal plasma fibrinogen concentration in cattle is 200 to 800 mg/dl.

EVALUATION OF COAGULATION

Coagulation tests are employed to diagnose various bleeding disorders. *Hemostasis* is normally achieved by complex interrelationships among vessel walls, platelets, and coagulation factors. *Coagulation factors* are plasma proteins, most of which are synthesized in the liver. Fibrin and aggregates of platelets make up the hemostatic plug, or clot, within the vessel lumen or wall.

The coagulation mechanism is usually divided into two pathways, extrinsic and intrinsic, both of which terminate in a common pathway leading to fibrin production. The *intrinsic pathway* of coagulation occurs intravascularly and is essential. The *extrinsic* or *tissue pathway* enhances coagulation. Various coagulation tests have been developed to evaluate the intrinsic and extrinsic pathways.

COAGULATION TESTS

Blood samples for coagulation tests should be collected carefully, with minimal tissue damage and minimal venous stasis. Samples should never be collected through indwelling catheters. The preferred anticoagulant for coagulation tests is sodium citrate. Samples for whole blood clotting time and activated coagulation time do not require an anticoagulant. Unless numerous coagulation tests are performed in the veterinary hospital laboratory, blood samples should be sent to nearby commercial laboratories for testing.

The blood should be placed in an ice bath at the time of collection and then centrifuged, and the plasma separated within 30 minutes of collection. The plasma can then be stored in an ice bath and is stable for most tests for 4 hours. If the sample is to be mailed to a commercial laboratory, the plasma should be rapidly frozen in dry ice, then packed in dry ice (about 10 lb) in a polystyrene container.

Coagulation tests that can be performed in a veterinary hospital laboratory include the following.

Whole blood clotting time

The whole blood clotting time (Lee-White method) is a test of the intrinsic clotting mechanism. The whole blood clotting time tests are not commonly performed, as the activated clotting time is more sensitive. Collect 3 ml of blood in a plastic syringe, noting the time blood first appears in the syringe (use a stopwatch). Place 1 ml of blood in each of three 10 × 75-mm tubes that have been rinsed with saline. Place the tubes in a 37°-C (98.6°-F) water bath or hold them in your hand. Tilt the first and then the second tube at 30-second intervals until coagulation occurs. Tilt the third tube in a similar manner. The time elapsed between the appearance of blood in the syringe and clot formation in the third tube is the clotting time. The normal whole blood clotting time for dogs is 2 to 10 minutes, horses 4 to 15 minutes, and cattle 10 to 15 minutes.

An alternative, more simple method is to collect the blood in a glass syringe and simply tilt the syringe back and forth until the blood clots. Blood normally clots in 2 to 10 minutes if a glass syringe is used.

Activated clotting time

The activated clotting time (ACT), another test of the intrinsic clotting mechanism, is the ideal screening test for use in veterinary practices. The ACT procedure uses diatomaceous earth as an activating agent. This shortens the normal clotting time, thus increasing the sensitivity of the whole blood clotting time. Commercially available ACT tubes are prewarmed in a 37°-C (98.6°-F) water bath. A plastic syringe is used to carefully draw 2 ml of blood, which is then injected into the ACT tube, and a stopwatch is started at the time of injection. The tube is inverted five times to mix and is replaced in the water bath for 1 minute, after which the tube is removed from the bath at 5-second intervals and tilted. The endpoint is the first evidence of clotting. Normal values are about 60 to 90 seconds. Severe thrombocytopenia (<10,000 platelets/μl) prolongs the activated clotting time, as do abnormalities associated with the intrinsic coagulation cascade.

Bleeding time

If an animal has a type of bleeding disorder that suggests inadequate platelets (petechiae, epistaxis, hematuria, etc.) but platelet numbers are adequate, the bleeding time should be determined.

A clean site devoid of hair (e.g., the nose) is chosen and a deep puncture is made with a lancet or #11 Bard Parker scalpel blade. Note the time when blood appears. Without touching the skin, a filter paper is used to remove the blood at 30-second intervals. The endpoint is when blood no longer appears from the puncture site. The normal bleeding time for domestic animals is 1 to 5 minutes. Bleeding time is prolonged with platelet defects (qualitative or quantitative), increased capillary fragility, and von Willebrand's disease.

More sophisticated platelet function tests for platelet aggregation or adhesiveness should be performed by large hospital or commercial laboratories.

ACTIVATED PARTIAL THROMBOPLASTIN TIME

The activated partial thromboplastin time (APTT) is another test of the intrinsic clotting mechanism. If the ACT is prolonged, citrated plasma should be taken to a reference laboratory for an APTT. Citrated plasma is incubated with an activator of Factor XII, platelet substitute (cephaloplastin). After addition of calcium, the time to form fibrin is exactly determined by manual or semi-automated methods using fibrometers. The APTT can also be used in conjunction with known factor-deficient plasmas to identify a specific factor deficiency. Citrated plasma is stable for 4 hours in an ice bath. Each laboratory should establish its own normal range, which should not exceed ±3 seconds from the mean (e.g., mean APTT of 17 seconds, with a normal range of 14 to 20 seconds). A variety of acquired and hereditary disorders, in addition to administration of heparin, can reduce one or more factors necessary for the normal intrinsic coagulation cascade.

ONE-STAGE PROTHROMBIN TIME

The one-stage prothrombin time (OSPT) is a test of the extrinsic clotting mechanism. Citrated plasma is added to a thromboplastin-calcium mixture and the time to form fibrin is exactly determined manually or with a fibrometer. The test is independent of platelet function.

The patient's citrated plasma, along with that of a normal control, should be placed in an ice bath and transported to the laboratory within 2 hours of collection. Each laboratory should establish its own normal values for OSPT. Duplicate determinations should agree within 1 second. The normal range for dogs is usually 7 to 10 seconds. The test should not be performed in the veterinary hospital laboratory unless it is needed fairly frequently. Commercial reagents with detailed instructions are available (General Diagnostics, Morris Plains, NJ).

A prolonged OSPT may be associated with severe liver disease, disseminated intravascular coagulation, or hereditary or acquired deficiencies of any factors of the extrinsic coagulation cascade. The test is very sensitive to vitamin K deficiency or antagonism (e.g., warfarin toxicity).

BONE MARROW EVALUATION

COLLECTION

A bone marrow aspiration biopsy is indicated in patients with unexplained blood findings suggesting marrow failure or neoplasia when it is not possible to make a diagnosis by careful examination of the peripheral blood. Indications include nonregenerative anemia, leukopenia, thrombocytopenia, possible lymphoproliferative or myeloproliferative disorders, and abnormalities of immunoproteins. Core biopsy is indicated when attempts to obtain an aspirate have been unsuccessful, as is often the case in patients with myelofibrosis, a condition in which the bone marrow becomes filled with fibrous connective tissue.

Bone marrow biopsy needles should be constructed of strong steel and have a short beveled point and a large hub for ease of use (Figure 2-14). Osgood and Rosenthal bone marrow biopsy needles (Becton-Dickinson, Rutherford, NJ)

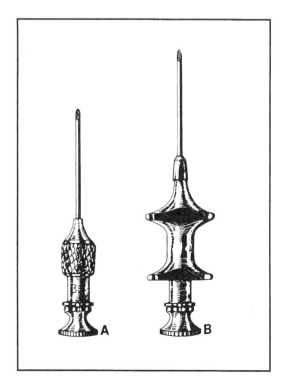

FIGURE 2-14. **A,** Osgood bone marrow biopsy needle. **B,** Rosenthal bone marrow biopsy needle. (From Banks WJ: *Applied veterinary histology,* ed 2, St Louis, 1993, Mosby.)

are quite satisfactory (16 to 18 gauge, 1 to $1\frac{1}{2}$ inch). They should be cleaned and autoclaved before each use. Conventional hypodermic needles may be satisfactory in cats with thin bones, but occlusion of the needle often prevents sample collection. Other required equipment includes clippers, soap, and skin disinfectant, a dry 12-ml syringe, local anesthetic, and microscope slides. A small tube containing EDTA is optional.

TECHNIQUE

The sites most commonly used in dogs and cats are the proximal end of the femur, the humerus, and the iliac crest. The iliac crest is usually used in cattle and horses. A local anesthetic (e.g., 2% lidocaine) injected into the skin, subcutaneous tissue, and periosteum is usually adequate. If the animal struggles, a short-acting general anesthetic may be required. If the femur is used, the animal should be placed in lateral recumbency, and the biopsy site prepared as for surgery. After infiltration with local anesthetic, the trochanteric fossa is located by placing the thumb on the greater trochanter (Figure 2-15). The needle is advanced toward the fossa with its long axis parallel to the long axis

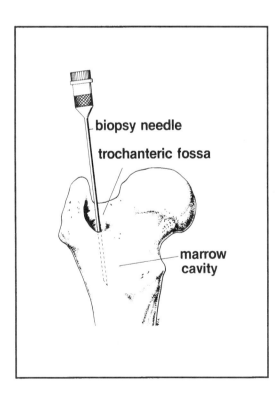

biopsy needle

trochanteric fossa

marrow cavity

FIGURE 2-15. Placement of a bone marrow biopsy needle in the trochanteric fossa of a dog. (From Banks WJ: *Applied veterinary histology,* ed 2, St Louis, 1993, Mosby.)

of the femur. The needle should be directed along the medial aspect of the greater trochanter until it encounters resistance.

When the needle has reached the cortex of the fossa, it should be rotated with short clockwise movements until it becomes firmly seated in bone. The leg can be stabilized as the needle is advanced by grasping the cranial aspect of the thigh and shaft of the femur and elevating the pelvic limb to a plane parallel to the table surface. The stylet should remain in the needle or the lumen may become clogged with bone. Advance the needle a few more millimeters, remove the stylet, and attach the syringe. Apply negative pressure only until marrow becomes visible in the syringe barrel. Aspiration of a large volume results in contamination of collected marrow with blood.

Release the negative pressure and remove the syringe. Place a small drop of marrow on each of several slides. Drop a second spreading slide gently on the marrow slide. The drop spreads rapidly between the glass surfaces. The slides are then pulled laterally, away from each other, while their surfaces are kept parallel (Figure 2-16). When placing the marrow directly on the slide, one must work very quickly, as the sample will clot within 60 seconds, rendering it useless. An alternative is to quickly place a few drops of collected marrow into an unstoppered commercial EDTA tube, which has had most of the EDTA

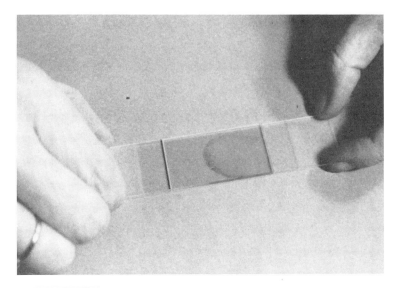

FIGURE 2-16. Bone marrow film preparation. A drop of marrow spread between two glass slides. The slides are about to be pulled laterally, away from each other.

shaken from it, thus preventing the marrow from clotting. Marrow films can then be made within the next few minutes.

If the iliac crest is used, the needle is placed on the superficial and dorsal portion and directed ventrally and medially. The needle should be firmly seated in bone and advanced several millimeters. Then proceed as described above. If a rib is used, the site of biopsy is usually located midway between the vertebra and the costal cartilage. Avoid damage to the intercostal artery, located caudal to each rib. If the sternum is used, position the biopsy needle so the long axis is perpendicular to the surface of the sternebrae and proceed as described above.

Bone marrow films should be stained as described for blood films.

EVALUATION OF BONE MARROW FILMS

A systematic approach should be used when evaluating a bone marrow film. The lower-power objective (10X) should be used to scan the entire slide. The number and degree of maturity of megakaryocytes should be noted, as well as the degree of overall cellularity and amount of fat (Figure 2-17). Red cell (*erythroid*) and white cell (*myeloid*) precursors should be identified, and the ratio of myeloid to erythroid cells (*M:E ratio*) estimated. While estimating this ratio, several fields in different areas of the film should be examined, as cells of one type are often seen together. It may be helpful to count 500 nucleated cells and classify them as erythroid or myeloid.

Erythroid and granulocytic precursors can usually be differentiated by their nuclear and cytoplasmic appearance (Plate 42). Nuclei of erythroid precursors tend to be round, with dark, coarse chromatin. These nuclei remain round

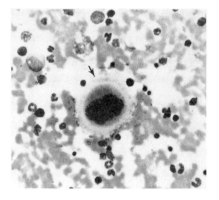

FIGURE 2-17.   Normal canine marrow film containing a megakaryocyte (*arrow*) and erythroid and myeloid precursors. (350X)

and become smaller as they mature. The nuclei of granulocytic precursors tend to be less perfectly round, elongating as they mature. The cytoplasm of erythroid precursors is deeply basophilic in more immature forms, becoming polychromatophilic and then pink as the cells mature. The cytoplasm of early granulocytic precursors contains pink primary granules; these disappear as the cell matures.

The completeness and orderliness of maturation in cells in both the erythroid and the myeloid series should be noted. Because blast cells divide to ultimately form 16 to 32 mature cells, about 80% of the granulocytic precursors should be the more mature forms (metamyelocytes, bands, neutrophils). About 90% of the erythroid series should be the more mature forms (rubricytes, metarubricytes). The erythroid series has complete maturation if significant numbers of polychromatophilic erythrocytes (reticulocytes) are present. Maturation of the myeloid series is complete if mature neutrophils are present. The presence and percentage of other types of cells (e.g., lymphocytes, plasma cells, macrophages) should be noted. *Erythrophagocytosis* (phagocytosis of RBCs by macrophages) and other unusual findings should be recorded.

MARROW CELL IDENTIFICATION

Descriptions of cells found within the marrow follow. Figures 2-18 and 2-19 illustrate examples of bone marrow films.

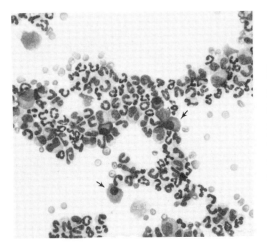

FIGURE 2-18.   Bone marrow film from a dog with granulocytic hyperplasia. Note that most of the precursors are myeloid. Plasma cells (*arrows*) appear to be present in increased numbers. Although rubricytic precursors appear to be decreased in number, the decrease is probably relative, as this dog is not anemic.

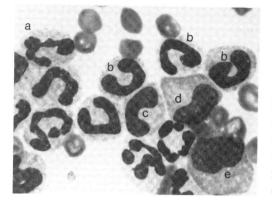

FIGURE 2-19. Bone marrow film from a dog with granulocytic hyperplasia. *a,* segmented neutrophil; *b,* band neutrophils; *c,* late metamyelocyte; *d,* early metamyelocyte; *e,* myelocyte. (1400X)

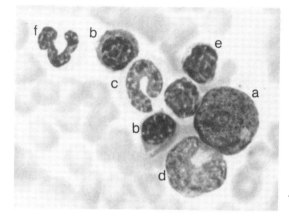

FIGURE 2-20. Normal bone marrow film. *a,* rubriblast; *b,* rubricyte; *c,* band neutrophil; *d,* metamyelocyte; *e,* lymphocyte; *f,* segmented neutrophil. (1400X)

ERYTHROCYTE PRECURSORS

RUBRIBLAST. Rubriblasts have a large, round nucleus, with royal-blue, stippled cytoplasm and a light-blue nucleolus (Figure 2-20).

PRORUBRICYTE. Prorubricytes are smaller than rubriblasts and have no nucleolus.

RUBRICYTE. Rubricytes are smaller than prorubricytes. Their nucleus contains dark clumps of chromatin and the cytoplasm becomes hemoglobin colored (Plate 42 and Figure 2-20).

METARUBRICYTE. Metarubricytes have a pyknotic nucleus, with cytoplasm that is more hemoglobin colored than that of rubricytes (Plate 42).

POLYCHROMATOPHILIC ERYTHROCYTE.   These are erythroid cells that have had their nucleus extruded. They are larger than mature erythrocytes. When they are stained with new methylene blue or brilliant cresyl blue, precipitated RNA is evident in the cytoplasm (reticulocyte).

GRANULOCYTE PRECURSORS

MYELOBLAST.   The nucleus of myeloblasts is not as round as that of rubriblasts and often is oval. One to two pale-blue nucleoli are present. The cytoplasm is blue-pink as contrasted to the royal-blue cytoplasm of rubriblasts (Plate 43).

PROGRANULOCYTE.   Small, pink granules can be seen in the cytoplasm of progranulocytes. A nucleolus may or may not be present (Plates 42 and 43).

MYELOCYTE.   The nucleus of myelocytes usually is oval and may be eccentric. The cytoplasm stains gray-blue (Figure 2-19 and Plate 43).

METAMYELOCYTE.   The nucleus of metamyelocytes becomes indented or kidney shaped, and their cytoplasm is less blue than that of myelocytes (Figures 2-19 and 2-20 and Plate 43).

BAND.   Band neutrophils have a horseshoe-shaped nucleus with slightly indented sides (Figures 2-19 and 2-20 and Plate 43).

Myelocytes, metamyelocytes, and bands may be either neutrophilic, eosinophilic, or basophilic. Eosinophil precursors contain distinct orange-pink granules, with basophilic cytoplasm. Basophil precursors contain purple or black granules.

PLATELET PRECURSORS

MEGAKARYOBLAST.   This cell is larger than other blast cells within the bone marrow. It contains two reddish nuclei and very basophilic, scanty cytoplasm.

PROMEGAKARYOCYTE.   The nuclei of promegakaryocytes partially divide and number 4, 8, 16, or 32. The nuclear lobes remain connected. The cytoplasm does not divide and consists of a rim around the nuclear mass.

MEGAKARYOCYTE.   The cytoplasm of megakaryocytes is abundant and pale blue and contains azurophilic granules. Mature megakaryocytes are very large (50 to 150 μ in diameter) (Plate 44).

PLATELET. Platelets (thrombocytes) are cytoplasmic structures of megakaryocytes. They vary in size and shape and contain azurophilic granules in a pale-blue background. Giant and cigar shapes are not uncommon, especially in cats.

OTHER CELLS OBSERVED IN BONE MARROW FILMS

LYMPHOCYTE. Small lymphocytes may be seen in bone marrow films, often comprising 10% to 15% of the total nucleated cells in cats.

PLASMA CELL. In a normal animal undergoing antigenic stimulation, plasma cells constitute less than 1% of the nucleated cells of bone marrow. Increased numbers are seen in animals with increased antibody production. Large numbers of immature or abnormal plasma cells in the bone marrow indicate multiple myeloma (a neoplasm of plasma cells). Plasma cells are transformed lymphocytes with abundant basophilic cytoplasm and a round, eccentric nucleus. The nuclear chromatin is usually clumped, resembling the nuclear pattern of rubricytes; they can be distinguished from rubricytes because plasma cells have a more abundant, more basophilic cytoplasm (Figure 2-18 and Plate 45). There is usually a well-defined perinuclear clear zone associated with the Golgi apparatus. Plasma cells are occasionally filled with round, clear, or pink structures called *Russell bodies.* The cell is then referred to as a *Mott cell.* Russell bodies are thought to be packets of immunoglobulin and are usually associated with intense antibody production.

MONOCYTE AND MACROPHAGE. These cells may be observed in bone marrow aspirates. Macrophages are best recognized when they contain phagocytized material, such as iron particles, nuclear material, and RBCs.

OSTEOBLAST. These cells are much larger than plasma cells but are somewhat similar. They have abundant basophilic cytoplasm, which is often vacuolated, and eccentric nuclei.

OSTEOCLAST. These are giant, multinucleated cells with abundant granular cytoplasm. Their nuclei are round and do not touch one another, unlike those of megakaryocytes.

MYELOPROLIFERATIVE AND LYMPHOPROLIFERATIVE DISORDERS
Leukemia, a neoplastic proliferation of hematopoietic cells within the bone marrow, is classified broadly into *myeloproliferative* and *lymphoproliferative.*

Diagnosis is based on finding characteristic blast cells in the blood and/or bone marrow and associated hematologic abnormalities. Specific cell types are identified by their morphologic appearance in Wright's-stained blood and bone marrow films and by their cytochemical staining properties, electron microscopic appearance, and monoclonal antibodies to surface antigens.

Myeloproliferative leukemia includes neoplastic proliferation of erythrocytes, granulocytes, monocytes, and megakaryocytes. *Lymphoproliferative leukemia* includes neoplastic proliferation of lymphocytes and plasma cells. Multiple cell lines may be neoplastic if the affected stem cell is multipotential; a common example is myelomonocytic leukemia, in which both neutrophils and monocytes have been neoplastically transformed.

MYELOPROLIFERATIVE DISORDERS.   Myeloproliferative disorders may involve primitive cells (poorly differentiated leukemia), RBCs (erythremic myelosis), granulocytes (granulocytic leukemia), or megakaryocytes (megakaryocytic leukemia) (Figure 2-21). Typically, normal marrow cells are displaced by proliferating immature cells. These disorders can occasionally be difficult to distinguish from marked erythroid regeneration or granulocytic hyperplasia in response to inflammation. A classification scheme similar to that used in humans has been described.[4]

Poorly differentiated leukemia is a proliferation of primitive, undifferentiated cells. These cells are large (12 to 20 μ), with a large, round, eccentric nucleus and basophilic to lavender cytoplasm. The nucleus may contain a nucleolus and the cytoplasm may contain pink granules. Cytoplasmic pseudopod-like structures

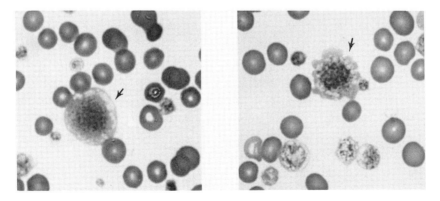

FIGURE 2-21.   Giant platelets (*arrows*) in peripheral blood from a cat with megakaryocytic leukemia. (1400X)

may project from the cells (Plate 46). If these structures break from cells, they may resemble giant platelets. Undifferentiated cells often have features of both erythroids and granulocytic precursors.

Erythremic myelosis is characterized by large numbers of early rubricytic precursors and decreased numbers of mature cells (polychromatophilic red cells). Although erythroid precursors may appear normal, they often have increased cytoplasm (megaloblastoid) as a result of asynchronous nucleus-cytoplasm maturation. Granulopoiesis is usually decreased (Plate 46). Increased numbers of nucleated erythroid precursors, which do not mature to polychromatophilic RBCs, are seen on blood films (Plate 47).

Granulocytic leukemia is usually characterized by an abnormal progression of maturation (large numbers of blasts, progranulocytes, myelocytes with few mature cells). Erythropoiesis is usually decreased.

Lymphoproliferative disorders. Tumors derived from lymphocytes or plasma cells are classified as lymphoproliferative neoplasms. Lymphoproliferative disorders are more common in domestic animals than are myeloproliferative disorders.

Lymphocytic leukemia (Plate 48) differs from malignant lymphoma (lymphosarcoma) primarily in anatomic distribution. Sarcomatous masses are present in lymphosarcoma but not in lymphocytic leukemia. However, about 10% to 25% of dogs and cats with lymphosarcoma develop leukemia. Lymphoproliferative disease arising in the bone marrow (lymphocytic leukemia) has a different biologic behavior, response to therapy, and prognosis. Lymphocytic leukemias are classified as either *chronic lymphocytic leukemia* or *acute lymphocytic leukemia*.

In *chronic lymphocytic leukemia,* the lymphocytes are small and appear well differentiated. This type of leukemia must be differentiated from physiologic lymphocytosis in excited cats, in which the absolute lymphocyte count may reach 20,000/μl, as well as from lymphocytosis induced by chronic antigenic stimulation, as seen in dogs with chronic ehrlichiosis.[5] *Lymphoblastic leukemia* is characterized by large numbers of lymphoblasts in the blood and bone marrow.

Plasma-cell myeloma (multiple myeloma) is a relatively rare lymphoproliferative neoplasm characterized by proliferation of plasma cells or precursors. As implied by the term "multiple myeloma," plasma cells proliferate at multiple sites in the bone marrow. While these plasma-cell proliferations may be diagnosed by examination of marrow films, they only infrequently result in plasma cells circulating in the blood. Although markedly increased numbers of plasma cells in the bone marrow (>20%) are often due to neoplasia, this proliferation may also be due to chronic antigenic stimulation.

An important diagnostic and clinical manifestation of plasma-cell myeloma is monocolonal gammopathy, which is detected by serum electrophoresis, a procedure performed in most diagnostic laboratories. Other diagnostic features include *Bence-Jones protein* (light chains of immunoglobulins) in the urine and radiographic evidence of osteolysis. Traditionally, two of these four diagnostic features are considered essential to diagnose plasma-cell myeloma. However, dogs with chronic ehrlichiosis may have monoclonal gammopathy and markedly increased numbers of plasma cells in the bone marrow. Fortunately, neoplastic plasma cells usually appear slightly abnormal or immature, with some multinucleated plasma cells present.

HEMOGRAMS IN SELECTED DISEASES

CASE 1

A 2-year-old Australian Shepherd was presented for acute onset of hematuria and depression. On physical examination, the dog had pale mucous membranes. The CBC results were as follows:

PCV: 11%
Hb: 4 g/dl
RBCs: $1.57 \times 10^6/\mu l$
MCV: 70 fl
MCHC: 36 g/dl
Total protein: 6.3 g/dl
WBCs: 32,000/μl
Segs: 24,000/μl
Bands: 1000/μl
Lymphs: 6000/μl
Monos: 3000/μl
Nucleated RBCs: 3000/μl
Platelets: 75,000/μl
Reticulocytes: 314,000/μl (20%)

The blood film demonstrated marked polychromasia and anisocytosis, with many spherocytes (Figure 2-22 and Plate 13). The serum was hemolyzed.

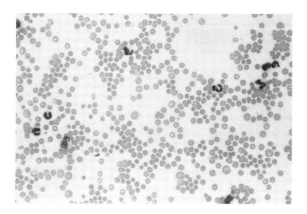

FIGURE 2-22. Canine blood film from Case 1. What is your diagnosis? (350X)

INTERPRETATION

A 20% reticulocyte count (314,000/μl) is evidence of a marked erythroid response. The anemia is regenerative, suggesting blood loss or blood destruction. Many spherocytes are diagnostic for immune-mediated hemolytic anemia. Neutrophilia, with a slight left shift, suggests an inflammatory response, which is typical in immune-mediated hemolytic anemia. Decreased platelets (immune-mediated thrombocytopenia) occur in about one third of affected patients. This case of immune-mediated hemolytic anemia exemplifies the necessity of careful evaluation of blood films; the many spherocytes were diagnostic.

CASE 2

An 8-year-old mixed-breed female dog was presented for evaluation of a mammary tumor, depression, hematuria, and gingival bleeding. The CBC results were as follows:

PCV: 16%
Total protein: 5.0 g/dl
WBCs: 50,000/μl
Segs: 44,000/μl (88%)
Bands: 3000/μl (6%)
Lymphs: 1000/μl (2%)
Monos: 1000/μl (2%)
Nucleated RBCs: 1000/μl (2%)
Platelets: markedly decreased on film, 20,000/μl
Polychromasia: 12%

There were numerous schistocytes (RBC fragments), and the neutrophils appeared toxic (basophilic vacuolated cytoplasm, Döhle bodies).

INTERPRETATION

The anemia is regenerative. The presence of schistocytes and decreased platelet numbers suggests disseminated intravascular coagulation (DIC), possibly secondary to the mammary tumor. An activated coagulation time, prothrombin time, activated partial thromboplastin time, and fibrin-degradation product determinations are needed to confirm DIC. The leukogram is evidence of the response to inflammation. The presence of toxic neutrophils suggests a bacterial or endotoxin component to the disease. An appropriate diagnosis is DIC secondary to a mammary tumor.

CASE 3

A 4-year-old Thoroughbred horse had been in a trailer accident 5 days previously and sustained severe lacerations and blood loss. The results of a CBC were as follows:

PCV: 18%
Total protein: 5.5 g/dl
WBCs: 15,000/µl
Segs: 13,500/µl
Bands: 500/µl
Lymphs: 500/µl
Monos: 500/µl
Platelets: adequate

No polychromasia was noted and there was an occasional Howell-Jolly body.

INTERPRETATION

Because horses do not release polychromatophilic RBCs (reticulocytes), even in the face of regenerative anemia, the lack of polychromasia is not meaningful. To determine if the anemia is regenerative, the MCV can be calculated (horses release larger cells in regenerative responses), which requires an RBC count. In addition, a bone marrow aspiration could be performed and reticulocytosis evaluated on the bone marrow film. Probably a more practical approach would be to perform the PCV on a weekly basis to determine if it is increasing.

Case 4

A 2-year-old Siamese cat was presented for evaluation of weight loss and anorexia. The CBC results were as follows:

PCV: 10%
Total protein: 8.5 g/dl
WBCs: 25,000/μl
Segs: 4000/μl (16%)
Bands: 1000/μl (4%)
Lymphs: 3000/μl (12%)
Nucleated RBCs: 17,000/μl (68%)
Corrected WBCs: 8000/μl
Reticulocytes: 0%
Platelets: slightly decreased

The neutrophils had toxic changes (blue, vacuolated cytoplasm, Döhle bodies).

Interpretation

Nucleated erythrocytes are early precursors (prorubricytes and rubricytes) (Plate 47). Many nucleated RBCs in conjunction with nonregenerative anemia (0% reticulocytes) suggest a myeloproliferative disorder (erythremic myelosis). A bone marrow aspiration and FeLV test are indicated. Note that the nucleated RBC count was included in the 100-cell differential count in this case. The corrected WBC count is obtained by subtracting the absolute number of nucleated RBCs from the observed WBC count. The diagnosis is myeloproliferative disorder (erythremic myelosis).

Case 5

A 1-year-old male Siamese cat was presented for evaluation of severe depression and anorexia of 3 days' duration. The CBC results were as follows:

PCV: 6%
Hb: 5.1 g/dl
RBCs: 2.27 × 10^6/μl
MCV: 22 fl
MCHC: 85 g/dl
WBCs: 6000/μl

Many Heinz bodies (80% of red cells affected) were suspected on Wright's-stained film and confirmed with new methylene blue stain (Plates 17 and 18). The blood was brown and very hemolyzed.

INTERPRETATION

Heinz bodies are the cause of hemolytic anemia. The hemolysis has resulted in a very high hemoglobin value, which has caused an erroneously high MCHC. Further questioning of the client revealed that the cat had been given two acetaminophen (Tylenol) tablets 36 hours previously. Acetaminophen acts as an oxidant of hemoglobin, resulting in Heinz body formation as well as methemoglobinemia, which resulted in the brown color of the blood. The diagnosis is Heinz body hemolytic anemia subsequent to acetaminophen toxicity.

REFERENCE VALUES

Tables 2-4, 2-5, and 2-6 contain reference ("normal") hematologic values for dogs, cats, horses, cattle, sheep, and pigs.[2]

CROSSMATCHING BLOOD FOR TRANSFUSION

A common treatment for anemia is transfusion of blood. To determine if the donor's and recipient's blood are immunologically compatible, crossmatching should be performed.

Red cell antigens are structures on the surface of RBCs from one animal that may react with antibodies in the plasma of another animal. These antigen-antibody reactions usually result in clumping or agglutination of RBCs. However, in some species, the antigen-antibody reaction is more likely to result in RBC lysis.

Although erythrocytes of common domestic animals possess antigens, naturally occurring antibodies, which are present in people, are relatively rare in animals. However, they do occur in cattle, sheep, and pigs. Once a transfusion has been given to an animal, antibodies against the RBC antigen (immune antibodies) are formed. However, because of the lack of naturally occurring antibodies, it has been a generally accepted principle in veterinary medicine that the first transfusion can be given without regard to the blood typing or crossmatching.

Table 2-4. Reference hematologic values for dogs and cats[2]

	Dogs RANGE (MEAN)	Cats RANGE (MEAN)
PCV (%)	37-55 (45)	24-45 (37)
Hemoglobin (g/dl)	12-18 (15)	8-15 (12)
RBC ($\times 10^6/\mu l$)	5.5-8.5 (6.8)	5-10 (7.5)
Total protein (g/dl)	6.0-7.5	6.0-7.5
WBC ($\times 10^3/\mu l$)	6.0-17.0 (11.5)	5.5-19.5 (12.5)
Differential, absolute		
Segs	60-77%; 3000-11,500 (7000)	35-75%; 2500-12,500 (7500)
Bands	0-3%; 0-300 (70)	0-3%; 0-300 (100)
Lymphs	12-30%; 1000-4800 (2800)	20-55%; 1500-7000 (4000)
Monos	3-10%; 150-1350 (750)	1-4%; 0-850 (350)
Eosinos	2-10%; 100-1250 (550)	2-12%; 0-1500 (650)
Basos	Rare	Rare
Platelets ($\times 10^5/\mu l$)	2.0-9.0	3-7 (4.5)
MCV (fl)	60-77 (70)	39-55 (45)
MCH (pg)	19-23	13-17
MCHC (g/dl)	32.0-36.0 (34.0)	30-36 (33.2)
Bone marrow M:E ratio	0.75-2.5:1 (1.2:1)	0.6-3.9:1 (1.6:1)

Although crossmatching may not be necessary with the first transfusion, subsequent transfusions require crossmatching. Breeding females, especially mares, should always be given properly matched blood to avoid sensitization that results in destruction of the foal's RBCs. Methods used for blood typing vary with the species.

Blood types

Dogs. There are at least eight different RBC antigens in dogs: DEA 1.1, 1.2, 3, 4, 5, 6, 7, and 8. DEA 1.1 and 1.2 are also referred to as "A" antigens, the ones of clinical significance. Because naturally occurring anti-A antibodies do

TABLE 2-5. Reference hematologic values for horses and cattle[2]

	HORSES RANGE (MEAN)	**CATTLE** RANGE (MEAN)
PCV (%)	32-52 (42)	24-46 (35)
Hemoglobin (g/dl)	11-19 (15)	8-15 (12)
RBC ($\times 10^6/\mu l$)	6.5-12.5 (9.5)	5-10 (7)
Total protein (g/dl)	6.0-8.0	6.0-8.0
WBC ($\times 10^3/\mu l$)	5.5-12.5 (9.0)	4.0-12.0 (8.0)
Differential, absolute		
Segs	30-65%; 2700-6700 (4700)	15-45%; 600-4000 (7000)
Bands	0-2%; 0-100 (2.0)	0-2%; 0-120 (20)
Lymphs	25-70%; 1500-5500 (3500)	45-75%; 2500-7500 (4500)
Monos	0.5-7%; 0-800 (400)	2-7%; 25-840 (400)
Eosinos	0-11%; 0-925 (375)	2-20%; 0-2400 (700)
Basos	0-3%; 0-170 (50)	0-2%; 0-200 (50)
Platelets ($\times 10^5/\mu l$)	1-6 (3.3)	1-8 (5)
MCV (fl)	34-58 (46)	40-60 (52)
MCH (pg)	15.2-18.6	14.4-18.6
MCHC (g/dl)	31-37 (35)	30-36 (32.7)
Bone marrow M:E ratio	0.94-3.76:1.0 (1.64:1)	0.31-1.85:1.0 (0.71:1)

not exist, the first transfusion of A-positive blood into an A-negative recipient does not result in a clinical reaction, but the transfused cells have a shortened life span (7 days). If a previously immunized A-negative dog receives A-positive blood, severe reactions occur in less than 1 hour.

Because there are no naturally occurring anti-A antibodies, crossmatching is of little value unless the animal has been previously sensitized with incompatible blood. A-negative dogs should be kept as blood donors to prevent reactions due to the A factor. Blood typing is performed at numerous veterinary teaching hospitals.

CATS. Blood groups of cats include A, B, and AB. Very few cats have group AB. The vast majority of cats in the United States have group A, which probably explains the low incidence of transfusion reactions in cats. Type-B cats

TABLE 2-6.   Reference hematologic values for sheep and pigs[2]

	SHEEP RANGE (MEAN)	PIGS RANGE (MEAN)
PCV (%)	24-50 (38)	32-50 (42)
Hemoglobin (g/dl)	8-16 (12)	10-16 (13)
RBC ($\times 10^6/\mu l$)	8-16 (12)	5-8 (6.5)
Total protein (g/dl)	6-7.5	6-7
WBC ($\times 10^3/\mu l$)	4-12 (8)	11-22 (16)
Differential, absolute		
Segs	10-50%; 700-6000 (2400)	28-47%; 3000-10,500
Bands	Rare	0-2%
Lymphs	40-75%; 2000-9000 (5000)	39-62%; 4300-13,700
Monos	0.6%; 0-750 (200)	2-30%; 220-2200
Eosinos	0.1%; 0-1000 (400)	0.5-11%; 0-2500
Basos	0-3%; 0-300 (50)	0-2%; 0-400
Platelets ($\times 10^5/\mu l$)	2.5-7.5 (4.0)	3.25-7.15 (5.2)
MCV (fl)	23-48 (33)	50-68 (63)
MCH (pg)	9-13	16.6-22
MCHC (g/dl)	31-38 (33.5)	30-34 (32)
Bone marrow M:E ratio	0.77-1.68:1 (1.1:1)	1.77 ± 0.52:1

are most likely to be purebred. Transfusing type-B cats with type-A blood may result in serious transfusion reactions and death. Thus blood for transfusion of purebred cats should be selected by crossmatching.

CATTLE.   Eleven blood groups have been described in cattle. Anti-J antibodies are the only common natural antibodies in cattle. It has been suggested that J-negative donors be used to minimize transfusion reactions. The lytic crossmatch is required because bovine and ovine erythrocytes have little tendency to agglutinate.

HORSES.   Sixteen blood antigens have been described in eight systems in horses. Naturally occurring antibodies do not exist, but antibodies may be present as a result of vaccinations containing equine tissue or transplacental immunization. Crossmatching should be done before the first transfusion in a horse, using both the lytic and agglutination procedures. Transfusion reactions in horses are commonly fatal.

CROSSMATCHING PROCEDURES

The following procedure can demonstrate both hemolysis and agglutination. Draw blood samples from both the donor and the recipient into individual clot tubes (no anticoagulant used). Centrifuge the clotted samples and transfer the serum to separate labeled tubes. Using cells from the recipient's and donor's clots, prepare an approximate 3% red cell suspension (percentage is not critical) in normal saline from each sample. Wash both of the suspensions three times with normal saline, centrifuging after each washing, until the supernatant is clear and colorless. After the final washing, redilute each tube of washed RBCs in saline, again to about a 3% cell suspension.

MAJOR CROSSMATCH. In a 12 × 75-mm test tube, place two drops of the recipient's serum and two drops of the donor's red cell suspension.

MINOR CROSSMATCH. In a 12 × 75-mm test tube, place two drops of the donor's serum and two drops of the recipient's red cell suspension.

Incubate the tubes in a 37°-C (98.6°-F) water bath for 30 minutes. Centrifuge the tubes for 2 minutes at 500 rpm. Examine the supernatant for hemolysis. Slight hemolysis of canine blood is nonspecific. Significant hemolysis in either of the crossmatched tubes indicates incompatibility and the necessity of choosing another donor.

After examining the supernatant for hemolysis, shake the tubes gently by tapping to detect grossly visible agglutination. If no agglutination is observed, transfer a small amount of the mixture to a microscope slide, apply a coverslip, and examine with the 10X objective for agglutination. Agglutination in either tube indicates incompatibility and necessity of choosing a new donor.

REFERENCES

1. Weiser: Hematologic techniques, *Vet Clin North Am* 11:189-208, 1981.
2. Jain: *Essentials of veterinary hematology,* Baltimore, 1993, Waverly.

3. Benjamin: *Outline of clinical pathology,* ed 3, Ames, IA, Iowa State University Press.

4. Jain, et al: Proposed criteria for classification of acute myeloid leukemias in dogs and cats, *Vet Clin Pathol* 20:63-82, 1991.

5. Weiser, et al: Granular lymphocytosis and hypoproteinemia in dogs with chronic ehrlichiosis, *JAAHA* 27:84-88, 1991.

BLOOD CHEMISTRY

J. Colville

CHEMICAL ASSAY OF SERUM, PLASMA, OR WHOLE BLOOD[1-6]

Many veterinary practices now own or lease chemistry analyzers to perform routine chemical assays in-house. Possibly nowhere more than in the laboratory is the veterinary technician more valuable to the practice.

Evaluation of chemical components of blood has become an important aid in formulating an accurate diagnosis, prescribing proper therapy, and monitoring the response to treatment. Most chemical assays measure either the level of a dissolved substance normally carried in the blood (plasma), or the amount of a substance not normally found in blood, which has been released into the blood from damaged or destroyed cells.

As the person most likely to be in charge of the laboratory, you must become familiar with the types of analytic instruments available (see Chapter 1), the variety of testing procedures used, and the rationale underlying the analyses.

The most important contribution you can make to the practice laboratory is to feel confident in your results when you hand them to the veterinarian. It is vitally important that the results are reliable. *In-vitro* results must reflect, as closely as possible, the actual *in-vivo* levels of blood constituents.

SAMPLE COLLECTION

Most chemical analyses require whole blood, plasma, or serum. Always check the test protocol for the type of sample required.

Whole blood.   Whole blood is made up of fluid and cells. The fluid component is plasma; the cellular component is made up of erythrocytes, leukocytes, and platelets.

A whole blood sample is obtained by withdrawing the blood into a suitable container with the proper anticoagulant to prevent clotting. As soon as the blood is collected, mix the blood and anticoagulant with a gentle rocking motion. Shaking the sample vigorously causes hemolysis, which in turn can affect the results of the assays when chemicals normally found within the erythrocytes are released into the plasma. If the assay will be delayed for over an hour after blood collection, refrigerate (0° to 4° C) the sample. When you are ready to run the analysis, warm the sample to room temperature (20° C) and remix gently. Whole blood should not be frozen.

Plasma.   Plasma is the fluid portion of whole blood in which the cells are suspended. It is made up of about 90% water and 10% dissolved constituents, such as proteins, carbohydrates, vitamins, hormones, enzymes, lipids, salts, waste materials, antibodies, and other ions and molecules. Procedure 3-1 describes obtaining a plasma sample.

Do not contaminate the sample with any cells from the bottom of the tube. Refrigerate the sample if you cannot centrifuge it within 1 hour. If heparinized plasma has been stored for some time after separation, centrifuge the sample again to remove any fibrin clots that might have formed. Plasma samples can be

---

Procedure 3-1.   Obtaining a plasma sample

1. Collect a blood sample in a container with the appropriate anticoagulant.
2. Mix the blood-filled container with a gentle rocking motion 12 times.
3. Make sure the container is covered to prevent evaporation during centrifugation.
4. Centrifuge (within an hour of collection) at 2000 to 3000 rpm for 10 minutes.
5. Using a capillary pipette, carefully remove the fluid plasma layer from the bottom layer of cells.
6. Transfer the plasma to a container labeled with the date, time of collection, patient's name, and case or clinic number.
7. Refrigerate or freeze as appropriate.

refrigerated or frozen. Freezing may affect certain test results, so check the test protocol before freezing a plasma sample.

SERUM.   Serum is plasma from which fibrinogen, a plasma protein, has been removed. During the clotting process, the soluble fibrinogen in plasma is converted to an insoluble fibrin clot matrix. When the clot forms, the fluid that is squeezed out around the cellular clot is serum. Obtaining a serum sample is described in Procedure 3-2.

Centrifuging at higher speeds than 2000 to 3000 rpm or for a prolonged time can result in hemolysis. Freezing may affect some test results, so check the test protocol before freezing a serum sample.

ANTICOAGULANTS

An anticoagulant is a chemical that, when added to a whole blood sample, prevents or delays clotting (coagulation) of the sample. Some anticoagulants may affect assays, so check the test procedure for the proper anticoagulant in which to collect the sample. For example, the sodium or potassium salt of an anticoagulant may affect the results of an electrolyte assay by adding sodium or potassium to the sample. The anticoagulant also may physically remove the

---

PROCEDURE 3-2.   Obtaining a serum sample

1. Collect a whole blood sample in a container that contains no anticoagulant.
2. Allow the blood to clot in its original container at room temperature for 20 to 30 minutes.
3. *Do not* refrigerate the blood until it has clotted.
4. Gently separate the clot from the container by running a wooden applicator stick around the wall of the container between the clot and the wall.
5. Cover the sample and centrifuge at 2000 to 3000 rpm for 10 minutes.
6. Using a capillary pipette, remove the serum from the clot.
7. Transfer the serum to a container labeled with the date, time of collection, patient's name, and clinic or case number.
8. Refrigerate or freeze the sample as appropriate.

constituent to be assayed. For example, an oxalate anticoagulant removes calcium from the sample, making it useless for calcium determinations. Other anticoagulants may inhibit certain enzymes and activate others.

HEPARIN.   Heparin is the anticoagulant of choice when plasma is required for analysis because it interferes least with chemical assays. Heparin is available as a sodium, potassium, lithium, or ammonium salt. It is thought to prevent clotting by preventing conversion of prothrombin to thrombin during the clotting processes.

To prevent clotting, heparin should be used at 20 units/ml of blood to be collected. The most convenient method for using heparin is to coat the inside walls of a syringe with liquid heparin before the sample is drawn from the patient. Vacuum collection tubes containing the proper amount of heparin are available commercially. These are most convenient when many heparinized samples are needed. The vacuum tubes have a limited shelf life, so they may not be practical for a practice that rarely needs heparinized plasma.

The major disadvantage of heparin is that it is relatively expensive. Also, heparin may interfere with some chemical assays. For example, it may cause falsely increased inorganic phosphorus levels in blood or may interfere with lactate dehydrogenase activity.

ETHYLENEDIAMINETETRAACETIC ACID.   EDTA is the anticoagulant of choice for hematologic studies because it does not alter cell morphology; it should not be used if plasma samples are to be subjected to chemical assays. EDTA is available as a sodium or potassium salt and prevents clotting by forming an insoluble complex with calcium, which is necessary for clot formation. To prevent clotting, EDTA is added at 1 to 2 mg/ml of blood to be collected. Vacuum collection tubes containing the proper amount of EDTA are commercially available.

The disadvantages of using EDTA for chemical assays are: it may interfere with color development in some alkaline phosphatase tests; it ties up metallic ions that may be necessary for enzyme activity; and it ties up calcium, making it unavailable for assay.

OXALATES.   Oxalates are available as sodium, potassium, ammonium, or lithium salts. They prevent clotting by forming insoluble complexes with calcium, which is necessary for clot formation. Potassium oxalate is the most commonly used oxalate salt. To prevent clotting, it is used at 1 to 2 mg/ml of blood to be collected. Vacuum collection tubes containing the proper amount of oxalate anticoagulant are available commercially.

The disadvantage of using oxalates is that they also may tie up metallic ions necessary for enzyme activity. Potassium oxalate may inhibit lactate dehydrogenase and alkaline phosphatase activity. Also, because it is a potassium salt, it cannot be used with blood samples to be assayed for potassium.

SODIUM FLUORIDE.   Sodium fluoride, best known as a glucose preservative, also has some anticoagulant properties. As an anticoagulant it is used at 6 to 10 mg/ml of blood to be collected. Vacuum collection tubes containing the proper amount of sodium fluoride for anticoagulation are available commercially. Sodium fluoride also can be added to other samples as a glucose preservative even if there is a different anticoagulant present. For glucose preservation, sodium fluoride is used at 2.5 mg/ml of blood.

SAMPLE VOLUME

The amount of blood collected from an animal depends on the quantity of serum or plasma required for the assay and the hydration status of the patient. For example, a well-hydrated animal with a PCV of 50% should yield a blood sample that is 50% cells and 50% fluid. A 10-ml blood sample should yield 5 ml of fluid. In dehydrated animals, hemoconcentration results in a smaller ratio of fluid to cells. A dehydrated animal with a PCV of 70% yields a blood sample that is 70% cells and 30% fluid. This means that only 3 ml of fluid will be obtained from a 10-ml blood sample.

As a rule of thumb, enough blood should be collected to yield enough serum, plasma, or whole blood to run all the planned chemical assays three times. This allows for technician error, instrument failure, or the need to dilute a sample without having to collect another sample from the animal.

FACTORS INFLUENCING RESULTS

Collection of a high-quality sample on which to perform an assay depends on a number of factors. Most adverse influences on sample quality can be avoided with careful consideration of sample collection and handling.

HEMOLYSIS.   When using a syringe for sample collection, avoid hemolysis. Hemolysis can result when a blood sample is drawn into a moist syringe, mixed too vigorously after sample collection, forced through a needle when transferring it to a tube, or frozen as a whole blood sample. A syringe must be completely dry before it is used, as water in the syringe can cause hemolysis. The needle from a syringe must be removed before transferring blood to a tube. Forcing blood through a needle may rupture cells. When transferring a blood sample to a tube, expel the blood slowly from the syringe without causing bubbles to form.

Hemolysis, regardless of cause, can greatly alter the makeup of a serum or plasma sample. For example, fluid from ruptured blood cells can dilute the sample, resulting in falsely lower concentrations of constituents than are actually present in the animal. Further, certain constituents, normally not found in high concentrations in serum or plasma, escape from ruptured blood cells, causing falsely elevated concentrations in the sample. Hemolysis can elevate levels of potassium, organic phosphorus, and certain enzymes in the blood. Hemolysis also interferes with lipase activity and bilirubin determinations. For this reason, plasma or serum is frequently the preferred sample over whole blood, and serum is frequently preferred over plasma.

CHEMICAL CONTAMINATION.   It is not necessary to use sterile tubes when collecting blood samples for routine chemical assays. However, the tubes must be chemically pure. Detergents must be completely rinsed from reusable tubes so they do not interfere with test results.

IMPROPER LABELING.   Serious errors may result if a sample is not labeled immediately after it is collected. The tube should be labeled with the date, time of collection, patient's name, and clinic number. Double-check the sample identification with the request form, if one is used, as you prepare the sample and perform the assay.

IMPROPER SAMPLE HANDLING.   Ideally, all chemical measurements should be completed within an hour of sample collection. Because this is not always possible, make sure samples are properly handled and stored so levels of their chemical constituents approximate those in the patient's body at the time of collection. It is especially important that samples not be allowed to become too warm. Heat can be very detrimental to a sample, destroying some chemicals and activating others, such as enzymes. If a serum or plasma sample has been frozen, be sure it is thoroughly mixed after thawing to avoid concentration gradients. Table 3-1 lists the recommended storage time limits of samples.

PATIENT INFLUENCES.   If practical, a sample should be obtained from a fasting animal. The blood glucose level can be elevated and the inorganic phosphorus

TABLE 3-1. Storage recommendations for various constituents in serum or plasma promptly separated from blood cells

CONSTITUENT	20° C	0°-4° C	−20° C	COMMENTS
Alkaline phosphatase	7 days	7 days	1 month	Levels may increase after storage; if frozen, thaw and leave at 4° C until analyzed
Albumin	1 week[1] 4 days[2]	1 month[1] 4 days[2]	2 months[1] 11 days[2]	
ALT (GPT)	2 days	1 week	Unstable	Is not stable during thawing
Amylase	1 month 1 month	7 months 1 month	2 months 1 month	
AST (GOT)	2 days	2 weeks	1 to several months	
Bilirubin	—	1 week	3 months	Protect from light; unstable at room temperature
BUN	8 hours	10 days	Several months	Bacterial contamination should be avoided; store at 4° C or −20° C if longer storage required
Calcium	10 days	10 days	10 days	Cork stopper increases calcium levels
Chloride	stable	stable	Stable	
Cholesterol	7 days	—	6 months	

Continued.

TABLE 3-1.—CONT'D.

CONSTITUENT	20° C	0°-4° C	−20° C	COMMENTS
CK	2 hours[3] 2 days[4]	6 hours[3] 1 week[4]	Unstable[3] 1 month[4]	Analyze ASAP as some isoenzymes are unstable
Creatinine	1 week	1 week	Stable	
Glucose	8 hours (24 hours[5])	72 hours	Stable	
Gamma-GT	2 days	1 week	1 month	
Inorganic phosphorus	—	1 week	3 weeks	
LDH[6]	Not recommended	1-3 days	1-3 days	Best to analyze ASAP
Sorbitol dehydrogenase	Not recommended	2 days[7]	Not recommended	
Total protein	1 week	1 month	Stable	
Uric acid	8 hours[8]	1 week	2 months	

1 – When analyzed using dye-binding methods.
2 – When analyzed using electrophoresis.
3 – "Nonactivated" CK. Does not thaw well.
4 – "Activated" CK.
5 – Sodium fluoride-preserved samples.
6 – LDH isoenzymes have varying stability times: LDH_1 = 1 month at all temperatures; LDH_2-LDH_5 = 10 days at 25° C; LDH_2 = 1 month at −20° C; LDH_3 = 1 month at −20° C; LDH_4 = less than 2 days at −20° C; LDH_5 = less than 8 days at −20° C.
7 – Levels drop appreciably. SDH not stable at any storage temperature.
8 – Recommended storage temperature if analyzed on the day of collection.

level decreased immediately after a meal. Also, postprandial (after-eating) lipemia results in a turbid or cloudy sample. Water intake need not be restricted.

ENZYMOLOGY

Enzymes are proteins produced inside cells. They induce chemical changes in other substances (called *substrates*) but are not changed themselves. An enzyme can speed up the rate of a biochemical reaction by acting as a catalyst to the reaction. Mostenzymes are formed and function intracellularly, so they are found in highest concentrations within cells. For this reason, the blood level of most enzymes is very low in a healthy animal. The blood level of an enzyme can be elevated if the enzyme has leaked out of damaged cells, or if the cells have increased production of the enzyme and the excess amount has leaked out of the cells into the blood.

The substance on which an *enzyme (E)* works is called a *substrate (S)*. Each enzyme (there are many) has a specific substrate. Each enzymatic reaction produces a specific *product (P)* from the interaction of substrate and enzyme. The reaction forms a product but no change in the enzyme.

$$S + E \rightarrow P + E$$

Because blood levels of enzymes are so low, it is difficult to directly measure enzyme concentrations. The assays performed to determine enzyme concentrations in blood indirectly measure the enzyme concentration present by directly measuring the enzymatic reaction.

ENDPOINT VS. KINETIC ASSAYS

Enzyme assay methods are classified as *endpoint* or *kinetic*. Using endpoint methods, the product formed from enzymatic action interacts with a reagent to produce a *color complex*. The amount of light absorbed by this color complex is proportional to the amount of color complex present, which indirectly reflects the concentration of the enzyme present in the sample. In other words, the more intense the color production, the more product that was produced because there was more enzyme present.

Kinetic methods measure the rate of the enzymatic reaction while it is in progress and usually involve serial measurements of the product concentration per unit of time. The rate of product formation, and hence the rate of the reaction, is proportional to the amount of enzyme present. Enzymes are most active when the substrate concentration is high and the product concentration is zero. If the enzyme concentration exceeds the substrate available, the enzyme activity is no longer proportional to the product formed (the substrate concentration has become a limiting factor) and the assay is invalid.

It is important that substrate concentrations be kept high enough so as not to invalidate the measurement. Test kits are manufactured so that a large amount of substrate is initially present in the system to avoid this problem. If the amount of enzyme present is doubled, the rate of the reaction is doubled and the amount of product formed is doubled, providing time is constant. If the amount of enzyme present is the same but the time is doubled, the amount of product doubles. From this it is evident that if both time and enzyme concentration are kept constant, the rate of the reaction can be determined.

FACTORS INFLUENCING ENZYME ACTIVITY

Enzyme activity can be inhibited by low temperatures, accelerated by high temperatures, and retarded by dehydration, ultraviolet light, and the salts of heavy metals (copper, mercury). Enzymes, being proteins, can be denatured by temperature and pH extremes or by organic solvents. Only a small change in its polypeptide chain structure may cause an enzyme to lose activity, so samples for enzyme assay must be handled with care.

Each enzyme has an optimum temperature at which it works most efficiently. This temperature is typically listed in the instructions accompanying the test kit or analyzer. Most assays are performed at temperatures between 30° C and 37° C (86° to 98.6° F). For every 10° C (18° F) above the optimal temperature, the enzymatic reaction doubles. It is important to closely monitor the incubator or water bath temperature used in enzyme assays.

COMPONENTS OF ENZYME ASSAYS

Enzyme assays use a number of components. The *substrate* is the substance acted on by the enzyme. A *buffer* keeps the pH of the system constant to ensure maximal enzyme activity. Sometimes an enzyme requires a *cofactor* or *coenzyme* to catalyze (accelerate) a reaction. These include various metals and vitamins that act by combining with the enzyme. In other situations a cofactor is not required, but an *activator* is. An *activator* does not directly take part in the reaction (as do coenzymes and cofactors) but enhances the catalytic (accelerating) activity of the enzyme.

It is important to regulate temperature during an enzyme analysis. In tests in which a "working substrate," which contains all the components except the reaction activator, is used, the mixture must be preincubated until it reaches the required temperature. In assays in which serum is added to the prewarmed test system, the serum must also be prewarmed. If refrigerated serum is added directly to the reaction cuvette, the temperature of the system is lowered, thereby altering the results.

Most enzyme analyses require serum as the sample. Many anticoagulants interfere with the activity of enzymes.

SELECTING A TEST METHOD

Selection of a test method for enzyme analysis depends on a number of factors. The system must be sensitive enough to detect small amounts of enzyme activity. Specificity is important because it is necessary to determine which tissues have been damaged, thus leaking enzymes into the blood.

A number of technical factors also should be considered. Is the method accurate and precise? How practical is it to perform, considering the instrumentation, technician time, and skill available in your laboratory? Cost also must be considered. Reagents should have an acceptable shelf life. Finally, results obtained from the method chosen should correlate with those of accepted reference methods.

UNITS OF MEASUREMENT

Enzyme concentrations are measured as units of activity. These units of measurement can be very confusing. One might assume that enzyme activity is proportional to the enzyme concentration, but this is true only under certain conditions.

It was the practice for each investigator who developed an enzymatic analytic method to assign his own unit of measurement to the results. These often reflected the developer's name: Bodansky, Somogyi, and Sigma-Frankel units. Because each of the assays was performed under differing conditions (pH, temperature), it became difficult to correlate results reported in one unit to those of another. To avoid this confusion, the International Union of Biochemistry established a unit of enzyme activity known as the International Unit (U or IU). Enzyme concentration is expressed as mU/ml, U/L or U/ml. An International Unit is defined as "that amount of enzyme, which, under given assay conditions, will catalyze the conversion of one micromole of substrate per minute." Box 3-1 shows how to convert various units to International Units.

Some laboratories have replaced the IU system with one better related to the Systeme Internationale (SI) set of basic units, which is based on the metric system. The *katal* then becomes the basic unit of enzyme activity. A katal is the amount of activity that converts one mole of substrate per second.

Box 3-1. Factors for converting various enzyme units to International Units (IU)

Alkaline phosphatase
>   Bodansky Units × 5.37 = IU/L
>   Shinowara-Jones-Reinhart Units × 5.37 = IU/L
>   King-Armstrong Units × 7.1 = IU/L
>   Bessey-Lowry-Brock Units × 16.67 = IU/L
>   Babson Units × 1.0 = IU/L
>   Bowers-McComb Units × 1.0 = IU/L

Amylase
>   Somogyi (saccharogenic) Units × 1.85 = IU/L
>   Somogyi (37° C; 5 mg starch/15 min/100 ml) × 20.6 = IU/L

Lipase
>   Roe-Byler Units × 16.7 = IU/L

Lactate dehydrogenase
>   Wroblewsky-La Due Units × 0.482 = IU/L
>   Wroblewsky-Gregory Units × 0.482 = IU/L

Transaminases
>   Reitman-Frankel Units × 0.482 = IU/L
>   Karmen Units × 0.482 = IU/L
>   Sigma-Frankel Units × 0.482 = IU/L
>   Wroblewsky-La Due Units × 0.482 = IU/L

Terms Used in Enzymology

Enzymes are usually named for the substrate on which they act or the biochemical reaction in which they participate. Most enzyme names end with the *-ase* suffix. For example, lipase is an enzyme that catalyzes biochemical reactions that result in the hydrolysis of *lipids* (fats) to fatty acids, and lactate dehydrogenase participates in a reaction that involves oxidation (dehydrogenation) of lactate to pyruvate.

Some enzymes found in different tissues occur as *isoenzymes.* An isoenzyme is one of a group of enzymes with similar catalytic activities but different physical properties. The serum concentration of an enzyme that occurs as isoenzymes is the total of the concentrations of all the isoenzymes present. By identifying which isoenzyme is present in the sample, the source of that particular isoenzyme can be identified. For example, serum alkaline phosphatase is found in many tissues, particularly osteoblasts and hepatocytes. If the total serum alkaline phosphatase level is found to be elevated, there is no way of knowing if the increase is from damaged bone cells or damaged liver cells. However, if the respective levels of the various isoenzymes of alkaline phosphatase are assayed, levels of the isoenzyme from the damaged tissue will be elevated, thus identifying the damaged tissue. The alkaline phosphatase assay performed in the practice laboratory is for *total* serum alkaline phosphatase because individual isoenzyme assay methods have not yet been developed for the practice laboratory.

REFERENCE RANGES

Reference ranges were formerly known as "normal values." The reference range for a particular blood constituent is a range of values derived when a laboratory has repeatedly assayed samples from a significant number of clinically normal animals of a given species. Numerous medicine and clinical pathology books list the reference ranges of blood constituents for domestic species. Alternatively, reference ranges can be formulated by local diagnostic laboratories or by your own practice laboratory.

The difficulty with establishing reference range values for any laboratory is that it is time consuming and expensive. If you wanted to establish a list of reference values for your laboratory, you would have to assay samples from a significant number of clinically normal animals; some investigators recommend analysis of at least 20 animals and others over 100 animals with similar characteristics. You would have to take into account the variety of breeds and species most often seen in your practice, the gender and sexual status (intact or neutered) of the tested animals, the environment (including husbandry and nutrition) in which these animals are kept, and your climate (drastic seasonal changes can affect assay results).

Reference ranges have not been included in the following discussions of blood constituents because of the variations found among different geographic areas. In some areas of the country or in different laboratories, the reference ranges may be wider or narrower than published ranges. It is up to each practice to decide which reference ranges most accurately reflect the values observed in its patients.

Sample preference varies with each instrument and each assay. One instrument may require whole blood as a sample for an assay. Another instrument may require heparinized plasma or serum. Sample preferences are not included in the following discussions.

Sample handling and special considerations are included in the following discussions as general guidelines. Always check the test protocol you are using for specific handling instructions or special considerations.

LIVER ASSAYS

The liver is the largest internal organ. It is a complex organ in terms of structure, function, and pathology. It has a multitude of functions, including metabolism (amino acids, carbohydrates, lipids); synthesis (albumin, cholesterol, plasma protein, clotting factors); digestion and absorption of nutrients (related to bile formation); secretion of bilirubin (bile); and elimination (detoxification of toxins, catabolism of certain drugs). All of these functions are run by enzymatic reactions.

No single test is superior to any other for detecting hepatic disease. New tests that will allow us to detect hepatic disease before the liver is severely damaged are always being evaluated.

ENZYMES ASSOCIATED WITH HEPATOCELLULAR DAMAGE

With this type of liver disease, the hepatocytes are damaged and enzymes leak out into the blood, causing a detectable rise in blood levels of enzymes associated with liver cells.

ALANINE AMINOTRANSFERASE (ALT)

RATIONALE.   This enzyme was formerly known as serum glutamic pyruvic transaminase (SGPT). In dogs, cats, and primates, the major source of ALT is the hepatocyte. For this reason it is considered a liver-specific enzyme in these species. In horses, ruminants, and pigs, there is not enough ALT in the hepatocytes for this enzyme to be considered liver-specific. Other sources of ALT are renal cells, cardiac muscle, skeletal muscle, and the pancreas. If any of these tissues is damaged, the blood level of ALT can rise. ALT is used as a screening test for liver disease because it is not precise enough to identify specific liver diseases. There is no correlation between the blood levels of the enzyme and the severity of hepatic damage.

SAMPLE HANDLING AND SPECIAL CONSIDERATIONS.   Avoid hemolysis and lipemia because they can artificially increase the enzyme concentration. Storage of samples at room temperature or in the refrigerator for 24 hours has no effect on results.

SAMPLE STABILITY.   Samples to be assayed for ALT can be stored for 2 days at 20° C and 1 week at 0° to 4° C. Samples should not be frozen.

ASPARTATE AMINOTRANSFERASE (AST)

RATIONALE.   This enzyme was formerly known as serum glutamic oxaloacetic transaminase (SGOT). AST is present in hepatocytes but also is found in significant amounts in many other tissues, including erythrocytes, cardiac muscle, skeletal muscle, the kidneys, and the pancreas. For this reason AST is not considered liver-specific. An increased blood level of AST may indicate nonspecific liver damage. It may also be caused by strenuous exercise or intramuscular injection. The most common causes of increased blood levels of AST are hepatic disease, muscle inflammation or necrosis, and spontaneous or artifactual hemolysis. If you encounter an elevated AST level, check your serum or plasma sample for grossly visible hemolysis, or spin a hematocrit tube of the patient's whole blood to check for hemolysis.

SAMPLE HANDLING AND SPECIAL CONSIDERATIONS.   Hemolysis and lipemia result in elevated blood concentrations of AST. AST levels are also elevated if the blood sample was stored before assay. Because the upper acceptable limit of AST concentration in horses is much higher than for other species, test methods developed for species other than horses may not be suitable for use in equine samples.

SAMPLE STABILITY.   Samples for AST analyses can be stored for 2 days at 20° C, for 2 weeks at 0° to 4° C, and for several months at −20° C.

SORBITOL DEHYDROGENASE (SD)

RATIONALE.   The primary source of SD is the hepatocyte. It is present in the hepatocytes of all common domestic species, but is especially useful for evaluating large animal (sheep, goats, swine, horses, cattle) liver damage. Large animal hepatocytes do not contain diagnostic levels of ALT, so SD offers a liver-specific diagnostic test. The plasma level of SD rises with hepatocellular damage or necrosis. SD assay can be used in all species to detect hepatocellular damage or necrosis, thus eliminating the need for other tests, such as ALT assay. The disadvantage of SD analysis is that SD is unstable in serum and its activity declines rapidly. Samples should be assayed for SD within 12 hours of collection.

Sample handling and special considerations. SD is an unstable enzyme and its activity deteriorates rapidly. Samples should be analyzed within 12 hours after collection. Hemolysis does not appear to affect results.

Glutamate dehydrogenase (GD)

Rationale. GD is found in high concentrations in the hepatocytes of cattle, sheep, and goats. Some investigators believe this is the enzyme of choice to analyze for hepatocyte damage or necrosis in cattle and sheep. GD could be the enzyme of choice for evaluating ruminant liver function, but no standardized test methodology has been developed for use in a veterinary practice laboratory.

Other enzymes in hepatocytes

Other enzymes in hepatocytes can leak out during liver damage or necrosis. However, these enzymes are seldom routinely analyzed in a veterinary practice laboratory because no standardized analyses have been developed. The analysis requires instrumentation not normally found in a practice laboratory, or not enough is known about the significance of an elevated serum level. Examples of such enzymes are arginase and ornithine carbamoyltransferase (OCT).

Enzymes associated with cholestasis

Blood levels of certain enzymes become elevated with biliary obstruction or a metabolic defect in liver cells.

Alkaline phosphatase (AP)

Rationale. Alkaline phosphatase is present as isoenzymes in many tissues, particularly osteoblasts, chondroblasts, and cells of the hepatobiliary system. Because AP occurs as isoenzymes in these various tissues, the source of an isoenzyme (location of the damaged tissue) can be determined by special analytic methods in commercial or research laboratories.

In young animals, most AP comes from osteoblasts and chondroblasts because of active bone development. In older animals, most AP comes from the liver as bone development stabilizes. Assay for AP in a practice laboratory determines the total blood AP concentration.

AP concentrations are most often used to detect cholestasis in dogs and cats. Because of wide fluctuations in normal blood AP levels in cattle and sheep, this test is not as useful for detecting cholestasis in these species.

SAMPLE HANDLING AND SPECIAL CONSIDERATIONS. Sample hemolysis or storage at room temperature for 24 hours has little effect on results. However, samples kept at room temperature for more than 24 hours may show an increased AP value. Do not use EDTA or oxalate anticoagulants.

SAMPLE STABILITY. Samples for AP analysis can be stored for 8 days at $20°$ C (a slight rise may be seen after 2 to 3 days), 8 days at $0°$ to $4°$ C, and 8 days at $-20°$ C.

GAMMA GLUTAMYLTRANSPEPTIDASE (GGT)

RATIONALE. Gamma glutamyltranspeptidase is sometimes referred to as gamma glutamyltransferase. GGT is found in many tissues, but its primary source is the liver. Cattle, horses, sheep, and goats have higher blood GGT activity than dogs and cats. Other sources of GGT include the kidneys, pancreas, intestine, and muscle cells. The blood GGT level is elevated with liver disease, especially with obstructive liver disease.

SAMPLE HANDLING AND SPECIAL CONSIDERATIONS. Hemolysis does not affect test results, but prolonged contact with erythrocytes may affect results.

SAMPLE STABILITY. Samples for GGT determination can be stored for 2 days at $20°$ C, 1 week at $0°$ to $4°$ C, and 1 month at $-20°$ C.

OTHER ENZYMES ASSOCIATED WITH CHOLESTASIS

Other enzymes that may be used in the future to evaluate cholestasis are guanase, leucine aminopeptidase (LAP), and 5'-nucleotidase (5'-ND). While these enzymes may be more specific for detecting cholestasis than those currently used (AP, GGT), no standardized test methodology has been developed.

Other tests of liver function

Various other tests can be used to evaluate liver function. Only bilirubin analysis will be discussed here. Other liver function tests are discussed in Chapter 8.

Bilirubin

RATIONALE.   Bilirubin is a metabolite of the heme portion of hemoglobin and as such is considered a waste product when erythrocytes die. It is removed from the plasma primarily by the liver. Until it is taken into the liver and conjugated with certain sugars, especially glucuronic acid (glucuronate), bilirubin is insoluble in water and must be bound to water-soluble albumin to stay in solution. After conjugation it becomes water soluble and is carried to the intestines by the blood, where it is converted to urobilinogen by bacterial enzymes. Some of the urobilinogen is resorbed back into blood and carried to the kidneys for elimination. The remainder of the urobilinogen is eliminated in feces.

Both unconjugated and conjugated bilirubin are found in plasma. Assays can directly measure *total bilirubin* (conjugated bilirubin plus unconjugated bilirubin) and conjugated bilirubin. *Conjugated bilirubin* is sometimes referred to as *direct bilirubin* because test methods directly measure the amount of conjugated bilirubin in the sample. *Unconjugated bilirubin* is sometimes referred to as *indirect bilirubin* because its concentration is indirectly calculated by subtracting the conjugated bilirubin concentration from the total bilirubin concentration of the sample.

Bilirubin is assayed to determine the cause of jaundice, to evaluate liver function, and to check the patency of bile ducts. Blood levels of conjugated (direct) bilirubin are elevated with hepatocellular damage or bile duct injury/obstruction. Blood levels of unconjugated (indirect) bilirubin are elevated with excessive erythrocyte destruction or defects in the transport mechanism that allows bilirubin to enter hepatocytes for conjugation.

SAMPLE HANDLING AND SPECIAL CONSIDERATIONS.   Hemolysis produces artificially low values if the diazo assay method is used (check the test protocol). Avoid using lipemic blood samples. Store samples in the dark because bilirubin is very light sensitive. Direct exposure to sunlight for an hour can decrease a sample's bilirubin level by up to 50%. Unconjugated bilirubin is more light sensitive than conjugated bilirubin.

SAMPLE STABILITY.   Samples for bilirubin determinations are not stable when stored at 20° C. Samples protected from light can be stored for 2 weeks at 0° to 4° C and up to 3 months at −20° C.

KIDNEY ASSAYS

The kidneys play a major role in maintaining homeostasis in animals. Their primary functions are to conserve water and electrolytes in times of a negative balance and increase water and electrolyte elimination in times of a positive balance; excrete or conserve hydrogen ions to maintain blood pH within normal limits; conserve nutrients, such as glucose and proteins; remove the end products of nitrogen metabolism, such as urea, creatinine and allantoin, so that blood levels of these end products remain low; produce renin (an enzyme involved in controlling blood pressure), erythropoietin (a hormone necessary for erythrocyte production), and prostaglandins (fatty acids used to stimulate contractility of uterine and other smooth muscle, lower blood pressure, regulate acid secretion in the stomach, regulate body temperature and platelet aggregation, and control inflammation); and aid in vitamin D activation.

Both urine and blood can be analyzed to evaluate kidney function. See Chapter 5 for urinalysis procedures and Chapter 8 for specific kidney function tests.

BLOOD UREA NITROGEN (BUN)

Some references use the term *serum urea nitrogen* (SUN) instead of blood urea nitrogen.

RATIONALE. Urea, a nitrogenous compound, is a product of amino acid breakdown in the liver. BUN levels are used to evaluate kidney function based on the ability of the kidney to remove nitrogenous waste (urea) from blood. This is not a very sensitive renal function test because about 75% of the kidney tissue must be nonfunctional before elevated values are detected. In healthy animals, urea is passively filtered out of plasma by the renal glomeruli. Some urea returns to the blood through the renal tubules but most is excreted in the urine. If the kidney is not functioning properly, sufficient urea is not removed from the plasma, leading to increased BUN levels.

SAMPLE HANDLING AND SPECIAL CONSIDERATIONS. Hemolysis has little effect on results. High-protein diets may cause an elevated BUN level because of increased amino acid breakdown, not because of decreased glomerular filtration. For this reason, an 18-hour fast is recommended before sample collection. Postprandial (after-eating) lipemia may result in a turbid final solution if a "wet" chemistry assay system is used.

Contamination of the blood sample with urease-producing bacteria (*Staphylococcus aureus, Proteus, Klebsiella*) may result in decomposition of urea and subsequently decreased BUN levels. To prevent this, analysis should be completed within several hours of collection or the sample should be refrigerated.

Sample stability. Samples for BUN determination can be stored for 8 hours at 20° C, 10 days at 0° to 4° C, and several months at −20° C.

CREATININE

Rationale. Creatinine is a metabolite of creatine. Creatine stores energy in muscles in the form of phosphocreatine. Creatinine is formed by decomposition of creatine in a nonenzymatic, irreversible reaction. Creatinine diffuses into most body fluids, including blood. If physical activity remains constant, the amount of creatine metabolism remains constant and the blood level of creatinine remains constant. The creatinine in blood is filtered through the glomeruli and eliminated in urine. Creatinine also can be found in sweat, feces, and vomitus and can be decomposed by bacteria.

Blood creatinine levels are used to evaluate renal function, based on the ability of the glomeruli to filter creatinine from blood and eliminate it in urine. Like BUN, creatinine is not a very accurate indicator of kidney function because nearly 75% of the kidney tissue must be nonfunctional before blood creatinine levels rise. Creatinine blood levels are not affected by a high-protein diet.

Sample handling and special considerations. Hemolysis has little effect on results.

Sample stability. Samples can be stored for 1 week at 30° to 37° C and almost indefinitely at −20° C.

PANCREAS ASSAYS

The pancreas is actually two organs, one exocrine and the other endocrine, held together in one stroma. The endocrine part of the pancreas is involved with carbohydrate metabolism through secretion into the blood of insulin (lowers blood glucose levels) and glucagon (elevates blood glucose levels). This is discussed later in this section and in Chapter 8.

The exocrine part of the pancreas secretes into the small intestine an enzyme-rich juice that contains enzymes necessary for digestion. The three primary pancreatic enzymes are trypsin, amylase, and lipase.

Trypsin

Rationale. Trypsin is a proteolytic enzyme that aids digestion by catalyzing the reaction that breaks down the proteins of ingested food. Trypsin activity is more readily detectable in feces than in blood. For this reason, most trypsin analyses are done on fecal samples. Trypsin is normally found in feces, and its absence is abnormal.

Two fecal test methods are used in the laboratory: the test tube method and the x-ray film test.

The *test tube method* involves mixing fresh feces with a gelatin solution. The test solution does not become a gel if there is trypsin present in the sample to break down the protein (gelatin). If trypsin is absent, the solution becomes a gel.

The *x-ray film test* uses the gelatin coating on undeveloped x-ray film to test for the presence of trypsin. A strip of x-ray film is placed in a slurry of feces and bicarbonate solution. If trypsin is present in the fecal sample, the gelatin coating is removed from the film upon rinsing with water. If there is no trypsin present, the gelatin coating remains on the film after rinsing.

The test tube method is considered more accurate than the x-ray film test in evaluating fecal trypsin proteolytic activity.

Sample handling and special considerations. Use fresh feces only. Fecal trypsin activity may be decreased if the patient has recently eaten raw egg whites, soybeans, lima beans, heavy metals, citrate, fluoride, or some organic phosphorus compounds. Trypsin activity may be increased by calcium, magnesium, cobalt, and manganese in the feces. Proteolytic bacteria in the fecal sample may result in false-positive (apparently normal) results, especially in older samples.

Sample stability. Do not use fecal samples more than 1 day old because proteolytic bacteria in the feces may cause false-positive results.

Amylase

Rationale. The primary source of amylase is the pancreas. Its function is to break down starches and glycogen in sugars, such as maltose and residual glucose. Increased levels of amylase appear in blood during acute pancreatitis, flareups of chronic pancreatitis, or obstruction of the pancreatic ducts.

Two amylase test methods are available: the saccharogenic method and the amyloclastic method.

The *saccharogenic method* measures production of reducing sugars as amylase catalyzes the breakdown of starch.

The *amyloclastic method* measures the disappearance of starch as it is broken down to reducing sugars through amylase activity.

The rise in blood amylase level is not always directly proportional to the severity of pancreatitis. Determinations of blood amylase and lipase activities are usually requested at the same time to evaluate the pancreas.

SAMPLE HANDLING AND SPECIAL CONSIDERATIONS. Do not use calcium-binding anticoagulants, such as EDTA, because amylase requires the presence of calcium for activity. Hemolysis may result in falsely elevated amylase levels. Lipemia may reduce amylase activity. The saccharogenic method is not recommended for canine samples because maltase in canine samples may artificially elevate assay results. Because normal canine and feline amylase values can be up to 10 times higher than those in humans, samples may have to be diluted if tests designed for human samples are used. Some investigators question the acceptability of "dry reagent" methods on canine samples.

SAMPLE STABILITY. Samples can be stored for up to 7 days at 20° C and up to 1 month at 0° to 4° C.

LIPASE

RATIONALE. The primary source of lipase is the pancreas. The function of lipase is to break down the long-chain fatty acids of lipids. Blood levels of lipase increase during episodes of pancreatitis. Test methods for determination of lipase levels are usually based on hydrolysis of an olive oil emulsion into fatty acids using the lipase present in patient serum. The quantity of sodium hydroxide required to neutralize the fatty acids is directly proportional to lipase activity in the sample. Most of these test procedures are time consuming.

Lipase assay may be more sensitive for detecting pancreatitis than amylase assay. The degree of lipase activity, like amylase activity, is not directly proportional to the severity of pancreatitis. Determinations of blood lipase and amylase activities are usually requested at the same time to evaluate the pancreas.

SAMPLE HANDLING AND SPECIAL CONSIDERATIONS. Do not use calcium-binding anticoagulants, such as EDTA. Hemolysis and lipemia should be avoided; however, hemolysis does not affect results of turbidimetric methods (check the test protocol).

SAMPLE STABILITY.   Samples for lipase assay can be stored for 1 week at 20° C and 3 weeks at 0° to 4° C.

GLUCOSE

RATIONALE.   The blood glucose level is used as an indicator of carbohydrate metabolism in the body. It also can be used as a measure of endocrine function of the pancreas. The blood glucose level reflects the net balance between glucose production (dietary intake, conversion from other carbohydrates) and glucose utilization (energy expended, conversion to other products). It also can reflect the balance between blood insulin and glucagon levels.

Glucose utilization depends on the amount of insulin and glucagon being produced by the pancreas. As the insulin level increases, so does the rate of glucose utilization, resulting in decreased blood glucose levels. Glucagon acts as a stabilizer to prevent blood glucose levels from becoming too low. As the insulin level decreases (as in diabetes mellitus), so does glucose utilization, resulting in increased blood glucose concentration.

SAMPLE HANDLING AND SPECIAL CONSIDERATIONS.   Serum and plasma must be separated from the erythrocytes immediately after blood collection. Glucose levels can drop 10% an hour if the sample of plasma is left in contact with erythrocytes at room temperature. Mature erythrocytes use glucose for energy, and, in a blood sample, they may decrease the glucose level enough to give false-normal results if the original sample had an elevated glucose level. If the sample originally had a normal glucose level, erythrocytes may use enough glucose to decrease the level to below normal or to zero. If the plasma cannot be removed immediately, the anticoagulant of choice is sodium fluoride at 6 to 10 mg/ml of blood. Sodium fluoride can be used as a glucose preservative with EDTA at 2.5 mg/ml of blood.

Refrigeration slows glucose utilization by erythrocytes. Hemolysis does not affect results. Because eating raises the blood glucose level and fasting decreases it, a 16- to 24-hour fast is recommended when possible for all animals, except mature ruminants, before the blood sample is collected.

SAMPLE STABILITY.   Samples for blood glucose determination can be stored for 8 hours at 20° C and 72 hours at 0° to 4° C. The stability of frozen samples has not been determined. Do not thaw and refreeze a sample more than once.

MISCELLANEOUS CHEMISTRY ASSAYS

CREATINE KINASE (CK)

RATIONALE. Creatine kinase was previously known as creatine phosphokinase (CPK). It is produced primarily in striated muscle cells and, to some extent, in the brain. It is considered one of the most organ-specific enzymes available for clinical evaluation. When skeletal muscle, including cardiac muscle, is damaged or destroyed, CK leaks out of the cells and produces an elevated blood CK level. Although the brain produces some CK, it is questionable as to how much CK from the brain actually enters the peripheral circulation.

CK is frequently assayed if an animal has an elevated blood AST level but shows no clinical signs of liver disease.

While the CK assay is an organ-specific assay, it cannot determine which muscle has been damaged or indicate the severity of the muscle damage. Anything that damages the muscle cell membrane can cause an increased blood CK level. Such damage may stem from intramuscular injections, persistent recumbency, surgery, vigorous exercise, electric shock, laceration, bruising, and hypothermia. Myositis and other myopathies also cause elevated blood CK levels.

CK levels in samples may be artificially increased by oxidizing agents (bleach), EDTA, citrate, fluoride, exposure to sunlight, or delay in assay.

SAMPLE HANDLING AND SPECIAL CONSIDERATIONS. Hemolysis does not affect results. CK is unstable, so samples should be assayed as soon as possible after collection. Keep the sample away from ultraviolet light.

SAMPLE STABILITY. CK is an unstable enzyme; analyze the sample as soon as possible. Samples must not be frozen.

LACTATE DEHYDROGENASE (LDH)

RATIONALE. LDH is produced by many tissues, including skin, kidney, muscle (including cardiac muscle), erythrocytes, and leukocytes. Although this enzyme is found in many tissues, it is not found in high enough concentrations in any one tissue to be considered organ- or tissue-specific. Cellular damage or necrosis in any of these tissues can elevate the blood LDH level.

LDH isoenzymes have been identified from different tissues, but assays for specific isoenzymes are not performed in the average veterinary practice laboratory. The LDH values reflect the total activity of all LDH isoenzymes and, therefore, are not organ- or tissue-specific. This enzyme is considered a nonspecific indicator of tissue necrosis.

SAMPLE HANDLING AND SPECIAL CONSIDERATIONS. Hemolysis, storing serum in contact with the clot or plasma in contact with blood cells, or using serum separator (cell separation) aids can falsely elevate LDH levels in samples. Sample storage below 10° C falsely decreases LDH values. Oxalate and EDTA anticoagulants inhibit LDH activity.

SAMPLE STABILITY. LDH appears to be most stable at room temperature or refrigerator temperature. Freezing the sample deactivates LDH. Because recommended storage times and temperatures vary, the sample should be analyzed as soon as possible after collection.

CHOLESTEROL

RATIONALE. Cholesterol is produced in almost every cell in the body and is especially abundant in hepatocytes, the adrenal cortex, ovaries, testes, and intestinal epithelium. The liver is the primary site of synthesis in most animals.

Cholesterol assay is sometimes used as a screening test for hypothyroidism. Thyroid hormone controls synthesis and destruction of cholesterol in the body. Insufficient thyroid hormone (hypothyroidism) results in hypercholesterolemia because the rate of cholesterol destruction is relatively slower than the rate of synthesis. Other diseases associated with hypercholesterolemia include hyperadrenocorticism, diabetes mellitus, and nephrotic syndrome. Dietary causes of hypercholesterolemia are rare but may include very high-fat diets or postprandial lipemia.

Note: Cholesterol by itself does not cause the grossly lipemic plasma seen after eating; triglycerides also are usually present. Administration of corticosteroids may also cause an elevated blood cholesterol concentration.

SAMPLE HANDLING AND SPECIAL CONSIDERATIONS. Check the test protocol for recommendations on sample handling. Hemolysis may elevate colorimetric test results. Fluoride and oxalate anticoagulants may elevate enzymatic method results.

SAMPLE STABILITY. Blood samples for cholesterol determinations can be stored for 48 hours at 20° C without separating serum or plasma from the cells.

Samples are very stable at 20° C if serum or plasma is removed from the cells and are stable for weeks at −20° C.

PLASMA PROTEIN ASSAYS

Plasma proteins are produced primarily by the liver and the immune system (consisting of reticuloendothelial tissues, lymphoid tissues, and plasma cells). Proteins have many functions in the body. They help form the structural matrix of all cells, organs, and tissues; they maintain osmotic pressure; they serve as enzymes for biochemical reactions; they act as buffers in acid-base balance; they serve as hormones; they function in blood coagulation; they defend the body against pathogenic microorganisms; and they serve as transport/carrier molecules for most constituents of plasma.

There are over 200 plasma proteins. Some plasma protein concentrations change markedly during certain diseases and can be used as diagnostic aids. Other protein concentrations change very little during disease. The most commonly assayed plasma proteins are albumin, fibrinogen, and globulins.

TOTAL PROTEIN

RATIONALE. Total *plasma* protein measurements include fibrinogen values. Total *serum* protein determinations measure all the protein fractions except fibrinogen, which is removed during the clotting process. The total protein concentration can be affected by altered hepatic synthesis, altered protein distribution, altered protein breakdown or excretion, dehydration, or overhydration.

Total protein concentrations are especially valuable in determining an animal's state of hydration. A dehydrated animal usually has a relatively elevated total protein concentration, while an overhydrated animal usually has a relatively decreased total protein concentration. Total protein concentrations are also useful as initial screening tests for patients with edema, ascites, diarrhea, weight loss, hepatic and renal disease, and blood clotting problems.

There are two commonly used methods for determining total protein levels: the refractometric method and the biuret method.

The *refractometric method* measures the refractive index of serum or plasma using a refractometer. This method is a good screening test because it is fast, inexpensive, and accurate.

The *biuret method* measures the peptide bonds of the protein in serum or plasma. This method is commonly used in analytic instruments used in the laboratory. It is a simple method and yields accurate results.

Serum is used if the total *serum* protein concentration is to be measured, and plasma is used if the total *plasma* protein concentration is to be measured. The total plasma concentration includes the fibrinogen concentration, while the total serum concentration does not.

SAMPLE HANDLING AND SPECIAL CONSIDERATIONS. Although moderate sample hemolysis does not affect results, marked hemolysis falsely increases total protein values. Do not use lipemic samples, especially if a refractometric method is used. Moderate icterus has no effect on the refractometric method. Heat, ultraviolet light, surfactant detergents, and chemicals can break down proteins, leading to artificially low results.

SAMPLE STABILITY. Information of sample stability is not available.

ALBUMIN

RATIONALE. Albumin is one of the most important proteins in plasma or serum. It makes up 35% to 50% of the total plasma protein in most animals, and any significant state of hypoproteinemia is most likely caused by albumin loss. Hepatocytes synthesize albumin, and any diffuse liver disease may result in decreased albumin synthesis. Renal disease, dietary intake, and intestinal protein absorption also can influence the plasma albumin level. Albumin is the major binding and transport protein in the blood and is responsible for maintaining osmotic pressure of plasma.

SAMPLE HANDLING AND SPECIAL CONSIDERATIONS. Hemolysis may increase the apparent albumin level if the bromcresol green method is used. Check the test protocol for the method used. Keep the sample covered to prevent dehydration, which can falsely elevate protein levels.

SAMPLE STABILITY. Samples for albumin determinations can be stored for 1 week (2 days on the clot has no effect) at 20° C, 1 month at 0° to 4° C, and indefinitely at −20° C.

GLOBULINS

RATIONALE. The globulins are a complex group of proteins. *Alpha globulins* are synthesized in the liver and primarily transport and bind proteins. Two important proteins in this fraction are high-density lipoproteins (HDL) and very low-density lipoproteins (VLDL). *Beta globulins* include complement (C_3, C_4), transferrin, and ferritin. They are responsible for iron transport, heme binding, and fibrin formation and lysis. *Gamma globulins* (immunoglobulins) are synthesized by plasma cells and are responsible for antibody production (immunity). Immunoglobulins identified in animals are IgG, IgD, IgE, IgA, and IgM. IgG antibodies comprise the most common viral, bacterial and toxin antibodies; it has been identified in all animals. IgE is involved in allergic and anaphylactic reactions; it has been identified in dogs. IgA is found in the secretions of the genitourinary, respiratory, and gastrointestinal tracts.

Serum protein assays can be performed with *serum protein electrophoresis*. The principle of electrophoresis is based on the migration patterns of the different serum protein fractions in an electrically charged field. A specific medium is used to trace the migration. The migration pattern depends on the electrical charge, size of the protein molecule, intensity of the electric field, and medium used. Electrophoretic techniques are not normally employed in a practice laboratory.

Because direct assay methods for globulins are often beyond the capabilities of a practice laboratory, indirect measurements are often used. The total *serum* protein concentration minus the albumin concentration gives an approximation of the total *serum* globulin concentration.

ALBUMIN-TO-GLOBULIN RATIO (A:G RATIO)

An alteration in the normal A:G ratio is frequently the first indication of a protein abnormality. The ratio is analyzed in conjunction with a protein profile. The A:G ratio can be used to detect increased or decreased albumin and globulin concentrations. Many pathologic conditions alter the A:G ratio.

The A:G ratio is determined by dividing the albumin concentration by the globulin concentration. In dogs, horses, sheep, and goats, the albumin concentration is usually greater than the globulin concentration (A:G ratio is > 1.00). In cattle, pigs, and cats, the albumin concentration is usually equal to or less than the globulin concentration (A:G ratio is <1.00).

FIBRINOGEN

RATIONALE.   Fibrinogen is synthesized by hepatocytes. It is the precursor of fibrin, the insoluble protein of blood clots. It is one of the factors necessary for clot formation. If fibrinogen levels are decreased, blood will not form a stable clot or will not clot at all. Fibrinogen makes up 3% to 6% of the total plasma protein content. Because it is removed from plasma by the clotting process, there is no fibrinogen in serum. Acute inflammation or tissue damage can

---

Procedure 3-3. Heat precipitation fibrinogen test

1. Fill two pairs of microhematocrit tubes (four tubes) with anticoagulated whole blood.
2. Spin one pair of tubes in a microhematocrit centrifuge.
3. Using a refractometer, read the total plasma protein concentration of each tube and average the values.
4. Heat the second pair of tubes in a 56° C incubator or water bath for 3 minutes. This will precipitate the fibrinogen.
5. After incubation, spin the second pair of tubes in a microhematocrit centrifuge.
6. Using a refractometer, read the total plasma protein concentration for each tube and average the values.
7. Calculate the fibrinogen value by subtracting the average total plasm protein value of the heated tubes from the average total plasma protein of the first (unheated) pair of tubes.

---

elevate plasma fibrinogen levels. The most common method of fibrinogen evaluation is the heat precipitation test (Procedure 3-3).

The fibrinogen value is calculated by subtracting the total plasma protein value of the heated tubes (this value should be the lower because fibrinogen has been removed from the plasma) from that of the unheated tubes.

Plasma is the only sample that can be used, as serum does not contain fibrinogen. EDTA plasma is preferred. Heparinized plasma may yield falsely low results.

Sample stability. Samples for fibrinogen determinations can be stored for several days at 20° C and several weeks at 0° to 4° C.

ELECTROLYTE ASSAYS

Electrolytes are the negative ions (anions) and positive ions (cations) of elements found in the fluids of all organisms. Some of the functions of electrolytes are maintenance of water balance, fluid osmotic pressure, and normal muscular and nervous functions. They also function in the maintenance and activation of several enzyme systems and in acid-base regulation.

Evaluation of electrolytes, such as sodium and potassium, was at one time not commonly performed in practice laboratories because of the special analytic instrumentation needed (e.g., flame photometer). With the advent of "dry reagent" chemistry analyzers, electrolyte assays can be routinely performed in the practice laboratory.

The most commonly analyzed electrolytes are calcium, inorganic phosphorus, potassium, sodium, chloride, and magnesium.

CALCIUM

RATIONALE.   More than 99% of the calcium in the body is found in bones. The remaining 1% or less has major functions in the body, including maintenance of neuromuscular excitability and tone (decreased calcium can result in muscular tetany), maintenance of activity of many enzymes, facilitation of blood coagulation, and maintenance of inorganic ion transfer across cell membranes.

Calcium in whole blood is almost entirely in plasma or serum. Erythrocytes contain very little calcium.

Calcium concentrations are usually inversely related to inorganic phosphorus concentrations. As a general rule, if the calcium concentration rises, the inorganic phosphorus concentration falls.

Hypercalcemia is an elevated blood calcium concentration. *Hypocalcemia* is a decreased blood calcium concentration.

SAMPLE HANDLING AND SPECIAL CONSIDERATIONS.   Do not use EDTA or oxalate anticoagulants, as they bind with calcium and make it unavailable for assay. Hemolysis results in a slight decrease in calcium concentration in samples as the fluid from the ruptured erythrocytes dilutes the plasma. Calcium concentrations can be increased if the sample comes in contact with cork stoppers.

SAMPLE STABILITY.   Samples for calcium determinations can be stored for 10 days at 20° C, 0° to 4° C, or −20° C.

INORGANIC PHOSPHORUS

RATIONALE.   Over 80% of the phosphorus in the body is found in bones. The remaining 20% or less has major functions, such as energy storage, release and transfer, involvement in carbohydrate metabolism, and composition of many physiologically important substances, such as nucleic acids and phospholipids.

Most of the phosphorus in whole blood is found within the erythrocytes as *organic phosphorus*. The phosphorus in plasma and serum is *inorganic phosphorus* and is the phosphorus assayed in the laboratory.

Inorganic phosphorus levels in plasma and serum provide a good indication of the total phosphorus in an animal. Plasma or serum phosphorus and calcium concentrations are inversely related. As phosphorus concentrations decrease, calcium concentrations increase.

Hyperphosphatemia is an increased serum or plasma phosphorus concentration. *Hypophosphatemia* is a decreased serum or plasma phosphorus concentration.

SAMPLE HANDLING AND SPECIAL CONSIDERATIONS.   Do not use hemolyzed samples, as the organic phosphorus liberated from the ruptured erythrocytes may be hydrolyzed to inorganic phosphorus. This results in a falsely elevated inorganic phosphorus concentration. The serum or plasma should be separated from the blood cells as soon as possible after blood collection and before the sample is stored.

SAMPLE STABILITY.   Samples for phosphorus determinations can be stored for 3 to 4 days at 20° C, 1 week at 0° to 4° C, and 3 weeks at −20° C.

SODIUM

RATIONALE.   Sodium is the major cation of plasma and interstitial (extracellular) fluid. It plays an important role in water distribution and body fluid osmotic pressure maintenance. In the kidney, sodium is filtered through the glomeruli and resorbed back into the body through the tubules in exchange, as needed, for hydrogen ions. In this manner, sodium plays a vital role in pH regulation of urine and acid-base balance.

Sodium concentrations are measured by *flame photometry* (usually not available in practice laboratories) or by "dry reagent" methods.

Hypernatremia refers to an elevated blood level of sodium. *Hyponatremia* is a decreased blood level of sodium.

SAMPLE HANDLING AND SPECIAL CONSIDERATIONS.   Do not use the sodium salt of heparin as an anticoagulant because it can falsely elevate the results. Hemolysis does not significantly alter results, but it may dilute the sample with erythrocyte fluid, causing falsely lower results.

SAMPLE STABILITY.   Information regarding sample stability for sodium analysis is not available.

POTASSIUM

RATIONALE. Potassium is the major intracellular cation. It is important for normal muscular function, respiration, cardiac function, nerve impulse transmission, and carbohydrate metabolism. In acidotic animals, potassium ions leave the intracellular fluid as they are replaced by hydrogen ions, resulting in elevated serum potassium levels (*hyperkalemia*). The serum potassium level also can be elevated in the presence of cellular damage or necrosis, which causes release of potassium ions into the blood. Decreased serum potassium levels (*hypokalemia*) can be associated with inadequate potassium intake, alkalosis, or fluid loss due to vomiting or diarrhea.

SAMPLE HANDLING AND SPECIAL CONSIDERATIONS. Plasma is the preferred sample because platelets can release potassium during the clotting process, causing artificially elevated potassium levels. Hemolysis should be avoided because the concentration of potassium within erythrocytes is higher than the concentration in plasma. Hemolysis releases potassium into the plasma, resulting in artificially elevated potassium levels. Do not refrigerate the sample until the plasma has been separated from the cells, as cooler temperatures promote loss of potassium from the cells without evidence of hemolysis. Do not freeze samples without first separating the blood cells, as the resulting hemolysis makes the sample unsuitable for testing.

SAMPLE STABILITY. Information on sample stability for potassium analysis is not available.

MAGNESIUM

RATIONALE. Magnesium is the fourth most common cation in the body and the second most common intracellular cation. Magnesium is found in all body tissues. More than 50% of the magnesium in the body is found in bones, closely related to calcium and phosphorus. It is an activator of enzyme systems and is involved in production and decomposition of acetylcholine. Imbalance of the magnesium:calcium ratio can result in muscular tetany from release of acetylcholine. Cattle and sheep are the only domestic animals that show clinical signs related to magnesium deficiencies.

Hypermagnesemia refers to an elevated blood magnesium level. *Hypomagnesemia* is a decreased blood magnesium level.

Sample handling and special considerations.   Anticoagulants other than heparin may artificially decrease the results. Hemolysis may elevate the results through liberation of magnesium from erythrocytes. Storage of sample without first separating out the blood cells does not appear to affect results. Unlike calcium concentrations, magnesium concentrations are not affected by contact with cork stoppers.

Sample stability.   Although values on the stability of magnesium after storage at room, refrigerator, and freezer temperatures are not available, we have found such samples to be very stable.

Chloride

Rationale.   Chloride is the predominant extracellular anion. It plays an important role in maintenance of water distribution, osmotic pressure, and the normal anion:cation ratio. Chloride is usually included in electrolyte profiles because of its close relationship to sodium and bicarbonate levels.

Hyperchloremia refers to an elevated blood chloride level. *Hypochloremia* is a decreased blood chloride level.

Sample preference.   Serum is the sample of choice. Heparinized plasma is preferred over EDTA plasma.

Sample handling and special considerations.   Hemolysis may affect test results by diluting the sample with erythrocyte fluid. Prolonged storage without first separating out the blood cells can cause slightly low results.

Sample stability.   Chloride samples are stable at room, refrigerator, and freezer temperatures if the serum or plasma is separated from the blood cells.

Bicarbonate

Rationale.   Bicarbonate is the second most common anion of plasma. It is an important part of the bicarbonate/carbonic acid buffer system and aids in transport of carbon dioxide from the tissues to the lungs. Both of these functions help keep the body pH in balance as acids and bases are continually introduced into the body. The kidney regulates bicarbonate levels in the body by excreting excesses after it has resorbed all that is needed. Bicarbonate levels are frequently estimated from blood carbon dioxide levels. The bicarbonate level is about 95% of the total carbon dioxide measured.

Arterial blood is the sample of choice for bicarbonate determinations. If plasma is used, lithium heparinate is the anticoagulant of choice.

Sample handling and special considerations. Chill the sample in ice water to prevent glycolysis from altering the acid-base composition. Freezing the sample results in hemolysis. Most test methods require incubation at 37° C.

Sample stability. Bicarbonate analysis should be completed as soon as possible.

References

1. Kaneko: *Clinical biochemistry of domestic animals,* ed 4, San Diego, 1989, Academic Press.

2. Willard, et al: *Small animal clinical diagnosis by laboratory methods,* Philadelphia, 1989, WB Saunders.

3. Tietz: *Fundamentals of clinical chemistry,* ed 2, Philadelphia, 1982, WB Saunders.

4. Henry: *Clinical diagnosis and management by laboratory methods,* ed 17, Philadelphia, 1984, WB Saunders.

5. Duncan: *Veterinary laboratory medicine, clinical pathology,* ed 3, Ames, Iowa, 1994, Iowa State University Press.

6. Sirois: *Veterinary clinical laboratory procedures,* ed 1, St Louis, 1995, Mosby.

Diagnostic Microbiology

M. Ikram

The veterinarian's ability to diagnose, evaluate, and manage microbial diseases is enhanced through use of laboratory tests. The accuracy and value of these tests depends on the abilities of the veterinary technician responsible for the laboratory. Veterinary technicians employed in veterinary clinics should be competent to perform such microbiologic procedures. A direct Gram stain of a clinical specimen sometimes permits tentative identification of an organism. More often, culture on an appropriate medium is essential for both tentative and final identification. In addition, subjective judgment is required for interpreting Gram stains, examining colonies on culture media, and interpreting medium changes and results of other biochemical tests.

EQUIPMENT AND SUPPLIES

THE LABORATORY

Ideally your practice facility should have a separate room for microbiologic procedures. The room should have good lighting and ventilation; a washable floor and limited traffic; at least two benches, one for processing the samples and a separate one for culture work, with smooth surfaces that are easily disinfected; gas and electrical outlets; ample storage space; and easy access to an incubator and a refrigerator.

MATERIALS FOR SUBMITTING SAMPLES TO A DIAGNOSTIC LABORATORY

The following materials should be kept on hand for submitting microbiologic samples to a diagnostic laboratory:

- Sterile cotton-tipped swabs
- Culturette swabs in transport medium
- Plastic specimen bags
- Sterile screw-capped containers (100 to 200 ml)
- Sterile screw-capped tubes or bottles (10 ml)
- Scissors, forceps, scalpel with blades (stored in 70% alcohol and flamed to sterilize)
- "Discard jar" containing disinfectant for contaminated instruments
- Small hacksaw to cut bone specimens
- Wooden tongue depressors for handling fecal specimens
- Bunsen burner (natural gas or propane gas)
- Racks to hold tubes and bottles
- Refrigerator
- "Cold packs" and polystyrene shipping containers

STAINS AND CULTURE SUPPLIES

Supplies for staining and culture of bacteriologic samples are discussed in the section on Bacteriology.

LABORATORY SAFETY

Most of the microorganisms encountered in the microbiology laboratory are potentially pathogenic. Therefore the safety of every person working in the laboratory depends on strict observance of rules that must be followed *to the letter.*

- *Wear a clean, long-sleeved, knee-length, white laboratory coat* to prevent contamination of street clothes and dissemination of pathogens to the general public.
- *Do not eat, drink, or smoke in the laboratory.*

- *Clean bench tops with disinfectant* at the beginning and end of the work period.
- *Tie back long hair* or tuck it inside your coat.
- *Avoid putting any object (pencil, fingers) in your mouth* while working in the laboratory. Do not moisten labels with your tongue.
- *Tape shut all containers of cultures of suspected or known pathogens* before disposal.
- *Treat spilled cultures with disinfectant* and allow contact for 20 minutes before cleaning up.
- *Flame wire loops contaminated with inocula immediately after use.*
- *Always observe aseptic technique when transferring or working with infectious agents or specimens.*
- *Make sure that the gas, water, and electrical appliances are turned off before leaving.*
- *Place contaminated materials (plates, test tubes, slides, pipettes, broken glass) in appropriate containers for disposal.*
- *Never use mouth pipetting in the microbiology laboratory.* Use automatic or bulb pipetting devices.
- *Wash your hands thoroughly before leaving the laboratory.*
- *Report all accidents promptly to the laboratory supervisor.*

BACTERIOLOGY

COLLECTING SPECIMENS

Proper collection of a specimen is of utmost importance to provide valuable diagnostic information. No matter how good the methods used in the laboratory, it is impossible to obtain satisfactory results with samples that are collected improperly.

The specimen selected must contain the organism causing the problem. Normal flora and contaminants can complicate sample collection and subsequent interpretation of results. The following guidelines should be kept in mind for proper specimen collection:

- *Obtain a complete history and sufficient clinical data to help select procedures most appropriate to isolate organisms that may be present.* Required data include the owner's name, clinic name, address, and phone number. Species, name, age, sex, number of animals affected or dead, duration of the problem, and major signs observed also should be included. The tentative diagnosis, organism suspected, any treatment given, and type of laboratory investigation required should be included in the record.

- *Collect the specimen aseptically.* Specimen contamination is the most common cause of diagnostic failure. The importance of aseptic collection of microbiologic specimens cannot be overemphasized. Collect samples as soon as possible following the onset of clinical signs.
- *Keep multiple specimens separate from each other to avoid cross contamination.* This is essential for intestinal specimens because of the normal flora found there.
- *Label the specimen container, especially if a zoonotic condition is suspected,* such as anthrax, rabies, leptospirosis, brucellosis, or equine encephalitis. Tissues in suspected zoonoses should be submitted in a sealed, leakproof, unbreakable container.
- *Contact the reference laboratory for advice on specimen collection.* If there is uncertainty on the most appropriate selection of specimen or a submission procedure, contact the laboratory for their suggestions.
- *Avoid hurrying to obtain results quickly at the expense of accuracy.*
- *Send the specimen to the diagnostic laboratory by the fastest possible means.* If the sample will be arriving during a weekend, inform the laboratory ahead of time so that arrangements can be made for pickup.
- *Discuss the results with the veterinarian promptly,* in a clear concise manner. Failure to do so reflects adversely on both the veterinarian and the laboratory.

Figure 4-1 shows the typical sequences of procedures used in processing microbiologic specimens.

ABORTION SPECIMENS

A good range of specimens is particularly important in cases of abortion. Specimens should include a small piece of placenta with one or two cotyledons, fetal stomach contents, amnionic fluid, and a piece of fetal liver, lungs, and spleen. For large animal fetuses aborted before 7 months of gestation, send the entire fetus. Pack the specimens in a leakproof container with several cold packs. If infectious bovine rhinotracheitis is suspected, submit pieces of lung and liver and a nasal wash.

Sometimes seroconversion coincident with abortion, as in bovine virus diarrhea or brucellosis, may provide more conclusive evidence of the cause than

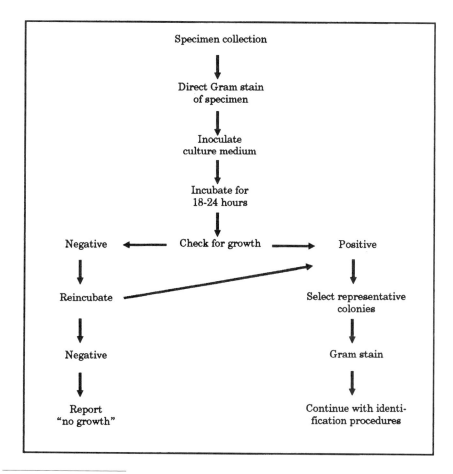

FIGURE **4-1.**   Sequence of procedures used in microbiologic examination.

isolation of pathogens. Thus, paired serum samples, one collected at the time of abortion and the other 10 to 14 days later, are required. If leptospirosis is suspected, a midstream urine sample and clotted blood sample should be submitted with placenta and fetal urine.

LEPTOSPIROSIS SPECIMENS
In diagnosing leptospirosis in cattle, a midstream urine sample is preferred to one collected by catheter. To induce cows to urinate, massage the vulva. Another method is to ask the farmer to hold the cows in a nearby corral until you arrive. When the cows are run into the shed, a few will urinate spontaneously. It is easiest to collect a midstream urine sample in a plastic container of about 200-ml capacity and then decant 20 ml of this into a

screw-capped bottle containing 1.5 ml of 10% formalin. This should be done within 10 minutes of collection or the *Leptospira* organisms may die and disintegrate. The formalin kills the leptospires but preserves their morphology.

When attempting to diagnose leptospirosis, collect paired blood and urine samples from clinically ill animals and from at least ten animals that have been in contact with them. *Handle suspected brucellosis and leptospirosis samples with caution.*

MILK SPECIMENS

Milk is cultured to identify the organisms that cause mastitis. If milk samples are not collected aseptically, microorganisms from the skin of the udder and from the air may contaminate the specimen, making culture results erroneous. If possible, collect milk samples from the cow after mastitis is noticed and before treatment is commenced. Culturing samples within 3 days of the last treatment usually results in a negative culture and meaningless findings. Do not wash the udder before obtaining samples unless it is very dirty. If the udder must be washed, use warm water and disinfectant at the recommended strength. Dry the udder and teats thoroughly with single-service paper towels.

Using 70% ethyl alcohol or 70% to 90% isopropyl alcohol, wipe the two teats farther from you first and then the two nearer teats. Be careful in swabbing the teat sphincter. Use sterile bottles or tubes with screw caps for collection. Dispatch Screw Cap Tubes (Gibco), with a small capped nozzle, are useful as the nozzle can be used for dispensing milk samples for culturing. Such containers as Whirl-Bags are not satisfactory.

Hold the collection tube as near to *horizontal* as possible. Discard the first few squirts of milk from each teat and then direct a little milk from each quarter into a separate tube that has been labelled. Sample the two teats nearer to you first and then those farther from you, so your arm does not accidentally brush against the disinfected teats before sampling. Collect the samples as quickly as possible, taking care not to contaminate the cap of the container. The forefinger should be held against the palm of the hand taking the sample, while the thumb is used to collect the milk. Screening of samples with the California mastitis test before culturing is recommended.

Refrigerate the milk samples as soon after collection as possible until they can be cultured. Do not freeze the samples. If mastitis due to *Mycoplasma* is suspected, ampicillin can be added at 1 to 10 mg/ml of milk sample to control contaminant bacteria. Keep these milk samples at room temperature so the *Mycoplasma* organisms can multiply in the sample. Another milk sample also should be taken without adding antibiotics so as to check for the more common mastitis-causing organisms, such as *Streptococcus agalactiae, Staphylococcus aureus, Streptococcus uberis, E. coli,* and *Nocardia.*

URINE SPECIMENS

Normal voided urine may contain small numbers of bacteria. It is important to differentiate these small numbers from significant bacteriuria. Urinalysis thus must be quantitative to yield meaningful results. Be careful to avoid contamination with preputial or vulvar flora. Ideally the vulva or prepuce should be thoroughly cleaned with detergent, after which at least 5 ml of a midstream sample are collected in a sterile tube. The presence of infection is determined from the number of organisms present. A bacterial count of $\geq 10,000/\mu l$ suggests an active infection. For diagnostic purposes, however, urine samples must be collected aseptically by catheter or cystocentesis. Midstream samples or samples collected by manual compression of the bladder are unacceptable.

Additional specimens should be submitted 72 to 96 hours after the start of antimicrobial therapy so as to monitor progress. Common pathogens isolated from urine samples include *E. coli, Staphylococcus aureus,* streptococci, *Proteus,* and *Pseudomonas.*

FECAL SPECIMENS

Feces should be collected in a fecal cup when freshly voided or directly from the rectum using aseptic precautions. In large animals, a disposable rubber glove or sleeve is useful. Once inverted and tied off, it can be submitted containing the specimen. In small animals, a sterile cotton swab can be used to collect samples from the rectum while avoiding contamination of the swab with anal skin microflora. A sample of at least 1 g is needed for bacteriologic examination.

It is important to remember that a single negative fecal culture does not rule out involvement of infectious agents (e.g., intermittent excretion of *Salmonella*); serial samples should be submitted. The most common organisms associated with intestinal infection are members of the family Enterobacteriaceae.

SPECIMENS FROM ABSCESSES AND WOUNDS

If the abscess has not ruptured, shave the area, swab liberally with alcohol, and allow it to dry. If the pus is liquid, a good sample can be obtained with a sterile syringe and wide-bore needle. When possible, obtain scrapings from the wall of the abscess, as causative organisms are more likely to be viable there. Collect several milliliters of material for culture rather than relying on a swab sample.

To culture wounds, the surrounding area should be disinfected and superficial debris lifted away. The surface of open wounds frequently contains contaminating bacteria. Gross observation of pus for color, odor, and presence of "sulfur granules" can be helpful, as is a direct smear for Gram staining. The swab must be taken near the edge of a wound, as the center frequently contains only necrotic debris. For draining abscesses, aspirate as deeply as possible, avoiding the surface of the wound. The most common pathogens involved with abscesses and wounds are *Staphylococcus, Streptococcus, E. coli, Proteus, Pseudomonas, Nocardia, Corynebacterium, Fusobacterium,* and *Clostridium.*

SPECIMENS FROM THE EYE

Organisms from the eye are often fastidious, such as *Moraxella* and *Streptococcus.* It is best to culture corneal scrapings, a swab rolled into the conjunctival sac, or lacrimal secretions collected with a sterile swab by applying the specimen directly onto a blood agar plate. If this is not possible, deposit the end of the swab into about 2 ml of sterile saline and culture within 2 hours of collection. Other pathogens isolated from the eye include *Staphylococcus, Pasteurella, Pseudomonas, Chlamydia,* and *E. coli.*

GENITAL SPECIMENS

CERVICOVAGINAL MUCUS ASPIRATE.   Cervival mucus may be collected in a sterile artificial insemination pipette introduced through a speculum. A syringe attached to the pipette by a short length of rubber tubing is used to aspirate the mucus. About 3 ml should be collected and expressed into vials containing Cary-Blair medium, a transport broth used for culture of *Campylobacter fetus* and other genital organisms. If *Taylorella (Hemophilus) equigenitalis* is suspected, use Amies' transport medium containing charcoal.

VULVAR SWAB.   The Culturette swab (Marion Scientific, Baxter) should be applied to the vulvar mucosa, particularly around the clitoral fossa. The swab is then cultured for *Ureaplasma diversum* and *Mycoplasma* species. Swabs that cannot be sent to the laboratory on the same day of collection should be stored at 4° C and shipped at 4° C with an ice pack. If the sample is to be held more than 2 days, it should be stored and shipped frozen at −70° C. *Mycoplasma* is very sensitive to drying; therefore, *do not submit dry swabs.* If mycoplasmal infection is suspected, tissue specimens are the preferred specimen. If swabs are submitted, they should only be submitted in Stewart agar medium (Star Swabs, Can Lab, and Fisher).

Specimens from the ear

Ear swabs are most often collected from dogs. Usually both ears should be individually swabbed, as comparison of the cultured organisms helps differentiate normal from abnormal flora. Organisms commonly involved in ear infections are *Staphylococcus aureus, Pseudomonas aeruginosa, Proteus, Streptococcus,* and *Malassezia pachydermatis (Pityrosporon canis).*

Culture of anaerobes

Because most anaerobes survive exposure to air for less than 20 minutes, collection of samples for anaerobic culture on swabs is completely useless. Acceptable anaerobic specimens include: blocks of tissue (2-inch cube minimum) in a closed sterile container; material placed in Becton-Dickinson's Anaerobic Specimen Collector; and pus and exudate collected in a sterile syringe, with the air expelled and the needle plugged with a rubber stopper or bent backward on itself.

Specimens should be cultured as soon as possible after collection. The specimen is inoculated onto a blood agar plate and into thioglycollate broth, which is a liquid medium used to grow anaerobes. The blood agar plates are put into an anaerobe jar, which provides an anaerobic environment during incubation. A self-contained system, such as a Gas Pack (Oxoid), can be used. A commercial anaerobe culture system, such as API Anaerobic System, is also available. In cases where demonstration of specific toxin is required, at least 20 ml of ileal contents or a loop of ileum with contents should be submitted.

Conditions in which isolation of anaerobes might be significant include soft-tissue abscesses, postoperative wounds, peritonitis, septicemia, endocarditis, endometritis, gangrene, pulmonary infection, and footrot in cattle, sheep, and swine. The isolated anaerobe may be the sole etiologic agent or a partner in a synergistic relationship with another bacterium. For example, liver abscesses seen at slaughter in otherwise healthy feedlot cattle commonly yield the anaerobe *Fusobacterium necrophorum* and the aerobe *Actinomyces (Corynebacterium) pyogenes.*

For conditions involving *Clostridium chauvoei, Cl. septicum, Cl. novyi,* and *Cl. sordellii,* most laboratories use the fluorescent antibody technique in diagnosis. Specimens include affected muscle and a rib containing bone marrow.

Interpreting results of bacteriologic tests

A diagnosis of the cause of a disease is based on clinical signs, gross pathologic observations, the organisms isolated, and the results of other laboratory tests. However, the significance of the isolated organisms depends on whether the samples were collected aseptically. Also important are how long after death the specimens were taken, and the interval between collection and examination of the specimens. The following should be borne in mind:

- *Some organisms, such as the Enterobacteriaceae, are ubiquitous, and their isolation might merely represent postmortem invasion of tissues, fecal contamination of samples, or soil contamination.*
- *Clostridium and other anaerobes are rapid postmortem invaders.* Bone marrow is often the last tissue to be invaded, so an unopened rib containing bone marrow can be a useful specimen.
- *Many organisms, such as Salmonella and Leptospira, are excreted by otherwise healthy animals.* A distinction must be made between subclinical infection and disease.
- *Mycobacterium paratuberculosis, Salmonella, and Leptospira are often excreted intermittently.* Therefore collection of serial samples following a negative result is justified.
- *The diagnosis of fungal infection must be made cautiously if the fungus is known to survive outside the animal body.* Histopathologic examination may determine whether the organism was present as a contaminant or was invading the tissue.

Table 4-1 summarizes bacterial pathogens of veterinary importance, species affected, resultant diseases or lesions, and specimens required for diagnosis.

Bacterial Cultures

Culture supplies

Supplies and equipment needed for culturing and identification of bacteria include:

- Small incubator, set at 37° C (98.6° F)
- Small autoclave for preparing culture media and sterilizing instruments and other equipment
- Refrigerator for storing media, reagents, and specimens
- Balance for weighing media in milligrams and grams
- Bunsen burner
- Inoculating needle holders, loops, and 22-gauge nichrome wire
- Waterproof marking pens

Text continued on p. 151.

Table 4-1. Summary of veterinary bacterial pathogens, animal species affected, resultant disease or lesions, and specimens for diagnosis

Organism	Species affected	Disease or lesion	Specimens
Actinobacillus			
A. lignieresi	Cattle, sheep	Granulomatous lesions containing pus; most commonly affects tongue (wooden tongue); found in rumen and on tongues of normal animals	Fresh tissue and pus
A. equuli	Foals, occasionally pigs and calves	"Sleepy foal" disease; abortion, navel illnesses	Fresh liver, spleen, bone marrow; abortion material
A. suis	Young pigs, foals	Fatal septicemia in animals <6 weeks; arthritis, pneumonia, or abscesses in older animals	Fresh liver, spleen, bone marrow; lung, pus
A. seminis	Sheep	Epididymitis in rams	Fresh semen, testes, epididymis
A. salpingitis	Chickens	Salpingitis and peritonitis in chickens; also isolated from cloaca of healthy chickens	Fresh affected tissue
A. pleuropneumoniae	Pigs	Fibrinous pleuropneumonia	Suspect tissue

Continued.

Table 4-1.—Cont'd

Organism	Species affected	Disease or lesion	Specimens
Actinomyces			
A. bovis	Horses, cattle	Poll evil and fistulous withers can occur as mixed infection with B. abortus, mandibular osteomyelitis	Fresh tissue, pus
A. suis	Pigs	Chronic granulomatous and suppurative mastitis in sows	Milk
A. viscosus	Hamsters, dogs	Periodontal disease; chronic granulomatous pleuritis	Fresh tissue, pus
A. pyogenes	Cattle, sheep, pigs	Suppurative mastitis and pneumonia	Milk, pus, tissue
Aeromonas			
A. hydrophila	Fish, reptiles, mammals, amphibians	Fish: generalized or localized infection, hemorrhagic septicemia; frogs: "red leg"; snakes: infectious stomatitis; mammals: neonatal infection in puppies; ubiquitous organism: may be primary or secondary pathogen	Fresh affected tissue
A. salmonicida	Trout, salmon	Furunculosis in trout and less commonly salmon	Fresh affected tissue or whole fish

BACILLUS

B. anthracis	Cattle, sheep, pigs, people	Anthrax, fatal septicemia in sheep, cattle, pigs; acute pharyngitis with hemorrhagic swelling of throat region	Fresh blood smear from ear vein; collect tissues with great caution
B. cereus	People, cats, dogs	Can cause food poisoning	Fresh fecal material
BACTEROIDES			
B. nodosus	Sheep	Foot rot in conjunction with *Fusobacterium necrophorum*	Fresh smear from lesion
B. melaninogenicus	Many species	Associated with other bacteria in such conditions as peritonitis, pericarditis, suppurative arthritis, and pneumonia	Fresh affected tissue
BORDETELLA			
B. bronchiseptica	Pigs, dogs, lab animals	Atrophic rhinitis in pigs; respiratory infection in dogs, associated with distemper virus; snuffles in rabbits and guinea pigs	Fresh nasal swabs or lungs

Continued.

Table 4-1.—Cont'd

Organism	Species affected	Disease or lesion	Specimens
Borrelia			
B. anserina	Poultry	Fowl spirochetosis, a fatal disease of chickens, turkeys, geese, and other fowl; acute septicemia, diarrhea, and anemia; transmitted by fowl ticks	Fresh blood, spleen, or liver smears
Other Borrelia species	Pigs, cattle	Associated ulcerative granuloma after trauma Enzootic/Foothill abortion	Fresh scrapings or biopsy material Fetal blood
Brucella			
B. abortus	Cattle, pigs, sheep, goats	Abortion; orchitis	Fresh fetal stomach contents, placenta, blood serum, milk, testes
	Horses	Chronic bursitis, fistulous withers, poll evil	Fresh material from lesions
B. melitensis	Goats, sheep, cattle	Abortion	As under B. abortus
B. ovis	Sheep	Abortion; epididymitis in rams	Fresh testes
B. suis	Pigs, occasionally cattle	Abortion; orchitis in boars	Fresh uterus, spleen, lymph nodes, semen, testes in boars
	Horses	Bursitis	Fresh material from lesions
B. canis	Dogs	Abortion (Beagles); infertility; epididymitis; orchitis	Fresh blood serum, lymph nodes, bone marrow

CAMPYLOBACTER

C. fetus ss fetus	Cattle	Abortion; infertility; fecal-oral route	Fresh vaginal mucus
C. fetus ss fetus	Sheep	Epizootics of abortion in sheep; oral infection; resides in intestine of cattle and sheep	Fetal stomach, cotyledons
C. fetus ss veneralis	Cattle	Abortion; infertility; venereal infection	Fresh vaginal mucus
C. fetus ss jejuni	Sheep, cattle	Epizootics of abortion; oral infection; healthy carriers, with organisms in intestinal tract	Rectal swabs or feces
C. sputorum ss mucosalis	Piglets	Pigs 2 to 6 weeks after weaning; hemorrhagic proliferative enteropathy; necrotic ileitis and watery diarrhea	Cannot be seen in fresh feces or ileal scrapings; need fixed ileal sections

CHLAMYDIA

Ch. psittaci (various strains)	Ewes	Enzootic abortion	Cotyledon, vaginal swab
	Cats	Feline pneumonitis (conjunctivitis, fever, ocular discharge)	Fresh conjunctival scrapings

Continued.

TABLE 4-1.—CONT'D

ORGANISM	SPECIES AFFECTED	DISEASE OR LESION	SPECIMENS
	Wild and domestic birds, people	Psittacosis/ornithosis—psittacine and other birds	Liver, spleen, kidney, lungs (can ship frozen)
	Cattle	Sporadic bovine encephalomyelitis; serofibrinous peritonitis is typical	Brain, fixed and fresh
	Sheep, calves, pigs (experimental infection in dogs)	Transmissible serositis (polyarthritis)	Synovial fluid or tissue; isolation/stained smears; diagnostic probability in neonates if arthritis is present without navel infection
	Cattle	Epizootic bovine abortion; tick transmitted; not demonstrated experimentally; may need other agents as well as *Chlamydia*	Cotyledon, vaginal swab, fetal lung and liver
CLOSTRIDIUM			
Cl. botulinum (Types A-G)	Many species	Botulism—types of most importance: A, B, & E—people; Cα—wild fowl, pheasants, chickens; Cβ—mink, cattle, horses (forage poisoning); D—cattle (South Africa); F—rare in people; G—unknown pathogenicity	Fresh serum obtained before death; at necropsy: heart, blood and intestinal contents; suspect feed; presence of toxin must be demonstrated

Cl. chauvoei	Cattle, sheep	Blackleg or blackquarter; gas gangrene	Fresh bone marrow in unopened rib; piece of affected muscle and heart
Cl. septicum	Cattle, sheep, horses, pigs	Malignant edema; gas gangrene/septicemia	As above
	Sheep	Braxy—infection of mucosa and submucosa of abomasum	Fresh and formalinized affected tissue
	Chickens	Necrotic dermatitis— gangrenous necrosis of skin; can be caused by Cl. novyi and Cl. perfringens, Type A	Fresh affected tissue
Cl. novyi (edematiens)			
Type A	Cattle, sheep	Gas gangrene of wounds; "big head" of rams, wounds due to fighting	Fresh rib with bone marrow; tissue with lesion; liver or whole carcass
Type B	Sheep, cattle	"Black disease"—necrotic hepatitis; follows fluke damage of liver	As above
Type C (Cl. bubalorum)	Buffalos (Indonesia)	Osteomyelitis	
(Cl. hemolyticum) (Cl. novyi Type D) Cl. perfringens Cl. welchii	Cattle, sheep	Bacillary hemoglobinuria or "red water disease"; infarcts of liver are characteristic	As above

Continued.

TABLE 4-1.—CONT'D

ORGANISM	SPECIES AFFECTED	DISEASE OR LESION	SPECIMENS
Type A	People	Food poisoning and gas gangrene; occasional cause of gas gangrene in animals	
Type B	Lambs	Lamb dysentery—severe enterotoxemia of neonates	
Type C	Sheep	"Struck"—acute intoxication	Fresh ileal contents for toxin demontration; fixed kidney and brain
	Calves, lambs, young pigs	Hemorrhagic enterotoxemia	
Type D	Sheep, occasionally goats, calves	Pulpy kidney disease—enterotoxemia, with focal symmetric encephalomalacia	
Type E	Lambs, calves	Reputed toxemia; not common	
Types A, C	Young chickens	Necrotic enteritis—acute enterotoxemia	Fresh liver and intestine for culture; fixed affected intestine
Cl. tetani	All species	Tetanus	Diagnosis usually based on clinical signs; fresh pus or tissue from invasion site if obvious

CORYNEBACTERIUM

C. bovis	Cattle	Found in mastitis milk samples; pathogenicity uncertain	Milk
C. pseudotuberculosis (*C. ovis*)	Sheep	Caseous lymphadenitis	Fresh and fixed affected lymph nodes
C. renale	Cattle	Cystitis, renal abscess	Fresh urine, kidney, bladder; fixed kidney
C. pilosum	Cattle	Cystitis	Fresh urine, bladder
Rhodococcus (*C.*) *equi*	Foals	Suppurative bronchopneumonia, multiple abscesses, arthritis	Fresh tissue, joints, abscess wall, lymph nodes
	Pigs	Abscesses in mandibular lymph nodes	Fixed affected tissues
	Cattle	Can be isolated from TB lesions	
Eubacterium (*C.*) *suis* (anaerobe)	Pigs	Cystitis and pyelonephritis in pigs; occurs in semen	Fresh urine, kidney, bladder, semen; fixed kidney, bladder
C. kutscheri (*C. murium*)	Mice, rats	Caseopurulent foci in lungs, lymph nodes, liver, kidney, skin	Fresh affected tissue

DERMATOPHILUS

D. congolensis	Cattle, horses, goats, sheep, polar bears	Dermatitis with scab formation and scab; fixed skin biopsy	Swab exudate, fresh plucked hair

Continued.

TABLE 4-1.—CONT'D

ORGANISM	SPECIES AFFECTED	DISEASE OR LESION	SPECIMENS
ERYSIPELOTHRIX			
E. rhusiopathiae (*E. insidiosa*)	Pigs	Diamond skin disease—septicemia, endocarditis, arthritis	Fresh liver, spleen, heart, synovial fluid
	Sheep, cattle,	Polyarthritis	Fixed skin, liver, kidney
	Turkeys, other birds	Septicemia	
ESCHERICHIA			
	Mainly young animals		
E. coli	Cattle, pigs	Calf scours; mastitis; piglet diarrhea; edema disease; hemorrhagic enteritis	Fresh feces, milk, urine, affected tissue
	Chickens	Air sacculitis; coligranuloma	Can be secondary agents and are rapid postmortem invaders
	Dogs	Urinary infections	
	Horses	Acute enterotoxemia in foals	
FRANCISELLA			
F. tularensis	People, wild animals, domestic	Necrotic foci in liver and spleen of wild rabbits and other animals	Fresh liver, spleen; lymph nodes are not involved

FUSOBACTERIUM

F. necrophorum (*Spherophorus necrophorus*)	Cattle	Principal agent of foot rot; necrobacillosis of liver in feedlot cattle (associated with *C. pyogenes*); calf diphtheria	Fresh pus or affected tissue; fixed affected tissue
	Sheep	Secondary invader in leg and lip ulceration; infectious bulbar necrosis (heel or foot abscess) in association with *C. pyogenes*	
	Goats	Associated with ulcerative stomatitis	
	Pigs	"Bull nose" —suppurative necrotic infection of nose and face; follows trauma	
	Horses	Involved in thrush	
	Fowl	Secondary invader of fowl pox virus lesions	

HEMOPHILUS

H. somnus	Cattle	Infectious thromboembolic meningoencephalitis; pneumonia and polyserositis	Fresh and fixed affected tissue

Continued.

Table 4-1.—Cont'd

Organism	Species affected	Disease or lesion	Specimens
H. suis and *H. parasuis* (*H. influenzae* var *suis*)	Pigs	Glasser's disease (polyserositis)	
H. gallinarum and *H. paragallinarum* (only need V factor)	Poultry	Fowl (infectious) coryza (nasal discharge and edema of face)	
H. hemoglobinophilus	Dogs	Commensal in prepuce	
Klebsiella			
K. pneumoniae	Pigs, cattle	Mastitis	Fresh milk
	Horses	Cervicitis and metritis, setpicemia in foals	Fresh liver, spleen, bone marrow
	Dogs	Pneumonia	Fresh lung
Leptospira			
L. interrogans	Cattle, sheep, pigs, horses	Cattle: hemoglobinuria and jaundice in calves; abortion, infertility, and agalactia in adults	Fresh kidney taken within 4 hours of death
L. pomona *L. hardjo*	Cattle	Pigs: abortion in late pregnancy; kidney lesions in young animals	Urine: 10 ml placed immediately in 1.5 ml of 10% formalin

Organism	Hosts	Disease	Specimens
L. grippotyphosa	Cattle, pigs, horses	Horses: fever, jaundice, occasionally abortion and periodic ophthalmia	Fixed kidney, liver
L. icterohemorrhagiae	Cattle, pigs, dogs	Dogs: acute hemorrhagic and icteric disease with *L. icterohemorrhagiae*	
L. canicola	Cattle, pigs, dogs	Uremia or inapparent with *L. canicola*	
L. bratislava	Pigs	Abortion, mummified fetus, stillbirth	Fresh and fixed kidney, uterus, placenta
LISTERIA			
L. monocytogenes	Cows, sheep, occasionally horses, dogs	Abortion; encephalitis	Fresh abortion specimens, brain or liver
	Rabbits, pigs, lambs, raccoons	Liver necrosis	Fixed affected tissues
	Chickens, turkeys, cage birds	Septicemia; necrotic foci in liver and pericardium	
MORAXELLA			
M. bovis	Cattle	Infectious keratoconjunctivitis (pink eye)	Fresh swab of eye discharges; plate directly on 5% ox blood agar if possible, or place swab in a little sterile saline for rapid transport to laboratory

Continued.

Table 4-1.—Cont'd

Organism	Species Affected	Disease or Lesion	Specimens
Mycobacterium			
M. bovis	Cattle, pigs, sheep, deer	Bovine-type tuberculosis; granulomas with caseation	Fresh and fixed lesions and affected tissue
M. avium	Pigs, poultry, horses, feral birds and animals	Avian-type tuberculosis; granulomas with caseation	
M. marinum	People, cold-blooded animals	"Swimming pool granuloma" in people	
M. lepraemurium	Rats	Rat leprosy—granulomas	
M. ulcerans	Cats	Skin granulomas that ulcerate	
M. paratuberculosis (M. johnei)	Cattle, sheep, goats	Johne's disease	Fresh feces, mesenteric lymph nodes, ileocecal valve or other affected gut; fixed intestine and mesenteric lymph nodes
Mycoplasma			
M. mycoides ss mycoides	Cattle	Contagious bovine pleuropneumonia	Fresh swabs containing exudates from eye, nostril, trachea, and genitalia should be placed in tubes of Mycoplasma broth, chilled to 2°-3° C and rapidly transported to the laboratory

Organism	Host	Disease	Specimen
M. bovis		Mastitis, arthritis, pneumonia	
M. dispar		Pneumonia (calves)	
M. bovigenitalis		Arthritis, vaginitis, seminal vesiculitis	
M. californicum		Mastitis	
M. canodense		Mastitis	
M. bovoculi		Keratoconjunctivitis	
M. agalactiae	Sheep, cattle	Contagious agalactia	Milk
M. conjunctivae		Keratoconjunctivitis	Eyes
M. capricolum		Mastitis, polyarthritis, pneumonia	Exudate, milk
M. ovipneumoniae	Sheep	Pneumonia	Serum, fresh lungs
M. mycoides ss mycoides	Goats	Polyarthritis, septicemia, mastitis, pneumonia	Milk, exudate, fresh lungs
M. mycoides ss capri		Contagious caprine pneumonia	
M. putrefaciens		Mastitis, arthritis	
M. hyorhinis	Pigs	Polyserositis, arthritis (baby pigs)	
M. hyopneumoniae		Enzootic (viral) pneumonia	
M. hyosynoviae		Polyarthritis (12-24 weeks old)	

Continued.

TABLE 4-1.—CONT'D

ORGANISM	SPECIES AFFECTED	DISEASE OR LESION	SPECIMENS
M. felis	Cats	Conjunctivitis	
M. cynos	Dogs	Pneumonia	
M. felis	Horses	Pleuritis	
M. gallisepticum	Chickens	Chronic respiratory disease	
M. synoviae	Chickens, turkeys	Infectious synovitis	
M. meleagridis	Turkeys	Air sacculitis, bursitis	
NOCARDIA			
N. asteroides	Cattle	Acute and chronic mastitis	Fresh milk or affected tissue
	Dogs, cats, other animals	Localized granulomatous lesions with or without lymph node involvement; generalized disease with pneumonia in dogs	Fixed lung or other affected tissue
PASTEURELLA			
P. multocida	Many animals	Frequently a secondary invader or opportunist; associated with shipping fever complex in cattle; snuffles in rabbits; enzootic pneumonia in pigs; primary cause: fowl cholera; hemorrhagic septicemia of cattle; severe mastitis in cattle and sheep	Fresh and fixed lung and spleen or other tissue with lesions

P. hemolytica	Cattle, sheep, pigs, goats, poultry	Associated with pneumonia, shipping fever in cattle; salpingitis of fowl
P. pneumotropica	Rodents	Pneumonia and abscesses
P. gallinarum	Chickens	Upper respiratory infection in chickens
P. anatipestifer	Ducklings	Septicemia in young ducks ("new duck disease")
PSEUDOMONAS		
P. aeruginosa	Many animals	Wound infections; bovine mastitis; otitis in dogs and cats; septicemia in chickens	Fresh swabs or affected tissue
P. pseudomallei	People, primates Cattle, sheep, horses, dogs, cats, rodents	Melioidosis or pseudoglanders Septicemia of abscesses in lungs, liver, spleen, lymph nodes, subcutis	Fresh pus, nodules, or abscess wall Fresh affected tissue
P. mallei	Horses, mules, donkeys	Glanders or farcy (eradicated in North America)	

Continued.

TABLE 4-1.—CONT'D

ORGANISM	SPECIES AFFECTED	DISEASE OR LESION	SPECIMENS
RICKETTSIA			
Ehrlichia canis	Dogs	Recurrent tick-borne fever	Blood smear (optimal time 2 weeks postinfection)
Ehrlichia equi	Horses	Fever and edema of legs (California)	Blood smears in febrile period
Ehrlichia risticii	Horses	Potomac horse fever	Blood or buffy coat smear, paired serum samples
Neorickettsia helminthoeca	Dogs	"Salmon poisoning"; carried by metacercariae of intestinal fluke (NW USA)	Fluke eggs in feces, smears of fluid aspirated from mandibular lymph nodes
Colesiota conjunctivae	Sheep	Contagious ophthalmia	Smears from conjunctival scrapings
SALMONELLA			
Over 1000 serotypes			
S. typhimurium	Cattle, sheep, pigs, horses, poultry	Acute septicemia, gastroenteritis	Fresh feces, mesentric lymph nodes
S. dublin	Cattle		
S. abortusequi	Horses	Abortion	Fetal fluid, fetus, fetal membranes
S. abortusbovis	Cattle	Abortion	

Organism	Animal	Disease	Specimen
S. bovismorbificans	Cattle	Enteritis	Feces
S. abortusovis	Sheep	Enteritis	Feces
S. choleraesuis	Pigs	Chronic enteritis	Feces
S. typhisuis	Young pigs		Feces
S. gallinarum	Chickens	Pullorum disease	Feces
S. pullorum			
S. arizonae	Chickens, turkeys	Septicema, enteritis	
S. enteritidis			
S. typhimurium	Chickens	Fowl typhoid	
SERPULINA (TREPONEMA)			
Serpulina (Treponema) hyodysenteriae	Pigs	Swine dysentery (catarrhal hemorrhagic enteritis)	Fresh rectal swabs taken by Culturette swabs; section of spiral colon (3-4 inches) in plastic bag; hold at 0-4° C and send to laboratory with ice packs as quickly as possible; DO NOT FREEZE
STAPHYLOCOCCUS			
S. aureus	Many animals	Suppurative wound infections; abscesses; mastitis	Fresh milk, wound, skin or abscess swabs

Continued.

Table 4-1.—Cont'd

Organism	Species Affected	Disease or Lesion	Specimens
S. epidermidis	Many animals	Usually nonpathogenic, but some strains can cause abscesses and skin infections	
S. intermedius	Dogs	Skin infections	
S. hyicus	Pigs	Exudative epidermitis; "greasy pig disease" or impetigo	
Streptococcus			
18 serogroups			
S. agalactiae (Group B)	Cattle, sheep, goats	Chronic mastitis	Milk, milk ducts
	Dogs	Neonatal septicemia	Exudate, urine,
	Cats	Kidney and urinary infections	uterine discharge
S. dysgalactiae (Group C)	Cattle	Mastitis (not a common cause)	
	Lambs	Polyarthritis	
S. equi ss equi (Group C)	Horses	Strangles, genital infection	Pus, lymph nodes, uterine or cervical swab
S. equi ss zooepidemicus (Group C)	Horses, cattle, pigs, poultry	Mastitis, abortion, naval infection	Milk, vulvar discharge
S. equi ss equisimilis (Group C)	Horses	Abscesses, endometritis	Pus, exudate
Enterococcus fecalis (Group D)	Many species	Endocarditis, mastitis	Feces, milk, urine

S. durans (Group D)		Urinary infection	
S. porcinus (Group E)	Pigs	Jowl abscess, lymphadenitis	Pus, lymph nodes
S. canis (Group G)		Neonatal septicemia, genital infection	Pus, serum
S. suis (Group R)	Weaner pigs	Meningitis, arthritis, pneumonia	Nasal discharge
S. uberis			
S. pneumoniae	Calves, primates	Pneumonia, meningitis	Nasal discharge, respiratory mucus
TAYLORELLA			
T. (Hemophilus) equigenitalis	Horses	Contagious equine metritis; possible abortion	Fresh cervical or uterine swabs; sheath swabs; place in Amies' transport medium
UREAPLASMA			
U. diversum	Cattle, turkeys	Vulvovaginitis, pneumonia	
VIBRIO			
V. metschnikovii	Chickens	Acute gastroenteritis in young chickens	Fresh section of small intestine or whole bird

Continued.

TABLE 4-1.—CONT'D

ORGANISM	SPECIES AFFECTED	DISEASE OR LESION	SPECIMENS
YERSINIA			
Y. pseudotuberculosis	Deer, birds, guinea pigs, sheep	Acute septicemic form or chronic with necrotic foci or abscesses through body; diarrhea	Fresh feces, intestine, lung, liver, spleen, lesions
Y. enterocolitica	Deer, birds, sheep, other animals	Enterocolitis	Fixed lung, liver, spleen, intestine, affected tissue

- Scalpels, scissors, forceps, and spatulas
- Pasteur pipettes and rubber bulbs
- Pipetting syringe for dispensing liquid media (e.g., Cornwall pipetting syringe)
- Culture media in plates and tubes
- Antimicrobial sensitivity discs (for antibacterials commonly used in the practice)
- Sensitivity disc dispenser (BBL, Oxoid, Difco)
- Distilled water
- Beakers, volumetric cylinders
- Flat-bottom flasks for preparing media from dehydrated powder
- Hot plate with a magnetic stirring facility (Fisher)
- Screw-capped bottles and tubes for storing media
- Racks for bottles and tubes
- Carbon dioxide jar (BBL, Oxoid) for isolation of microaerophiles (alternatively, a 1-lb canning jar with a 1-inch piece of candle provides an atmosphere of about 2% carbon dioxide)
- Disinfectant solution for wiping down bench surfaces
- Soap, paper towels, and paper towel dispenser
- Plain, sterile, cotton-tipped swabs
- API, Minitek, Enterotube II, and Bactube identification systems (Hoffman-La Roche)
- Organisms for quality control (Difco) (see discussion following)
- Disposal bin lined with autoclavable bags for disposal of cultures and other contaminated materials.

QUALITY-CONTROL CULTURES

Some cultures are required in a laboratory for quality-control purposes. Various procedures and supplies must be monitored as to quality and accuracy, including antibacterial susceptibility tests, media, biochemical tests, and certain tests for identification, such as the zone of beta hemolysis around *Staphylococcus aureus* for the CAMP test. A selection of control organisms can be obtained on discs from Difco Laboratories (Box 4-1). Media not containing fermentable sugars, such as trypticase soy agar (BBL) and maintenance medium (Difco), are suitable for maintaining fewer fastidious organisms, such as *Staphylococcus aureus* and Enterobacteriaceae. The bacteria can be stab inoculated into a tube of medium and subcultured about every 2 months.

Streptococcus, Pasteurella, and *Actinobacillus* die quickly on culture plates. Streptococci can be kept in a tube of cooked meat broth and subcultured about

Box 4-1. Commercial firms supplying microbiologic products

American Scientific Products[2]
1430 Wantegan Rd
McGaw Park, IL 60085
(800) 233-4362

Analylab Products[11]
Div Ayerst Laboratories
15620 Industrial Pkwy
Cleveland, OH 44135
(800) 645-7035

Baxter Diagnostic[1,2,3]
Canlab Div
2390 Argentia Rd
Canada Mississauga, Ontario L5N 3P1
(800) 668-4666

BBL Microbiology Systems[1,6,7,12,14]
Div Becton, Dickinson
POB 243
Cockeysville, MD 21030
(800) 638-8663

Burroughs Wellcome[10]
Wellcome Reagent Div
Order Dept, POB 1887
Greenville, NC 27834
(919) 758-3436 (Ext 2285/6)

Difco Laboratories[1,3,6]
POB 1058A
Detroit, MI 48232
(313) 961-0800

Fisher Scientific Company[2,3,6]
Corporate Headquarters
711 Forbes Ave
Pittsburgh, PA 15219
(412) 562-8300

General Scientific Products[2]
8741 Landmark Rd
POB 26509
Richmond, VA 23261
(804) 264-7560

Gibco Products[1,3,8,9]
3175 Staley Rd
Grand Island, NY 14072
(800) 828-6686

Hoffman-La Roche[15,16]
401 The West Mall, Ste 700
Etobicoke, Ontario M9C 5J4
Canada
(800) 268-0482
(416) 620-2800 Collect

Johns Scientific[1,2]
175 Hanson St
Toronto, Ontario
Canada
(800) 268-4410

Marion Scientific[4]
9233 Ward Pkwy
Kansas City, MO 64114
(800) 821-7772

NCS Diagnostic[17]
130 Matheson Blvd
Mississauga, Ontario L4Z 1Y6
Canada
(800) 268-2857

Oxoid USA[1,6,7]
9017 Red Branch Rd
Columbia, MD 21045
(410) 997-2216

Pitman-Moore[13,18]
421 E. Hawley St
Mundelein, IL 60060
(708) 949-3300

Sigma Chemical Co[5]
POB 14508
St. Louis, MO 63178
(800) 325-3010

1 - Dehydrated and prepared culture media in plates and tubes.
2 - General laboratory supplies, equipment.
3 - Staining kit sets.
4 - "Culturette" swabs.
5 - Chemicals, laboratory antibiotics, dyes for staining.
6 - Antibiotic sensitivity discs.
7 - Anaerobic and carbon dioxide systems.
8 - Distilled water.
9 - Sterile blood.
10 - "Streptex" for Lancefield grouping.
11 - API identification system.
12 - Minitek identification system.
13 - Canine brucellosis diagnostic test.
14 - Products obtained through distributors, such as Fisher Scientific or American Scientific.
15 - Bactube.
16 - Enterotube II.
17 - Virology supplies.
18 - Dermatophyte test medium.

every 4 weeks. *Pasteurella* and *Actinobacillus* remain viable if mixed with about 0.5 ml of sterile whole blood in a small tube and stored in a deep freeze at $-10°$ C or lower. Otherwise these two genera should be subcultured on blood agar about every 3 days.

Control cultures can be kept at room temperature in screw-capped tubes but preferably in a refrigerator at $4°$ C, as this reduces the metabolic rate of the organisms.

CULTURE MEDIA

Culture medium (plural, *media*) is any material, solid or liquid, that can support the growth of microorganisms. For bacteriology, culture media can be purchased as dehydrated powder or as prepared agar plates or ready-to-use media for biochemical tests. Most of the commonly used media can now be obtained already prepared from supply houses. This is probably most convenient for a small laboratory because preparation time is saved, the manufacturers attend to quality control, and small quantities can be obtained.

BASIC NUTRIENT MEDIA. Nutrient media typically contain peptone, salt, dextrose, water, meat extract, and a solidifying agent, such as agar or gelatin.

- *Peptone* is partially hydrolysed protein that can be readily metabolized by bacteria to provide amino acids and other simple nitrogenous compounds. It is the principal nutrient of the medium and is needed for growth. It has some buffering action and contains a considerable amount of inorganic salts.
- *Salt* is added to adjust the osmotic pressure of the medium so that it is isotonic for the bacterial cell.
- *Dextrose* serves as a source of carbon and energy for bacteria.
- *Water* is added to provide food material in solution form that can be used by bacteria. Usually distilled water is used to ensure the uniformity of different batches of media.
- *Meat extract* provides water-soluble carbohydrates, nitrogen, and vitamins.
- *Solidifying agents* include agar and gelatin. Agar is a dried extract of sea algae known as agarphytes. It is a long-chain nonnutrient polysaccharide that is not attacked by bacteria. It is available as a fine, almost colorless powder. For solid medium, add 1.5% agar; for semi-solid medium, add 0.1% to 0.5%, depending on the degree of solidity required. Agar is a liquid at $>42°$ C and a solid at $\leq42°$ C; this is an important consideration when preparing media.

- *Gelatin* is a protein obtained from animal tissues. It solidifies when present in medium at 12% to 30% concentration. It has two disadvantages: It melts at 28° to 31° C and therefore will not remain solid at 37° C (the usual temperature of bacterial incubation). Also, bacteria themselves attack the gelatin and liquefy it.

ENRICHED MEDIA.   Enriched media are formulated to meet the requirements of the most fastidious pathogens. They are essentially basic nutrient media with extra nutrients added, such as blood, serum, or egg. Examples include blood agar and chocolate agar.

SELECTIVE MEDIA.   Selective media contain antibacterial substances, such as bile salts or antibacterials that inhibit or kill all but a few types of bacteria. They facilitate isolation of a particular genus from a mixed inoculum. Examples of selective media are brilliant green agar and MacConkey agar.

DIFFERENTIAL MEDIA.   Differential media allow bacteria to be differentiated into groups by biochemical reactions on the medium. Simmons' citrate is a differential medium.

ENRICHMENT MEDIA.   These are liquid media that favor growth of a particular group of organisms. They either contain nutrients that encourage growth of the desired organisms or contain inhibitory substances that suppress competitors. Examples include tetrathionate broth and selenite broth.

SYNTHETIC MEDIA.   These are prepared exclusively from pure chemical substances, and their exact chemical composition is known. They are used mainly in experimental work, but a few used for biochemical tests might be included in this category. An example is Koser citrate broth.

PREPARATION OF CULTURE MEDIA

The major firms supplying prepared and dehydrated media are BBL, Difco, Gibco, and Oxoid (Box 4-1). If you are preparing media from dehydrated powder or granules, always follow the manufacturer's instructions. The following directives are not meant to be comprehensive but emphasize important points for beginners preparing media that cannot be obtained commercially:

- *Use clean glassware* rinsed free of detergents and other chemicals. The glassware need not be sterile unless sterilized medium is being decanted into it.

- *Weigh out the appropriate amount* of dehydrated medium, place in a flask, and add distilled water. Always use distilled water, as this is free from chlorine and heavy-metal ions that can inhibit bacterial growth. Containers of distilled water can be obtained commercially.
- *Prepare the medium in a container about twice the final volume of the medium.* This allows adequate mixing and allows for frothing of the medium during heating.
- *Media that do not contain agar can usually be dissolved with gentle agitation.* Dehydrated media containing agar, however, are best dissolved by bringing the mixture to a boil, with continuous stirring using a glass rod or a hot plate that incorporates a magnetic stirrer system. Caking at the bottom of the flask may occur if stirring is not adequate.
- *Once dissolved, dehydrated media are usually sterilized in an autoclave or pressure cooker* at 121° C (15 lb pressure) for 15 minutes. However, some media contain ingredients that cannot tolerate this high temperature, and the manufacturer's instructions indicate the medium should be sterilized at 118° C or 115° C for a slightly longer time. Some selective media, such as brilliant green agar, can be sterilized by boiling for about a minute.
- *Agar media should be cooled, preferably in a water bath, to 50° to 56° C before the plates are filled.* Remember that agar solidifies at 42° C. One liter of liquid agar medium usually makes 70 to 100 agar plates.
- *Some additives to media may not tolerate boiling or autoclaving* and so must be added after the media have been autoclaved and cooled. These additives must, of course, be sterile. Blood and serum are collected aseptically, while certain dyes and sugars are sterilized by passing them through a membrane filter of 0.2-μ pore size to remove bacteria.
- *Commercial dehydrated media often contain buffering agents* that keep the pH within a desired range (usually pH 6.8 to 7.2). However, as part of quality-control procedures, or if you are preparing a medium from basic ingredients, the pH of cooled media should be checked. This is best done using an electronic pH meter, but pH paper strips can also be used. The pH is adjusted by adding drops of 1-N or 0.1-N NaOH or HCl.
- *After the poured plates are set, allow them to dry at room temperature,* or at 37° C for a few hours, to ensure that there is no surface moisture when you use them. The plates can then be placed in sealed plastic bags and stored in a refrigerator.

Blood agar.   This enriched medium supports the growth of most bacterial pathogens. Trypticase soy agar, blood agar base, Columbia agar, or Eugon agar may be used. The last two base media have extra nutritive value. Bacterial colony size is often larger than when trypticase soy agar is used as the blood agar base.

The blood agar base, such as trypticase soy agar or Columbia agar, is prepared in the usual manner, sterilized and cooled to 50° to 56° C. Sterile blood is added at 5% to 7%. Sheep blood is usually used because ovine blood accurately reflects hemolytic reactions, and it is available commercially. The blood can be collected aseptically from a healthy animal using a human donor set; otherwise use 10% sodium citrate solution at a 1:10 ratio as an anticoagulant.

If the blood has been stored in the refrigerator, warm the blood to room temperature or to 37° C in the incubator before adding it to the agar base. This avoids thermal shock to the red blood cells. Mix the blood and agar base together well before pouring the plates. If bubbles form on the surface of the poured plates, quickly pass a low Bunsen flame across the surface of the plates before the agar sets.

Blood agar should be bright red. A brownish-red color may indicate one or more of the following problems:

- The blood is too old and the red blood cells are hemolyzing.
- The blood was added to the agar base when the medium was too hot.
- Inadequate mixing of the blood with the agar base has prevented oxygenation of the red blood cells.
- Thermal shock has caused hemolysis because refrigerated blood was not warmed before adding it to the molten agar.

If the blood agar plates are contaminated, examine them to decide whether the contaminant bacterial colonies are throughout the medium or just on the surface. If colonies are evident throughout, the blood itself is probably contaminated and should be discarded. If the colonies are only on the surface of the medium, the plates were probably accidentally contaminated after pouring.

Blood agar acts as an enrichment medium as well as a differential medium because four distinct types of hemolysis can be detected on blood agar.

- *Alpha (α) hemolysis* refers to partial hemolysis that creates a narrow band of greenish or slimy discoloration around the bacterial colony.
- *Beta (β) hemolysis* refers to complete hemolysis that creates a clear zone around the bacterial colony.

- *Gamma (γ) hemolysis* produces no change in the appearance of the medium and no hemolysis around colonies.
- *Delta (δ) hemolysis,* also called double-zone hemolysis, consists of a zone of hemolysis surrounded by a narrow zone of hemolysis around a bacterial colony.

MacCONKEY AGAR. This is a selective and differential medium. It contains crystal violet, which suppresses growth of Gram-positive bacteria, and bile salts that are selective for Enterobacteriaceae, and a few other bile salt-tolerant Gram-negative bacteria. Growth or no growth on MacConkey agar can be used as a test for primary identification of Gram-negative genera.

The indicators in MacConkey agar are lactose and neutral red. Lactose-fermenting organisms, such as *E. coli, Enterobacter,* and *Klebsiella* species produce acid from lactose and grow as pinkish-red colonies on this medium. Bacteria that cannot ferment lactose attack the peptone in MacConkey agar, producing an alkaline reaction and colorless colonies. Clinical specimens for routine isolation are usually separately cultured on both blood and MacConkey agars.

Examination of both blood and MacConkey agar cultures, inoculated with the same clinical specimen, can yield considerable information. For example, no growth on the MacConkey agar plate but good growth on the blood agar plate suggests that the isolated pathogen is probably Gram positive.

CHOCOLATE AGAR. If *Hemophilus* infection is suspected, specimens should also be inoculated on a chocolate agar plate in addition to blood and MacConkey agar plates. In this very nutritive medium, hemolyzed red blood cells have released the "V" and "X" growth factors required by *Hemophilus.* Hemolytic activity cannot be observed on chocolate agar. Growth of all *Hemophilus* species is enhanced by increased CO_2 tension; some require 10% CO_2 for growth.

BRAIN-HEART INFUSION BROTH. This is a useful, general purpose broth used to increase the number of organisms (pre-enrichment) before they are plated on solid medium. For example, it can be difficult to isolate *Listeria* from brain specimens, especially those from cattle, without pre-enrichment. Pieces of the patient's medulla and brainstem are finely cut up or homogenized, and a 10% to 20% suspension is made in the infusion broth. This is refrigerated at 4° C for up to 12 weeks. Subcultures are made on blood agar and MacConkey agar after 1, 3, 6, and 12 weeks of incubation.

There is generally no difficulty in isolating *Listeria* from abortion cases or from animals with the visceral forms of listeriosis. Specimens from these can be plated directly onto solid medium. Streptococci appear to be especially susceptible to desiccation. When a swab sample is the only specimen available, the likelihood of isolating streptococci can be enhanced by pre-enrichment. The swab is placed in about 10 ml of infusion broth and incubated at 37° C for 24 hours. A loopful of broth can then be plated out on solid medium.

If you are testing the sterility of dried milk powder, bone meal, or other substances that may have been subjected to heat treatment in processing, the sample should first be placed in nutrient broth for 24 hours at 37° C and then plated out on agar medium. If you are attempting to isolate salmonellae from these samples, place about 1 ml of broth into 10 ml of tetrathionate broth for another 24 hours' incubation at 37° C before plating on selective medium.

When culturing blood samples, about 1 ml of the patient's blood sample is added to nutrient broth or a special blood culture medium, which can be obtained commercially. Because a patient's blood contains many substances that are inhibitory to bacteria, adding the blood sample directly to broth dilutes the effect of these natural inhibitors.

MANNITOL SALT AGAR. This is not usually used routinely but is a highly selective medium for staphylococci and could be used to isolate *Staphylococcus aureus* from contaminated specimens. The medium has a high salt content (7.5%) and contains mannitol and the pH indicator phenol red. Staphylococci are salt tolerant. *Staphylococcus aureus,* but usually not *Staphylococcus epidermidis,* ferments mannitol. The resulting acid turns *Staphylococcus aureus* colonies and the surrounding medium yellow.

PURPLE BASE AGAR WITH MALTOSE. This medium is used for presumptive identification of staphylococci. *Staphylococcus aureus* ferments maltose and changes the medium's color from purple to yellow. *Staphylococcus intermedius* produces a slight color change and *Staphylococcus hyicus* produces no color change (does not ferment maltose).

HEKTOEN ENTERIC AGAR. Hektoen enteric agar has a high carbohydrate and peptone content to counteract the inhibitory effects of the bile salts and indicators also in the medium. It only slightly inhibits growth of *Salmonella* and *Shigella* yet still inhibits accompanying microorganisms.

Lactose-positive colonies are differentiated from lactose-negative colonies by the indicators bromthymol blue and acid fuchsin. Added carbohydrate, such as sucrose or salicin, which is fermented more easily than lactose, also further differentiates organisms. The combination of thiosulfate with ferric ammonium citrate causes hydrogen sulfide-producing colonies to become black.

The following summarizes the typical appearance of the more important bacteria on Hektoen enteric agar:

ORGANISM	COLONY APPEARANCE
Shigella, Providencia	Green, moist, raised colonies
Salmonella, Proteus	Blue-green, with or without a black center
Coliforms (rapid lactose fermenters)	Salmon-pink to orange, surrounded by a zone of bile precipitate

BISMUTH SULFITE AGAR.   In this selective medium, freshly precipitated bismuth sulfite acts with brilliant green to suppress growth of coliforms while permitting growth of salmonellae. Sulfur compounds provide a substrate for hydrogen sulfide production. The metallic salts in the medium stain the colony and surrounding medium black or brown in the presence of hydrogen sulfide.

Atypical colonies may appear if the medium is heavily inoculated with organic matter. Such a situation may be prevented by suspending the sample in sterile saline and using the supernatant for inoculation.

The freshly prepared medium has a strong inhibitory action and is suitable for heavily contaminated samples. Storing the poured plates at 4° C for 3 days causes the medium to change color to green, making it less selective with small numbers of salmonellae being recovered.

The typical appearance of colonies of important bacteria on bismuth sulfite agar is as follows:

ORGANISM	COLONY APPEARANCE
Salmonella typhi	Black "rabbit-eye" colonies, with surrounding black zone and metallic sheen after 18 hours; uniformly black after 48 hours' incubation
Other *Salmonella* species	Variable colony appearance after 18 hours (black, green, or clear and mucoid); uniformly black colonies seen after 48 hours, often with widespread staining of the medium and a pronounced metallic sheen
Other organisms (coliforms, *Serratia*, *Proteus*)	Usually inhibited but occasionally dull green or brown colonies with no metallic sheen or staining of surrounding medium

UREA TUBES.   Urea slants are streaked with inoculum and incubated overnight at 37° C. Urea medium is a peach color. If the bacteria hydrolyze the urea in the medium, ammonia production turns the medium to a pink color. A negative result produces no color change.

SULFIDE-INDOLE-MOTILITY TUBES.   The tube of sulfide-indole-motility medium is inoculated with a straight stab to a depth of about 1 inch. Care is taken to withdraw the wire out along the same line as on entry (see Figure 4-6). Hydrogen sulfide production is indicated by blackening of the medium. Indole production requires addition of 5 drops of Kovac's reagent to the top of the medium. If tryptophan has been broken down to indole by the bacteria in the tube, a red ring immediately forms on top of the medium.

INDOLE SPOT TEST.   This is a new test to detect indole production. A drop of para-dimethyl amino cinnamaldehyde (DMCA) is placed on a piece of filter paper. A drop of the test culture is then applied with an applicator stick or loop. A green or blue-green color indicates indole production.

SIMMONS' CITRATE TUBES.   Simmons' citrate medium differentiates bacteria according to their use of citrate. Only the slant surface in inoculated. If bacteria use the citrate in the medium, a deep blue color develops. The unchanged medium is green.

TETRATHIONATE BROTH.   This is an enrichment broth for isolation of *Salmonella*. It is prepared according to the manufacturer's instructions. The suspension is mixed thoroughly and heated to sterilize it. The cooled medium is aseptically dispensed in 10-ml quantities into sterile tubes or bottles. An iodide solution must be added to the tetrathionate broth base, at 0.2 ml iodide/10 ml broth base, immediately before use. The iodide solution is made from 6 g of iodine and 5 g of potassium iodide ground together in a mortar. Add the water gradually until a solution is obtained. The solution must be stored in a container whose lid does not contain rubber, as the solution attacks rubber.

SELENITE BROTH.   This is another enrichment broth for *Salmonella* isolation. It is prepared by mixing 23 g of selenite in 1 L of distilled water and boiling to sterilize. Avoid excessive heating. Do not sterilize the solution in an autoclave. Dispense the sterile solution into sterile tubes to a depth of at least 5 cm.

TRIPLE SUGAR-IRON AGAR.   This is a composite medium for presumptive identification of salmonellae and for initial differentiation of enteric bacteria (Figure

4-2). The essential ingredients of the medium are 1% lactose; 1% sucrose (or saccharose); 0.1% glucose (dextrose); an indicator system for hydrogen sulfide production; and pH indicator, phenol red, that colors the uninoculated medium red. All enterobacteria ferment glucose, and the small amount (0.1%) is attacked preferentially and rapidly. At an early stage of incubation, both slant and butt turn yellow due to acid production. However, after the glucose is metabolized under aerobic conditions and provided the organism cannot ferment lactose or sucrose, the slope reverts to the red (alkaline) condition. The butt, under anaerobic conditions, remains yellow (acidic). To allow this reaction, the triple sugar-iron agar must always be used in tubes with loose caps or plugged with sterile cotton.

If the organism can ferment lactose and/or sucrose as well as the glucose, these are then attacked with resulting acid production, and the medium turns yellow (acidic) throughout. Lactose and sucrose are present in 1% quantities to maintain acidic conditions in the slant, which remains yellow. With organisms that produce hydrogen sulfide, blackening of the medium is partly superimposed on the other reactions. The triple sugar-iron slants should be read after about 16 hours' incubation at 37° C. After longer incubation the blackening tends to reach the bottom of the tube and obscures the yellow butt.

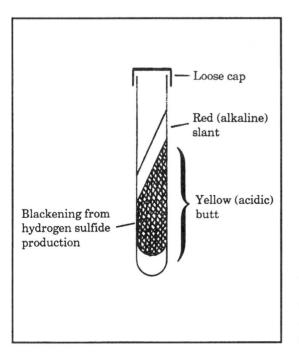

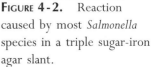

FIGURE 4-2. Reaction caused by most *Salmonella* species in a triple sugar-iron agar slant.

To summarize the reactions of *Salmonella* in triple sugar-iron agar:

- Alkaline (red) slant and alkaline (red) butt: none of the sugars have been attacked.
- Alkaline (red) slant and acidic (yellow) butt: glucose fermentation only.
- Acidic (yellow) slant and acidic (yellow) butt: glucose attacked as well as lactose and/or sucrose.
- Blackening along stab line and through medium: hydrogen sulfide production.

The triple sugar-iron slant is stab inoculated with a single colony from the selective medium, using a straight inoculating wire. Take the wire right down to the bottom of the agar and, on withdrawing the wire, streak the agar slant. The inoculating wire still contains enough bacteria to incoulate a tube of lysine decarboxylase broth. When searching for salmonellae, at least two suspicious colonies should be individually tested in triple sugar-iron agar per brilliant green plate. Incubate the triple sugar-iron tubes, with loose caps, at 37° C for 16 to 24 hours.

LYSINE DECARBOXYLASE BROTH.   This medium examines the ability of an organism to decarboxylate the amino acid, lysine, to the alkaline end-product, cadaverine. The uninoculated medium is usually yellowish purple. Initially, the enterobacteria preferentially ferment the small amount of glucose (0.1%) in the medium. Acid is produced and the indicator, bromocresol purple, turns the medium yellow. However, on further incubation, bacteria that can decarboxylate lysine produce cadaverine, and this alkaline byproduct turns the medium purple (lysine positive). With organisms unable to attack lysine, the medium remains yellow (lysine negative).

LYSINE IRON AGAR.   Lysine iron agar is a sensitive medium for detection of both *Salmonella* and *Arizona* organisms. The medium is tubed, sterilized, and slanted so that a short slant and deep butt are formed. It is inoculated with a straight needle by stabbing to the base of the butt and streaking the slant. The caps of the tubes must be replaced loosely so that aerobic conditions prevail on the slant. Incubate at 37° C overnight.

Cultures that rapidly produce lysine decarboxylase cause an alkaline reaction (purple color) throughout the medium. Organisms that do not decarboxylase lysine produce an alkaline slant and acidic butt (yellow color).

Cultures that produce hydrogen sulfide cause an intense blackening in the medium.

Due to determination of the lysine, *Proteus* and *Providencia* cultures produce a red slant over an acidic butt.

METHYL RED.   Glucose phosphate peptone medium tests the ability of an organism to produce large quantities of acidic end-products (methyl red positive) or to produce acetylmethylcarbinol (*Voges Proskauer positive*). The test medium is inoculated and incubated at 37° C for 24 to 48 hours. About 5 drops of the methyl red reagent are mixed in the test medium and the test is read immediately. A positive methyl red test is bright red and a negative is yellow. If the methy red test is negative, the *Voges Proskauer test* can be performed in the same tube. One ml of 40% KOH and 3 ml of a 5% solution of alpha-naphthol in absolute ethanol are added to the tube, and the contents are mixed and allowed to stand for 15 to 30 minutes. A pink color, becoming crimson, indicates production of acetylmethycarbinol (*Voges Proskauer positive*). Most enterobacteria are methyl red positive or Voges Proskauer positive, but not positive to both tests.

INOCULATING CULTURE MEDIA

ASEPTIC TECHNIQUE.   When inoculating media and handling the specimen, care must be taken to prevent contamination. Aseptic (sterile) technique must be used as follows:

- When obtaining samples from a cadaver or excised organs, sear the surface of the organ or tissue with a flamed spatula before it is cut open for sample collection.
- Keep culture plates closed unless inoculating or removing colony specimens for testing.
- When transferring samples from or to a tube, flame the tube neck before and after transfer of material (Figure 4-3). Also, do not put the cap down. Instead, hold it between your last two fingers (Figure 4-4).
- When flaming an inoculation loop or wire, put the near portion of the wire in the flame first and then work toward the contaminated end. Placing the contaminated end into the flame first could result in splattering of bacteria, causing aerosol contamination.
- When the specimen collected is a liquid, inoculate a very small quantity of well-mixed samples at the edge of the plate with a sterile swab or bacteriologic loop. Some labs use pre-sterilized glass rods for streaking samples because Bunsen burners are not always available, and glass rods are autoclavable. If the specimen has been initially collected on a swab, this is streaked directly onto the plate.

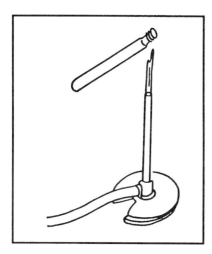

FIGURE 4-3. Flaming the neck of a culture tube before transfer of a sample.

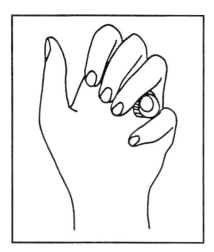

FIGURE 4-4. Culture tube cap is held between the last two fingers during transfer of a sample.

STREAKING CULTURE PLATES.   There are several methods of streaking an agar plate, but the so-called "quadrant" streak method is probably the best (Figure 4-5). In Figure 4-5, area A is the primary streak or "well" of the plate. The bacteriologic loop may or may not be flamed and cooled before making streaks B, C, and D. This depends on your estimate of the number of bacteria present in the specimen. It is a good practice to employ two loops, one of which is flamed and cooling while the other is being used.

Each streaked area is overlapped only once or twice to avoid depositing excessive numbers of bacteria in an area. Otherwise, the resultant colonies are

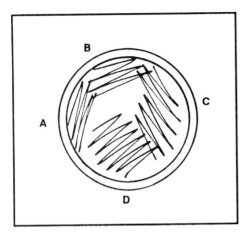

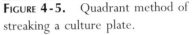

Figure 4-5.   Quadrant method of streaking a culture plate.

not discrete and isolated. Isolated colonies typically grow in area D of the plate (Figure 4-5).

It is important to use the entire plate, keeping the streak lines close together to include as many streaks as possible, and taking care not to overlap the other streak lines. If several types of colonies grow on the plate, subculture each colony onto separate plates and repeat the procedure until a pure culture is obtained.

A convenient system of reporting growth on culture plates is as follows:

Slight growth (in areas of initial streaking only	+1
Low moderate	+2
High moderate	+3
Heavy (growth in all areas of streaking)	+4

For opportunistic pathogens, growth should be 3+ or 4+, and organisms should be seen in direct smears at 2+ or higher levels before pathogenic significance is attached to their presence.

Inoculating slants.   If agar slants are used, only the surface of the slant may be inoculated, or the butt and the surface may both be inoculated. To inoculate only the surface of the slant, use a straight flamed wire to obtain a colony of bacteria from the primary isolation plate. Streak the surface of the slant in the form of an **S** shape (Figure 4-6).

To inoculate both the butt and slant, stab the butt of the slant with the tip of the inoculating wire and carefully withdraw it up the same insertion path. Then streak the surface of the slant in an **S** shape (Figure 4-6). There will be

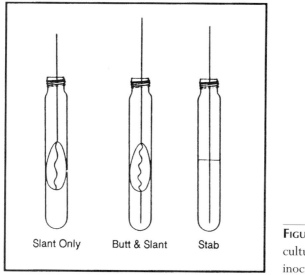

Slant Only   Butt & Slant   Stab

FIGURE 4-6. Inoculation of culture tubes with an inoculating wire.

enough bacteria on the wire to inoculate the surface even after stabbing the butt. Replace the tube's cap loosely.

INCUBATING CULTURES

For pathogens that can invade the internal organs of an animal, the optimum growth temperature is usually near 37° C. For some fish pathogens, skin pathogens (such as dermatophytes), and environmental organisms, the optimum growth temperature is lower. Care should be taken to maintain the incubator temperature at 37° C, which is the optimum temperature, as bacterial growth cannot occur above this temperature.

Incubation time depends on the generation time of individual bacterial species and the type of medium on which they are growing. For routine cultures, plates should be incubated for 48 hours, with plates examined after 18 to 24 hours of incubation. Such organisms as *Nocardia* may take 72 hours before colonies are visible. The culture plates should be inverted during incubation so that moisture does not collect on the surface of the agar, as this can cause clumping of colonies.

Some pathogens require carbon dioxide for growth in the culture atmosphere. A candle jar may be used for this purpose. The plates are placed in a large jar, a lit candle is put on top of the plates, and the jar is sealed. The candle flame soon dies, leaving a decreased amount of oxygen and increased carbon dioxide in the jar's atmosphere. (*Note:* This does not create an anaerobic

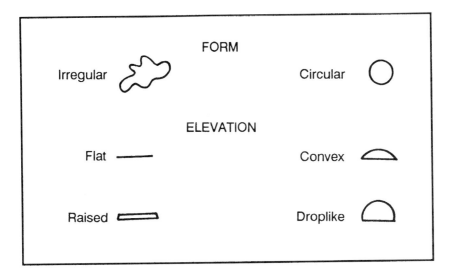

FIGURE 4-7.   Bacterial colonies may be characterized by their form and elevation.

condition.) The plates are incubated for 18 to 24 hours and then checked for growth. If there is no growth, the plates are reincubated in the candle jar for another 18 to 24 hours and rechecked for growth. Larger laboratories may have incubators that automatically monitor temperature, CO_2 and O_2 levels, and humidity.

COLONY CHARACTERISTICS

An experienced technician can recognize several bacteria based on gross observation of the colonies alone. Various colony characteristics can help identify the bacterium involved (Figure 4-7). These include size (in millimeters or described as pinpoint, medium, large), color (yellow, white, gray, cream, etc), density (opaque, transparent), elevation (raised, flat, convex, droplike), form (circular, irregular), consistency (buttery, brittle, sticky), odor (pungent, sweet, etc.), and any hemolysis (alpha, beta, gamma).

BACTERIAL STAINING

Two commonly used stains are Gram stain and acid-fast stain. Stained smears may be directly examined for bacteria (presence, numbers, type). Information obtained from a direct smear may help in determining the suitability of the specimen for identification, the predominant organism in a mixed specimen, the appropriate medium for culture, and the appropriate antibacterials for sensitivity testing. Staining kits for Gram and Ziehl-Neelsen (acid-fast) stains are available commercially (Box 4-1).

STAINING SUPPLIES

Supplies needed for staining include:

- Microscope with built-in light source and low-power, high-dry, and oil-immersion objectives
- Glass microscope slides (3 × 1 inches)
- Coverslips (22 × 22 mm)
- Bacterial loop holders and loops
- Gram stain kit
- Difco TB stain kit (acid-fast staining)
- Staining rack or two glass rods, joined at the ends by rubber tubing
- Dropper or squeeze bottles for stain solutions

PREPARING STAINING SOLUTIONS

GRAM STAIN. Gram staining is performed with crystal violet, Gram's iodine, decolorizer, and dilute carbol fuchsin.

Crystal Violet

crystal violet	2.0 g
ethanol 95% (vol/vol)	20.0 ml
ammonium oxalate	0.8 g
distilled water	80.0 ml

First dissolve the crystal violet powder in the ethanol, then dissolve the ammonium oxalate in the distilled water. To aid dissolving, agitate both mixtures in a bath of hot water. Mix the two solutions.

Gram's Iodine (mordant)

iodine crystals	1.0 g
potassium iodide	2.0 g
distilled water	200.0 ml

Grind the iodine and potassium iodide together in a mortar. Add distilled water slowly. If necessary, agitate in a bath of hot water to aid dissolving.

Decolorizer
  ethanol 95% (vol/vol)
Dilute Carbol Fuchsin (counterstain)
    concentrated carbol fuchsin   10.0 ml
    distilled water   90.0 ml

ZIEHL-NEELSEN OR ACID-FAST STAIN. Acid-fast staining uses carbol fuchsin, acid alcohol, and methylene blue or brilliant green.

Concentrated Carbol Fuchsin
    basic fuchsin   1.0 g
    ethanol 95% (vol/vol)   10.0 ml
    ammonium oxalate   5.0 g
    distilled water   100.0 ml

Dissolve the basic fuchsin in the ethanol, then add the phenol dissolved in the water. Mix and allow to stand for a few days before filtering into a container.

Acid-Alcohol (decolorizer)
    concentrated hydrochloric acid   8.0 ml
    ethanol 95% (vol/vol)   97.0 ml

Add the acid to the alcohol.

Methylene Blue (counterstain)
    methylene blue   8.0 g
    ethanol 95% (vol/vol)   300.0 ml
    distilled water   1300.0 ml
    potassium hydroxide   0.13 g

If using Loeffler's methylene blue, exclude the potassium hydroxide.

Brilliant Green (alkaline, alternative counterstain)
    brilliant green   1.0 g
    sodium hydroxide 0.01%   100.0 ml

MODIFIED ZIEHL-NEELSEN STAIN. Modified Ziehl-Neelsen stain uses carbol fuchsin, acetic acid, and methylene blue.

Dilute Carbol Fuchsin (same formula as for Gram stain)
Acetic Acid (decolorizer)
    concentrated acetic acid   1.0 ml
    distilled water   200.0 ml
Methylene Blue (same formula as for Ziehl-Neelsen stain)

KINYOUN STAIN.   This stain contains basic fuchsin, phenol, and ethanol.

    basic fuchsin   4.0 g
    phenol   8.0 ml
    ethanol 95%   20.0 ml
    distilled water   100.0 ml

Dissolve the basic fuchsin in ethanol and add the water slowly while stirring. Then add the phenol.

FLUORESCENT ACID-FAST STAIN.   This stain uses auramine 0, phenol, acid-alcohol, and potassium permanganate.

    auramine 0   0.1 g
    phenol   3.0 ml
    ethanol 95%   10.0 ml
    distilled water   87.0 ml

Dissolve 0.1 g of auramine 0 in 10 ml of 95% ethyl alcohol. Mix 3 ml of liquefied phenol in 87 ml of distilled water. Combine first with the second solution.

Acid-Alcohol (decolorizer)
    hydrochloric acid   0.5 g
    (6 ml of 1-M HCl)
    ethyl alcohol 70%   100.0 ml

Add 0.5 g of hydrochloric acid to 100 ml of 70% ethyl alcohol, and mix.

Potassium Permanganate (counterstain)
    potassium permanganate   0.5 g
    distilled water   100.0 ml

Add 0.5 g of potassium permanganate to 100 ml of distilled water and mix well.

DMSO ACID-FAST STAIN.   This stain uses basic fuchsin, ethyl alcohol, phenol, glycerol, DMSO, and malachite green.

Primary Stain

basic fuchsin (certified pure crystals)	4.0 g
ethyl alcohol 95%	25.0 ml
phenol 3%	100.0 ml

Dissolve the basic fuchsin in ethyl alcohol, then add the phenol. Mix well, then add:

glycerol	25.0 ml
DMSO, reagent grade	25.0 ml
distilled water	160.0 ml

Allow stain to stand for at least 30 minutes, then pass through coarse filter paper.

Combination Decolorizer and Counterstain

malachite green (96% dye content) (stock solution: 6 g/100 ml distilled water)	200.0 ml
glacial acetic acid 99.5%	30.0 ml
glycerol	50.0 ml

GIEMSA STAIN.   Giemsa stain is made from Giemsa powder, glycerol, and methanol.

Giemsa powder	1.0 g
glycerol	66.0 ml
absolute methanol	66.0 ml

Giemsa powder is allowed to dissolve in the glycerol at 55° to 60° C for about 2 hours. Methanol is added and mixed thoroughly. For use, one part of this stock solution is mixed with 40 to 50 parts of neutral distilled water buffered to pH 6.8.

FILTERING STAINING SOLUTIONS

After a staining solution is prepared, it should be filtered into a clean container before use. Commercially prepared staining solutions may require filtering if a precipitate forms.

QUALITY CONTROL

Each time a clinical specimen is stained, also stain a sample from the control cultures. This serves to check on the quality of your staining procedures and materials.

GRAM STAINING PROCEDURE

Gram staining is used to categorize bacteria as Gram positive or Gram negative, based on their cell wall structure.

PROCEDURE.   The sample should be applied thinly on the slide. Swab specimens can be rolled lightly onto the slide. Touching the sterile wire to one colony on the plate is usually sufficient to obtain enough bacteria for application to the slide. The colonies should be young (24-hour culture), as older colonies may not yield proper results, and the stained bacteria often become excessively decolorized.

Bacterial samples from plates are gently mixed in a drop of water or saline on the slide. If the sample is obtained from inoculated broth, two to three loopfuls are spread onto the slide. A sample may also be directly smeared onto a slide, such as from tissue or an abscess.

Regardless of how the specimen is transferred onto the slide (swab, pipette, wire), care must be taken not to destroy the organisms.

The sample droplet on the slide should be encircled using a wax pencil to help find the area after staining. After the material has dried on the slide, it is passed through a flame two or three times, specimen side up. Take care not to overheat the slide. This can be tested on the back of the hand. The slide should feel warm but not hot. Heat fixing prevents the sample from washing off and helps preserve cell morphology. It also kills the bacteria and renders them permeable to stain.

The Gram staining procedure is as follows:

- Place the slide on a staining rack over a sink.
- Pour crystal violet solution onto the smear. Let stand 30 seconds.
- Rinse gently with water (tap water is acceptable).
- Pour iodine solution onto the smear. Let stand 30 seconds.
- Rinse gently with water.
- Wash the smear with decolorizer until no more purple color washes off (usually 10 seconds or less). Do not over-decolorize.
- Rinse with water and replace on the rack.
- Pour basic fuchsin or safranin onto the smear. Let stand 30 seconds.
- Rinse with water.
- Air dry or blot between sheets of paper towel.
- Examine microscopically with the 100X oil-immersion lens.

INTERPRETING GRAM STAINS.   Bacteria that retain the crystal violet-iodine complex and stain purple are termed *Gram positive*. Those that lose the crystal violet or purple color and stain red by safranin or basic fuchsin are classified as *Gram negative.*

The morphology of the bacteria on the smear is also important to note. The bacteria may be bacilli, cocci, coccobacilli or spiral, and arranged randomly or in pairs, chains, or clusters.

Sometimes an organism may stain both Gram positive and negative. This is called a *Gram-variable reaction.* This may occur due to excessive decolorization, an overly thick smear, excessive heat fixation, old cultures, or poor quality of stain.

Determining the Gram stain reaction is an important step in the identification process. It takes practice to perform the procedure properly and interpret the results correctly. To ensure proper staining quality, known (control) Gram-positive and Gram-negative organisms should be stained at least once a week and with each new batch of stain. These control organisms can be kept growing in the laboratory (see Quality Control above).

THE KOH TEST.   In the event of a Gram-variable reaction, a quick way to check the Gram reaction is with the potassium hydroxide (KOH) test. The procedure is as follows:

- Place a loopful (or two, if necessary) of 3% KOH solution on a slide.
- Remove a generous quantity of surface growth from the culture and transfer it to the drop of KOH.
- Stir the specimen into the KOH drop with a loop and then slowly and gently lift the loop. After a maximum of 2 minutes of stirring (usually 30 seconds), Gram-negative organisms develop a mucoid appearance and produce a sticky strand when the drop is lifted with the loop. If the organisms are Gram positive, the mixture stays homogeneous and does not form a strand on lifting.
- Record the reaction as Gram negative (sticky strand and mucoid mass formed) or Gram positive (no sticky strand or mucoid mass formed).

ACID-FAST STAIN

This stain is used to detect mycobacteria *(Mycobacterium bovis, M. avium, M. paratuberculosis)* and *Nocardia.* Of the various types of acid-fast stains, some are better for mycobacteria and some for *Nocardia.*

ZIEHL-NEELSEN ACID-FAST STAIN.   This method uses carbol fuchsin stain, acid-alcohol decolorizer, and methylene blue counterstain.

A thin smear is prepared. The slide is air dried and heat fixed by passing the slide, specimen side up, through a flame. This process fixes the specimen to the slide and helps preserve bacterial cell morphology. Ziehl-Neelsen staining is done as follows:

- Flood the slide with carbol fuchsin stain and heat over the flame until the stain steams. Remove the slide from the heat and let it set for 5 minutes.
- Rinse with water (tap water is acceptable).
- Decolorize with acid-alcohol for 1 to 2 minutes until the red color is gone.
- Rinse with water.
- Counterstain with methylene blue for 30 seconds.
- Rinse with water and dry over gentle heat.

Acid-fast bacilli (mycobacteria) are stained red, while nonacid-fast microorganisms stain blue.

MODIFIED ZIEHL-NEELSEN STAIN WITH BRILLIANT GREEN.   This staining is done as follows:

- Flood the slide with carbol fuchsin for 3 minutes, heat, and then rinse with water.
- Decolorize with acid-alcohol for 3 minutes exactly.
- Rinse with water.
- Counterstain with brilliant green (alkaline) for 3 minutes.

The advantage of the alkaline brilliant green counterstain is that it is almost impossible to overstain the smear.

MODIFIED ZIEHL-NEELSEN STAIN WITH METHYLENE BLUE.   This very useful procedure stains bacteria that are partially acid-fast. These organisms resist decolorization by 0.5% acetic acid but not by acid-alcohol. *Brucella, Nocardia asteroides,* and *Chlamydia* can be stained with this modified Ziehl-Neelsen stain.

- Flood the smear with dilute carbol fuchsin for 10 minutes.
- Decolorize with 0.5% acetic acid for 20 to 30 seconds.
- Rinse with water.
- Counterstain with methylene blue for 2 minutes.
- Rinse and dry.

Brucella and *Chlamydia* stain bright red and are observed as clumps in smears made from fetal stomach contents and cotyledons from abortion cases. *Nocardia asteroides,* in pus or deposits from mastitic milk, are usually in the filamentous phase and some filaments stain red.

KINYOUN ACID-FAST STAIN.   This stain is useful when *Nocardia* infection is suspected.

- Flood a fixed smear with the stain and let it set for 3 minutes. No heating is required.
- After staining, follow the Ziehl-Neelsen acid-fast stain procedure.
- A brilliant green counterstain is sometimes used instead of methylene blue.

Nocardia organisms are partially acid-fast and are partially stained red. If counterstained with brilliant green, *Nocardia* stains red while other organisms stain green.

FLUORESCENT ACID-FAST STAIN.   This is a fluorescent stain for acid-fast bacilli. After staining a smear with fluorescent dyes, such as auramine 0 and rhodamine, fluorescent microscopy reveals acid-fast bacilli glowing a yellow-orange color against a dark brown color. This method is commonly used for staining *Mycobacterium* species of mammalian origin. The procedure is as follows:

- Heat fix the smear.
- Stain the smear for 15 minutes at room temperature.
- Rinse with tap water.
- Decolorize for 2 minutes with acid-alcohol.
- Rinse with tap water.
- Counterstain with potassium permanganate for 3 minutes.
- Rinse with tap water.
- Air dry.
- Examine with a fluorescent microscope for fluorescent bacilli.

DMSO-ACID-FAST STAIN.   This is a popular method for staining *Mycobacterium* species of avian origin. The procedure is as follows:

- Prepare smears and heat fix.
- Stain with carbol fuchsin-DMSO solution for 2 minutes exactly.
- Rinse with water.
- Counterstain and decolorize in glacial acetic acid malachite green solution for 2 minutes. If an even background of green/blue-green is not obtained, the slide should be returned to the solution for an additional 1 or 2 minutes.

- Rinse in tap water.
- Air dry and examine with the oil-immersion lens.

GIEMSA STAIN

This stain is used to detect spirochetes and rickettsiae and to demonstrate the capsule of *Bacillus anthracis* and the morphology of *Dermatophilus congolensis.*

- Fix the smear in absolute methanol for 3 to 5 minutes and air dry.
- Dip the smear in diluted stain for 20 to 30 minutes. The staining time may be extended as indicated by results. For *Borrelia anserina,* gently heat the smear while it is covered with Giemsa stain. Stain for 4 to 5 minutes.
- Rinse with water.
- Air dry and examine for purplish blue-stained bacteria.

SPECIFIC DIAGNOSTIC PROCEDURES EMPLOYING STAINED SMEARS

A summary of the main diagnostic uses of stained smears is given in Table 4-2, but a few useful procedures are discussed here in greater detail.

ABSCESSES, SUPPURATIVE EXUDATES, AND DISCHARGES. It is usually helpful to make a Gram-stained smear from this type of material, even if you intend to attempt to isolate the causative organism. When possible, obtain scrapings from the wall of the abscess, as organisms are often absent or not viable in the center of these lesions. It is also advisable to prepare wet preparations, as fungi such as *Blastomyces* or *Cryptococcus* may be involved. These are discussed in the section on Mycology. The most common pyogenic organisms are summarized in Table 4-2.

STREPTOTHRICOSIS. *Dermatophilus congolensis* causes an infection of the superficial layers of the skin and is characterized by serous scabs, often along the back. Although most animals and people seem to be susceptible, the condition is seen mainly in horses, sheep, and cattle.

Specimens should consist of hair plucked from the lesions. These characteristically come away with a considerable amount of scab at the end. When making stained smears from the scab material, use a scalpel to shave off a few bits of scab into a drop of distilled water on a slide. Allow the flakes of scab to soften for a few minutes in the water, then make a smear using another slide in a scissor action. Take care not to break up the pieces of scab too much or the characteristic filaments of *Dermatophilus* may be broken up into less diagnostic Gram-positive cocci (zoospores).

Text continued on p. 183.

TABLE 4-2. Diagnostic uses of stained smears

DISEASE AND SPECIES AFFECTED	SPECIMEN	CAUSATIVE ORGANISM	APPEARANCE IN STAINED SMEARS
GRAM STAIN			
Abscesses or suppurative conditions	Pus or exudates		
Many animal species		*Staphylococcus aureus*	Gram-positive cocci, often in clumps
Sheep, cattle		*Actinomyces (Corynebacterium pyogenes)*	Pleomorphic Gram-positive
Sheep, goats		*Corynebacterium pseudotuberculosis*	All forms, from rods to cocci
Many animal species, group C in horses		Streptococci	Gram-positive cocci, can be in chains
Dogs, cats (bite wounds)		*Pasteurella multocida*	Gram-negative rods
Many animal species		*Pseudomonas aeruginosa*	Gram-negative rods
Cattle, sheep, pigs (foot abscesses)		*Fusobacterium necrophorum*	Slender, long, Gram-positive rods, often with pointed ends

Continued.

TABLE 4-2.—CONT'D

DISEASE AND SPECIES AFFECTED	SPECIMEN	CAUSATIVE ORGANISM	APPEARANCE IN STAINED SMEARS
Actinobacillosis (wooden tongue) and actinomycosis (lumpy jaw) Cattle	Granules from pus	*Actinobacillus lignieresi* *Actinomyces bovis*	Gram-negative rods Gram-positive, filamentous and branching
Clostridial enterotoxemia Pulpy kidney in lambs	Scraping from small intestine of a recently dead animal	*Clostridium perfringens*, Type D	Large numbers of Gram-positive, short thick rods (presumptive evidence only)
Colibacillosis Calves, pigs, lambs <1 week of age	Scraping from small intestine of a recently dead animal	Enteropathogenic strains of *E. coli*	Numerous Gram-negative rods (presumptive evidence only)
Nocardiosis and actinomycosis Dogs	Pus and granules	*Nocardia asteroides*, *Actinomyces viscosus*	Both Gram-positive, filamentous and branching; *Nocardia* is modified Ziehl-Neelsen positive
Strangles Horses	Pus	*Streptococcus equi*	Gram-positive cocci, can be in chains

Streptothricosis Many species susceptible; seen mainly in sheep, cattle, horses	Scabs	*Dermatophilus congolensis*	Large Gram-positive cocci (zoospores) arranged two or more across in branching filaments
Urinary tract infections Dogs, cats	Very fresh and carefully collected urine	*E. coli, Proteus, Enterobacter, Staphylococcus aureus*, fecal streptococci, *Pseudomonas aeruginosa*	Bacteriuria indicated by ≥1 organism(s) per oil-immersion field

DILUTE CARBOL FUCHSIN (SIMPLE) STAIN

Campylobacter infections			
infertility in cattle	Vaginal mucus	*Campylobacter fetus* ss *venerealis*	Comma-shaped rods that can be in short chains resembling seagulls
Abortion in sheep, cattle	Fetal stomach, cotyledons	*Campylobacter fetus* ss *fetus*	
Foot rot in sheep	Material from lesion	*Fusobacterium (Bacteroides) nodosus*	Rods with knobbed ends (must be present for a diagnosis of foot rot)
		Fusobacterium necrophorum	Long slender rods, often with pointed ends

Continued.

TABLE 4-2.—CONT'D

DISEASE AND SPECIES AFFECTED	SPECIMEN	CAUSATIVE ORGANISM	APPEARANCE IN STAINED SMEARS
Swine dysentery	Feces or scrapings from colon	*Serpulina (Treponema) hyodysenteriae*	Numerous long (7 μ) but fine spiral organisms
Various necrotic lesions	Material from lesions	*Fusobacterium necrophorum*	Long slender rods, often with pointed ends
MODIFIED ZIEHL-NEELSEN STAIN			
Brucellosis			
Cattle	Vulvar discharge, cotyledons, fetal stomach contents	*Brucella abortus*	Small, red coccobacilli in clumps
Sheep	Cotyledons, fetal stomach contents	*Brucella ovis*	Small, red coccobacilli in clumps
Dogs	Vulvar discharge	*Brucella canis*	Small, red coccobacilli in clumps
Sows	Fetal stomach contents, vulvar discharge	*Brucella suis*, occasionally *Brucella abortus*	Small, red coccobacilli in clumps
Chlamydial diseases			
Cats	Conjunctival scrapings in feline pneumonitis	*Chlamydia psittaci*	Small coccobacilli in clumps; stain red

Sheep, cattle	Fetal cotyledons from bovine and ovine abortions		Similar to *Brucella* but usually smaller and do not grow on conventional media
Sheep, pigs, calves	Joint fluid in polyarthritis		
Nocardiosis			
Dogs	Pus and granules	*Nocardia asteroides*	Long, branching filaments, many staining red
Bovine mastitis	Sediment from centrifuged milk		

ZIEHL-NEELSEN (ACID-FAST) STAIN

Acid-fast granulomas			
Cats	Scrapings from lesions	Unknown *Mycobacterium* spp	Large numbers of red, acid-fast rods
Jchne's disease or paratuberculosis			
Cattle, sheep, goats	Feces, ileocecal valve smear, mesenteric lymph nodes	*Mycobacterium paratuberculosis*	Fairly short, red, acid-fast bacteria in clumps; must be in clumps to be diagnostic for Johne's disease

Continued.

Table 4-2.—Cont'd

Disease and species affected	Specimen	Causative organism	Appearance in stained smears
Tuberculosis			
Avian	Suspect lesions	*Mycobacterium avium* ss *avium*	Large numbers of acid-fast organisms; stain red and are often beaded
Swine	Suspect lesion, often in cervical lymph nodes	*Mycobacterium avium* ss *avium* or *Mycobacterium bovis*	Fewer organisms present
Giemsa Stain			
Anthrax			
Cattle, sheep	Blood smear from ear vein	*Bacillus anthracis*	Purplish, square-ended rods, often in chains; surrounded by a capsule
Spirochetosis			
Fowl	Whole blood taken during febrile stage (3-5 days after infection); collect from several birds	*Borrelia anserina*	Helical organisms, 6-30 μ long, 0.2-0.3 μ wide, with 5-8 spirals

Leave the crystal violet stain on the smear for only 2 seconds. The organism is intensely Gram positive and if it is stained too deeply, it may be difficult to see the characteristic filaments composed of individual zoospores arranged in lines, two or more zoospores across. A definitive diagnosis of streptothricosis can usually be made from stained smears alone.

NOCARDIOSIS AND ACTINOMYCOSIS IN DOGS. Infections caused by *Nocardia asteroides* and *Actinomyces viscosus* are fairly common in dogs. The conditions can be clinically indistinguishable, and thoracic and a subcutaneous forms are seen in both. Differentiation of these diseases is important because the antibacterial susceptibility of the organism differs. *A. viscosus* is usually sensitive to penicillin, but *N. asteroides* is not.

Smears made from thoracic fluid or serosanguineous pus from subcutaneous abscesses can be stained by the Gram or modified Ziehl-Neelsen method. If granules are present in the pus, crush them on the slide using a scalpel. Both *A. viscosus* and *N. asteroides* appear as long, Gram-positive, branching filaments in smears stained by the Gram method. However, *N. asteroides,* but not *A. viscosus,* is partially acid-fast and some of the filaments of *N. asteroides* stain red in smears stained by the modified Ziehl-Neelsen method.

ACTINOMYCOSIS AND ACTINOBACILLOSIS IN CATTLE. Infections caused by *Actinomyces bovis* in cattle can affect bone as well as soft tissue, whereas those caused by *Actinobacillus lignieresi* affect soft tissue only. Both conditions often occur as suppurating abscesses in the jaw region. Granules characteristically occur in pus from abscesses caused by both organisms.

Wash several granules free from pus in distilled water and crush them gently onto a slide. Spread the crushed material to make a thin smear and stain using the Gram method. *Actinomyces bovis* appears as long, branching, Gram-positive filaments, whereas *A. lignieresi* is a moderate-sized, Gram-negative rod.

ACID-FAST GRANULOMAS IN CATS. This condition in cats is manifested as small granulomatous skin lesions, often on the feet, that tend to ulcerate. They are caused by an unidentified *Mycobacterium* species. A smear can be prepared from scrapings of the lesions or from a biopsy. Smears stained by the Ziehl-Neelsen method show numerous slender, often beaded, red-staining (acid-fast) rods. However, Kinyoun modification of the Ziehl-Neelsen stain is recommended because no heating is required. If the smear is stained with the fluorescent acid-fast stain, small fluorescent bacilli are seen on microscopy. A DMSO acid-fast stain is useful for *Mycobacterium* species of avian origin.

Mastitis. Mastitis may be caused by bacterial or mycotic organisms. Several laboratory tests are available to diagnose mastitis, including the California mastitis test, somatic cell count, and milk culture (see Chapter 12). A quick check to detect bacteria can be done by preparing a thin smear of mastitic milk. The smear is heat fixed and stained with Gram stain or methylene blue.

The most common microorganisms involved with mastitis are *Staphylococcus aureus, Streptococcus agalactiae, Streptococcus uberis, E. coli, Corynebacterium,* and *Pseudomonas aeruginosa.*

Clostridial enterotoxemia. The main clinical signs of clostridial enterotoxemia are diarrhea and often death in circumstances precipitating an intestinal disturbance. Lamb dysentery caused by *Clostridium perfringens* type B does not occur in North America. Type-C enterotoxemia affects neonatal lambs, pigs, and calves. Type-D enterotoxemia, usually seen in feeder lambs, is commonly referred to as "pulpy kidney disease."

The clinical diagnosis can be supported by demonstration of clostridia (large, Gram-positive rods) in stained smears from the small intestinal mucosa of a recently dead lamb. Clostridial organisms are not present in large numbers in the small intestine of healthy animals. Postmortem invasion of the small intestine by clostridia, however, can be rapid.

Fresh ileal contents can be submitted to a laboratory for confirmation. Demonstration and identification of the toxin are necessary for definitive diagnosis.

Colibacillosis. This disease mainly affects calves, pigs, and lambs under a week of age. Enteropathogenic *E. coli* strains invade the small intestine, where they adhere to mucosal epithelial cells. Gram-stained smears from the small intestinal mucosa disclose large numbers of Gram-negative rods that are not present in healthy animals. This observation is only significant if the examination is made on a sick animal immediately after death, as postmortem invasion of the small intestine by *E. coli* is rapid. An indirect fluorescent antibody test is available for identification of *E. coli* K-99 antigen (see Chapter 9).

Urinary tract infections. These are most commonly seen in dogs and cats. They can be caused by *E. coli, Proteus, Enterobacter, Staphylococcus aureus,* fecal streptococci, or *Pseudomonas aeruginosa.* A rapid check for bacteria can be done by Gram staining a smear of a drop of fresh midstream urine. The presence of ≥ 1 bacterium per oil-immersion field in fresh, aseptically collected urine strongly suggests a urinary infection. This should be confirmed by bacterial cultures.

PRIMARY IDENTIFICATION OF BACTERIA

With experience, you can learn to identify pathogenic bacteria using a systematic approach (Figure 4-8).

The specimens are first streaked onto a primary medium, such as blood agar and MacConkey agar. The plates are incubated for 18 to 24 hours and then examined for growth. If an incubated plate has colonies, one must decide if the bacteria should be identified.

Most Gram-positive and Gram-negative organisms grow on blood agar. Gram-positive organisms usually do not grow on MacConkey agar, but this agar supports growth of most Gram-negative organisms. It is preferable to select the colony from the routine blood agar plate rather than from MacConkey agar. The danger in subculturing from a selective medium like MacConkey agar is that there may be inhibited organisms present as microcolonies on the plate. One of these could inadvertently be the colony of interest.

With comparatively few tests, an organism may be identified to the genus level with a fair degree of certainty (Tables 4-3 and 4-4).

GRAM STAIN

With a stained smear prepared from a pure culture or a single colony, organisms that have retained the crystal violet-iodine complex and that stain blue-purple must be regarded as Gram positive. If there is a Gram-variable or a doubtful reaction, perform the KOH test.

SIZE, SHAPE, ARRANGEMENT

There is considerable variation in the size of bacteria. The bacteria most frequently studied in the laboratory range from 0.5 to 1 μ in width and 2 to 5 μ in length. Coccoid forms range from 0.75 to 1.2 μ in diameter. Rod forms have a width of 0.1 to 2 μ and a length of 2 to 5 μ. Spirochetes are 3 to 5 μ long.

Bacteria can be organized into four groups according to their shape (Figure 4-9):

- *Coccus.* These are spherical cells, such as *Staphylococcus aureus.* This organism causes mastitis in animals.
- *Bacillus.* These are shaped like rods or cylinders, such as *Bacillus anthracis.* This organism causes anthrax in animals and people.
- *Spiral.* These usually occur singly and can be subdivided into loose spirals, such as *Borrelia anserina,* which causes avian borreliosis, tight spirals, such as *Leptospira pomona,* which causes red water disease in

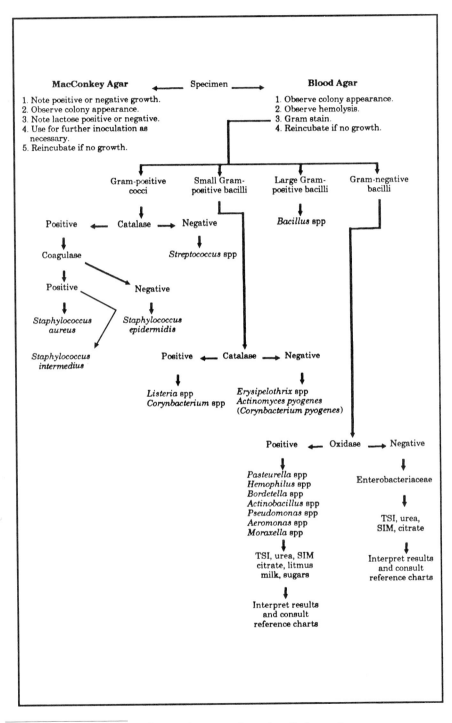

Figure 4-8. Flow chart of procedures used to identify bacteria.

TABLE 4-3. Primary identification of Gram-positive bacteria

CHARACTERISTICS	IDENTIFICATION												
Shape	C	C	C	C	B	B	B	B	B	B	B	B	B
Acid-fast	−	−	−	−	−	−	−	−	−	+	−	−	−
Spores	−	−	−	−	−	−	−	−	−	−	−	+	+
Motility	−	−	−	+	+	−	−	−	−	−	−	V	V
Growth in air	+	+	+	+	+	+	+	−	+	+	+	+	−
Catalase	+	+	−	−	+	+	+	−	−	V	+	+	−
Oxidase	−	−	−	−	−	−	−	−	−	−	−	V	−
Glucose (acid)	V	+	+	+	+	+	−	+	+	+	+	V	V
O-F test													
Oxidation	+	−	−	−	−	−	−	−	−	+	+	+	−
Fermentation	−	+	+	+	+	+	+	+	+	N	−	+	+
Micrococcus	x												
Staphylococcus		x											
Streptococcus			x	x[1]									
Listeria					x								
Corynebacterium						x	x[2]	x[3]	x[4]				
Erysipelothrix									x				
Lactobacillus									x				
Actinomyces								x	x[5]				
Mycobacterium										x			
Nocardia										x[6]	x		
Bacillus					x[7]	x[7]	x[7]				x[7]	x	
Clostridium									x[7]				x

1 - Some group-D streptococci
2 - *Rhodococcus (Coryn.) equi*
3 - *Eubacterium (Coryn.) suis*
4 - *Actinomyces (Coryn.) pyogenes*
5 - *A. viscosus*
6 - *N. asteroides* (partially acid fast)
7 - Asporogenous variants

C = Coccus
B = Bacillus
V = Variable among species
+ = >80% of strains positive
− = >80% of strains negative
N = Not tested
O = Oxidation
F = Fermentation

TABLE 4-4.   Primary identification of Gram-negative bacteria

CHARACTERISTICS	IDENTIFICATION																		
Shape	C	C	B	B	B	B	B	B	B	B	B	B	B	B	B	B	B	B	B
Motility	−	−	−	V	−	−	−	+	−	+	+	−	+	−	−	−	+	−	−
Growth in air	+	+	+	+	+	+	+	+	+	+	+	+	+	+	(+)	(+)	(+)	(+)	−
Growth on MacConkey agar	−	−	V	+	+	−	−	+	+	+	−	V	+	−	−	−	−	−	−
Catalase	+	+	+	+	+	+	+	+	+	+	V	+	+	+	+	+	V	V	V
Oxidase	+	+	−	−	+	+	+	+	+	+	−	+	+	+	+	−	+	−	−
Glucose (acid)	V	−	+	+	+	+	+	+	+	+	+	+	−	−	−	−	−	V	V
O-F test																			
Oxidation	+	−	+	−	−	−	−	−	−	+	+	+	−	−	−	−	−	N	−
Fermentation	−	−	−	+	+	+	−	+	+	−	+	−	−	−	−	−	−	N	+
Neisseria	x																		
Branhamella		x																	
Acinetobacter			x																
Enterobacteriaceae				x															
Actinobacillus					x														
Pasteurella					x[1]	x	x[2]												
Aeromonas								x	x[3]										
Pseudomonas										x									
Chromobacterium											x								
Flavobacterium												x							
Alcaligenes fecalis													x						
Bordetella bronchiseptica													x						
Moraxella bovis														x					
Brucella															x	x[4]			
Campylobacter																	x		
Hemophilus																		x	
Bacteroides																			x

1 - *P. hemolytica*
2 - *P. anatipestifer*
3 - *A. salmonicida*
4 - *B. ovis* and *B. neotomae*

( ) = 5-10% CO_2 required by some strains
C = Coccus
B = Bacillus
+ = >80% of strains positive
− = >80% of strains negative
V = Variable among species
N = Not tested
O = Oxidation
F = Fermentation

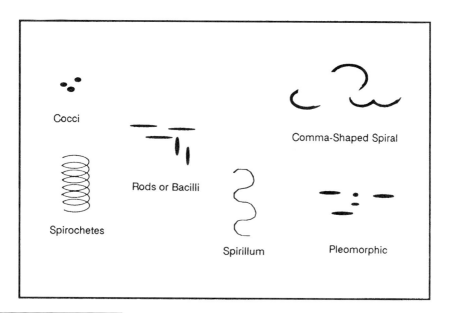

FIGURE **4-9.**   Bacterial cell morphology.

cattle, and comma-shaped spirals, such as *Campylobacter fetus* ss *fetus,* a cause of abortion in cattle.

- *Pleomorphic.* In this category the shape may range from cocci to rods.

Bacteria are found in a variety of arrangements. Some grow as single cells, whereas others remain attached after dividing and form chains or clusters. Many exhibit patterns of arrangement that are important for their identification (Figure 4-10):

- *Single.* Some bacteria occur singly, such as spirilla (singular: spirillum) and most bacilli (singular: bacillus).
- *Pairs.* Some bacteria occur in pairs, such as *Streptococcus pneumoniae* (diplococcus).
- *Clusters or Bunches.* Some bacteria occur in clusters, bunches, or groups. For example, *Staphylococcus aureus* forms grape-like clusters.
- *Chains.* Some organisms grow in short or long chains, such as *Streptococcus* species.
- *Palisades.* Some organisms can be arranged in a palisade or Chinese letter pattern, such as *Corynebacterium* species.

With pleomorphic organisms, such as *Corynebacterium,* it can sometimes be difficult to judge whether the organism is a coccus or a bacillus. If the

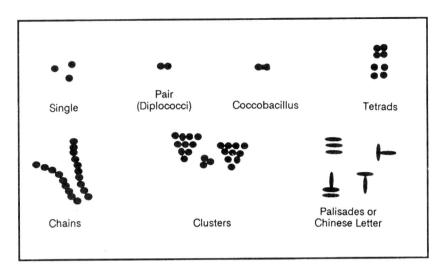

FIGURE 4-10. Bacterial cell arrangement.

Gram-stained smear was made from a pure culture and any of the cells present are definitely rod-shaped, the organism must be regarded as a bacillus for purposes of identification.

SPORES

When cultured, a few genera of bacteria form intracellular refractile bodies called *endospores* or, more commonly, *spores*. Organisms in the genera *Bacillus* and *Clostridium* are spore formers. Spores vary in size, shape, and location in the cell and may be classified as follows (Figure 4-11):

- *Central*. Present in the center of the cell, such as *Bacillus anthracis*.
- *Subterminal*. Present near the end of the cell, such as *Clostridium chauvoei*.
- *Terminal*. Present at the end or pole of the cell, such as *Clostridium tetani*.

It is not usually necessary to carry out a special spore stain, as the endospores can be visualized as nonstaining bodies with Gram stain.

OTHER STAINING PROCEDURES

It is not necessary to do a Ziehl-Neelsen, Kinyoun acid-fast, or fluorescent acid-fast stain unless *Mycobacterium* involvement is suspected. The modified Ziehl-Neelsen stain is useful if searching for *Brucella* or to differentiate between

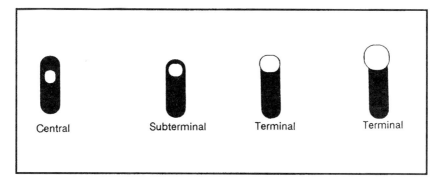

| Central | Subterminal | Terminal | Terminal |

FIGURE **4-11.** Bacterial endospores.

Nocardia asteroides (modified Ziehl-Neelsen positive) and *Actinomyces viscosus* (modified Ziehl-Neelsen negative). Both appear as Gram-positive bacilli in a smear from colonies on agar.

MOTILITY

Two methods are commonly used to test motility. First, a young broth culture can be examined microscopically. A moderately heavy suspension is made in a few milliliters of nutrient broth incubated for 2 to 3 hours at room temperature. A loopful of this culture is placed on a microscope slide under a coverslip and examined with the high-dry objective. If the bacteria are obviously motile, with individual cells moving backward or forward among other cells, the answer has been obtained. Be careful, however, not to mistake Brownian movement for true motility. Brownian movement is the shifting of cells or particles, with little movement relative to each other.

If the organisms are nonmotile on microscopic examination, motility media should be used. Two tubes of a motility medium, such as sulfide-indole-motility (SIM) medium (BBL), are stab inoculated. One tube is incubated at 37° C and the other at room temperature for 24 to 48 hours. Some organisms, such as *Providencia rettgeri,* tend to be motile at ambient temperature but not at 37° C. If growth is restricted to the stab inoculation line, the organism is nonmotile. If there is diffuse growth throughout the medium, the bacterium is motile. To interpret the results, hold the tubes against a good light and compare the inoculated tubes with an uninoculated one.

The SIM medium is unsuitable for motility testing of organisms that produce hydrogen sulfide in this medium, as the blackening that results can make the motility test difficult to read.

Catalase test

The catalase test is done on Gram-positive cocci and small Gram-positive bacilli. It tests for the enzyme catalase, which acts on hydrogen peroxide to produce water and oxygen. A small amount of a colony from a blood agar plate is placed on a microscope slide and a drop of catalase reagent (3% hydrogen peroxide) is added. If the colony is catalase positive, gas bubbles are produced. No bubble production indicates a negative result.

It is important not to transfer any blood agar with the colony, as blood agar itself can produce a slightly positive reaction. A positive reaction also may occur if a mixed colony is sampled, that is, one with both catalase-positive and catalase-negative organisms growing together. This is why it is important to streak the plate carefully to obtain isolated colonies. Staphylococci can be used as catalase-positive controls and streptococci as catalase-negative controls.

Coagulase test

The coagulase test is done on catalase-positive, Gram-positive cocci. *Staphylococcus aureus* produces coagulase, an enzyme that coagulates plasma. The test is used to differentiate between coagulase-positive *Staphylococcus aureus, Staphylococcus intermedius,* and coagulase-negative *Staphylococcus,* such as *Staphylococcus epidermidis* or *Staphylococcus saprophyticus.*

Tube coagulase test. Lyophilized plasma (purchased from a medical supply house) is diluted according to the manufacturer's directions. About 0.5 ml is placed in a test tube and inoculated with a loopful of the organism from a noninhibitory medium, such as blood agar. This is incubated at 37° C and read hourly for 4 hours. A negative reaction is indicated by no clot formation, while a positive reaction is indicated by clots. If the test result remains negative, the sample is incubated again for 24 hours and then read.

Slide coagulase test. The slide coagulase test is a rapid screening test that detects surface-bound coagulase or clumping factor. Over 95% of coagulase-producing staphylococci possess clumping factor.

A loopful of staphylococci from a colony is first emulsified in a drop of water or saline solution to yield a thick suspension. A drop of fresh rabbit or human plasma is then added and stirred with a sterile loop. A positive reaction is indicated by clumping within 5 to 20 seconds.

The Staphyloslide (BBL) agglutination test and Staphaurex (Wellcome) are also commercially available. Staphyloslide detects a cell wall polypeptide clumping factor. Staphaurex is based on latex agglutination to detect protein A, independent of clumping factor.

Staphylococci that yield a negative slide result should be tested with the tube test to confirm the results.

OXIDASE ACTIVITY

This test depends on the presence of cytochrome C oxidase in bacteria. A drop of 1% tetramethyl-p-phenylenediamine is added to a piece of filter paper in a Petri dish. The filter paper must be damp but not saturated. A short streak of the sample is made on the filter paper using a glass rod or the end of a Pasteur pipette that has been bent into a hook. The sample should be applied with a gentle rubbing action. Do not use a nichrome bacteriologic loop, as any traces of iron may give a false-positive result.

In a positive test, the reagent is reduced to a deep purple color within 60 seconds. If the color-change reaction takes longer than this, the test should be regarded as negative. Note that oxidase reagent tends to be unstable and becomes discolored with time. It should be discarded if it becomes dark purple.

Pseudomonas aeruginosa can be used as an oxidase-positive control and *E. coli* as an oxidase-negative control.

ACID PRODUCTION FROM GLUCOSE

A tube of 1% glucose in peptone broth, containing a pH indicator, is inoculated and incubated for 24 to 48 hours at 37° C. For fastidious organisms, such as *Streptococcus,* about 5 drops of sterile serum should be added to the peptone water medium or growth may not occur.

OXIDATION-FERMENTATION TEST

This test is designed to assess whether carbohydrates are destroyed by oxidation or fermentation. Conventional commercial tubes of media are really only suitable for testing such organisms as enterobacteria, *Pseudomonas,* or *Aeromonas.* Other organisms may not grow in the medium. However, the basal medium can be enriched with 2% serum or 0.1% yeast extract.

Before use, two tubes of oxidation-fermentation medium, with loosened caps, should be heated in a beaker of boiling water to drive off dissolved oxygen. After steaming for a few minutes, the tubes are cooled rapidly under cold running water. Both tubes of media are stab inoculated with the test organism, using a straight wire. Immediately a layer of paraffin oil should be added to a depth of about 1 cm on the top of one of the tubes. Incubate at

37° C for up to 14 days, though 24 to 48 hours is usually sufficient. The pH indicator in the medium is usually bromthymol blue. This gives the uninoculated medium a green color, turning yellow when acid is produced by the organism's attack on the glucose in the medium. Table 4-5 summarizes the results of the oxidation-fermentation test.

Oxidative organisms, such as *Pseudomonas,* only attack the glucose, with resultant acid production at the surface of tubes not sealed by paraffin oil.

Identification of Bacteria in Specimens

Enterobacteriaceae

After death, organisms in this family rapidly invade tissues surrounding the intestines. If the animal has been dead for some hours, the presence of enterobacteria in tissues outside of the bowels must be interpreted with caution. However, enterobacteria isolated from a recently dead animal, from aseptically obtained mastitic milk samples, and from carefully collected feline or canine urine samples may be regarded as significant.

Remember that septicemia due to *E. coli* is rare in animals more than a week of age. The carrier state of *Salmonella* infections is common, and the organisms can be excreted by apparently healthy animals.

Figure 4-12 contains a flow chart for presumptive identification of Enterobacteriaceae.

Culture characteristics.   The colonies of the various enteric bacteria on blood agar are not sufficiently distinctive to aid in their identification. There are exceptions. Colonies of *Proteus vulgaris* and *P. mirabilis* swarm over a blood agar

Table 4-5.   Interpretation of the oxidation-fermentation test

	BACTERIUM		
PREPARATION	ENTEROBACTERIA AEROMONAS	PSEUDOMONAS	ALCALIGENES FECALIS
Tube without oil	Yellow	Yellow	Green
Tube with oil	Yellow	Green	Green
Reaction	Fermentation	Oxidation	No reaction

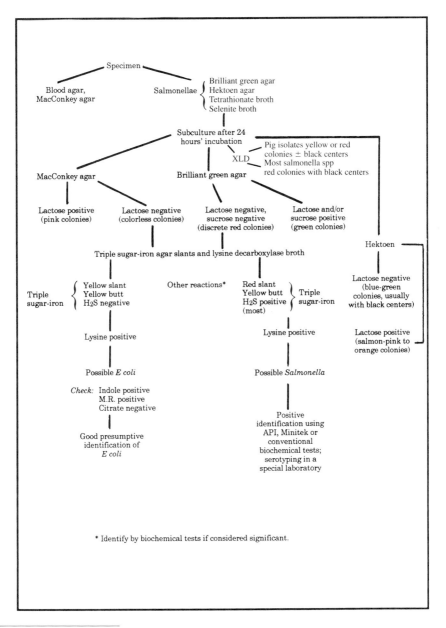

FIGURE 4-12.   Flow chart for identification of Enterobacteriaceae.

plate. The bile salts in MacConkey agar restrict this swarming although it can occur after 72 hours' incubation or if there is moisture on the surface of the MacConkey agar. *Klebsiella, Enterobacter,* and a few strains of *E. coli* produce very mucoid colonies, particularly pronounced after 48 hours' incubation. Table 4-6 shows a short list of reactions for quick differentiation of these three bacteria.

Some strains of *E. coli* can be hemolytic, but this is now thought not to correlate with pathogenicity. *Serratia marcescens* produces an orange-red pigment if incubated at ambient temperatures, but few strains produce pigment at 37° C.

ISOLATION OF SALMONELLAE FROM FECAL AND TISSUE SAMPLES.   When attempting to isolate salmonellae, specimens should be inoculated into an enrichment broth, such as tetrathionate and/or selenite and also onto selective media, such as brilliant green, Hektoen, and MacConkey agars. A subculture is made on selective media after 24 and 48 hours' incubation of the enrichment broth at 37° C. If the specimens came from pigs or poultry, the more fastidious salmonellae, such as *S. choleraesuis, S. typhisuis, S. pullorum,* and *S. gallinarum,* must be considered. These salmonellae are often inhibited by brilliant green agar and do not grow in tetrathionate broth. However, selenite broth and Hektoen, bismuth sulfite, and MacConkey agars usually grow them.

IDENTIFICATION OF SALMONELLA COLONIES.   Plates are examined for typical *Salmonella* colonies. On MacConkey agar, they are lactose nonfermenters and appear colorless. On bismuth sulfite agar, they appear as black colonies surrounded by dark halos and/or colonies with a distinct metallic sheen.

On Hektoen agar, salmonellae are lactose nonfermenters and form blue-green colonies, usually producing hydrogen sulfide (black or dark colonies with black centers). *Salmonella arizonae* may appear as a lactose fermenter

TABLE 4-6.   Reactions for presumptive identification of *Klebsiella, Enterobacter,* and *E. coli*

	OBSERVATION			
BACTERIUM	INDOLE	METHYL RED	CITRATE	MOTILITY
E. coli	+	+	−	+
Klebsiella	−	±	+	−
Enterobacter	−	−	+	+

(yellow colonies) and may or may not produce hydrogen sulfide. On brilliant green agar, salmonellae form pink colonies surrounded by bright red medium and on XLD colonies they are red with black centers.

Suspect colonies are inoculated into a few drops of urea medium. Only urease-negative colonies are used to inoculate triple sugar-iron agar, lysine-iron slants, decarboxylate lysine broth, and malonate broth. This is to determine if the isolates produce typical biochemical reactions for salmonellae. A blood agar plate is also inoculated so the suspect salmonellae are available for poly "o" testing if results of biochemical tests warrant it. Table 4-7 shows typical reactions of Enterobacteriaceae in lysine-iron agar.

The chances of isolating salmonellae are increased if two tubes of enrichment broth are inoculated per specimen. A tube of tetrathionate broth and a tube of selenite broth should be used. Fecal and tissue samples should be added in 5% to 10% quantities to the enrichment broth. Excessive amounts of inocula inhibit rather than aid the selectivity of enrichment broths.

Selenite broth can be purchased as a prepared tubed medium. Tetrathionate is obtained as a dehydrated tetrathionate broth base.

Table 4-8 summarizes differentiation of Gram-negative bacteria. Notice that not all *Salmonella* strains produce hydrogen sulfide in triple sugar-iron agar. *Salmonella choleraesuis* does not form hydrogen sulfide, but the variant *S. choleraesuis* var *kunzendorf* does. *Salmonella typhisuis,* which only causes disease in young pigs, is exceptional in that it is lysine negative.

Enterobacteriaceae can be finally identified using API or Enterotube and Minitek biochemical systems.

PRESUMPTIVE IDENTIFICATION OF *E. COLI*. A variety of tests can be used for quick identification of *E. coli*. The pink colonies (lactose positive) that *E. coli* forms on MacConkey agar can be tested in triple sugar-iron agar and lysine decarboxylase broth. The appearance in triple sugar-iron agar is a yellow slant and yellow butt, with no hydrogen sulfide production but often considerable gas production that can disintegrate the agar slant. Most *E. coli* strains are lysine positive.

Three other test results give a strong presumptive identification of *E. coli:* hydrogen sulfide negative, motility positive, and indole positive in sulfide-indole-motility medium; methyl red positive; and citrate negative.

ORGANISMS FROM MASTITIC MILK SAMPLES

Many organisms, including fungi, can cause mastitis. Milk culture can be used to diagnose clinical mastitis, but its main use is in detecting subclinical mastitis. Subclinical mastitis is difficult to diagnose because there are no clinical signs.

TABLE 4-7.   Reactions of Enterobacteriaceae in lysine iron agar

GENUS AND SPECIES	SLANT	BUTT	GAS	HYDROGEN SULFIDE
Escherichia	K	K or N	− or +	−
Shigella	K	A	−	−
Salmonella	K	K or N	−	+ (−)
typhi	K	K	−	+ or −
paratyphi-A	K	A	+ or −	− or +
Arizona	K	K or N	−	+ (−)
Citrobacter	K	A	− or +	+ or −
Edwardsiella	K	K	− or +	+
Klebsiella	K or N	K or N	+ or −	−
Enterobacter				
cloacae	K or N	A	+ or −	−
aerogenes	K	K or N	+ (−)	−
hafniae	K	K or N	− or +	−
Serratia	K or N	K or N	−	−
Proteus				
vulgaris	R	A	−	− (+)
mirabilis	R	A	−	− (+)
morganella	K or R	A	−	−
Providencia	R	A	−	−

An alkaline or neutral reaction in the butt of this medium indicates decarboxylation.
K = alkaline
N = neutral
A = acidic
R = red (oxidative deamination)
From Edwards, Ewing: *Identification of enterbacteriaceae,* Dubuque, IA, 1989, Burgess Publishing.

Two main tests are employed to detect subclinical mastitis before resorting to culture procedures.

CALIFORNIA MASTITIS TEST (CMT).   This is a qualitative screening test that can be used as a "cowside" test. The test is based on gel formation when the test reagent reacts with DNA in somatic cells. As the cell count of the milk increases, the gelling action increases. Therefore the test provides an indirect

TABLE 4-8.   Reactions of Gram-negative bacteria on triple sugar-iron slants and in lysine decarboxylase broth

REACTIONS ON TSI SLANT	ORGANISMS EXPECTED AND LYSINE REACTION		
	LYSINE POSITIVE	LYSINE NEGATIVE	LYSINE VARIABLE
Acidic slant Acidic butt No H$_2$S No gas (reaction may be weak)	*Serratia* spp *Aeromonas* *hydrophila* ss *proteolytica*	*Aeromonas hydrophila* ss *anaerogenes* *Erwinia* spp *Actinobacillus* spp *Shigella sonnei* *Pseudomonas* *pseudomallei*	*Pasteurella* spp *E. coli* "inactive" *Pseudomonas* spp (some)
Acidic slant Acidic butt No H$_2$S Gas in butt (strong reaction)	*E. coli* *Enterobacter* *aerogenes* *Enterbacter* *gergoviae* *Klebsiella* spp	*Cedecea* spp *Rahnella* spp *Aeromonas hydrophila* ss *hydrophila* *Enterobacter cloacae* *Providencia* (some)	*Kluyvera* spp
Acidic slant Acidic butt H$_2$S produced Gas in butt	*Arizona* (some)	*Citrobacter* (some) *Proteus vulgaris*	
Alkaline slant Acidic butt No H$_2$S No gas	*Obesumbacterium* spp	*Shigella* spp *Providencia* spp *Yersinia* *pseudotuberculosis* *Xenorhabdus* spp *Pasteurella multocida* (some)	
Alkaline slant Acidic butt No H$_2$S Gas in butt	*Salmonella* *choleraesuis* *Salmonella sendai* *Salmonella* *abortus-equi* *Hafnia alvei*	*Salmonella typhisuis* *Salmonella paratyphi A* *Morganella morganii*	

Continued.

Table 4-8.—Cont'd

	Organisms expected and lysine reaction		
Reactions on tsi slant	Lysine positive	Lysine negative	Lysine variable
Alkaline slant Acidic butt H₂S produced No gas	*Salmonella pullorum* (some) *Salmonella gallinarum* *Salmonella typhi*		
Alkaline slant Acidic butt H₂S produced Gas in butt	*Salmonella* serovars (most) *Arizona* serovars (most) *Edwardsiella tarda*	*Citrobacter* spp *Proteus vulgaris* (some) *Proteus mirabilis* *Salmonella typhisuis* (some)	

From Carter: *Diagnostic procedures in veterinary bacteriology and mycology,* Springfield, IL, 1984, Charles C Thomas.

measure of the cell count. The degree of gel formation is scored negative, trace, 1, 2, or 3.

To perform the CMT, about 2 ml of milk are placed in each of the four cups on the CMT paddle, and an equal amount of reagent is added. The paddle is gently rotated for about 10 seconds in a circular pattern to mix the milk and reagent. A score is then assigned for each quarter, according to the chart of grading and interpretation (Table 4-9).

Precautions to be considered in this test are as follows:

- *DNA in somatic cells deteriorates upon standing.* If the test is to be used as a laboratory test, the milk samples should be kept refrigerated but not for more than 48 hours. Unrefrigerated milk cannot be tested accurately after about 12 hours.
- *White blood cells tend to migrate with milk fat.* Therefore, thorough mixing of samples just before testing is essential.
- *CMT reaction must be scored 10 to 15 seconds after mixing starts.* Weaker reactions fade thereafter.

Direct somatic-cell count. This can be performed by counting somatic cells using a microscope or with an electronic cell counter (Coulter counter). In either case, the results are reported as the number of cells per milliliter of milk.

TABLE 4-9.   Grading of California mastitis test results

SYMBOL	MEANING	VISIBLE REACTION	INTERPRETATION
−	Negative	Mixture remains liquid with no evidence of a precipitate.	0-200,000 cells/ml 0-25% PMNs
T	Trace	Slight precipitate forms and is seen to best advantage by tipping the paddle back and forth and observing the mixture as it flows over the bottom of the cup. Trace reactions tend to disappear with continued movement of the fluid.	150,000-500,000 cells/ml 30-40% PMNs
1	Weak positive	A distinct precipitate but no tendency toward gel formation. With some samples the reaction is reversible. With continued movement of the paddle, the precipitate may disappear.	400,000-1,500,000 cells/ml 40-60% PMNs
2	Distinct positive	Mixture thickens immediately, with some suggestion of gel formation. As the mixture is swirled, it tends to move toward the center, leaving the bottom of the outer edge of the cup exposed. When the motion is stopped, the mixture levels out again and covers the bottom of the cup.	800,000-5,000,000 cells/ml 60-70% PMNs

Continued.

TABLE 4-9—CONT'D

SYMBOL	MEANING	VISIBLE REACTION	INTERPRETATION
3	Strong positive	Gel formation causes the surface of the mixture to become convex. Usually a central peak remains projecting above the main mass after the motion of the paddle has been stopped. Viscosity is greatly increased, so that there is a tendency for the mass to adhere to the bottom of the cup.	Cell number generally $>5,000,000$/ml 70-80% PMNs
+	Alkaline milk pH 7.0 or over	This notation should be added to the CMT score when the reaction is distinctly alkaline, as indicated by a contrasting deeper purple color.	An alkaline reaction reflects depressed secretory activity as a result of inflammation or in drying-off of the gland.
y	Acidic milk	Bromcresol purple is distinctly yellow at pH 5.2. This notation should be added to the score when the mixture is yellow.	Distinctly acidic milk in the udder is rare. When encountered, it indicates fermentation of lactose by bacterial action within the gland.

PMN = polymorphonuclear leukocyte

MILK CULTURE.   Only positive milk samples identified by CMT or direct somatic-cell count should be cultured. The milk sample is inoculated on blood agar and MacConkey agar and incubated at 37° C for 24 hours. Milk samples are also incubated simultaneously. If the cultures show minimal or no growth after 24 hours of incubation, a subculture is made on the blood and MacConkey agar plates from the incubated milk samples. The subcultured plates and the original culture plates are incubated for 24 hours at 37° C. A rapid but presumptive identification of the organism can be made on colonial morphology, followed by confirmatory tests:

- *Staphylococcus aureus* forms moderate-sized (3-mm) colonies. Colonies of bovine strains are yellow, surrounded by a double zone of hemolysis. This organism does not grow on MacConkey agar.
- *E. coli* forms pink colonies on MacConkey agar and glistening colonies on blood agar, with an unpleasant odor.
- *Klebsiella pneumoniae* colonies become very mucoid after 48 hours' incubation. Growth on MacConkey agar is also mucoid.
- *Enterobacter aerogenes* cannot be distinguished from *Klebsiella* on colony appearance.
- *Streptococcus* forms small (1-mm) colonies resembling dew drops. *Streptococcus agalactiae* strains may produce a clear zone of beta hemolysis. Streptococci are the only bacteria that grow on Edwards' medium. Hence, their growth on Edwards' medium is one of the methods of detecting streptococci associated with mastitis.
- *Pseudomonas aeruginosa* forms large colonies that usually produce a bluish-green pigment on both blood and MacConkey agars. Many strains produce a characteristic and not unpleasant odor.
- *Actinomyces (Corynebacterium) pyogenes* forms very small colonies surrounded by a zone of clear hemolysis. At 16 to 24 hours' incubation, the hemolytic effect is often seen before the colonies become visible. There is no growth on MacConkey agar.
- *Nocardia asteroides* colonies are not usually visible until after 48 to 72 hours' incubation. The colonies become powdery and are intensely white and adherent to the medium. This organism does not grow on MacConkey agar.
- *Pasteurella multocida* forms moderately sized, nonhemolytic colonies that produce a characteristically sweetish odor. The colonies have a superficial resemblance to those of enterobacteria, but there is no growth on MacConkey agar.

CONFIRMATORY TESTS. *Staphylococcus aureus* appears as Gram-positive cocci, often arranged in clusters resembling "bunches of grapes." The coagulase test is the most definitive test for pathogenicity of staphylococci. It distinguishes *Staphylococcus aureus* from *Staphylococcus epidermidis,* which can occasionally be hemolytic. However, only Gram-positive and catalase-positive cocci should be subjected to the coagulase test. Also, any degree of clotting of the plasma in 3 to 4 hours is regarded as a positive finding. Known coagulase-negative and coagulase-positive staphylococci should be used as controls. Commercial systems, such as ApiStaph-Ident and Minitek, can be used to identify staphylococci.

Presumptive identification of *E. coli, Klebsiella,* and *Enterobacter* can be made using a few biochemical tests (triple sugar-iron, lysine, sulfide-indole-motility, methyl red, and citrate), as indicated in the previous section. *Serratia marcescens* occasionally causes mastitis. Only a few strains produce the orange-red pigment at 37° C. If, however, the inoculated plates or subcultures are left at room temperature, the pigment may be observed. The API, Enterotube, or Minitek commercial kit system should be used for complete identification of enterobacteria.

The colony appearance of mastitis-causing streptococci, with their ability to hydrolyze esculin, can be a useful first step in their identification (Figure 4-13). Gram-positive, catalase-negative colonies are streaked on Edwards' or esculin blood agar. Browning of Edwards' or esculin blood agar, as a sequel to hydrolysis, can be seen with greater clarity if the culture plates are examined under an ultraviolet (Wood's) lamp. A uniform blue glow is evident on uninoculated plates containing esculin and on plates in which the streptococci have not hydrolyzed the esculin. A dark-brown coloration of colonies and the surrounding medium indicates streptococci that attack esculin.

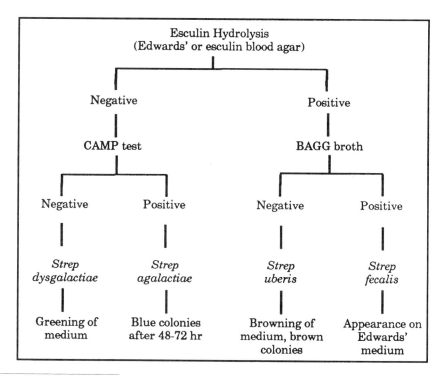

Figure 4-13.   Differentiation of streptococci using esculin hydrolysis.

Ruminant red blood cells, partially lysed by the beta-hemolysin of *Staphylococcus aureus* at 37° C, are completely hemolyzed in the presence of Lancefield group-B streptococci, including *Streptococcus agalactiae*. This is the basis of the CAMP test, used to identify *Streptococcus agalactiae*.

The CAMP test uses a blood agar plate prepared with sheep or cattle red blood cells containing esculin. A thin streak is made down the center of the agar plate using a *Staphylococcus aureus* strain that produces a good zone of partial hemolysis. Several suspect *Streptococcus agalactiae* strains can be tested on one plate. The streptococci to be tested are streaked at right angles to the *Staphylococcus aureus* streak, bringing them within 1 to 2 mm of the *Staphylococcus aureus* streak. Include a known *Streptococcus agalactiae* streak on every plate as a control. The plates are incubated at 37° C for 24 hours.

An arrow of enhanced, complete hemolysis indicates a positive test for *Streptococcus agalactiae* (Figure 4-14). About 5% of *Streptococcus uberis* strains and an occasional strain of *Streptococcus dysgalactiae* produce a small zone of hemolysis close to the *Staphylococcus aureus* streak, but the reaction is rounded and weak. *Streptococcus uberis* can be distinguished from *Streptococcus agalactiae* by the color of its colonies and brown discoloration of the medium.

BAGG broth (BBL) is a buffered azide glycerol broth for detection of enteric streptococci, such as *Streptococcus fecalis*. These Lancefield group-D streptococci may occasionally cause mastitis, but they are often present in milk samples as contaminants and must be distinguished from *Streptococcus uberis*. BAGG broth is inoculated with the test streptococcus and incubated, in addition to a control broth containing a known *Streptococcus fecalis* culture, for 48 hours at 37° C. Cloudiness in the broth, with a color change from purple to yellow, indicates a positive result. BAGG broth inoculated with *Streptococcus*

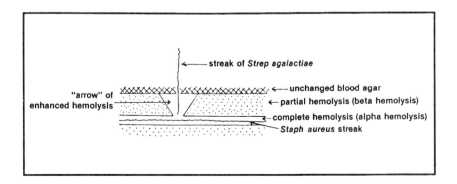

FIGURE 4-14.   CAMP test for *Streptococcus agalactiae*.

uberis remains clear and purple (negative). Commercial test kits, such as Rapid Strep, are available.

Figure 4-13 provides a flow chart for identification of some streptococci.

Pseudomonas aeruginosa can usually be identified by the large colonies, blue-green pigment, and characteristic odor it produces. If there is doubt, carry out the tests listed under the section on Primary Identification of Bacteria, with inoculation of a tube of tech agar (BBL), which is designed to enhance pyocyanin production by *P. aeruginosa* strains. *Pseudomonas aeruginosa* is the only *Pseudomonas* species that produces the blue-green pigment, pyocyanin.

In Gram stains, *Actinomyces (Corynebacterium) pyogenes* appears as a highly pleomorphic Gram-positive organism, showing all forms, from cocci to rods that tend to occur in palisade and "Chinese character" arrangements. A useful confirmatory test is to inoculate the center of a Loeffler serum slant (Oxoid) heavily with the test organism. *Actinomyces (Corynebacterium) pyogenes* is the only *Corynebacterium* species that can cause a pit in the serum slant after 24 hours' incubation at 37° C. *Corynebacterium bovis* occurs commonly in milk samples, but there is doubt regarding the organism's pathogenicity. It forms small, white, dry, nonhemolytic colonies that are often confined to the initial streak, where there is a milk residue.

Nocardia asteroides can usually be presumptively identified by its appearance on blood agar. It is a Gram-positive, moderate-sized rod. If the milk sample is centrifuged, modified Ziehl-Neelsen staining reveals a branching, filamentous organism, with some filaments staining red (positive). If a centrifuge is not available, take some material with a Pasteur pipette from the very bottom of the tube and make a smear.

Streptomyces is a common, nonpathogenic soil and air organism with colonies quite similar to those of *Nocardia*. However, most strains of *Streptomyces* have an unmistakable earthy odor, are likely to form filaments in the milk sample, and are negative on modified Ziehl-Neelsen staining.

With experience, a presumptive identification can be made from the characteristic odor of *Pasteurella multocida* and from its failure to grow on MacConkey agar. The organism can be identified to the genus level by carrying out the tests listed under Primary Identification (see previously). In addition, *P. multocida* is a good indole producer. *Pasteurella pneumotropica* also forms indole but is unlikely to be associated with mastitis. If there is any doubt, identify the organism using the API or Minitek systems or Enterotube.

Organisms from urine samples
In contrast to methods used for milk samples, methods of culturing urine samples emphasize procedures for determining the number of bacteria present.

However, isolation and identification of pathogenic bacteria also are important when determining the cause of urinary infection.

Culture fresh urine samples. Samples that cannot be cultured within 2 hours after collection should be refrigerated. Streak a blood agar plate with the urine sample using a 0.001-ml calibrated loop (Figure 4-15).

After the plates are incubated at 37° C for 18 to 24 hours, colonies are counted. A bacterial count of less than 10,000 is usually considered insignificant. A commercial Bactube Kit method is also available. For positive identification and differentiation of bacteria, the colonies are subjected to Gram staining, culturing for isolation, and biochemical tests.

IDENTIFICATION OF OTHER ORGANISMS FROM ROUTINE CULTURES

The organisms mentioned here are those commonly isolated from cultures of abscesses and samples from urinary tract, respiratory tract, and other lesions. Several conditions, mentioned in the section on Staining, can be diagnosed with some certainty by examination of stained smears only. Confirmatory biochemical tests are more conveniently carried out using the API or Minitek systems in a small laboratory, rather than stocking a large range of conventional biochemical media. Complete information on the methodology of the API and Minitek systems can be obtained from the manufacturer (Box 4-1). Charts, tables, computerized coding systems, or characterization profiles, designed to

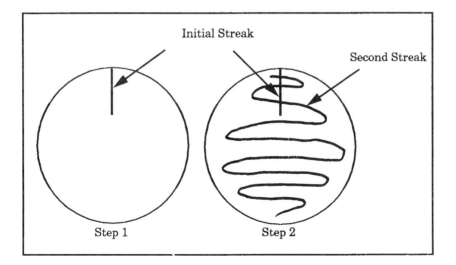

FIGURE **4-15.**   Procedure for streaking a urine culture plate. Short, straight initial streak is followed by a second, curved streak covering the remainder of the plate. Do not flame the loop between the first and second streaks.

be used only with the system for which they were produced, are also available. It is important to remember that the results of biochemical tests in the miniaturized systems may vary among the systems and may also be different from results obtained by conventional test methods.

Most species of *Actinomyces* are anaerobic, except *A. viscosus,* which can cause granulomatous pleuritis in dogs. This condition must be differentiated from nocardiosis, which has similar clinical signs and gross pathologic changes. These two diseases can usually be diagnosed with the aid of staining.

Actinobacillus is a Gram-negative bacterium that grows on MacConkey agar. It is fermentative, oxidase and catalase positive, and nonmotile. It tends to be comparatively species specific, *A. lignieresi* mainly affecting cattle, *A. equuli* foals, *A. suis* pigs and foals, and *A. seminis* causing epididymitis in rams. Epididymitis due to *Brucella ovis* can be clinically similar to an *A. seminis* infection, but chronic cases due to *A. seminis* are often very purulent. The organism is unreactive biochemically and modified Ziehl-Neelsen negative. *Brucella ovis* is seen as clumps of red, modified Ziehl-Neelsen-positive rods in smears from lesions. A few biochemical reactions can be used to differentiate the three main *Actinobacillus* species (Table 4-10).

Aeromonas hydrophila, a Gram-negative, opportunistic pathogen, is most commonly isolated from fish and reptiles but occasionally infects mammals. It is often strikingly hemolytic on blood agar and produces an offensive odor. It grows well on MacConkey agar but is catalase and oxidative positive, whereas the enterobacteria are oxidase negative. Its colonies can resemble those of *Pseudomonas.* Both genera are motile, but *Aeromonas* is fermentive and *Pseudomonas* is oxidative.

TABLE 4-10. Reactions used to differentiate the three main *Actinobacillus* species

	A. *LIGNIERESI*	A. *EQUULI*	A. *SUIS*
Clear hemolysis on blood agar	−	(−)	(+)
Esculin hydrolysis	−	−	+
Urease production	+	+	+
Salicin (acid)	−	−	+
Mannitol (acid)	+	+	−
Trehalose (acid)	−	+	+

( ) = some exceptions

The typical clumps of red *Brucella* coccobacilli are seen in smears stained with modified Ziehl-Neelsen or Koster stain from lesions or, with abortions, from fetal stomach contents. *Brucella ovis* and *B. abortus* require CO_2 for growth, but *B. canis* and *B. suis* do not. Other than *B. ovis,* they are rapid urease producers. *Brucella abortus* gives a positive result in 2 hours and *B. canis* and *B. suis* in a half hour. Selective media are desirable for the brucellae because of the large number of contaminant bacteria present in specimens, as in uterine discharges and cotyledons. Isolation of these organisms is best attempted in a specialized laboratory. A slide agglutination test is available for canine brucellosis (see Chapter 9).

Bordetella bronchiseptica is a respiratory pathogen that may be isolated from pigs with atrophic rhinitis. It may also be a secondary invader in dogs with distemper and a cause of respiratory infections in rabbits (one cause of "snuffles") and guinea pigs. *Bordetella bronchiseptica* is a small Gram-negative rod that grows on MacConkey agar. It is motile, oxidase and catalase positive, citrate and urease positive, and indole negative. It reduces nitrates and does not attack carbohydrates. Most strains are hemolytic on blood agar.

Many conditions caused by *Campylobacter fetus* ss *fetus,* such as abortions in cattle and sheep, can be diagnosed by stained smears. Culture is necessary to confirm the diagnosis. As these are fastidious organisms, culture is best done in a specialized laboratory.

Corynebacterium organisms are pleomorphic Gram-positive rods. *Actinomyces (Corynebacterium) pyogenes* is invariably hemolytic, with pinpoint colonies after 24 hours' incubation. A useful identifying feature of *Actinomyces pyogenes* is its ability to "pit" a Loeffler's serum slope after 24 hours' incubation. *Rhodococcus (Corynebacterium) equi* is nonhemolytic and very unreactive against carbohydrates. However, after 48 hours' incubation, the colonies are characteristically mucoid and salmon pink, both increasing with incubation time. A short list of biochemical reactions for the corynebacteria of veterinary interest is given in Table 4-11. Corynebacteria are rather fastidious, so the sugar reactions should be carried out in cystine trypticase agar (BBL) base medium.

Dermatophilus congolensis is so characteristic in stained smears (see Staining) that it is usually unnecessary to do cultures. Some stains require CO_2 for primary isolation (a candle jar is satisfactory), but all strains grow aerobically on subculture. Small, rough, hemolytic colonies appear after 48 hours' incubation. The colonies are embedded in the medium.

Erysipelothrix rhusiopathiae and *Listeria monocytogenes,* both moderate-sized, Gram-positive rods, are superficially similar in Gram-stained smears and in culture. They must also be distinguished from nonpathogenic *Erysipelothrix*-like

Table 4-11. Some biochemical reactions for corynebacteria of veterinary interest

	Hemolysis	"Pitting" Loeffler's	Catalase	Urease	NO₃ Red	Glu	Acid in Lact	Malt
Actinomyces (Coryn.) pyogenes	+	+	−	−	−	+	+	+
Coryn. renale	V	−	+	V	V	+	V	V
Rhodococcus (Coryn.) equi	−	−	+	V	+	−	−	−
Coryn. pseudotuberculosis	V	−	+	V	V	+	V	+
Coryn. bovis	−	−	+	−	−	−	−	−
Coryn. kutscheri (Coryn. murium)	−	−	+	V	+	+	−	+
Coryn. suis (anaerobic)	−	−	−	+	−	V	−	+

Glu = glucose
Lact = lactose
Malt = maltose
V = variable reaction, depending on strain

organisms and from nonpathogenic *Listeria* species. The major differentiating characteristics are given in Table 4-12.

On blood agar, colonies of *L. monocytogenes,* beta-hemolytic streptococci, and *Actinomyces (Corynebacterium) pyogenes* have a similar appearance. They form small colonies, surrounded by an entire edge and a clear zone of hemolysis. After 24 hours' incubation, young colonies of *E. rhusiopathiae* usually have a narrow zone of partial hemolysis that progresses to a slight zone of clear hemolysis after 48 hours' incubation.

In Gram-stained preparations from colonies, *L. monocytogenes* has many coccal cells, and care is needed not to mistake it for a streptococcus. Rough colonies of *E. rhusiopathiae* can yield small coccobacilli and short, filamentous forms.

"Tumbling" motility is characteristic of *L. monocytogenes.* This can be seen in a wet preparation of a broth culture incubated at room temperature for 2 to 3 hours. Individual cells suddenly tumble over and over before moving off again normally. When grown in a semi-solid medium, *Listeria* produces a characteristic umbrella-shaped growth. The API 20s Kit is available commercially for identification of *L. monocytogenes.*

TABLE 4-12.   Major differentiating characteristics of *Erysipelothrix* and *Listeria*

	ERYSIPELOTHRIX RHUSIOPATHIAE	ERYSIPELOTHRIX-LIKE ORGANISMS	NONPATHOGENIC LISTERIA SPP	LISTERIA MONOCYTOGENES
Clear hemolysis	−(24 hr)	−	−	+
Oxidase	−	−	−	−
Catalase	−	−	+	+
Motility	−	−	+	+(25° C)
Hydrogen sulfide in triple sugar-iron	+(2-5 days)	+	−	−
Esculin hydrolysis	−	+	+	+
"Bottle brush" in gelatin	+(3-5 days)	+	−	−

The hydrogen sulfide production by *E. rhusiopathiae* in triple sugar-iron stab cultures is meager and just along the stab line but is very characteristic for the organism. The "bottle brush" appearance of colonies in gelatin takes several days to develop and occurs mainly with the rough strains of the organism. Esculin hydrolysis can be tested on esculin blood agar or on esculin slants that are available commercially. Browning of the medium, seen more clearly under ultraviolet light, is a positive reaction.

Listeria monocytogenes is easily isolated from abortion specimens and abscesses, but a cold enrichment technique is required to recover the organism from brain specimens (see Bacteriologic Cultures previously).

Most *Hemophilus* organisms require X and/or V factors for growth. The exceptions are *H. somnus* and *H. (Taylorella) equigenitalis,* though their growth is enhanced by the X factor. Colony growth of *Hemophilus* species is increased in an atmosphere with 5% to 10% CO_2.

Chocolate agar (BBL) is the medium of choice. In an emergency, a fresh blood agar plate, supplying some X factor, and a streak of *Staphylococcus aureus* (V factor), grows many of the organisms. There is a greater chance of isolating *H. somnus* if generous amounts of tissue are pre-enriched in brain-heart infusion broth and plated after 24 hours' incubation.

Hemophilus organisms form small, circular colonies, usually needing 48 hours' incubation at 37° C before they are visible. *Actinomyces (H) pleuropneumoniae (parahemolyticus)* is isolated from swine and is often hemolytic. The other two species of *Hemophilus* isolated from swine include *H. parasuis* and *H. suis*. To differentiate between the species, the organism is grown on blood agar and requirements for X and V factors are determined. If the organism requires V factor, it establishes satellite colonies around the *Staphylococcus* streak. The requirement for both X and V factors can be tested by streaking the suspect organism on trypticase soy agar (with almost no X or V factors) and adding discs containing X, V, and combined XV factors (Oxoid or BBL) to the surface of the agar. Satellite colonies grow around the disc containing the required growth factor(s).

Table 4-13 summarizes the characteristics of *Hemophilus* spp. As shown in Table 4-13, *H. suis* requires both X and V factors, while *Actinomyces (H.) pleuropneumoniae* requires only V factor. A urea test is used to differentiate these two species. *Actinomyces (H.) pleuropneumoniae* is urease positive, while *H. suis* is urease negative.

Moraxella bovis is a small, aerobic, nonmotile, Gram-negative coccobacillus associated with keratoconjunctivitis in cattle. It produces oxidase, and some strains are catalase positive. *Moraxella bovis* does not attack carbohydrates but is weakly proteolytic and slowly liquefies gelatin and pits Loeffler's serum slants. Colony variants are common; hemolytic/nonhemolytic and rough/smooth colonies occur. Subcultures may produce a mixture of colony variants, giving the impression of impure cultures.

Isolation of *M. bovis* is more likely if a swab of lacrimal secretions or discharge is plated directly on blood agar. Failing this, place the swab in a little sterile saline and plate out within 2 hours of collection.

When *Nocardia asteroides* is suspected, it is always worthwhile to stain a smear from the original specimen with modified Ziehl-Neelsen stain. Observation of modified Ziehl-Neelsen-positive filaments and the characteristic colonies gives a presumptive identification (see Staining and Identification of Organisms from Bovine Mastitis Samples).

Pasteurella organisms have an affinity for the respiratory system, though *P. multocida* can be associated with bovine mastitis and with cat and dog bites. The fermentation of carbohydrates should be tested using CTA-based media (BBL). A few reactions for identification of the *Pasteurella* species are listed in Table 4-14.

Pseudomonas aeruginosa is the main veterinary pathogen in the *Pseudomonas* genus, with the exception of the exotic species *P. mallei* and *P. pseudomallei.* Identification of *P. aeruginosa* is discussed under Bovine Mastitis.

Streptococcus, a Gram-positive coccus, forms small, circular colonies. On blood agar, a streptococcus species may be beta-hemolytic (total hemolysis), alpha-hemolytic (partial hemolysis), or gamma-hemolytic (no hemolysis).

TABLE 4-13. Characteristics of *Hemophilus* species

SPECIES	FACTOR REQUIRED		REQUIRED CO_2	PRINCIPAL HOST	DISEASE	SPECIMEN
	X	V				
H. suis	+	+	+	Swine	Glasser's disease	Joint fluid
H. parasuis	−	+	+	Swine	Secondary invader in swine influenza	Lungs
Actinomyces (H.) pleuropneumoniae	−	+	(+)	Swine	Pleuropneumonia	Lungs, pleura
H. gallinarum	+	+	+	Chickens	Infectious coryza	Nasal discharge and/or trachea
H. paragallinarum	−	+	+	Chickens	Infectious coryza	As above
H. somnus	(+)	−	+	Cattle	Meningoencephalitis, polyarthritis, etc	Brain, joint fluid, lungs
Taylorella (H.) equigenitalis	(+)	−	+	Horses	Contagious equine metritis	Cervical swabs

( ) = not required but enhances growth

TABLE 4-14. Reactions for identification of *Pasteurella* species

	P. MULTOCIDA	*P. HEMOLYTICA*	*P. GALLINARUM*	*P. PNEUMOTROPICA*
Hemolysis (blood agar)	−	+	±	−
Growth: MacConkey agar	−	±	−	−
Indole	+	−	−	+
Urease	−	−	−	+
Glucose	+	+	+	+
Lactose	−	+	−	+
Sucrose	+	+	+	+
Mannitol	±	+	−	−
Salicin	−	+	−	−
Esculin hydrolysis	−	±	−	−

TABLE 4-15. Differential reactions for Group-C streptococci

	STREP. EQUI	*STREP. ZOOEPIDEMICUS*	*STREP. EQUISIMILIS*
Trehalose	−	−	+
Sorbitol	−	+	−
Lactose	−	+	±
Maltose	+	±	+

Lancefield grouping can be carried out by the conventional acid-extraction method, or more conveniently using the Streptex latex test (Burroughs Wellcome), which covers groups A, B, C, D, F, and G.

Among the most important streptococci are those of group C from horses. These must be differentiated when a decision must be made regarding vaccination against strangles (*Streptococcus equi* ss *equi* infection). Table 4-15 lists biochemical tests that can be carried out using CTA-based media (BBL) or peptone water sugars with about 5 drops of sterile serum added per 5 ml of medium.

Coagulase-positive staphylococci have been placed into three biotypes, with *Staphylococcus aureus* the parent biotype. *Staphylococcus intermedius* has been isolated from dogs with pyoderma and mastitis and from pigeons, mink, and horses. *Staphylococcus hyicus* has been recovered from pigs with polyarthritis, the skin of pigs with and without exudative epidermitis ("greasy pig disease"), the intact skin and mange lesions in cattle, and cows with mastitis. It is probably sufficient to establish that a *Staphylococcus* is coagulase positive, as this correlates well with pathogenicity (see Identification of Bacteria from Bovine Mastitis Samples). However, a test employing a purple agar base (BBL), with 1% maltose added, can be used to differentiate the three bio-types (Table 4-16).

Yersinia organisms are now members of the Enterobacteriaceae. The general characteristics of *Y. pseudotuberculosis* and *Y. enterocolitica* are lactose-negative (colorless) colonies on MacConkey agar, oxidase negative but catalase positive, does not produce hydrogen sulfide in triple sugar-iron agar, urease positive but phenylalanine negative, and motile at room temperature but not at 37° C. These are the two *Yersinia* species of greatest veterinary interest, but *Y. pestis,* the plague bacillus, is enzootic in wild rodents in 17 western states. *Yersinia pestis* is urease negative and nonmotile.

Yersinia pseudotuberculosis can usually be isolated from caseous lesions on primary inoculation of solid media. However, attempted isolation of *Yersinia* spp, particularly *Y. enterocolitica,* from feces should employ a cold-enrichment process (see Culture Methods). Table 4-17 summarizes reactions used to differentiate *Yersinia* spp.

TABLE 4-16. Differentiation of three species of staphylococci

	TUBE COAGULASE TEST	PIGMENTATION OF COLONY	PURPLE AGAR BASE WITH 1% MALTOSE
Staph. aureus	+	+	Diffuse yellow color around colonies in 12-24 hours
Staph. intermedius	+	−	Yellow to yellow-green under colonies in 48-72 hours*
Staph. hyicus	+	−	Diffuse alkaline (purple) reaction around colonies

*Not reliable for *Staph. intermedius* strains from species other than dogs.

Table 4-17. Differential reactions of *Yersinia* species

	Y. PESTIS	*Y. PSEUDOTUBERCULOSIS*	*Y. ENTEROCOLITICA*
Indole	−	−	±*
Urease	−	+	+
Ornithine decarboxylase	−	−	+
Esculin hydrolysis	−	+	−
Rhamnose	−	+	(−)
Sorbitol	−	−	+
Sucrose	−	(−)	+
Salicin	+	+	−

*Most European strains are negative but most American strains are positive.
( ) = some exceptions

ANTIMICROBIAL SUSCEPTIBILITY TESTING

When bacteria are isolated from a patient, an antimicrobial test is done to determine the susceptibility or resistance to antimicrobial drugs. The results of this test can indicate which antimicrobial to use in treatment. Ideally, the specimen used for antimicrobial susceptibility testing should be taken from the animal before treatment begins. The veterinarian may begin treatment before obtaining susceptibility results but then may change to a more appropriate drug when the results are available.

Use fresh clinical samples for a direct susceptibility test. It is best to first isolate the suspected pathogen and then do the susceptibility testing. This ensures that the test is done on the causative organism, rather than on a mixed floral specimen or a contaminant. A Gram stain is done on the isolate to determine which antimicrobial discs to use. Some antimicrobials are more effective against Gram-positive or Gram-negative bacteria. Groups of antimicrobials may be tested according to the disease being investigated, such as respiratory disease or mastitis. The organisms typically causing each disease tend to respond to certain groups of antimicrobials.

AGAR DIFFUSION METHOD

The agar diffusion method for antimicrobial susceptibility testing is most commonly employed and uses paper discs impregnated with antimicrobials. It is quantitative and requires measurement of zone sizes to give an estimate of antimicrobial susceptibility. The concentration of drug in the disc is chosen to correlate with serum and tissue levels of the drug in the treated animal.

Diffusion methods in common use include the U.S. Food and Drug Administration (FDA) method; standardized disc susceptibility method, which is a modified Bauer-Kirby technique; the International Collaborative Study (ICS) standardized disc technique; and the Stokes disc method. The FDA susceptibility test will be described here. It is designed for testing the antimicrobial susceptibility of rapidly growing aerobic pathogens, such as Enterobacteriaceae, staphylococci, and *Pseudomonas*.

CULTURE MEDIA FOR ANTIMICROBIAL SUSCEPTIBILITY TESTING

Mueller-Hinton agar gives the most reproducible results and is suitable for testing both antibiotics and sulfonamides. Ensure that there is no gross moisture on the agar surface or on the lid before use. Plates can be checked for sterility by incubating two or three from a batch at 37° C for 24 hours.

Some organisms, such as streptococci, do not grow sufficiently well on plain Mueller-Hinton agar for a test to be read. In these cases, Mueller-Hinton agar plus 5% blood must be used. However, having departed from the standardized FDA method, the zone sizes must be interpreted with caution. For example, the zone sizes for novobiocin are smaller if the medium contains blood. Most streptococci are still susceptible to penicillin.

INOCULUM PREPARATION AND INOCULATION OF PLATES

A pure culture should be used for susceptibility testing. However, if there are well-spaced colonies on the plate inoculated from an original specimen, it is permissible to use these. With a sterile loop, touch just the surface of three or four of them and place them in saline or broth to make a suspension. If bacteria are taken from just the surface of the colony, there is less likelihood of picking up an unseen contaminant growing at the base of the colony. Always take more than one colony of a bacterial species, as a single colony may represent a variant that has a susceptibility pattern different from that of the parent strain.

Under no circumstances is it justifiable, with veterinary specimens, to carry out an antimicrobial susceptibility test using the original inoculum. This is because the chance of only one bacterial species being present in the specimen is minimal. Completely erroneous results are obtained if a susceptibility test is carried out with a mixed inoculum containing more than one species.

A correct inoculum density is an important aspect of getting reproducible results. The "lawn" of cells that grows up after inoculation should be evenly distributed. Extremes in inoculum concentration must be avoided. Several methods can be used to obtain a correct inoculum.

The FDA advocates use of a 2- to 8-hour broth culture, incubated at 37° C, to produce a bacterial suspension of moderate turbidity. The culture is prepared by inoculating 4 to 5 ml of nutrient broth, such as trypticase soy broth or brain-heart infusion, with bacteria obtained by touching the surface of 3 to 4 similar-appearing colonies. The incubated broth is diluted with sterile saline or distilled water to a controlled density, equivalent to 0.5 McFarland standards attained by adding 0.5 ml of 1.17% $BaCl_2$-2 H_2O solution to 99.5 ml of 0.36-N sulfuric acid.

Another method is to dilute an overnight broth culture in saline to the turbidity density described above. This is usually a 1 : 50 dilution of the overnight broth culture.

A rapid method that gives good results is to make a suspension of three to seven well-spaced colonies in about 2 ml of sterile saline or distilled water. The turbidity thus obtained should be equivalent to 0.5 McFarland barium sulfate turbidity standards.

The Prompt Veterinary Sensitivity Standardizing System (BBL) has been developed to rapidly standardize the inoculum density, making it equivalent in performance to the 0.5 McFarland standard. This precludes the incubation period, periodic checking of the inoculum density, and turbidity adjustment by dilution. Thus the system enables one to obtain precise, reliable sensitivity results with a more efficient use of time and less chance of human error.

The Prompt System consists of a plastic vial with a snap top containing 1 ml of saline and a separate inoculator wand. The inoculator wand is a polypropylene rod attached to a cap. At the tip of the rod is a cavity for picking up a controlled number of organisms (5 to 10 colonies) from the primary culture plate.

After picking up the colonies, the top is snapped off the plastic vial, the wand is placed firmly into the vial, and the contents are mixed. This gives the inoculum density equivalent to the 0.5 McFarland standard.

Inoculation of the plates, using the inoculum prepared by either of the above methods, is carried out by saturating a sterile cotton swab with the bacterial suspension. Excess moisture is removed from the swab by rotating it against the side of the tube above the level of the fluid. The bacterial suspension is streaked evenly over the surface of the agar medium with the swab. The agar medium is streaked successively in three directions, and then the swab is run around the circumference of the plate to ensure that the entire surface is covered (Figure 4-16).

Inoculated plates should be allowed to dry for 15 to 30 minutes at room temperature before applying the antimicrobial discs.

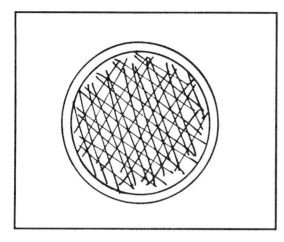

FIGURE 4-16. In antimicrobial susceptibility testing, the sample is incubated in trypicase soy broth. Then a swab sample is streaked in several directions onto Mueller-Hinton agar.

ANTIMICROBIAL DISCS

Use the range of antimicrobial discs that correspond to the drugs most commonly employed in the practice. The antimicrobial content in a disc is indicated in Table 4-18. Only one disc representative of the tetracyclines and one for the sulfonamides are necessary because of the phenomenon of cross-resistance. For example, if the bacterial species is resistant to one of the tetracyclines, it is usually resistant to all members of the group.

Always keep antimicrobial discs in the refrigerator (4° C) when they are not being used and put them back as soon as possible after use. Never use outdated discs. The potency of the antimicrobial discs can be monitored with control organisms of known sensitivity patterns.

Place the antimicrobial discs on the inoculated agar surface with a disc dispenser or sterile forceps that have been flamed and cooled between each use and gently press down on each disc to ensure contact with the surface. The discs should be no closer than 10 to 15 mm to the edge of the plate and sufficiently separated from each other to avoid overlapping of the zones of inhibition. The spacing can be carried out using sterile forceps with the plate over a template, or by using a disc dispenser. One type of disc dispenser delivers eight different antimicrobial discs onto a standard 100-mm-diameter plate, and another can dispense 12 discs onto a 150-mm Petri dish (BBL, Difco).

Put the plates in the incubator at 37° C within 15 minutes after placing the discs on the inoculated agar. Incubate the plates aerobically and upside down. Keep the plates in stacks of four or less, as plates in the center of a tall stack take longer to reach incubation temperature.

Table 4-18.   Interpreting inhibition zone size with the FDA standardized disc method

		Inhibition zone diameter (mm)		
Antimicrobial	Disc content	Resistant organisms (#)	Susceptible intermediate	Organisms susceptible
Ampicillin[a]: for Gram negatives and enterococci	10 μg	≤11	12-13	≥14
Ampicillin[a]: for staphylococci and penicillin G-susceptible organisms	10 μg	≤20	21-28	≥29
Ampicillin[a]: sulbactam for Gram-negative enterobacteria, staphylococci, and *Hemophilus* spp	10 μg	≤19	—	≥20
Bacitracin	10 units	≤8	9-12	≥13
Carbenicillin: for *Proteus, E. coli*	100 μg	≤17	18-22	≥23
Carbenicillin: for *Pseudomonas aeruginosa*	100 μg	≤13	14-16	≥17
Cephalothin[b]	30 μg	≤14	15-17	≥18
Chloramphenicol	30 μg	≤12	13-17	≥18
Clindamycin	2 μg	≤14	15-20	≥21
Colistin	10 μg	≤8	9-10	≥11
Enrofloxacin	5 μg	≤17	18-21	≥22
Erythromycin	15 μg	≤13	14-17	≥18
Gentamicin	10 μg	≤12	13-14	≥15
Kanamycin	30 μg	≤13	14-17	≥18
Methicillin[c]	5 μg	≤9	10-13	≥14
Nalidixic acid	30 μg	≤13	14-18	≥19

Neomycin	30 µg	≤12	13-16	≥17
Nitrofurantoin	300 µg	≤14	15-16	≥17
Novobiocin[d]	30 µg	≤17	18-21	≥22
Novobiocin[e]	30 µg	≤14	15-16	≥17
Penicillin G for staphylococci[f]	10 units	≤20	21-28	≥29
Penicillin G for other bacteria[f]	10 units	≤20	12-21	≥22
Polymyxin B	300 units	≤8	9-11	≥12
Rifampin: for *Neisseria meningitidis*	5 µg	≤24	—	≥25
Hemophilus spp		≤16	17-19	≥20
Streptomycin	10 µg	≤11	12-14	≥15
Sulfonamides	250 or 300 µg	≤12	13-16	≥17
Tetracycline[g]	30 µg	≤14	15-18	≥19
Tilmicosin	15 µg	≤11	12-16	≥15
Tobramycin	10 µg	≤12	13-14	≥15
Trimethoprim-sulfa	1.25 µg 23.75 µg	≤10	11-15	≥16
Vancomycin	30 µg	≤9	10-11	≥12

a - Use for testing susceptibility to ampicillin and hetacillin.
b - Use when susceptibility to cephalothin, cephaloridine, cephalexin, cefazolin, cephacetrile, cephradine, cefaclor, and cephapirin is observed.
c - Use for testing susceptibility to all penicillinase-resistant penicillins.
d - Not applicable to a medium containing blood.
e - Use when the test medium contains blood.
f - Use for testing susceptibility to all penicillinase-susceptible penicillins except ampicillin and carbenicillin.
g - Use for testing susceptibility to all the tetracyclines.

READING THE ZONES OF INHIBITION

The plates should be read after a constant period, most satisfactorily after overnight incubation (18 to 24 hours). Prolonged incubation can alter the size of the zone of inhibition with antimicrobials that are not stable at 37° C or at best make the zones hard to read. If rapid results are imperative, the diameters of the zones of inhibition may be read after 6 to 8 hours' incubation. These results should be confirmed by reading them again after overnight incubation.

Measure the diameter of each inhibition zone (including the diameter of the disc) from the underside of the plate, using calipers, transparent ruler, or template. The zones are measured and recorded to the nearest millimeter. IfMueller-Hinton agar with blood has been used, the zone size must be read from the top surface, with the lid of the plate removed.

INTERPRETATION OF ZONE SIZES

Table 4-18 lists some of the commonly used antimicrobials and gives the suggested interpretation of zone sizes with the FDA standardized disc method. The zone sizes are divided into two major categories: resistant and susceptible to the particular antimicrobial agent. The latter category is subdivided into intermediate susceptibility and susceptible. For predictive purposes, a resistant organism is not likely to respond to therapy with the drug. A susceptible organism is susceptible to ordinary doses of the antimicrobial. Intermediate susceptibility implies that the organism is susceptible to ordinary doses when the drug is concentrated in the urine or tissues, or the antimicrobial can be used for treatment of systemic infections if a high dosage is safe.

The zone size alone is not indicative of the efficacy of an antimicrobial. Some drugs, such as vancomycin and colistin, do not readily diffuse through agar and give small inhibition zones, even when the test organism is fully susceptible. Therefore direct comparisons of zone diameter, produced by unrelated antimicrobials, are misleading and should not be made.

CONTROL ORGANISMS

Susceptible reference organisms, such as *Staphylococcus aureus,* American Type Culture Collection (ATCC) 25923, and *E. coli,* ATCC 25922, should be put up regularly, preferably in parallel with each batch of antimicrobial susceptibility tests. These control organisms are used to check such factors as the growth-supporting capability of the medium, potency of antimicrobial discs, and other variable conditions that can affect results.

LIMITATIONS OF THE TEST

The FDA method is designed for rapidly growing bacteria. Caution is needed if testing anaerobes or slow-growing organisms, for which the criteria for interpreting zone diameters have not yet been established with certainty. In general, the zone diameters are somewhat larger, for an equivalent minimal inhibitory concentration, with slow-growing organisms than with rapid growers.

Some rare strains of staphylococci are resistant to methicillin and other penicillinase-stable penicillins. The routine test cannot be relied on to detect these strains, but they can be detected by incubation of an additional susceptibility test plate, containing a methicillin disc, at 30° C. A reduced zone diameter, or no zone, surrounding the methicillin disc on the plate incubated at 30° C is presumptive evidence of methicillin resistance.

SEROLOGIC EXAMINATION

Serologic procedures are widely used in veterinary diagnostic laboratories for positive identification of bacteria that are apparently identical in their morphology and physiology. These procedures are faster and more economical than culture methods. Many serologic procedures can be performed without much difficulty at the veterinary clinic.

SAMPLE COLLECTION

Blood samples for serologic testing must be collected in sterile tubes. Samples collected in EDTA, heparin, or sodium citrate are satisfactory. If samples are to be sent to a diagnostic laboratory, send freshly collected blood cooled to 4° C when it is clotted. It is best to separate the clot from the serum and to send serum samples instead of whole blood. If the serum is to be kept for several days before shipping (waiting for a convalescent sample), the serum must be separated from the clot and stored frozen. Early separation of serum from the clot prevents hemolysis. Hemolyzed blood samples are unsatisfactory because hemolysis makes interpretation of results difficult.

If paired serum samples are submitted, mark them as "acute" and "convalescent" with dates of sample collection.

SEROLOGIC TESTS

AGGLUTINATION TEST.   Agglutination refers to clumping of bacteria caused by a specific antibody. In this procedure, serum containing specific antibodies is added to a standard suspension of antigen (bacteria). The resulting degree of agglutination (clumping) or lack of agglutination is then assessed. The agglutination test is one of the most commonly employed tests in diagnosis of bacterial infection. The test may be performed on glass slides or plastic cards or in tubes. The slide and card tests are commonly used as screening tests. In the tube agglutination test, the reagent and serum sample are mixed in a test tube.

The most common serologic test performed in veterinary clinics and at cattle sales is the Brewer card test. The test is performed by mixing stained *Brucella* organisms with serum from an animal. The card is then rocked for a few minutes. A positive reaction is characterized by clumping or agglutination and possibly clearing of the color stain. Clumps may gather around the edge of the card, producing a "ring."

The milk ring test detects *Brucella* antibodies in the milk of infected cows. The procedure is performed by adding to the milk sample a suspension of *Brucella* bacteria stained with dye and then thoroughly mixing it. As the cream rises, a mass of agglutinated, dyed bacteria floats upward with the cream and forms a ring.

For diagnosis of brucellosis in dogs, a commercial kit is available (see Chapter 9).

PRECIPITATION TEST.   Precipitation is a reaction between a soluble antigen and a soluble antibody, forming an insoluble precipitate. Lancefield classification or grouping of hemolytic streptococci is based on such a precipitation reaction or test. Once streptococci are classified to a particular group by precipitation testing, the species can be identified by using a battery of biochemical tests to detect different sugars. Streptococci of groups B, C, and E are the most frequently encountered streptococci in veterinary medicine.

FLUORESCENT ANTIBODY TECHNIQUE.   This is used to detect and localize antigens. Almost any antigen, whether fixed in tissues or in live cell suspension, can be detected by this method. In this procedure, a specific antibody is labelled with a fluorescent dye. The labelled antibody is then added to cells or tissues. If the antibody is specific to the antigen being tested for, a stable complex forms and is evident under fluorescent microscopy.

This procedure is very useful to detect very small numbers of bacteria. It is also useful if two bacterial species are morphologically and physiologically identical, and cultural procedures are time consuming and expensive.

Some bacterial species routinely evaluated with this technique include *Clostridium chauvoei, Clostridium septicum, E. coli* (K99), *Leptospira, Fusobacterium necrophorum,* and *Listeria monocytogenes.* The fluorescent antibody technique is also used for identification of viruses (see the section on Virology later in this chapter).

MYCOLOGY

SUPPLIES AND EQUIPMENT

A separate room and incubator should be used for fungal culture, as spores tend to contaminate plates put up for bacteriologic culture. If an incubator is inadvertently contaminated with fungal spores, swab the interior thoroughly with 70% ethyl or isopropyl alcohol or place a bowl of water and one of alcohol at the bottom of the incubator and leave the incubator empty of plates for 24 hours, with the door shut, at 37° C.

In addition to those mentioned in the Bacteriology section, supplies and equipment required for mycology include 20% potassium hydroxide, lactophenol cotton blue, and India ink. It is convenient to store these reagents in dropper bottles. A Wood's lamp (ultraviolet light 3650 angstroms), wooden-handled mycology needles, clear cellophane tape, and culture media are also needed.

FUNGAL CULTURES

Fungi that can invade tissue grow at body temperature (37° C). Using this temperature for incubation of primary cultures inhibits many contaminant saprophytic species. The exception to this is when examining specimens for dimorphic fungi, such as *Blastomyces* and *Histoplasma.* These organisms produce sporulating mycelia at 25° C and in their saprophytic phase, but appear as budding yeast cells in 37° C cultures and in animal tissue. Cultures should be incubated, in parallel, at both temperatures.

Cultures for dermatophytes, or ringworm fungi, are incubated at 25° to 30° C. The exception here is the slow-growing *Trichophyton verrucosum,* which can tolerate incubation at 37° C. At this temperature, *T. verrucosum* is less likely to be overgrown by contaminant fungi.

Because many pathogenic fungi, such as *Candida albicans* and *Aspergillus fumigatus,* are ubiquitous, tissue sections showing invasion are mandatory for definitive diagnosis of a mycotic infection. Occasionally, myceliate fungi or yeasts may appear on blood agar plates put up for bacteriology. These, of course, may be contaminants, but it is worthwhile to submit some of the original specimen, in 10% formalin, for histopathologic examination. It is also useful to examine a potassium hydroxide (KOH) wet preparation for fungal elements.

KOH PREPARATION.   A small amount of material is scraped from the lesion or tissue and placed in a drop of 20% KOH on a microscope slide. A coverslip is placed on the preparation and pressed down gently to spread the preparation. This is left to clear in a moist chamber for a few hours or overnight. The chamber can be a Petri dish with a moist filter at the bottom. The slide is placed on a bent glass rod.

Lactophenol cotton blue stain is a mounting medium used to stain fungal preparations on microscope slides. This medium is especially useful for preparing cellophane tape mounts (see Chapter 7). Its components are as follows:

Liquefied phenol	25.0 ml
Lactic acid	20.0 ml
Glycerol	40.0 ml
Cotton blue	0.05 g
Distilled water	15.0 ml

Dissolve the cotton blue in distilled water using a magnetic stirrer. Add the rest of the ingredients and stir well. Filter the solution into a stock bottle. The prepared solution has a shelf life of 1 year. It should be refiltered if the dye precipitates.

FUNGAL SUBCULTURES

Subcultures for identification or referral to another laboratory can be made in several ways:

YEASTS.   These organisms can be streaked out on blood agar or Sabouraud dextrose agar, as for bacteria.

MYCELIATE FUNGI PRODUCING SPORES.   Cut crosshatches into the center of a Sabouraud dextrose agar plate with a few shallow cuts from a sterile scalpel. Using the same scalpel, collect some of the spores from the center of the colony to be subcultured and press them gently into the cross-hatched agar.

MYCELIATE FUNGI NOT PRODUCING SPORES.   Cut a small (1 cm^2) square of agar from the center of a Sabouraud dextrose agar plate with a sterile scalpel. Take a square of the same size from the edge of the colony to be subcultured. This is made to fit snugly into the hole in the agar. It is always advisable to take material for subculture from the edge of a fungal colony, as the old mycelia at the center of the colony may not be viable.

Mycology is time consuming and requires experience and rather specialized techniques. In a small laboratory it might be advisable to rely on the simplified techniques described in this section, supplemented by referral of specimens to a larger laboratory for histopathologic examination and culture.

Table 4-19 contains a list of pathogenic fungi of veterinary importance.

Text continued on p. 232.

TABLE 4-19. Summary of pathogenic fungi, species affected, disease or lesions caused, and specimens for diagnosis

ORGANISM	SPECIES AFFECTED	DISEASE OR LESION	SPECIMENS
Microsporum		Ringworm	Fresh plucked hair and skin scrapings from edges of lesions; send to laboratory in paper envelopes
M. canis	Dogs, cats		
M. distortum	Dogs, cats, horses, pigs		
M. gallinae	Chickens, turkeys		
(*T. gallinae*)	("white comb")		
M. gypseum	Horses, cats, dogs, other species		
M. nanum	Pigs		
M. persicolor	Voles, bats, dogs		
Trichophyton			
T. equinum	Horses, donkeys		
T. erinacei	Hedgehogs, dogs, people		
T. mentagrophytes	Most animal species		
T. rubrum	Primarily people, but also dogs, cats		
T. simli	Poultry, monkeys		
T. verrucosum	Primarily cattle		
Candida albicans	Chickens, turkeys, other birds	Infection of mouth, crop, esophagus	Fresh affected tissue or scrapings from affected tissue

Continued.

TABLE 4-19.—Cont'd

Organism	Species affected	Disease or lesion	Specimens
Some other *Candida* spp (such as *C. tropicalis*) can cause lesions	Dogs Cats Calves, foals	Mycotic stomatitis Enteritis of kittens Infections of oral and intestinal mucosae	Fixed affected tissue
	Cattle Horses	Mastitis Genital infections—both sexes	Most common after extensive antibiotic therapy
	Pigs	Infection of esophagus and stomach	
Malassezia pachydermatis (*Pityrosporon canis*)	Dogs	Chronic otitis externa	Fresh ear swabs
Cryptococcus neoformans	People, dogs, cats (infection frequently affects nervous systems)	Subacute or chronic affected tissue	Fresh nasal discharge, milk
Cryptococcus neoformans (worldwide distribution)	Cattle	Sporadic cases of mastitis	Fixed affected tissue, brain, lung

Coccidioides immitis (SW USA and South America; occurs in soil)	People, horses, cattle, sheep, dogs, cats, captive feral animals	Disease characterized by granulomas, often in bronchial and mediastinal lymph nodes and lungs; can cause lesions in brain, liver, spleen, kidneys	Fresh and fixed lesions and affected tissue
Histoplasma capsulatum (NE, central, and S central USA; occurs in soil)	People, dogs, cats, sheep, pigs, horses	Disease that generally affects reticuloendothelial system; dogs, cats: ulcerations of intestinal canal; enlargement of liver, spleen, lymph nodes; TB-like lesions	Fresh and fixed lesions or affected tissue
Histoplasma farciminosum (Mediterranean, Asia, Africa, and part of Russia)	Horses, mules, donkeys	Epizootic lymphangitis, African farcy, or Japanese glanders	Fresh pus and discharges from lesions
Blastomyces dermatitidis (USA, Canada, and Africa; occurs in soil)	People, dogs, cats, sea lions	Granulomatous lesions in lungs and/or skin and subcutis	Fresh and fixed lesions and affected tissue

Continued.

TABLE 4-19.—CONT'D

ORGANISM	SPECIES AFFECTED	DISEASE OR LESION	SPECIMENS
Sporothrix schenckii	People, horses, dogs, pigs, cattle, fowl, rodents	Subcutaneous nodules or granulomas that eventually discharge pus; can include involvement of bones and visceral organs	Fresh and fixed pus, granulomas
Rhinosporidium seeberi (not yet cultured *in vitro*)	Horses, dogs, cattle, people	Characterized by polyps on the nasal and ocular mucous membranes	Fresh nasal discharge and polyps; fixed polyps
Aspergillus A. *Fumigatus* main pathogen; potentially pathogenic A. *flavus* A. *nidulans* A. *niger*	Many animal species and birds	Fowl: air sac infection; diffuse and nodular forms in lungs; "brooder pneumonia" in chicks and poults; cattle: occasional mycotic abortion and mastitis; horses: guttural pouch mycosis; dog: infection of nasal chambers	Fresh deep scrapings or affected tissue Abortions: see text
A. *flavus* A. *parasiticus* A. *ochraceus*	Ducklings, domestic birds, pigs, dogs	Aflatoxicosis; affects liver and sometimes kidneys	Suspect food product

Organism	Host	Disease	Specimen
A. clavatus	Pigs	Hemorrhagic disease; profuse hemorrhage in many tissues, jaundice, and liver lesions	
	Cattle	Trembling syndrome: *A. flavus* and *A. fumigatus* toxins; abortion; toxins of *A. ochraceus* cause fetal death; hyperkeratosis lesions on muzzle and mouth from *A. clavatus* toxins	
Petriellidium boydii (*Allescheria boydii*)	Cattle	Abortion, mastitis	Fresh milk, uterine discharges, affected tissue
	Equidae	Abortion, metritis, infertility	Fixed affected tissue
	People, other animals	Mycetoma; progressive disease of subcutis	

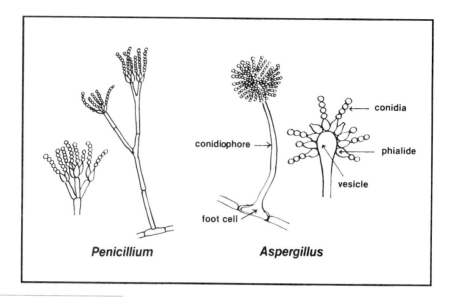

FIGURE **4-17.** Fruiting heads of *Penicillium* and *Aspergillus*.

FUNGI CAUSING DEEP MYCOSES

SPECIMEN COLLECTION

Frozen tissue should be submitted for fungal culture. The tissue containers should be marked "Caution," as fungi causing mycoses in animals are potential zoonotic agents. Do not send swab samples unless a yeast infection is suspected. Such fluids as blood, cerebrospinal fluid, or aspirates should be submitted in screw-cap tubes.

ASPERGILLUS

These organisms are essentially saprophytes, but some *Aspergillus* species can be opportunistic pathogens, causing both infections and toxicosis. *Aspergillus fumigatus* is estimated to be responsible for 90% to 95% of cases of aspergillosis.

The diagnosis of aspergillosis is based on several observations. Examination of a KOH wet preparation of the original specimen reveals septate hyphae. A colony of *A. fumigatus* grows rapidly, often appearing in 24 to 48 hours. It is flat and at first white and floccose. As conidia develop, the colony rapidly becomes bluish-green and powdery. Old cultures have a characteristic grayish, "smoky" cast.

Some *Aspergillus* colonies bear a strong resemblance to those of certain *Penicillium* species. A cellophane-tape preparation is made to examine the fruiting heads of the suspect colony. This is done by taking about 2 ½ inches of clear cellophane tape and pressing the center of the tape, sticky side down, onto the center of the colony. The tape, with hyphae and fruiting heads adhering to it, is placed with the sticky side down on a microscope slide, with a drop of lactophenol cotton blue on it. The tape acts as its own coverslip. The slide preparation is examined under low power or high dry if necessary.

Aspergillus fumigatus has a vesicle resembling an inverted flask (Figure 4-17). The single row of phialides is borne on the upper half of the vesicle in a crowded parallel fashion. Phialides are produced simultaneously in *Aspergillus* species, whereas with *Penicillium* species there is successive production.

A tissue sample should be placed in 10% formalin and referred for histopathologic examination. Septate hyphae are seen invading the tissue and causing a tissue reaction.

CANDIDA ALBICANS

This yeast is often a commensal on normal mucous membranes. *Candida* infections most commonly occur after prolonged antibiotic therapy. The diagnosis of candidiasis is based on several findings.

In wet mounts from scrapings from lesions, thin-walled oval and budding yeast cells (2 to 6 μ in diameter) and occasionally pseudohyphae are present. Gram-stained smears disclose intensely Gram-positive oval yeast cells. *Candida albicans* grows on blood agar or Sabouraud dextrose agar as white, smooth colonies with a yeast-like odor. The colonies are not unlike those of micrococci and appear after 24 to 48 hours of incubation.

Presumptive identification of *Candida albicans* can be made on its ability to produce germ tubes in bovine serum. A light inoculum of the yeast is made in 0.5 ml of serum incubated at 37° C for 2 hours. In a drop of the inoculated serum examined under the low-power or high-dry objective, the germ tubes appear as small sprouts developing from the yeast cells, without a constriction at their points of origin.

Definitive identification is based on fermentation and carbohydrate assimilation tests. Chlamydospore formation on cornmeal agar or chlamydospore agar is also characteristic of *Candida albicans*. Histopathologic examination reveals yeast cells and pseudohyphae in tissue, causing an inflammatory reaction. A commercial system, such as API Yeast Ident, can be used to identify *Candida albicans*.

MALASSEZIA PACHYDERMATIS

Malassezia pachydermatis (Pityrosporon canis) is one of the most common causes of otitis externa. It is readily observed in Gram-stained smears of exudate as an oval or bottle-shaped, small budding cell. Wet mounts with 10% NaOH show clusters of thick-walled, rounded budding cells. The organism can be cultured on Sabouraud dextrose agar at 25° C. Addition of olive oil or coconut oil before inoculation enhances growth.

CRYPTOCOCCUS NEOFORMANS

Cryptococcus is seen most commonly in dogs and cats and occasionally in horses. In all three species the organism usually causes a progressive paranasal infection that does not respond to antibiotic therapy. In such cases, infection due to *Cryptococcus* or *Aspergillus fumigatus* should be considered.

In clinical cases of cryptococcosis, yeast cells can be seen in wet mounts of the purulent nasal discharge. A little of the discharge is mixed on a slide in a drop composed of distilled water and India ink. The proportion of India ink to water is arbitrary and can be adjusted, but a ratio of 1:2 is usually satisfactory. A coverslip is added and the preparation is examined under low-power and high-dry magnifications. The characteristic and strikingly large capsules of *Cryptococcus neoformans* show up well by this method. Material should be sent to a reference laboratory for confirmation by culture.

BLASTOMYCES DERMATITIDIS

Blastomycosis is almost always seen in dogs or people. It occurs most commonly in the northcentral and southeastern states of the United States. Granulomatous, discharging ulcers or abscesses usually form in the lungs with subsequent spread to other tissues and organs, including the skin. If material from these lesions, collected by syringe or scalpel, is examined on a wet mount made in 20% KOH, the characteristic yeast form of the organism can be seen. The cells of this dimorphic yeast are large (8 to 15 µ in diameter), oval or spherical, and thick walled. The single bud is connected to the mother cell by a wide base. This characteristic, together with the thick walls of the cells, is typical of *Blastomyces*. Immunologic tests and mouse inoculation can be used for identification; however, material from the granolomatous nodules should be submitted to a laboratory for confirmation by culture.

HISTOPLASMA CAPSULATUM

In the central United States, histoplasmosis is the most frequently encountered systemic infection in dogs. It is less common in other species, in which the infection can be subclinical. The disease should be suspected in dogs with chronic, intractable coughing and diarrhea. The cells of this dimorphic yeast are small (1 to 3 µ in diameter) and rarely found extracellularly and so are difficult to see in clinical material. Smears from tissue can be stained by the Giemsa or

Wright's method and examined under oil immersion. The organisms occur intracellularly, usually in monocytic cells, as small oval cells surrounded by a halo. The exoantigen test is an immunodiffusion test used by some laboratories for rapid identification of *Blastomyces dermatitidis, Histoplasma capsulatum,* and *Coccidioides immitis.* Confirmation should be made by submitting material for histopathologic examination and culture.

DERMATOPHYTES

Dermatophytes cause superficial mycoses. Ringworm can often be diagnosed by clinical signs. However, ringworm can manifest itself in several forms: subclinical or inapparent, which is quite common in young kittens and rodents; typical ringed lesions; and nodular or tumorous lesions called *kerions.* Ringworm lesions may have to be differentiated from other conditions that include mite or ectoparasite infestations; *Dermatophilus congolensis* infections in horses, cattle and sheep; pityriasis rosea, of unknown etiology, in pigs; and lesions due to hypersensitivity, especially in dogs.

Dermatophytes can be classified as to the habitat in which they are most likely to be found: *anthropophilic,* confined to people; *zoophilic,* parasites of animals; and *geophilic,* normally existing as free-living saprophytes in the soil. Of the 15 known geophilic species, five may occasionally be opportunist pathogens, and only one, *Microsporum gypseum,* commonly causes lesions in animals. These geophilic species pose a certain difficulty in diagnosis, as they must be differentiated from zoophilic species.

SPECIMEN COLLECTION

Hair should be plucked from the periphery of the lesion. A Wood's lamp may help detect hairs that are fluorescent although not all ringworm organisms cause fluorescence. Hairs cut with scissors give disappointing results, as the arthrospores are often at the base of the hairs and remain on the animal. Skin scrapings are taken with a blunt scalpel from the lesion's edge. Continue scraping until blood is just drawn.

Specimens from pigs, particularly, are often contaminated with saprophytic fungi. Lesions can be swabbed with 70% isopropyl alcohol and allowed to dry before specimens are taken.

Collect hairs and skin scrapings in paper envelopes. The specimens tend to stay drier and less contaminated in envelopes than when placed in a closed container.

DIAGNOSIS OF RINGWORM

WOOD'S LAMP EXAMINATION.   Hair samples from dogs and cats, or the animals themselves, should be examined under the Wood's (ultraviolet) lamp. Hairs infected with *Microsporum canis, M. distortum,* or *M. audouinii* (anthropophilic) may fluoresce a clear apple green under the Wood's lamp in a darkened room. About 60% of positive cases involving *M. canis* fluoresce. This seems to depend on whether the fungus has reached the right growth stage to produce fluorescence. No fluorescence on Wood's lamp examination does not rule out the possibility of ringworm infection.

DIRECT MICROSCOPY.   To establish a diagnosis of ringworm, the fungus must be demonstrated in the hairs by direct microscopy. This is particularly essential with geophilic species, such as *M. gypseum.* Its presence in culture alone may simply represent contamination from soil.

A few selected hairs and a little of the skin scrapings are placed in a drop of 20% KOH on a microscope slide. A coverslip is applied with gentle pressure and the preparation is gently heated and allowed to set for 10 to 15 minutes. Another procedure is to leave the preparation in a moist chamber for a few hours or overnight before examination.

Examine the wet preparation under the low-power objective and then under high dry for chains of the highly refractile arthrospores that sheathe infected hairs. These are at the roots of the hairs. The arthrospores of *Trichophyton verrucosum* (cattle) are particularly large (5 to 10 μ), whereas those of *M. canis* are about 2 to 3 μ.

Also mange mites can be observed in the cleared preparations. If scab material is present in samples from cattle, sheep, or horses, make a Gram-stained smear for *Dermatophilus congolensis.*

CULTURE.   *Trichophyton verrucosum* requires thiamin and inositol for growth, and *T. equinum* requires nicotinic acid. These growth factors can be supplied by adding yeast extract to the medium. Phytone yeast extract agar (BBL) is available in dehydrated powder form and supports growth of these two dermatophytes. It contains streptomycin and chloramphenicol, which control bacterial contaminants but not fungi. If you are routinely involved with dermatophyte specimens from horses or cattle, then prepared plates can be used, such as Mycosel agar (BBL) or Mycobiotic agar (Gibco). These contain chloramphenicol to suppress bacterial growth and cycloheximide to control saprophytic fungi. Dermatophytes are resistant to both antimicrobial agents.

Sabouraud dextrose agar is a more conventional medium for culture of dermatophytes. The low pH of about 5.6 inhibits most bacterial contaminants, but many saprophytic fungi grow on it. Prepared plates of Sabouraud dextrose agar are offered by BBL, Difco, Gibco, and Oxoid. An alternative would be to prepare Sabouraud dextrose agar from dehydrated powder and add Oxoid's SR75 Dermasel supplement, which contains cycloheximide and chloramphenicol. Shallow cuts with a sterile scalpel are made at eight separate sites on the agar plate. A few of the plucked hairs and/or skin scrapings are pushed gently into the agar at these sites.

The temperature of incubation should be 25° to 30° C for optimum growth of dermatophytes. If the temperature is consistently lower than 23° to 24° C, growth is slow and atypical. Although dermatophytes can be grown at a warm ambient temperature, incubating at 28° to 30° C is ideal for growth. For *T. verrucosum,* 37° C is recommended for more rapid growth; this temperature also suppresses growth of saprophytic fungi. Cultures should be incubated for up to 3 weeks for most dermatophytes and up to 6 weeks for the slower-growing species, such as *T. verrucosum.*

To avoid drying of the cultures, tape can be used to seal the plates. The tape should be removed and reapplied every 3 to 4 days, as dermatophytes are strict aerobes. The plates are incubated right side (lid) up to prevent spores from being liberated as the plates are opened.

IDENTIFICATION OF DERMATOPHYTES

Dermatophytes can usually be identified by colony morphology and by microscopic examination of colonies for macroaleuriospores (old name: macroconidia). Many dermatophytes have characteristically pigmented colonies (Table 4-20).

Suspect colonies should be microscopically examined for macroaleuriospores. A drop of lactophenol cotton blue is placed on a microscope slide. Some material from the center of the colony is teased out in the liquid using flamed mycology needles. The preparation is covered by a coverslip and examined under low-power and high-dry objectives. An easier way to examine for macroaleuriospores is to use the cellophane-tape method (see *Aspergillus fumigatus* above).

Some dermatophytes, such as *M. canis* and many *Trichophyton* species, are poor or slow macroaleuriospore producers. Any present will be found at the center of the colony. If none are seen on initial examination, it is worthwhile reincubating the culture or transferring a piece of thallus aseptically to cereal agar. Growth on this medium usually induces production of macroaleuriospores.

TABLE 4-20. Colony characteristics, macroaleuriospores, and main host(s) of some commonly isolated dermatophytes

DERMATOPHYTE AND MAIN HOST(S)	COLONY CHARACTERISTICS	MICROSCOPIC CHARACTERISTICS	
Microsporum canis Dogs, cats, occasionally other species	Comparatively rapid growth; flat colony; surface white and silky at center, with bright yellow periphery; reverse side is yellow	Some strains are poor producers of macroaleuriospores; when present, 8- to 15-celled, spindle-shaped and older spores ending in a distinct knob	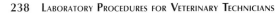
Microsporum gypseum Horses, wild rodents, occasionally other species	Comparatively rapid growth; colony flat, with irregularly fringed border; surface is coarsely powdery, light ochre to cinnamon brown; reverse is brownish yellow	Numerous macroaleuriospores; boat-shaped, 3- to 9-celled, walls rough, shorter, broader than those of *M. canis*	
Microsporum distortum Dogs, less common in cats	Growth comparatively rapid; colony flat with tendency to develop radial grooves; surface velvety or fluffy, white to tan; reverse is whitish to yellowish tan	Macroaleuriospores usually numerous and characteristically distorted	
Microsporum nanum Pigs, rare in other animals	Growth comparatively rapid; surface at first white and cottony, becoming granular, buff-colored; reverse is brownish red; colonies of some strains have fringed borders	Numerous macroaleuriospores; pear-shaped, 2-3 cells with relatively thin walls, characteristic for *M. nanum*	

Organism / Host	Colony characteristics	Microscopic characteristics
Trichophyton mentagrophytes Many species; most commonly dogs, guinea pigs, wild rodents, horses, pigs	Growth rapid; colony type varies from flat, granular and tan, rather like *M. gypseum*, to heaped and cottony white; reverse is yellowish to orange-brown	Granular colonies have numerous macroaleuriospores, cigar-shaped with 2-6 cells; often no macroaleuriospores from heaped colonies
Trichophyton verrucosum Cattle	Growth very slow, none may be obvious for 2 weeks; colony small, velvety and white; can later become heaped and folded	Macroaleuriospores are very rare, but at 37° C, thick-walled, rounded chlamydospores can be numerous
Trichophyton equinum Horses, less common in other animals	Growth quite rapid; colony flat, white at first with yellow in peripheral growth, later becoming velvety and cream to tan; reverse can be yellowish in young colony but later becomes dark brown	Macroaleuriospores are rare; if present they are the typical cigar shape of the *Trichophyton* genus

Development of macroaleuriospores may be monitored by preparing a slide culture as follows:

- Place a sterile piece of filter paper on the bottom of a sterile Petri dish. Wet the filter paper with sterile water.
- Place a bent glass rod on the filter paper (Figure 4-18).
- Pass a microscope slide through a flame several times to sterilize it. Then place the slide on the glass rod.
- Aseptically cut and remove a 1 × 1-cm block of the desired agar and place the agar block on the flamed slide.
- Inoculate the four sides of the agar block with spores or mycelial fragments of the fungus.
- Place the lid on the Petri dish and seal with Parafilm.
- Incubate at 28° C and check periodically under the microscope for growth and sporulation. Once sporulation has occurred, use forceps to

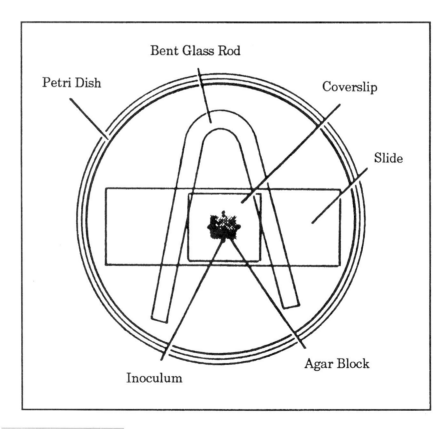

FIGURE 4-18. KOH preparation of a fungal sample.

carefully remove the coverglass from the agar block (do not slide it off; flip it off).

- Apply a drop of 95% ethanol to wet the fungus. Place a drop of lactophenol cotton blue on a clean slide, lower the coverslip onto it, and examine with the microscope.

A dermatophyte test medium in kit form is available from Difco and Pitman-Moore. This is a modified Sabouraud agar with a pH indicator, phenol red. Any dermatophytes present produce alkaline metabolites that change the yellowish medium to red, usually within 14 days.

With veterinary specimens, which contain numerous contaminant fungi, it is unwise to use dermatophyte test medium as the sole culture procedure. The slant provides too small an area on which to place clinical material. Some contaminant fungi also change the color of the medium, although not to the dark red produced by dermatophytes. However, this color change by dermatophytes masks the characteristic pigmentation of their colonies, which is used for identification.

Dermatophyte test medium can be used as a supplementary identification method, with the suspect dermatophyte subcultured onto the medium. Cut a small hollow in the middle of the dermatophyte test medium slant with a sterile scalpel. Using the same scalpel, cut a piece of mycelium from the edge of the colony and fit it snugly into the hollow in the dermatophyte test medium slant. Incubate the medium at 25° to 30° C for 7 to 14 days. A distinct red color in the medium indicates that the fungus may be a dermatophyte.

NONPATHOGENIC GEOPHILIC DERMATOPHYTES

The following three dermatophytes, which occur in soil, are common contaminants of animal hairs. They are considered nonpathogenic but must be differentiated from dermatophytes capable of causing ringworm:

- *Microsporum cookei.* The surface of the colony is cream colored and powdery, but the reverse is purple-red. Macroaleuriospores are abundant and very similar to those of *M. gypseum.*
- *Trichophyton ajelloi.* The surface of the colony is powdery and a rich orange-buff color. The reverse of the colony is violet-black although some strains have a pale yellow reverse. The abundant microaleuriospores are cigar shaped.
- *Trichophyton terrestre.* The colony has a powdery to granular surface, white to cream yellow in color. The reverse is pinkish or yellow. The macroaleuriospores are slender and pencil shaped.

SEROLOGIC DIAGNOSIS OF MYCOSES

Serologic diagnosis of mycoses in animals has received very little attention, although in people such tests are used to aid diagnosis and prognosis. Unfortunately, serologic diagnosis is not available to veterinarians through most human diagnostic laboratories. Most tests in human medicine are for systemic mycoses. These are *in vitro* procedures, including complement fixation, agglutination, and sometimes the precipitin test. Fluorescent antibody techniques have been developed for many fungi, usually to identify isolates rather than to measure antibody.

In vivo skin tests (delayed reaction, 24 to 48 hours) are used in human medicine for diagnosis of histoplasmosis, blastomycosis, coccidioidomycosis, and sporotrichosis. These tests also should be applicable to animals. Skin tests and exoantigen immunodiffusion tests for histoplasmosis have been used in dogs.

Recently, an agar gel immunodiffusion (AGID) test has been used on serum samples from dogs to confirm *Aspergillus fumigatus* infection of the nasal cavity. It is likely that AGID tests also will have application in diagnosing fungal upper respiratory infections in horses.

VIROLOGY

Virologic techniques are performed in specialized laboratories. They include histopathologic and serologic examination, electron microscopy, and attempted isolation and identification of the virus. Contact the diagnostic laboratory to check what facilities are available, what samples are preferred, and whether a transport medium is considered necessary. Table 4-21 indicates the types of specimens usually collected for diagnosis of the more common viral diseases of domestic animals. If an exotic (reportable) disease is suspected, the proper authorities should be notified and no clinical material removed from the farm.

Many of the viral diseases encountered can be diagnosed on clinical and pathologic grounds. Serologic tests are available for most viral diseases. These usually require paired serum samples collected 2 to 3 weeks apart, early in the disease and on recovery. A rising antibody titer indicates recent infection by the virus. Collection of serum samples from contact animals is worth considering, as these animals are more likely to have low initial titers to the virus.

Virus isolation is expensive and time consuming and may only provide a diagnosis after the animals have recovered or died. There are, however, instances when isolation and identification of a virus should be attempted: to

Text continued on p. 249.

TABLE 4-21. Common viral infections of domestic animals

VIRUS	DISEASE OR LESION	SPECIMENS
CATTLE		
Bovine herpesvirus 1	Infectious bovine rhinotracheitis and infectious pustular vaginitis	Mucosal scrapings; whole aborted fetus or fresh and fixed fetal kidney and liver; paired serum samples
Bovine herpesvirus 2	Bovine mammillitis; dermatitis, often hemorrhagic, of udder and teats, muzzle lesions in sucking calves	Vesicular fluid from early lesions or deep scrapings from older lesions; fixed biopsy; scabs of no value
Alcelaphine herpesvirus 1	Malignant catarrhal fever	Fixed liver, brain, kidney, lymph nodes, adrenals, and lesions from alimentary tract
Flavivirus	Bovine virus diarrhea-mucosal disease	Fresh spleen, lymph nodes and blood clot; serum; fixed portions of lesions
Retrovirus	Bovine leukosis	Lesions, fresh and fixed; EDTA blood
Picornaviruses	Enteroviruses: possible involvement in neonatal disease	Feces and serum
	Rhinoviruses: upper respiratory tract infection	Nasal mucosal scrapings
	Foot and mouth disease virus: lesions	Vesicular fluid; serum
Parvovirus	Diarrhea in young calves	Feces
Reoviruses	Respiratory and enteric conditions in young calves	Nasal mucosal scraping; feces; serum
	Bovine rotavirus: associated with diarrhea in young calves	Feces

Continued.

TABLE 4-21—CONT'D

VIRUS	DISEASE OR LESION	SPECIMENS
Adenoviruses	May cause upper respiratory tract infections	Nasal scrapings
Paramyxovirus	Parainfluenza 3: upper respiratory tract infections and occasionally pneumonia Rinderpest virus: profuse diarrhea	Nasal scrapings; whole blood; lung Serum
Papilloma virus	Papillomas (warts)	Fixed and fresh excised tumors
Poxviruses	Pseudocowpox (paravacinia, milker's nodules); dermatitis on udder and teats with "horseshoe" scab formation Papular stomatitis: ulcers in buccal cavity and lips, mainly in calves	Deep scrapings of early lesions Deep scrapings of several oral ulcers; fixed tissue from lesion

HORSES

Herpesvirus	Herpesvirus 1: rhinopneumonitis; abortion	Nasal scraping; fresh, whole aborted fetus or fresh and fixed fetal liver; kidney and lung
	Herpesvirus 2: upper respiratory tract of normal horses; pathogenicity uncertain Herpesvirus 3: coital exanthema; venereal vulvitis or balanitis	Deep scrapings of lesions
Papilloma virus	Papillomas (warts)	Fresh and fixed excised tumors
Orthomyxovirus	Influenza virus: upper respiratory tract infection and occasionally pneumonia	Nasal scrapings; lung; whole blood

Paramyxovirus	Parainfluenza; upper respiratory tract infection	Nasal scrapings from very early cases; serum
Picornavirus	Rhinoviruses: upper respiratory tract infection, mainly in young horses	Nasal scrapings and exudates
Togaviruses	Arteritis; edema of the limbs and eyes; abortion	Nasal or conjunctival exudates in transport medium (Hanks' with antibiotics and 1% bovine albumin; store at $-20°$ C)
	Western, eastern, and Venezuelan equine encephalomyelitis	Fresh and Fixed brain

SHEEP

Herpesvirus	Adenomatosis: chronic progressive lung disease in sheep >4 yr; no metastases	Fixed lung lesion
Paramyxovirus	Parainfluenza 3: signs referable to respiratory tract, with pneumonia in young animals	Nasal scrapings very early in disease; isolation often difficult from pneumonic lesions; serum
Picornavirus	Foot and mouth disease	Vesicular fluid; serum
Togavirus (closely related to BVD virus of cattle)	Border disease of lambs or "hairy shaker" disease: neonatal condition; hairy coat, nervous signs, poor growth	Serum
Poxvirus	Contagious pustular dermatitis; orf; scabby-mouth disease	Scabs and scrapings from young lesions; fixed lesions
Rotavirus	Diarrhea in lambs	Feces and serum

Continued.

Table 4-21 —Cont'd

Virus	Disease or Lesions	SPECIMENS
Pigs		
Herpesvirus	Inclusion-body rhinitis (porcine cytomegalovirus): deaths in pigs <2 wk old; subacute in older pigs	Whole, recently dead pig carcass or sick live pig; head of older pigs or fixed nasal mucosa
	Pseudorabies (Aujeszky's disease): respiratory infections and abortions	Lesions from recently dead pigs; serum
	Vesicular disease	Vesicular fluid
Picornavirus	Talfan or Teschen's disease: porcine poliomyelitis	Fresh and fixed whole brain; serum
	Encephalomyocarditis: sudden death in pigs >12 wk old	Recently dead pigs or fresh heart, spleen; fixed heart and brain; serum
	SMEDI viruses: stillbirths, mummification, embryonic deaths, infertility	Aborted fetuses; serum
	Enteroviruses: possible involvement in neonatal diarrhea	Feces; serum
	Foot and mouth disease	Vesicular fluid; serum
Parvovirus	Reproductive failure	Freshly aborted fetuses, especially mummified fetuses; serum
Rotavirus	Acute gastroenteritis in piglets	Feces
Orthomyxovirus	Influenza A: bronchopneumonia and lung edema	Respiratory exudates or lung; serum
Coronaviruses	Transmissible gastroenteritis: vomiting and diarrhea in sows and young pigs	Live affected piglets or fresh and fixed small intestine; serum; feces are valueless
	Hemagglutinating encephalomyelitis: vomiting, wasting, and constipation in young pigs	Live affected piglets or fresh and fixed brain; serum

Cats

Herpesvirus 1	Herpesvirus serotype 1: rhinotracheitis; occasionally abortion in queens and some fatalities in neonates	Nasal scrapings early in disease
	Herpesvirus-induced feline urolithiasis	Diagnosis by clinical signs
Parvovirus	Panleukopenia or feline infections enteritis: congenital abnormalities, such as cerebellar hypoplasia	Fresh spleen, fixed portions of intestine, lymph nodes, thymus, bone marrow; EDTA blood

Dogs

Herpesvirus	Deaths in neonatal pups; may be cause of "fading puppy syndrome"; rhinitis and pharyngitis in pups >6 wk old; vaginitis and abortion	Whole puppy carcass or fresh and fixed kidney, spleen, lungs, liver and nasopharynx; serum
Rhabdovirus	Rabies	Consult with state veterinarian
Papilloma virus	Oral papillomas (warts)	Fixed and fresh excised tumors
Paramyxoviruses	Canine distemper (hard-pad disease)	Fresh whole lung; fixed lung, brain, bladder, kidney, liver, gallbladder
	Parainfluenza: upper respiratory tract infection	Respiratory exudates
Adenoviruses	Infectious canine hepatitis (canine adenovirus 1): Rubarth's disease; hepatitis and death, especially in young pups	Whole puppy carcass or fresh nasopharyngeal scraping, and fresh and fixed lung, kidney, spleen, liver, brain; feces and urine from live pups; serum

Continued.

TABLE 4-21—CONT'D

VIRUS	DISEASE OR LESION	SPECIMENS
	Canine adenovirus 2: upper respiratory tract infection; occasionally causes pneumonia (infectious tracheobronchitis)	Nasal swab and scrapings; fresh and fixed lung
Parvoviruses	Enteritis, myocarditis, leukopenia; closely related to feline panleukopenia virus	Fresh feces; serum; mesenteric lymph nodes; ileum; spleen
Coronavirus	Vomiting, diarrhea	Feces
Reovirus	Reovirus (1 and 2) infection: usually mild upper respiratory infection	Nasal exudate; feces
Rotavirus	Gastroenteritis in young pups	Feces

BIRDS, POULTRY

Herpesvirus	Infectious laryngo-tracheitis: severe dyspnea, coughing	Tracheal exudate
	Marek's disease: nervous signs, paralysis	Liver, lungs, tissues, blood, bone marrow
Retrovirus	Avian leukosis: tumorous enlargement of liver and spleen	Spleen, liver
Picornavirus	Encephalomyelitis, paresis, sitting on hock	Brain, gizzard, spinal cord
Reovirus	Infectious bursal disease, swelling of cloacal bursa, edema	Feces, kidney, bursal tissue
Paramyxovirus	Paramyxovirus I: Newcastle disease	Exudate, serum
Poxvirus	Respiratory/nervous signs Fowl pox: Nodules in skin, heavy scabs	Vesicular fluid, scab scrapings

establish the identity of a viral disease not previously seen in a practice; to discover the exact agent when serologic and other tests have given equivocal results; to find the immunologic type of a virus in an epizootic; and to verify the etiologic agent if a public health problem is involved.

Isolation of a virus from a diseased animal does not necessarily mean the virus caused the disease, as many viruses can persist in animals without clinical signs of illness. Some other pathogen or condition could have been responsible for the disease. Virus isolation is most successful when specimens are collected early in the active infectious phase of the disease.

Viruses vary greatly in their ability to remain viable in tissues and exudates. Contamination with bacteria greatly decreases the success of attempted virus isolation. The general rules are:

- Collect specimens that are likely to contain large numbers of virus particles.
- Take specimens from live or very recently dead animals, even if this means sacrificing an affected animal.
- Collect specimens aseptically.
- Keep specimens at 4° C and get them to a laboratory in the shortest time possible.

COLLECTION OF SPECIMENS

Viruses are often present in the nasal or pharyngeal secretions early in the acute stage of respiratory diseases. Take mucosal scrapings rather than just swabs of the secretions. Sterile wooden tongue depressors are useful for mucosal scrapings. Attempted isolation from blood samples might be considered in generalized catarrhal diseases that tend to have a viremic stage. Poxviruses can often be demonstrated by electron microscopy in fluid from early vesicular lesions and sometimes in scabs from early lesions.

Do not neglect to also select specimens for indirect studies, such as serologic, hematologic, histologic, and bacteriologic examinations. Viral diseases are often complicated by pathogenic bacteria acting as secondary invaders. These can often turn a mild viral infection into a serious disease. Specimens for histopathologic examination should consist of thin sections of tissue placed immediately into 10% formalin. Sections for histologic examination must never be frozen, as this causes tissue artifacts that may be difficult to differentiate from a pathologic process.

Tissue samples for attempted virus isolation should be 2-inch cubes that contain both diseased and normal tissue, if possible. Obtain mucosal scrapings instead of merely swabs. Sterile screw-capped containers should be used for collection, using a separate container for each sample. Employ strict asepsis and label the containers carefully.

SUBMISSION OF SAMPLES

Specimens should be refrigerated (4° C) when possible, as virus titers decrease as temperature increases. If the specimens will be delivered to the virology laboratory within 24 hours, they can be stored at 4° C and packed with coolant packs or ice in a polystyrene-insulated carton for shipment. If there will be more than 24 hours' delay, snap freezing at −70° C and shipping on dry ice is desirable, except for specimens of suspected parainfluenza and influenza virus, in which case the integrity of these viruses is best preserved at −20° C. Specimens must be shipped in airtight containers to prevent entry of CO_2 into the container. CO_2 gas from the dry ice can lower the pH of fluid, killing any pH-labile viruses.

Small pieces of tissue, fecal material, or mucus can be preserved in vials filled with 50% glycol and stored at 4° C. A virus transport medium is available commercially (NCS Diagnostics). Because viruses vary in their longevity, it is best to contact a reference laboratory for recommendations on the appropriate transport medium and sampling procedure.

Fecal materials and fluids often are submitted for electron microscopic examination. A fixative, such as universal or 10% buffered neutral formalin, should be added to the sample at a maximum of 1:1 fixative to sample to prevent overdilution of virus particles.

For urine samples, send approximately 5 ml in a sterile container. Do not use virus transport medium. Keep the specimen chilled if it is to arrive at the laboratory within 24 hours of collection; otherwise, freeze at −70° C and ship frozen.

If blood samples have been collected for serologic examination, leave them at room temperature and allow the clot to retract; then refrigerate them. Do not freeze blood samples, as freezing causes hemolysis and may render serum samples useless for serologic examination.

CELL CULTURE

To demonstrate the presence of a virus in a specimen, the virus is grown (isolated) in the laboratory or the virus antigens or antibodies are assayed. Unlike bacteria, which can be grown on nutrient agar, viruses need living cells in which to grow and replicate.

The tissue cells are placed into a suitable glass bottle or chamber containing a medium rich in nutrients. The cells settle and begin to grow in a confluent monolayer across the surface of the container.

Various types of cells have been used for tissue culture of viruses. Most animal cells can be grown *in vitro* for some generations, but some cells divide indefinitely and are used for virus isolation. These cells are called *continuous cell lines* and are of a single type of cell. Continuous cell lines, such as those from fetal kidney, embryonic trachea, skin and other cells, are derived from monkeys, dogs, cattle, pigs, cats, mice, hamsters, rabbits, and other animals. The virus specimen is commonly inoculated into a primary culture of cells derived from the same species of animal from which the specimen was taken.

After the cell culture has been inoculated with the virus specimen and incubated, the cell culture is examined. If the virus is present, cell damage may be visible as the virus particles invade the tissue cells. This damage is referred to as a *cytopathic effect*. Different types of cytopathic effects are used to identify viruses. Some viruses cause cell lysis, while others cause the cells to fuse and form syncytiae (sheets) and giant cells. An inclusion body is another type of cytopathic effect that may be seen.

EMBRYONATED EGG CULTURES

Embryonated eggs are a valuable medium for cultivation of viruses. Although embryonated eggs are very convenient for growing viruses, the range of viruses that can be grown in them is somewhat limited.

Canine distemper virus and poxviruses are grown on chorioallantoic membranes, producing pox lesions that are visible to the naked eye. Influenza virus grows initially in the amnionic sac and then in the allantoic cavity, causing death of the embryo in 48 to 72 hours. Newcastle disease virus grows in the allantoic cavity, causing death of the embryo in 48 to 72 hours.

SEROLOGIC EXAMINATION

Clinical signs and cell culture examination may identify the virus to a family level and perhaps to the genus and species level as well, but definitive identification requires serologic procedures based on immunologic principles. Sometimes these serologic procedures may be used on the specimens directly, which saves the time and expense of cell culture.

DIRECT IMMUNOFLUORESCENCE

In this type of test, an antibody to a specific virus, such as rabies virus, is labelled with a fluorescent dye and is added to the specimen. If virus antigen is present in the specimen, the antibody binds to it (Figure 4-19). If the virus antigen is not present, the antibody is washed away in the rinsing step of the

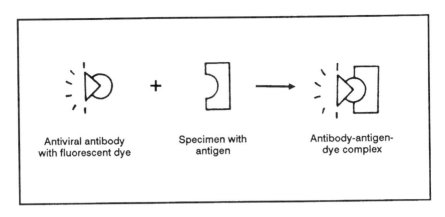

FIGURE **4-19.** With direct immunofluorescence, antiviral antibody labeled with a flourescent dye is added to the specimen, forming an antibody-antigen-dye complex.

procedure. Upon microscopic examination, any antibody-antigen complex is visible as fluorescence.

INDIRECT IMMUNOFLUORESCENCE

An indirect procedure using two antibodies is also used. Antiviral antibodies, called *immunoglobulins,* are produced in an animal, such as a rabbit. The second antibody is an antirabbit immunoglobulin labeled with the fluorescent dye. The second antibody binds to the first antibody, which binds to any virus antigen in

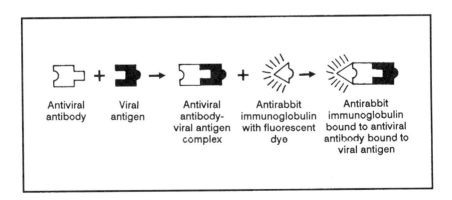

FIGURE **4-20.** With indirect immunofluorescence, antibody forms a complex with the virus anitgen, which then binds with antirabbit immunoglobin and the fluorescent dye.

the specimen (Figure 4-20). This complex is then detected on microscopic examination.

If no virus antigen is present in the specimen, there is no binding and the unbound dye is washed away. This technique has some advantages over the direct fluorescent technique, including increased sensitivity. An example of a disease diagnosed by this method is cryptosporidiosis.

RADIOIMMUNOASSAY

In this procedure, the label is a radioactive element, such as iodine. This radioactive label is attached to an antiviral antibody that combines with virus antigen in the specimen (Figure 4-21). A gamma counter is needed to detect the presence of the antibody-antigen complexes. Thyroid hormone levels are measured by this method.

ENZYME-LINKED IMMUNOSORBENT ASSAY

This type of test (ELISA) uses test trays containing antibody-coated wells. The sample is added to the wells and any virus antigen binds to the antibody. A second antiviral antibody is then added; this antibody is enzyme-labeled. If virus was present in the sample and was bound to the antibody that coated the well, the second antibody also binds to the virus. When a substrate that reacts with the enzyme is added, the resultant color change is proportional to the amount of virus antigen present in the sample (Figure 4-22). If there was no virus in the

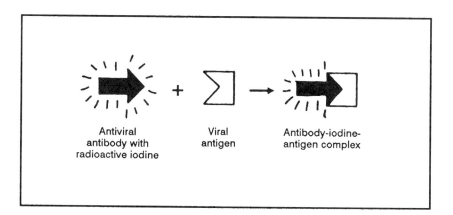

FIGURE **4-21.** In radioimmunoassay, antiviral antibody labeled with a radioactive element, such as iodine, is added to the specimen, forming an antibody-iodine-antigen complex.

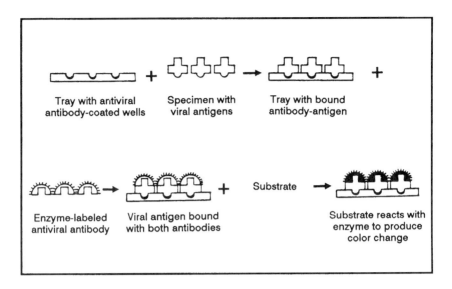

FIGURE 4-22.   With enzyme-linked immunosorbent assay, viral antigens bind with antibody in the test wells, an enzyme-labeled antiviral antibody is added, and finally a substrate is added to produce a color change.

sample, the second antibody is washed away in the rinsing process and no color change is seen. Feline leukemia virus is detected with this method.

IMMUNODIFFUSION

With immunodiffusion, antigen in the specimen and antibody are placed into separate wells in agar. They diffuse into the agar and form a visible band of precipitation when they combine (Figure 4-23). If no band forms, there is no virus antigen present in the sample. Bovine leukemia virus is detected by immunodiffusion.

COMPLEMENT FIXATION

Complement is a series of enzymes in normal serum that combine with an antibody-antigen complex to cause lysis of cells, destruction of bacteria, and other immune responses. In complement fixation, complement becomes "fixed" when it combines with an antibody-antigen complex. The complement fixation test is used to detect viral antibodies in a serum sample, as in anaplasmosis.

The patient's serum sample is heated to inactivate its complement. A known amount of complement is added to the serum. A known amount of virus

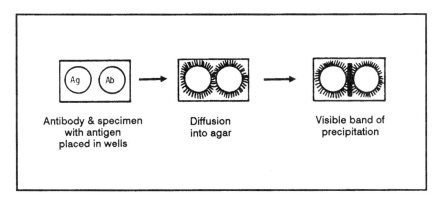

Figure 4-23.   In immunodiffusion, antigen and antibody in separate wells diffuse out into the agar and form a visible precipitate where they meet.

antigen is then added and this mixture is incubated to allow fixation of the complement if virus antibodies are present in the serum. Sensitized RBCs (RBCs that have complexed with anti-RBC antibodies) are then added and the mixture is incubated. If virus antibody is present in the serum, viral antibody-viral antigen complexes are formed and there is no lysis of the RBCs. Complement was "fixed" and was not available to lyse RBCs. If no virus antibody is present in the serum, complexes of anti-RBC antibody–RBC antigen and complement are formed, and the RBCs are lysed (Figure 4-24).

VIRUS NEUTRALIZATION IN CELL CULTURE
Two types of virus neutralization techniques are used: inhibition of cytopathic effects and plaque reduction. Before doing these tests, it must be known that the virus in the sample causes cytopathic effects or plaque formation. By using a specific antibody, the virus can then be identified. Bovine virus diarrhea is diagnosed by virus neutralization.

INHIBITION OF CYTOPATHIC EFFECTS.   A specific antibody to a particular virus is incubated with a specimen that contains the unidentified virus. Cell culture tubes are then inoculated with this mixture and checked daily for cytopathic effects. Complete inhibition of cytopathic effects is considered a positive virus neutralization test and indicates the identity of the virus. The virus in the specimen formed a complex with the added antibody and was unable to cause cytopathic effects. If cytopathic effects are produced, the particular virus tested is ruled out.

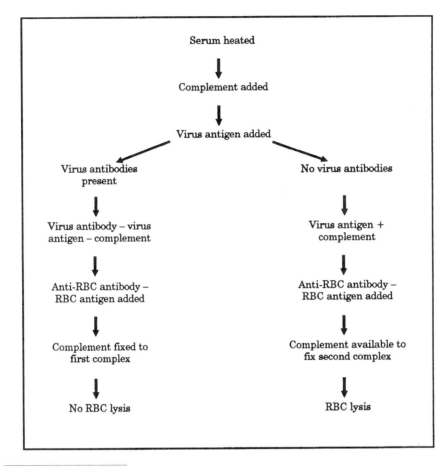

FIGURE 4-24. Complement fixation test shows no RBC lysis if virus antibody is present.

PLAQUE REDUCTION. The specimen containing the unidentified virus is incubated with antibody for a particular virus. Cell culture tubes are then inoculated with this mixture and incubated again. An agar medium containing a dye is added and incubated, and the culture is observed daily for the presence and numbers of plaques, which are necrotic cells surrounded by living cells. Necrotic cells do not pick up the dye and are colorless, while living cells are stained by the dye. An 80% or greater reduction of plaque counts is positive and confirms the identity of the virus. The specific antibody has formed a complex with the virus, preventing it from forming plaques.

Electron microscopy

The two basic techniques for routine diagnostic use of electron microscopy are negative staining of virus particles and thin-sectioning of virus-infected cells. Electron microscopy can be used to identify viruses to the family level and sometimes to the genus or species level. Parvovirus can be detected by electron microscopy.

Negative staining. A virus suspension made from a clinical sample is mixed with a heavy-metal stain. The heavy-metal atoms surround the virus particles. The electron beam of the electron microscope passes through the virus particles but cannot pass through the metal atoms. This gives the appearance of a "negative stain," that is, the virus is light and "unstained" and the surrounding background of metallic atoms is dark and appears "stained."

Thin sectioning. This technique uses the intact virus-infected cells, which are examined with the electron microscope. It gives a more reliable diagnosis than simple negative staining of the clinical sample because tissues from the animal or inoculated tissue cell culture are used, and the virus and the cell it is infecting are both preserved for examination. This complex procedure consists of several preparatory steps and includes the negative-staining step.

Immunoelectron microscopy

With this technique, monoclonal or polyclonal antibodies are added to a virus suspension made from the clinical specimen. If the corresponding virus antigens are present in the suspension, antibody-antigen complexes form. The suspension is centrifuged and combined with a heavy-metal stain and then applied to an electron microscope grid for examination using the negative-staining procedure.

Antibody is added to increase the likelihood of seeing virus particles. The complexes or aggregates are more easily seen than a few individual virus particles, especially when virus concentration is low. Coronavirus may be detected by this method.

Direct detection of viral nucleic acid

In this research technique, DNA strands of a virus are separated and one of the strands is labeled with a radioactive isotope or a nonradioactive label. The labeled "probes" are added to separated strands of viral DNA from cells infected with the unknown virus. Under appropriate conditions, the two strands combine with each other if they are from the same virus. Because one of the strands is labeled, it can be detected and the identity of the virus is confirmed.

RECOMMENDED READING

Carter: *Diagnostic procedures in veterinary bacteriology and mycology,* ed 4, Springfield, IL, 1984, Charles C Thomas.

Carter, Chengappa: *Essentials of veterinary bacteriology and mycology,* ed 4, Philadelphia, 1991, Lea & Febiger.

Castro, Heuschele: *Veterinary diagnostic virology,* St Louis, 1992, Mosby.

Cottral: *Manual of standardized methods for veterinary microbiology,* Ithaca, NY, 1978, Comstock Publishing.

Fenner et al: *Veterinary virology,* Orlando, 1987, Academic Press.

Ikram, Hill: *Microbiology for veterinary technicians,* St Louis, 1991, Mosby.

Quinn et al: *Clinical veterinary microbiology,* St Louis, 1994, Mosby.

URINALYSIS

J.G. Zinkl

Urinalysis is a relatively simple, rapid, and inexpensive laboratory procedure. With a minimal investment in laboratory equipment and reagents, the veterinary technician can perform a complete urinalysis that provides a wealth of information regarding not only the urinary tract, but other body systems as well.

SPECIMEN COLLECTION

The first step in performing a urinalysis is proper collection of a urine sample. It is of utmost importance that this be done carefully to ensure meaningful results. There are four basic methods for collecting a urine sample: cystocentesis, catheterization, expressing the bladder, and natural voiding of the urine (urination). The two preferred methods are cystocentesis and catheterization; these methods provide optimum samples for all aspects of urinalysis by avoiding contamination from the distal genital tract and external areas. It may be easier to collect samples by voiding or expression of the bladder, but urine collected in these ways may be of limited diagnostic value. Except for cytologic examination, it is best to perform a urinalysis on preprandial morning samples. Morning samples tend to be the most concentrated, which increases the chances of finding abnormalities.

VOIDED SAMPLE

The simplest sample to obtain is the voided sample, collected as the animal urinates. A sample collected in this manner is not satisfactory for bacteriologic examination, as it is often contaminated during urination. Occasionally, voided samples contain increased white blood cell counts due to contamination from

259

inflammatory lesions of the distal genital tract. Results of other evaluations are unaffected.

A voided sample is collected in a clean, although not necessarily sterile, container. Before collection, the vulva or prepuce should be washed to decrease contamination of the sample. A mid-urination (mid-stream) sample is best, as there is less chance that it will be contaminated. Sometimes the initially voided urine is collected as a precaution against not being able to collect a mid-urination sample.

Dogs may begin to urinate and then stop when collection is attempted. Chances of success may be increased by attaching a paper cup to a long pole and collecting the sample without disturbing the animal. A voided sample from a cat is difficult to obtain. Occasionally, cats urinate into an empty litter pan in a cage devoid of papers. Cows may be stimulated to urinate by rubbing a hand or dry hay ventral to the vulva in a circular fashion. Horses may be stimulated by rubbing a wet, warm cloth on their ventral abdomen.

EXPRESSING THE BLADDER

Urine may be collected in small animals by manual compression of the bladder. Samples obtained in this manner are usually unsatisfactory for bacteriologic culturing. As for collection of a voided sample, the external genitalia should be cleaned before bladder expression. With the animal standing or in lateral recumbency, one palpates the bladder in the caudal abdomen. Urine is expelled with gentle, steady pressure. Care must be taken not to exert too much pressure and injure or rupture the bladder. One must be patient, as relaxation of the bladder sphincters often takes a few minutes. This method should never be used on animals whose urethra may be obstructed.

In large animals, urination may be stimulated by maintaining pressure on the bladder through the rectal wall while performing rectal palpation.

CATHETERIZATION

Catheterization is the insertion of a catheter into the bladder via the urethra. Catheters of rubber, plastic or metal may be used. As with the previous two methods of collection, the external genitalia should be cleaned before the procedure. Sterile catheters should always be used and sterile gloves worn. Care must be taken to maintain sterility and prevent trauma to the urinary tract. The catheter should pass easily through the urethra. A small amount of sterile, water-soluble lubricating jelly, such as K-Y Jelly (Johnson & Johnson), should be placed on the tip of the catheter. Care must be taken to avoid trauma to the sensitive urethral mucosa. The distal end of many catheters is designed for attachment to a syringe, and urine can be collected with gentle aspiration. Collection into a sterile syringe is especially advantageous if bacteriologic culture is anticipated. Often the first portion of the sample obtained is discarded because of possible contamination as the catheter was advanced through the distal urethra (Procedure 5-1).

CYSTOCENTESIS

Cystocentesis is often used to collect sterile urine samples from dogs and cats (Figure 5-1 and 5-2). This is only done when the bladder is full, to avoid damage to other internal organs. Sometimes as much urine as possible is removed from the bladder to prevent pressure on the bladder wall and leakage of urine though the hole created by the needle. However, unless the bladder is markedly extended, a volume sufficient to perform urinalysis and possibly culture (5 to 10 ml) can be removed without damaging the bladder or causing urine to leak through its wall (Procedure 5-2).

All of the above methods of collection are satisfactory for qualitative analysis. However, for quantitative analysis, a 24-hour sample must be collected. Recently, ratios of certain urine constituents (e.g., protein) to creatinine have been used to obtain data that can be interpreted in a similar manner to 24-hour urinary excretions.

QUALITY ASSURANCE

Quality assurance begins with proper specimen identification and handling. All samples should be labeled immediately after collection, and urinalysis should be performed soon after the sample is collected. Reagent strips and tablets must be kept in tightly sealed bottles, and outdated reagents must be replaced with fresh reagents. Reactions for most constituents in urine can be checked against available controls (e.g., Chek-Stix: Miles Laboratories; Uritrol: Harleco; Liquid Urine Control: Alta Diagnostics: Laguna Hills, CA). In addition, urine samples with distinct reactions for certain constituents can sometimes be preserved and used as positive controls. The results obtained from control samples and

PROCEDURE 5-1.   Methods for catheterization of the urinary bladder

MALE DOGS

1. The patient is placed in a standing position, and the operator should stand on the right side of the patient. Catheterization can also be performed with the patient in lateral recumbency. (Left-handed technicians should stand on the left side of the dog. All the activities should be performed with the opposite hand in the directions given below.)
2. Retract the prepuce with the right hand.
3. Gently clean the tip of the penis with a dilute solution of benzalkonium chloride. Dry the tip of the penis with cotton sponges.
4. Apply a small amount of sterile gel (K-Y jelly) to the lead end of a sterile polypropylene urinary catheter (5-, 8- or 10-French). Place the catheter in the external orifice of the penis. The catheter can be wrapped to prevent contamination.
5. Slowly advance the catheter until urine flows from the end or urine can be aspirated with a syringe.
6. Immediately label the syringe or tube with patient identification information using indelible ink.

FEMALE DOGS

1. The patient is placed in a standing position on a table, and the operator should stand behind the patient.
2. An assistant holds the tail up so that it does not interfere with the procedure. The assistant can also support and restrain the patient.
3. Clip or comb any long hair around the vulva so that it will not touch the catheter.
4. Clean and dry the vulva as above.
5. Gently dilate the vulva with a vaginal or nasal speculum to see the urethral orifice.
6. Place the tip of a lubricated, sterile catheter (reusable metal bitch, 10-French, or Foley catheter) in the orifice.
7. Slowly advance the catheter until urine flows from the end or urine can be aspirated with a syringe.
8. Immediately label the syringe or tube with patient identification information using indelible ink.

MALE CATS

1. The patient is restrained in dorsal recumbency, and the operator should stand on the right side or behind the patient.
2. With the fingers of the left hand, retract the prepuce and extrude the penis.
3. Clean and dry the penis as above.
4. Insert a lubricated, 3.5-French catheter or a Sovereign tom cat catheter into the external orifice.
5. Gently advance the catheter using a rotary motion until urine flows from the end or urine can be aspirated with a syringe.
6. Immediately label the syringe or tube with patient identification information using indelible ink.

FEMALE CATS

1. The patient is restrained in sternal recumbency, and the operator should stand to the rear of the patient.
2. Clean and dry the external surface of the vulva as above.
3. Advance a small bitch catheter or a lubricated, 5-, 8- or 10-French catheter into the vagina while exerting gentle downward pressure on the catheter tip.
4. Because this is a blind procedure, gently advance the catheter and retract it until it enters the urethra.
5. Slowly advance the catheter until urine flows from the end or urine can be aspirated with a syringe.
6. Immediately label the syringe or tube with patient identification information using indelible ink.

MALE HORSES

1. Both stallions and geldings can be catheterized to obtain urine.
2. The operator, whether right- or left-handed, should stand on the left side of the patient because horses are used to being handled from this side. Foals may be placed in lateral recumbency.
3. Retract the prepuce and expose the tip of the penis.
4. Wash and dry the tip of the penis.
5. Insert into the urethral orifice a lubricated, 22- to 32-French rubber catheter of sufficient length to reach the bladder.
6. Slowly advance the catheter until urine flows from the end of the catheter into an appropriate collecting vessel.
7. Immediately label the vessel or tube with patient identification information using indelible ink.

FEMALE HORSES

1. The operator stands to the rear of the patient. For safety the horse should be in a stanchion that allows the operator access to the vulva.
2. Wash and dry the vulva.
3. Guide a metal mare catheter, held under the index finger, into the urethral orifice through the vulva into the vagina.
4. Slowly advance the catheter until urine flows from the end of the catheter into an appropriate collecting vessel.
5. Immediately label the vessel or tube with patient identification information using indelible ink.

MALE CATTLE

Male cattle are difficult or impossible to catheterize.

FEMALE CATTLE

1. The operator stands to the rear of the patient. The cow should be restrained in a head stanchion or a chute. Calves can be placed in lateral recumbency for ease of catheterization.
2. Wash and dry the vulva.
3. Guide a catheter into the urethral orifice using a speculum or by holding it under the index finger.
4. As often as necessary, gently move and probe the urethral orifice to advance the catheter because cows have a urethral diverticulum near the orifice into which the catheter frequently passes.
5. Slowly advance the catheter until urine flows from the end of the catheter into an appropriate collecting vessel.
6. Immediately label the vessel or tube with patient identification information using indelible ink.

made-up controls should be plotted to determine if observer drift or reagent decomposition is occurring. Technicians gain confidence when they obtain results that are consistent from day to day. Further, veterinarians feel more confident in results that are generated in a laboratory that has a quality assurance program.

SPECIMEN PRESERVATION

Ideally, samples should be analyzed within 30 minutes of collection to avoid post-collection artifacts and degenerative changes. If immediate analysis is not

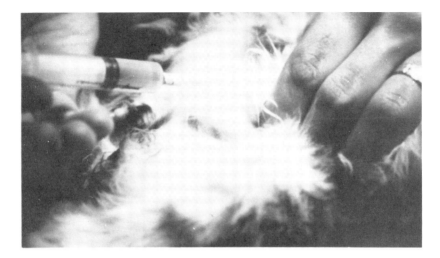

FIGURE 5-1.   Cystocentesis in a cat.

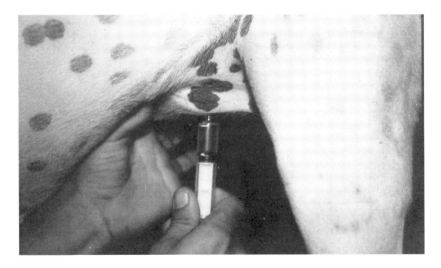

FIGURE 5-2.   Cystocentesis in a dog.

possible, refrigeration will preserve most urine constituents for an additional 6 to 12 hours. Samples should be warmed to room temperature before evaluation. Cytologic features tend to deteriorate rapidly in urine. If cytologic evaluation is to be performed, the urine should be centrifuged immediately and 1 to 2 drops of the patient's serum or bovine albumin added to the sediment to preserve cell morphology.

PROCEDURE 5-2. Methods for antepubic cystocentesis

EQUIPMENT

No specialized equipment is needed for obtaining urine by cystocentesis.

1. Sterile 1- or 1.5-inch, 22- or 23-gauge needles (never larger than 20-gauge needles) should be used.
2. Sterile 5- or 10-ml syringes (although occasionally large amounts of urine may be aspirated for therapeutic reasons) are sufficient for urinalysis.

METHOD

The method is similar for dogs and cats and only slightly different for males and females.

1. If the operator is right handed, the patient is placed in a standing position with its head toward the operator's left. (For a left-handed operator, all the activities should be performed with the opposite hand in the directions given below.) Very small animals and most cats may have to be placed in lateral recumbency to provide sufficient space to operate a syringe.
2. In most dogs and cats the caudoventral abdomen is relatively free of hair. Occasionally, a small amount of hair must be clipped from the area into which the needle will be inserted.
3. Clean the area with soap and water and dry with a cotton sponge.
4. Palpate the bladder and gently hold in place against the ventrolateral abdominal wall with the left hand.
5. Insert the needle in a caudodorsal direction toward the midline.
   - For male dogs, insert the needle caudal to the umbilicus and to the side of the sheath.
   - For female dogs and for cats, insert the needle on the ventral midline caudal to the umbilicus.
6. Gently aspirate urine into the syringe. Occasionally it may be necessary to slightly alter the position of the needle by gently turning the syringe to maintain urine flow.
7. Immediately label the syringe or tube with patient identification information using indelible ink.
8. If urine is not obtained, completely withdraw the needle and use another sterile needle and syringe to attempt the process again.

Decreased glucose and bilirubin concentrations, increased pH due to bacterial breakdown of urea to ammonia, crystal formation with increased sample turbidity, disintegration of casts and RBCs (especially in dilute or alkaline urine), and bacterial proliferation may occur in samples allowed to stand for long periods at room temperature. Crystals may form in refrigerated samples.

Refrigerated urine should be warmed to room temperature before determining the specific gravity and before microscopic evaluation of crystals. If a sample is to be mailed to an outside laboratory or held for longer than 6 to 12 hours, it may be preserved by addition of one of the following: 1 drop of 40% formalin in 1 oz of urine; toluene sufficient to form a layer on top of the sample; a single thymol crystal; or 1 part 5% phenol to 9 parts urine. If formalin is to be used as a preservative, chemical tests should be performed before addition of formalin because it interferes with some chemical analyses, especially that for glucose. Formalin, however, is the best preservative for formed elements in urine.

GROSS EXAMINATION

Gross examination includes all of the observations that can be made without the aid of a microscope or chemical reagents (Procedure 5-3).

URINE VOLUME

Information concerning the amount of urine passed is often provided by the animal's owner. However, owners may mistake frequent urination (*pollakiuria*) for increased urine production (*polyuria*). Therefore it is important to obtain an estimate of the amount of urine an animal is producing. Many factors influence the amount of urine produced, including water intake, environmental temperature, food intake, level of physical activity, size of the animal, and species. Observing a single urination is not reliable for estimating urine output of an animal. Ideally, twenty-four-hour urine volume should be determined. However, this is often impractical. Observing an animal in its cage or outdoors may provide a rough estimate of the volume of urine being produced. Table 5-1 lists the approximate daily urine production for common domestic species.

Polyuria, the production of excessive amounts of urine, occurs with intake of excessive amounts of water (*polydipsia*). Usually, with polyuria the urine is

PROCEDURE 5-3.   Routine urinalysis procedure

REAGENTS AND MATERIALS

Refractometer

Multistix or other urinalysis strips

3% sulfosalicylic acid

Ictotest tablets and pads

Glass microscope slides (1 × 3 inches) and coverslips (22 × 22 mm)

Microscope with at least 10X and 40X objectives

Automatic pipettes and tips (100 µl)

Calibrated 12-ml, conical centrifuge tubes

Either 10 × 75-mm or 12 × 75-mm glass test tubes

Test tube rack

Parafilm

Distilled or deionized water

Centrifuge capable of 2000 rpm

METHOD

1. Prepare a worksheet with patient identification, date, time, and method of urine collection. Worksheets in which data can be recorded next to the test method are extremely helpful for organization, efficiency, and completeness.

2. Record color, appearance, and odor of sample (if any). Record volume of urine obtained for analysis and estimate of total volume if the sample was obtained in a manner so that the bladder was completely emptied. Make sure the sample is at room temperature before proceeding with further evaluation.

3. Label two calibrated centrifuge tubes and pour 5 ml of urine into one tube. Occasionally, it may be necessary to use smaller volumes. However, a standard volume of 5 ml should be used if possible. (Consistency in the volume used will allow comparison and reproducibility in results of sedimentation and microscopic evaluation.) Record on the urinalysis form the volume of urine being used.

4. Centrifuge the sample using a consistent time and speed for reproducibility and adequate sedimentation (generally, 1500 to 2000 rpm [approximately 100 G] for 5 minutes). Record the volume of sediment. Pour off the supernatant into the second centrifuge tube for biochemical analysis and refractive index. Leave a small amount of urine in the tube and resuspend the sediment pellet in this urine.

5. Determine and record specific gravity using the refractometer (see Procedure 5-4). Make sure the refractometer is cleaned between samples.

6. Biochemical analysis by reagent strip methods requires timing and proper handling of both the sample and the reagent strips. Reagent strips have buffers and other chemicals on the reaction pads that can be overwhelmed by excess urine, contaminated by flow between pads, and altered by prolonged exposure to oxygen. Make sure the reagent strips are not outdated and close the container tightly immediately after use. Dip the strip quickly into urine supernatant and lightly tap the edge of the strip to remove excess urine without allowing the pads to touch any object or urine to run between pads. Read the reaction pads at appropriate times comparing color changes to the charts provided. Record the semi-quantitative results on the urine worksheet. The remaining supernatant should be retained for further biochemical testing (tablet tests, sulfosalicylic acid turbidimetry, etc.) (see protein determination by sulfosalicylic acid and bilirubin by Ictotest, Procedures 5-5 and 5-6).

7. Using the original tube with sediment, resuspend the pelleted material in the remaining small amount of urine and place either 1 to 2 drops of unstained urine on a microscope slide for evaluation with reduced condenser lighting or place desired stain in with suspension, mix well, and evaluate stained urine. Record results of low-power findings (10X objective) and high-power findings (40X objective): crystal, cells, casts, bacteria, etc. A thorough and routine slide evaluation will allow for consistent and reproducible results.

pale and has a low specific gravity. Polyuria occurs in many diseases, including nephritis, diabetes mellitus, diabetes insipidus, pyometra in dogs and cats, and liver disease. It is also seen following administration of diuretics, corticosteroids, or fluids.

Oliguria, a decrease in urine output, occurs with acute nephritis, fever, shock, decreased fluid intake, high environmental temperature, heart disease and dehydration. *Anuria,* the complete lack of urine production, could be considered extreme oliguria. Anuria may be seen in complete urethral obstruction and in urinary bladder rupture. Anuria should not be diagnosed unless no urine is voided for about 12 hours and the animal is in a normal state of hydration.

Table 5-1. Normal daily urine production for common domestic species

Species	Daily urine output (ml/lb)
Dogs	12-30
Cats	4.5-9
Cattle	8-20
Horses	2-8
Swine	2-14
Sheep, goats	4.5-18

Color

The normal yellow color of urine is due to the presence of pigments called urochromes. Often the degree of yellow coloration correlates with the urine's concentration. Colorless urine usually has a very low specific gravity and is often associated with polyuria. Dark yellow to yellow-brown urine generally has a high specific gravity and may be associated with oliguria. Yellow-brown or greenish urine that produces a greenish-yellow foam when shaken is likely to contain bile pigments. Red or reddish-brown urine indicates the presence of RBCs (*hematuria*) or hemoglobin (*hemoglobinuria*). Urine that is brown when voided may contain myoglobin (*myoglobinuria*) excreted during conditions that cause muscle cell lysis (e.g., exertional rhabdomyolysis in horses). Some drugs may alter the color of urine; red, green, or blue urine may be observed.

Transparency

Normal urine is clear when voided, except equine urine. Normal equine urine is cloudy due to calcium carbonate crystals and, rarely, mucus secretion by the kidneys. Transparency is noted as clear, cloudy, or flocculent. Clear samples usually do not have much sediment on centrifugation. Cloudy samples usually contain large particles, and they usually yield a significant amount of sediment on centrifugation. Urine may become cloudy while standing due to bacterial multiplication or crystal formation. Substances that cause urine to be cloudy include RBCs, WBCs, epithelial cells, casts, crystals, mucus, fat, and bacteria. Flocculent samples contain suspended particles that are sufficiently large to be seen with the naked eye.

ODOR

The odor of urine is not highly diagnostic but may sometimes be helpful. The urine of male cats, goats, and pigs has a strong odor. An ammonia odor may occur with cystitis caused by bacteria that produce urease (e.g., *Proteus*) that has metabolized urea to ammonia. Occasionally samples that are left standing may develop an ammonia odor due to bacterial growth. A sweet, fruity odor indicates ketones and is most commonly found with diabetes mellitus, acetonemia in cows, and pregnancy disease in ewes.

FOAM

A small amount of white foam can be produced by shaking a sample of normal urine. Urine containing large amounts of protein tends to form a greater quantity of foam that lasts longer than normal. Yellow-greenish foam indicates the presence of bile pigments in the sample.

SPECIFIC GRAVITY

Specific gravity is defined as the weight (density) of a quantity of liquid as compared with that of an equal amount of distilled water. The specific gravity of urine is determined by the number and molecular weight of dissolved solutes. The specific gravity of urine from polyuric patients tends to be low, and that of urine from oliguric patients tends to be high. Table 5-2 lists the reference ranges for urine specific gravity for normal domestic species.

There are several methods to determine the specific gravity of urine.

REFRACTOMETER.   The refractometer or total solids meter (Figure 5-3) is a device that can be used to approximate specific gravity (relative density) of urine and other body fluids. The refractometer determines the refractive index of a fluid: the ratio of the velocity of light in air to the velocity of light in a solution. Light waves bend as they pass through the medium in which they travel. This bending is measured by the refractometer. The refractive index of a fluid is influenced by the same factors that determine specific gravity and therefore provides an estimate of urine specific gravity. Because the density of a fluid is influenced by temperature, refractometers should be temperature corrected to allow accurate and reproducible results. Advantages of the

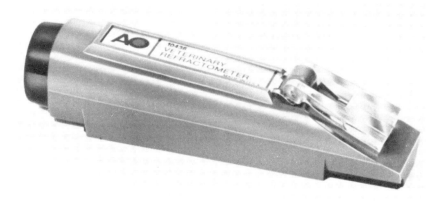

FIGURE 5-3. Refractometer or total solids meter. (Courtesy A.O. Reichert Scientific Instruments.)

refractometer are that it is easy to use and only a few drops of urine are needed (Procedure 5-4).

URINOMETER. The urinometer is a less expensive but less desirable method for determining urine specific gravity. It is a more cumbersome instrument that requires a large volume of urine (approximately 10 ml) and, in general, provides less reproducible results than a refractometer. The urinometer floats in a vessel containing urine, and the specific gravity is read at the bottom of the meniscus (Figure 5-4). The vessel should be deep enough for the urinometer to float and wide enough so that the urinometer does not cling to the sides of the vessel. The urine should be at room temperature, as the urinometer is calibrated at about 20° C (68° F). If the urine is too warm, the reading will be erroneously low; cold urine produces artificially high readings. When the urine volume is insufficient to use the urinometer, it can be diluted with distilled water and the true specific gravity determined in a manner similar to that for more concentrated samples using the refractometer.

REAGENT STRIPS. Several reagent strips have been developed to determine urine specific gravity. These seem to be the least reliable method for determination of specific gravity. With urine of high specific gravity (>1.030), the strips often show a reaction for a lower specific gravity, or the reaction is inconsistent with those shown on the container label.

Procedure 5-4. Determining urine specific gravity by refractometry

1. Centrifuge the urine at 100 to 200 G for 5 minutes. (It is important to use centrifuged urine because suspended materials in the urine will cause the line in the refractometer to be indistinct rather than sharp.)
2. Place a drop of urine on the glass plate, close the plastic cover, and determine the specific gravity from an internal scale. (Some older refractometers may only have a scale for refractive index. In this case the specific gravity is determined from charts provided with the instrument.)
3. Occasionally the specific gravity will be greater than the upper range of the refractometer. When that occurs, the following steps will allow the determination of the specific gravity.
   - Pipette 0.5 ml of urine into a tube.
   - Pipette 0.5 ml of distilled or deionized water into the tube.
   - Gently mix the urine and water.
   - Remove a small portion of the mixture and determine the specific gravity of the mixture.
   - Multiply the numbers after the decimal point by 2 to determine the specific gravity of the urine.
   - Example: Initial reading is above the scale.

     The 1:1 dilution reads 1.036.
     .036 $\times$ 2 = .072
     The true urine specific gravity is 1.072.

4. Record the results.

Table 5-2 lists the urine specific gravity for normal domestic species. The specific gravity of normal urine varies from one specimen to another, depending on eating and drinking habits, environmental temperature, and when the sample was collected. An early morning sample tends to be the most concentrated.

Causes of altered urine specific gravity. Increased urine specific gravity is seen with diminished water intake, increased fluid loss through sources other than urination (sweating, panting, or diarrhea), and increased excretion of urine

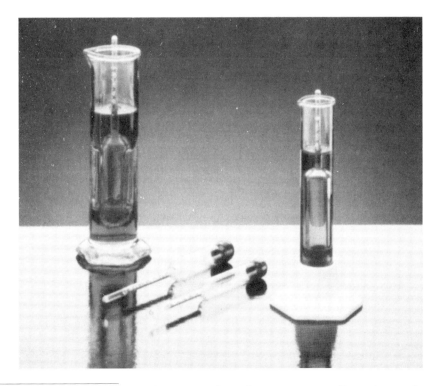

FIGURE 5-4.   Urinometers. The one on the right requires a smaller volume of
urine than the one on the left. (Courtesy Becton-Dickinson.)

solutes. Decreased water intake in animals with normal renal function rapidly
causes increased urine specific gravity. Dehydration increases urine specific
gravity. Increased urine specific gravity is often seen in acute renal disease.
Shock also increases urine specific gravity.

Decreased urine specific gravity is seen in diseases in which the kidneys
cannot resorb water and with increased fluid intake, such as with polydipsia or
excessive fluid administration. Pyometra, diabetes insipidus, psychogenic polydipsia, some liver diseases, certain types of renal disease, and diuretic therapy
result in decreased urine specific gravity.

Isosthenuria occurs when the urine specific gravity approaches that of the
glomerular filtrate (1.008 to 1.012). Frequently, animals with chronic renal
disease produce isosthenuric urine. In animals with kidney disease, the closer
the specific gravity is to isosthenuric, the greater the amount of kidney function

TABLE 5-2. Urine values for common domestic species

	DOGS	**CATS**	**HORSES**	**CATTLE**	**SWINE**	**SHEEP**
Volume (L/day)	0.04-2	0.075-0.2	3-10	6-25	2-6	0.05-2
Specific gravity	1.025 (1.018-1.045)	1.030 (1.020-1.040)	1.035 (1.020-1.050)	1.015 (1.005-1.040)	1.015 (1.010-1.030)	1.030 (1.020-1.040)
pH	5.2-6.8	6-7	7-8.5	7-8.5	6-8.5	6-8.5
Glucose	None	None	None	None	None	None
Protein	None/trace	None/trace	None	None/trace	None/trace	None/trace
Bilirubin	None/trace	None/trace	None	None/trace	None	None/trace
Ketones	None	None	None	None/trace	None	None

that has been lost. When these animals are deprived of water, their urine specific gravity usually remains in the isosthenuric range.

ASSAYS FOR CHEMICAL CONSTITUENTS

Testing for various chemical constituents of urine has been greatly simplified by the advent of reagent tablets or paper reagent strips impregnated with appropriate chemicals. There are reagent strips that test for numerous constituents simultaneously, and there are strips for individual tests. The two primary manufacturers of the reagents are Miles Inc., Diagnostic Division, Elkhart, IN, and Boehringer Mannheim Corporation, Diagnostic Laboratory Systems Division, Indianapolis, IN. Urine is added to these tablets or strips are dipped in the urine sample and the color changes are noted at specific intervals (Figures 5-5 and 5-6). The concentration of various constituents is determined by comparing the resulting colors with color charts supplied by the manufacturer (e.g., Clinitek 100, Miles Laboratories). It is important to carefully follow the manufacturer's directions. Reflectant spectrometry instruments are available to automate evaluation and recording of data. These instruments eliminate the errors associated with individual differences in color perception.

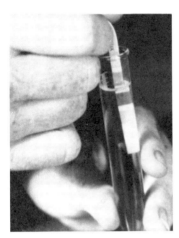

FIGURE 5-5. Urine being tested with a combination dipstick.

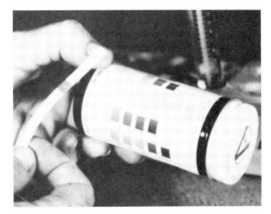

FIGURE 5-6. After the dipstick is dipped in the urine, the resultant color changes are compared with those on the container, each of which indicates a specific urine constituent.

pH

pH expresses the concentration of hydrogen ion (H^+). Essentially this is a measure of the degree of acidity or alkalinity of urine. A pH above 7.0 is *alkaline,* while a pH below 7.0 is *acidic.* It is important that proper technique be employed for accurate results. The pH of samples left standing open at room temperature tends to increase due to loss of CO_2, while delays in reading the reaction may lead to color changes and false readings. If samples containing urease-producing bacteria are left standing, the pH usually increases.

The pH of a healthy animal's urine depends largely on its diet. Plant diets usually cause alkaline urine, while high-protein cereal diets or diets of animal origin cause acidic urine. Therefore, herbivores normally have alkaline urine, carnivores acidic urine, and omnivores either acidic or alkaline urine, depending on what was ingested. Many dog foods contain substantial amounts of plant material that may cause the urine to be slightly alkaline. Nursing herbivores have acidic urine from consumption of milk. Table 5-2 lists the normal urine constituents and characteristics, including pH, for common domestic species.

Urine pH is usually measured with reagent strips. Decreased pH (acidity) may be due to several factors, including fever, starvation, high-protein diet, acidosis, excessive muscular activity, or administration of certain drugs. Increased pH (alkalinity) may be caused by alkalosis, infection of the urinary tract with urease-producing bacteria, use of certain drugs, or by urine retention, as occurs with urethral obstruction or bladder paralysis.

PROTEIN

Protein is usually absent or present only in trace amounts in normal urine obtained by catheterization or cystocentesis. In healthy animals, plasma proteins that pass into the glomerular filtrate are resorbed in the renal tubules before the filtrate reaches the renal pelvis. However, voided samples or those obtained by expressing the bladder may contain additional protein due to secretions that may contaminate urine during its passage along the urinary tract. Occasionally, trauma to the urinary tract resulting from cystocentesis, catheterization, or bladder expression may cause sufficient bleeding to result in a trace of protein in the urine. The relationship of any protein measured in the urine and possible leakage through the renal glomeruli must be interpreted in light of the collection method, urine concentration, rate of urine formation, and contributions from any hemorrhage or inflammation noted by sample analysis.

Protein levels in urine can be measured by several methods.

PROTEIN DETERMINATION BY REAGENT TEST STRIPS. Urine dipsticks allow semiquantitative measurement of protein in urine by progressive color changes on the reaction pad. These reactions can be converted to a semiquantitative measurement based on charts provided. The accuracy of these methods is variable. Reagent strips primarily detect albumin and are much less sensitive to globulins. False-positive results may also occur in alkaline urine. However, reagent strip analysis is a rapid, convenient and reasonably accurate method of determining urinary protein levels. Protein measurements that are considered excessive or pathologic should be confirmed by sulfosalicylic acid turbidimetry or by specific biochemical analysis.

PROTEIN DETERMINATION BY SULFOSALICYLIC ACID TURBIDIMETRY. Sulfosalicylic acid turbidity determines urine protein levels by acid precipitation. The resultant turbidity is proportional to the concentration of protein. Results are compared with levels in prepared standards and thus can be reported in semiquantitative units. The advantage of this method is that it is equally sensitive to albumin and globulins. It is quite useful to confirm strip methods, especially in alkaline urine. Extremely alkaline urine may titrate the acid and decrease the amount of protein precipitated (Procedure 5-5).

Very dilute urine may yield a false-negative result because the protein concentration may be below the sensitivity of the testing method. However, a trace amount of protein in a very dilute sample may be clinically significant because dilute urine often occurs when a large volume of urine is being produced, such as in a patient with chronic renal failure.

PROCEDURE 5-5.   Determination of urine protein concentration by the sulfosalicylic acid test

1. Prepare 3% sulfosalicylic acid in distilled or deionized water by dissolving 30 g of sulfosalicylic acid in 1 L of water.
2. Place 1 ml of urine supernatant in two 10 × 75-mm glass test tubes.
3. Add 3 ml of 3% sulfosalicylic acid to one of the tubes and 3 ml of water to the other tube. (If the volume of urine is insufficient, the ratio of 1 part urine to 3 parts reagents must be maintained in order to properly quantitate the reaction.)
4. Mix by inversion.
5. Compare the sulfosalicylic acid tube and the water tube. There should be no turbidity in the water tube. Determine the results as follows:

Negative	=	No visible turbity
Trace	=	Barely visible turbity
1+	=	Distinct turbidity but able to read black typing on a white background through the tube
2+	=	Moderate turbidity and unable to read black typing on a white background through the tube
3+	=	Heavy turbidity with fine granulation and cloudiness
4+	=	Heavy and floculant turbidity

6. Record the results.

Occasionally a small amount of protein is found in the urine of normal animals. Transient proteinuria may be due to a temporary increase in glomerular permeability, allowing excessive protein to enter the filtrate. This is due to increased pressure in the glomerular capillaries and can be found with muscle exertion, emotional stress, or convulsions. Occasionally a small amount of urine protein is found after parturition, during the first few days of life, and during estrus. The presence of protein in the urine is usually abnormal and is primarily due to disease of the urinary tract (or possibly the genital system).

In most cases, *proteinuria* indicates disease of the urinary tract, especially of the kidneys. Both acute and chronic renal diseases lead to proteinuria. Acute nephritis is characterized by marked proteinuria with leukocytes and casts, while in chronic renal disease the degree of proteinuria is qualitatively less. However, in chronic renal disease, urine output is usually excessive with low specific gravity; therefore, the total protein excreted is actually quite significant. The ratio of urine protein to creatinine is used to determine the degree of protein loss in chronic renal disease.

Multiple myeloma, a cancer of plasma cells, may produce large quantities of protein that can leak through the glomerulus. In patients with myeloma, proteins may be passed in the urine because they have damaged the glomerulus or because they are the so-called "light chains," which freely pass through the glomerular filter. Often these proteins do not react with the protein pad on dipsticks, and the sulfosalicylic acid method is necessary to detect them.

Mild proteinuria is seen with passive congestion of the kidneys, as in congestive heart failure or any other impediment of blood flow from the kidneys. Proteinuria of renal origin can also be caused by trauma, tumors, renal infarcts or nephrosis due to drugs and chemicals, such as sulfonamides, lead, mercury, arsenic, or ether.

Inflammation of the urinary or genital tract may cause proteinuria of postrenal origin. Proteinuria may also be seen with traumatic catheterization.

GLUCOSE

The presence of glucose in urine is known as *glucosuria* or *glycosuria*. The amount of glucose in the urine depends on blood glucose levels, as well as the rates of glomerular filtration and tubular resorption. Glucosuria usually does not occur in normal animals unless the blood glucose level exceeds the renal threshold (approximately 170 to 180 mg/dl for dogs). At this concentration, tubular resorption cannot keep up with the glomerular filtration of glucose, and glucose passes into the urine.

Glucosuria occurs in diabetes mellitus due to a deficiency of insulin or an inability of insulin to function. Insulin is necessary to transport glucose into body cells, and a deficiency causes hyperglycemia and spilling of glucose into the urine. A high-carbohydrate meal may lead to blood glucose levels exceeding the renal threshold and thus glucosuria. Because of this, a period of fasting is recommended before urine glucose concentration is determined. Fear, excitement, or restraint, especially in cats, often causes hyperglycemia and glucosuria due to epinephrine release. Glucosuria often occurs after IV administration of fluids containing glucose and occasionally after general anesthesia. Occasionally, glucosuria is found in hyperthyroidism, Cushing's disease, and chronic liver disease. A rare condition called renal glucosuria can occur when the blood glucose concentration is in the normal range. Renal glucosuria is due to reduced resorption of glucose in the renal tubules.

False positives for glucose may be seen after use of various drugs, including ascorbic acid (vitamin C), morphine, salicylates (e.g., aspirin), streptomycin, penicillin, chloramphenicol, and oxytetracycline.

Various reagent test strips are available for detecting glucose in urine. Clinitest Reagent Tablets (Ames) are also available. These tablets detect any sugar in the urine, whereas the test strips detect only glucose.

KETONES

Ketones include acetone, acetoacetic acid, and beta-hydroxybutyric acid. Ketone bodies are formed during catabolism of fatty acids. Normal animals have very small amounts of ketones in the blood. Conditions characterized by altered carbohydrate metabolism may result in excessive amounts of fat catabolism to provide energy. When this is not accompanied by sufficient carbohydrate metabolism, the excess ketones spill into the urine (*ketonuria*).

A common cause of ketonuria is ketonemia (ketosis) in lactating cows and pregnant ewes and cows. In ewes, this condition is called pregnancy toxemia and is seen when the ewe is carrying twins. Ketosis is associated with hypoglycemia and is caused by carbohydrate intake insufficient to meet energy requirements. Body fat is then rapidly metabolized, resulting in ketonemia and ketonuria.

Ketosis frequently occurs in diabetes mellitus. Because the animal lacks the insulin necessary for carbohydrate metabolism, fat is broken down to meet the animal's energy needs and excess ketones are excreted in the urine. Ketones are important sources of energy and are normally produced during fat metabolism. Problems develop, however, when excessive ketones are produced. Ketones are toxic, causing CNS depression and acidosis. Acidosis due to ketonemia is termed *ketoacidosis.*

Ketosis also occurs with high-fat diets, starvation, fasting, long-term anorexia, and impaired liver function. With a high-fat diet, a relatively low percentage of energy needs is met by carbohydrates, so a great amount of fat is used to meet energy needs. In the fasting, starved, or anorexic animal, body fat is used to meet energy needs, producing a greater than normal amount of ketones. With liver damage, impaired carbohydrate metabolism leads to fat serving as the main energy source, especially when the damaged liver cannot store adequate amounts of glycogen.

MEASUREMENT OF URINE KETONE CONTENT. Urinary ketones are detected using urinary reagent strips with a ketone reagent pad or with separate reagent tablets (Acetest Reagent Tablets, Ames). The color intensity is roughly proportional to the concentration of urine ketones. These methods are most sensitive to acetoacetic acid and less sensitive to acetone and do not detect beta-hydroxybutyric acid.

BILE PIGMENTS

Bile pigments that are commonly detected in urine are bilirubin and urobilinogen. Only conjugated bilirubin is found in urine, as unconjugated bilirubin does not pass through the glomerulus into the renal filtrate because it is bound to albumin and is not water soluble. Normal dogs, especially males, occasionally have bilirubin in their urine because of a low renal threshold for conjugated bilirubin and the ability of their kidneys to conjugate bilirubin. Many normal cattle also have small amounts of bilirubin in their urine. Bilirubin is usually not found in the urine of cats, pigs, sheep, and horses.

Bilirubinuria is seen in a number of diseases, including obstruction of bile flow from the liver to the small intestine. Bilirubinuria results from accumulation in hepatic cells of conjugated bilirubin that is regurgitated into the blood and excreted in the urine. Conditions causing biliary obstruction include calculi in the bile duct, tumors in the area of the bile duct, acute enteritis, pancreatitis, and obstruction of the upper intestinal tract. Bilirubinuria also occurs in liver disease. When conjugated, bilirubin enters the bloodstream after being released from damaged liver cells and passes into the urine.

Hemolytic anemia may also cause bilirubinuria, especially in dogs. In hemolytic anemia the liver's ability to excrete the excess bilirubin may be exceeded, resulting in regurgitation of conjugated bilirubin into the blood and ultimately bilirubinuria. In dogs, unconjugated bilirubin from hemoglobin catabolism in the mononuclear phagocytic system can be conjugated in the kidney and passed in the urine.

Bilirubinuria is detected with the Ictotest (Ames) (Procedure 5-6). A diazo compound in the tablet reacts with bilirubin to produce a blue or purple color. The speed with which the color changes and the degree of color change indicate the amount of bilirubin present. Reagent strips are less sensitive than Ictotest tablets. Urine to be tested for bilirubin must not be exposed to light because bilirubin is broken down by short-wave light. False-negative results for bilirubin occur in urine that is exposed to sunlight or artificial light.

In the intestines, bacteria convert bilirubin to *stercobilinogen* and *urobilinogen*. The bulk of these products is excreted in the feces, but some is resorbed into the bloodstream and excreted by the liver into the intestinal tract. A small

---

PROCEDURE 5-6.   Ictotest for bilirubin in urine

1. Place 10 drops of urine supernatant onto the square absorbent test mat supplied with the Ictotest.
2. Place an Ictotest reagent tablet in the center of the mat.
3. Carefully place a large drop of water in the center of the tablet and allow it to bubble for a few seconds.
4. Place a second drop of water on the tablet so that it overflows onto the reagent pad.
5. After 60 seconds, observe the area of the pad around the tablet for color change.
6. Determine the results as follows:

Negative	=	No change or pink to red color
1+	=	Definite blue to purple color
2+	=	Medium blue to purple color
3+	=	Dark purple color after only 30 seconds
4+	=	Dark purple color develops immediately

7. Record the results.

amount of resorbed urobilinogen is excreted by the kidneys into the urine. It is normal to have urobilinogen in the urine sample.

The reliability of screening tests for detection of urobilinogen is questionable due to the instability of urobilinogens. It is absolutely necessary to use fresh urine because urobilinogen is rapidly converted (oxidized) to urobilin in samples left standing. Urobilin does not react with the reagent strips and false-negative results occur when there is a significant delay between sample collection and testing for urobilinogen.

A decreased amount or total absence of urobilinogen in urine may indicate bile duct obstruction. If bile cannot reach the intestine, urobilinogen cannot be produced by bacteria. In conditions with polyuria, the urine may be so dilute that urobilinogen goes undetected. Broad-spectrum oral antibiotics may alter the intestinal flora so that urobilinogen is not produced, even though bilirubin is present.

Increased urine urobilinogen may be found with hemolysis, which increases bilirubin excretion into the intestines and thus increases amounts of urobilinogen produced by intestinal bacteria. Occasionally, hepatocellular damage decreases the liver's ability to remove urobilinogen from the portal circulation after it has been resorbed from the intestinal tract, and abnormally large amounts of urobilinogen enter the urine.

BLOOD

Tests for blood in urine detect *hematuria* (the presence of intact RBCs in urine), *hemoglobinuria* (the presence of free hemoglobin in urine), and *myoglobinuria* (the presence of myoglobin in urine). Hematuria, hemoglobinuria, and myoglobinuria can occur simultaneously. The presence of one does not rule out the others.

HEMATURIA.   Hematuria is usually a sign of disease somewhere in the urogenital tract, while hemoglobinuria usually indicates intravascular hemolysis. Some systemic conditions may also cause hematuria. In very dilute or highly alkaline urine, erythrocytes often lyse to yield hemoglobin. Therefore hemoglobinuria may not be due to hemoglobin entering the urine via the glomerulus. Ghost cells (the shells of lysed RBCs) may be seen on microscopic examination of sediment if the source of hemoglobin is lysis of RBCs.

Moderate to large amounts of blood impart a cloudy red, brown, or wine color to the urine. Similar colors, but with a transparent appearance that remains after centrifugation, indicate hemoglobinuria. With minute amounts of blood in the urine, a visible color change is usually not evident. *Occult* (hidden) *blood* occurs when the urine is not obviously discolored by blood but blood is detected by chemical analysis. For a further discussion of hematuria, see the section on microscopic examination of urinary sediment.

Hemoglobinuria. Hemoglobinuria is usually due to intravascular hemolysis. Hemoglobin from RBCs broken down intravascularly (*hemoglobinemia*) is normally bound to the plasma protein haptoglobin. When hemoglobin is bound to haptoglobin, it does not pass through the glomerular membrane. If intravascular hemolysis overwhelms haptoglobin's binding ability, hemoglobinemia leads to hemoglobinuria because free hemoglobin filters through the glomerular membrane. Hemoglobinuria is indicated by a positive test for hemoglobin although no RBCs are observed in the urine sediment, or the degree of the reaction is greater than can be accounted for by the numbers of RBCs in the sediment.

Hemoglobinuria may be seen with many conditions causing intravascular hemolysis, including autoimmune hemolytic anemia, isoimmune hemolytic disease of neonates, incompatible blood transfusions, severe burns, leptospirosis, babesiosis, systemic lupus erythematosus, certain heavy-metal toxicities (copper, mercury), ingestion of certain poisonous plants, conditions that result in severe hypophosphatemia, postparturient hemoglobinemia in cattle, and the idiopathic hemoglobinuria of cattle that occurs after they drink large quantities of very cold water.

If the urine is dilute or very alkaline, hemoglobinuria can originate from lysis of RBCs in the urine. This must be considered hematuria, as intact RBCs were present initially. Often ghost RBCs can be found when hemoglobinuria is due to release of hemoglobin from RBCs in the urine. True hemoglobinuria is due to hemoglobinemia.

Because the test for blood in the urine detects hemoglobinuria, hematuria, and myoglobinuria, one must also consider urine sediment examination, history, physical examination findings, and additional laboratory procedures to determine the cause of the positive test for blood in the urine.

Myoglobinuria. Myoglobin is a protein found in muscle. Muscle damage causes release of myoglobin into the blood. Myoglobin passes through the glomeruli and is excreted in the urine. Urine containing myoglobin is very dark brown to almost black. If a positive occult blood test in urine is due to myoglobin, no intact RBCs are seen in the urinary sediment and the plasma is not red. Myoglobinuria is frequently seen in horses with exertional rhabdomy-olysis (*azoturia*).

When the test for blood in the urine is positive, hemoglobinuria can presumptively be differentiated from myoglobinuria by evaluating the color of plasma and urine simultaneously. If the plasma is red and the urine is red or brown, hemoglobinuria is most likely. If the plasma is clear and the urine is brown, myoglobinuria is likely. Because myoglobin is not bound to serum proteins, it readily crosses the glomerular capillaries, and it appears in urine when plasma concentrations are insufficient to cause a color change. On the other hand, because hemoglobin is attached to haptoglobin, it must reach high levels in the blood before there is sufficient free hemoglobin to cross the glomerular membranes. The high concentration of haptoglobin-bound hemo-globin causes the noticeable change in plasma color.

Many reagent test strips detect hematuria, hemoglobinuria, and myoglobi-nuria. Occultest Reagent Tablets (Ames) is a sensitive test to detect blood in urine. A drop of urine is placed in the center of a filter paper square. The tablet is placed on the drop of urine and 2 drops of water are then placed on the tablet, so the water runs over the tablet and onto the filter paper. Appearance of a blue color on the filter paper surrounding the tablet within 2 minutes indicates blood. Any color change occurring after 2 minutes is of no significance. Hematest Tablets (Ames) are designed to detect occult blood in feces but can be used with urine. However, they are more expensive and less sensitive than Occultest Reagent Tablets. The urine must contain a considerable amount of blood before a positive reaction is determined. As with other urine chemical tests, the test for hemoglobin should be performed on the supernatant of centrifuged urine. Hematuria and hemoglobinuria can sometimes be differentiated by comparing the reactions of centrifuged and uncentrifuged urine.

Hemoglobin and myoglobin can be differentiated on the basis of their different molecular weights and different solubility in ammonium sulfate. The most reliable method for differentiating hemoglobin and myoglobin is separa-tion of myoglobin by centrifugal-assisted filtration. Because myoglobin has a molecular weight of approximately 16,000 D and hemoglobin has a molecular weight of approximately 64,000 D, they can be separated by centrifugal-assisted filtration using special tubes that allow the smaller myoglobin mol-ecules to pass through the filter and prevent passage of hemoglobin molecules. Myoglobin and hemoglobin can also be differentiated by their differences in solubility in an 80% saturated solution of ammonium sulfate. Hemoglobin

PROCEDURE 5-7. Methods to differentiate hemoglobinuria from myoglobinuria

These tests are only performed on samples that have previously tested positive for hemoglobin. Usually they are only performed in animals that appear to have muscular disease.

CENTRIFUGATION-ASSISTED FILTRATION

1. Place 0.5 ml of urine supernatant in the sample reservoir of a microcon-30 microconcentrator tube.
2. Centrifuge for 15 minutes at 3000 rpm.
3. Remove the sample reservoir.
4. Record the color of the filtrate and compare it to the original urine supernatant.
5. Test the filtrate for hemoglobin and compare the results to those of the urine supernatant.
6. If the test is positive, myoglobin is present. If the positive reaction is qualitatively less than that in the original sample, both myoglobin and hemoglobin are present.

AMMONIUM SULFATE PRECIPITATION

1. Add 2.8 g of $(NH_4)_2 SO_4$ to 5 ml of urine supernatant.
2. Vigorously shake the tube until the $(NH_4)_2 SO_4$ dissolves.
3. Centrifuge the mixture at 100 rpm for 10 minutes.
4. Test the supernatant for hemoglobin and compare the results with those of the urine supernatant.
5. If the test is positive, myoglobin is present. If the positive reaction is qualitatively less than that in the original sample, both myoglobin and hemoglobin are present.

precipitates in an 80% saturated ammonium sulfate solution, but myoglobin does not. However, differentiating hemoglobinuria from myoglobinuria on the basis of their ammonium sulfate solubility is of questionable reliability (Procedure 5-7).

NITRITE. Some bacteria contain enzymes that reduce nitrate to nitrite in the urine. The presence of nitrite in urine suggests bacteriuria. However, a negative nitrite test does not indicate that bacteria are absent. To detect nitrate-reducing bacteria, the diet must contain nitrate that can be excreted in the urine and the urine must be retained in the bladder for sufficient time for organisms to produce detectable concentrations of nitrite. Because animals with urinary tract infections usually urinate frequently, this test is often negative even when bacteria are present. Microscopic examination remains the best screening test to detect bacteria in urine. Conversely, positive nitrite results should be confirmed with microscopic examination or culture of urine. The nitrite test should be considered a screening test only. It does not substitute for microscopic examination of the urine sediment.

LEUKOCYTES. Presumptive evidence of leukocytes (WBCs) in urine can be obtained with the leukocyte reaction of certain reagent strips. However, many false-negative reactions occur, and microscopic evaluation is necessary to confirm a positive result.

MICROSCOPIC EXAMINATION OF URINE SEDIMENT

Microscopic examination of urine sediment is extremely important, especially for recognizing diseases of the urinary tract. It must be a part of every urinalysis. Many abnormalities in a urine sample cannot be detected with reagent test strips or tablets, but often a specific diagnosis can be made by observation of the urine sediment. In addition, urine sediment examination is occasionally an aid in diagnosing systemic disease.

Except in horses, normal urine does not contain a large amount of sediment. Small numbers of epithelial cells, mucus threads, RBCs, WBCs, hyaline casts, and crystals of various types can be found in the urine of normal animals. The urine of horses usually has large amounts of calcium carbonate crystals. As previously indicated in the section on urine collection, bacteria and aberrant substances may be present in a urine sample that has been contaminated during collection.

The best samples for sediment examination are morning samples or samples collected after several hours of water deprivation. Because such samples are more concentrated, the chances of finding formed elements are increased. It is important that urine for sediment examination be fresh. If a voided sample is collected, a mid-stream sample is preferred because it is less likely to be contaminated by debris from the external genital surfaces, such as cells and bacteria. Urine collected by cystocentesis is the best sample for microscopic examination. As discussed previously, many changes occur in a sample as it ages. If the sample cannot be examined immediately, it should be refrigerated or preserved.

For semiquantitative measurements of the formed elements in urine, the volume of urine used and the volume of sediment obtained should be recorded. If a sufficient volume has been obtained, 5 ml of a well-mixed sample should be placed in a graduated, conical centrifuge tube and centrifuged for 3 to 5 minutes at approximately 100 G (about 1000 to 2000 rpm, depending on the radius of the centrifuge). The procedure should be standardized for a particular centrifuge to yield uniform results. Some centrifuges, such as the Clay-Adams Triac, are calibrated to provide the proper force over sufficient time to completely sediment the formed elements in the urine. After centrifugation, the volume of sediment is recorded and the supernatant is gently poured off, leaving about 0.3 ml of urine adhered to the sides of the tube. This remaining urine is allowed to run down the inside of the centrifuge tube, and the sediment is resuspended by gently flicking the bottom of the centrifuge tube.

The sediment may be examined stained or unstained (Procedure 5-8). To examine an unstained sediment, a small drop of the suspended sediment is placed on a clean glass slide, covered with a coverslip, and examined immediately. Subdued light that partially refracts the elements must be used to examine unstained urine sediment. Proper lighting is achieved by partially closing the microscope's iris diaphragm and adjusting the condenser downward. Phase-contrast microscopy provides far better distinction of elements than does reduced illumination using bright-field microscopy. Microscopes with phase-contrast capabilities are only slightly more expensive than bright-field microscopes, and they can also be used for routine microscopy. The light path of a phase-contrast microscope must be properly adjusted to take full advantage of its capabilities.

Stained sediment may also be examined. Satisfactory stains include Sternheimer-Malbin stain (Sedi Stain: Becton Dickinson, Rutherford, NJ) or 0.5% new methylene blue containing a small amount of formalin. One drop of stain is mixed with the suspended sediment before placing a drop of sediment on a slide. The amount of illumination is less critical when examining a stained specimen than with an unstained one although reduced illumination also aids visualization of substances by providing contrast.

The specimen is scanned under low power (10X objective) to gain an impression of what is present and to identify larger elements, such as casts or aggregates of cells. The entire area under the coverslip should be examined because casts tend to migrate to the edge of the coverslip. Casts and crystals are

---

PROCEDURE 5-8.   Microscopic examination of urine sediment

1. Place a small drop of suspended urine sediment on a glass slide and cover with a 22 × 22-mm coverslip.
2. Place the slide on the microscope and swing the 10X lens into place.
3. Reduce the light intensity and lower the substage condenser.
4. Focus on the material on the slide.
5. Scan the slide and identify larger elements, such as casts and crystals. Both the center and edges of the slide should be examined.
6. Swing the 40X lens into place and readjust the light, if necessary.
7. Identify formed elements, including RBCs, WBCs, epithelial cells (and their type), casts, crystals, and bacteria.
8. Evaluate the sediment as follows:
   • Crystals and casts—numbers per low-power field (LPF)
   • Cells (and sometimes casts and crystals)—numbers per high-power field (HPF)
   • Bacteria and sperm

Rare	=	Only 2 or 3 seen on scanning several HPF
1+	=	Less than 1/HPF
2+	=	1-5/HPF
3+	=	6-20/HPF
4+	=	Greater than 20/HPF

9. Record the results.

---

identified and reported as the number observed per low-power field. High power (40X objective) is necessary to accurately identify most objects, to detect bacteria, and to differentiate cell types. Epithelial cells, RBCs, and WBCs are reported as the average number observed per high-power field (HPF). Bacteria are reported as few, moderate, or many, and their morphology (cocci, bacilli) is noted.

The amount of sediment can be accurately measured with calibrated slides (UriSystem Slides: Fisher Scientific, Pittsburgh, PA). A more refined version has ruled areas similar to that of a hemocytometer. Such systems are rarely used to evaluate urine samples from animals.

CONSTITUENTS OF URINE SEDIMENT

Various cells, microorganisms, urinary casts, fat, crystals, and contaminating artifacts may be found in urine sediment.

RBCs (ERYTHROCYTES)

Erythrocytes may have several different appearances, depending on the urine concentration and time elapsed between collection and examination. Red blood cells are small. In a fresh sample, RBCs usually have smooth edges and appear yellow to orange, but they can be colorless if their hemoglobin has diffused out during standing (Figure 5-7). In concentrated urine, RBCs shrink and crenate. Crenated RBCs have ruffled edges and are slightly darker. Crenated RBCs may even appear granular due to membrane irregularities. In dilute or alkaline urine, RBCs swell and may lyse. Swollen RBCs have smooth edges and are pale yellow or orange. Lysed RBCs may appear as colorless rings (shadow cells or ghost cells) that vary in size. However, lysed RBCs, especially when due to marked alkalinity, usually dissolve and cannot be found on microscopic examination. Normally, urine sediment contains less than 2 to 3 RBCs/HPF (high-power field).

Because mammalian RBCs contain no nucleus, they can be confused with fat globules and yeast. However, their light yellow to orange color usually allows them to be differentiated from these other elements. Further, variation in RBC size is minimal, whereas fat globules vary in size. To accurately differentiate RBCs from these other constituents, acetic acid is allowed to

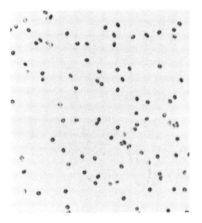

FIGURE 5-7. Red blood cells in canine urine. (160X)

diffuse under the coverslip by placing a small amount of 2% acetic acid next to the coverslip. If the structures disappear, they are RBCs because none of the other structures mentioned will dissolve in acetic acid.

Erythrocytes in urine usually indicate bleeding somewhere in the urogenital tract or occasionally in the genital system. A voided sample from a female in proestrus or estrus or after parturition may be contaminated with RBCs. Both females and males with inflammatory conditions in the genital system may have RBCs in urine collected by free catch or expression of the bladder, but not in samples collected by catheterization. Even the slight trauma that occurs from catheterization, cystocentesis, and manual expression of the bladder can slightly increase the number of RBCs in the sediment. Generally, cystocentesis does not cause much increase in RBC numbers. It is important to note the method of urine collection on the laboratory report to help determine the significance of RBCs in urine.

WBCs (LEUKOCYTES)

Very few WBCs are found in the urine of animals without urinary or genital tract disease. Leukocytes are spherical and have a granular appearance; they are larger than RBCs and smaller than renal epithelial cells (Figure 5-8). The granular appearance is due to the fact that most WBCs in urine are neutrophils, which contain large numbers of lysosomes. With phase-contrast microscopy and in stained sediment, the polymorphic nucleus of neutrophils can often be seen. Leukocytes are usually in very low numbers in urine (0 to 1/HPF). Finding

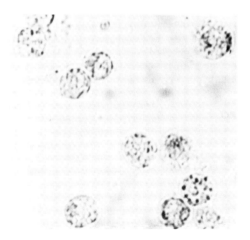

FIGURE 5-8. White blood cells in canine urine. (500X)

more than 2 to 3 WBCs/HPF indicates inflammation somewhere in the urinary or genital tracts. Excessive WBCs in the urine is termed *pyuria.* Pyuria is indicative of nephritis, pyelonephritis, cystitis, urethritis, or ureteritis.

Epithelial cells

Three types of epithelial cells may be found in urinary sediment.

Squamous epithelial cells.   Squamous epithelial cells, derived from the distal urethra, vagina, vulva, or prepuce, are occasionally found in voided samples. Their presence is usually not considered significant. They are the largest of the epithelial cells, and the largest cells found in urine sediment. They are flat cells with a homogeneous appearance. They often have straight edges and distinct corners. They may show a small, round nucleus (Figures 5-9 and 5-10). Squamous epithelial cells are not normally seen in samples obtained by cystocentesis or catheterization.

Transitional epithelial cells.   Transitional epithelial cells come from the bladder, ureters, renal pelvis, and proximal urethra. They are usually round, but they may be pear shaped or caudate. They are granular, have a small nucleus, and are larger than WBCs (Figures 5-10, 5-11, and 5-12). Occasional transitional cells (0 to 1/HPF) may be found in urinary sediment due to sloughing of old cells, but an increased number suggests cystitis or pyelone-

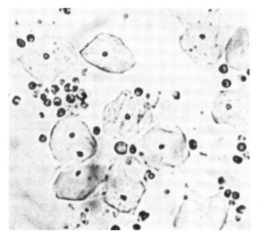

Figure 5-9.   Squamous epithelial cells in canine urine. (400X)

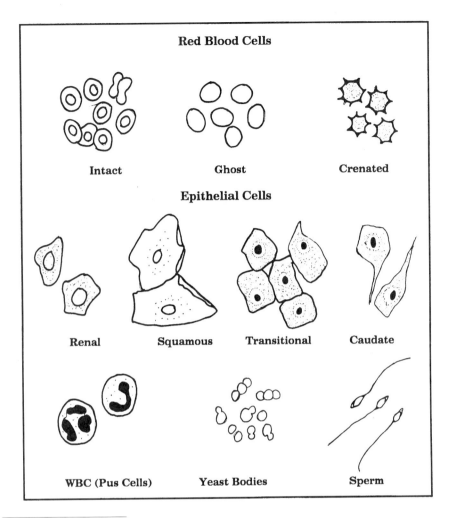

Red Blood Cells

Intact Ghost Crenated

Epithelial Cells

Renal Squamous Transitional Caudate

WBC (Pus Cells) Yeast Bodies Sperm

FIGURE **5-10.**   Cell types that may be found in urine.

phritis. Increased numbers may also be seen if catheterization was used to obtain the sample.

RENAL EPITHELIAL CELLS.   Renal epithelial cells are the smallest epithelial cells seen in urine. They originate in the renal tubules. They are only slightly larger than WBCs and are often confused with them. Renal epithelial cells are generally round and contain a large nucleus (Figures 5-10 and 5-13). They are rarely found (0 to 1/HPF). Increased numbers of these cells occurs in diseases of the kidney parenchyma.

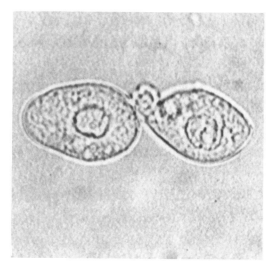

FIGURE 5-11. Transitional epithelial cells in canine urine. (500X)

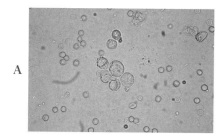

A

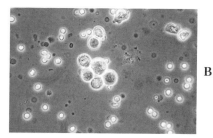

B

FIGURE 5-12. Cluster of bladder epithelial cells and numerous RBCs. **A,** Bright-field microscopy. **B,** Phrase-contrast microscopy.

MICROORGANISMS

A variety of microorganisms may be found in urine sediment, including bacteria, fungi, and protozoa. Normal urine is free of bacteria, but it may be contaminated from the vagina, vulva, or prepuce during urination. Normal samples collected by cystocentesis or catheterization do not contain bacteria. Because bacteria often proliferate in urine that has been left standing for some time, especially at room temperature, it is important to examine a fresh sample or immediately refrigerate the sample. Bacteria are very small and can only be identified at higher magnifications (Figure 5-14). They may be round (cocci) or

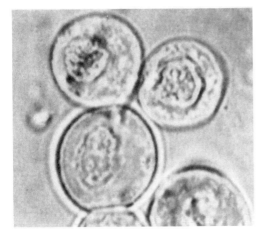

FIGURE 5-13.   Renal epithelial cells in canine urine. (500X)

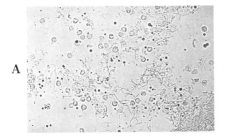

A

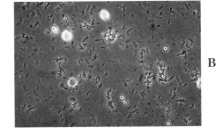

B

FIGURE 5-14.   Bacteria and leukocytes. **A,** Bright-field microscopy. **B,** Phase-contrast microscopy.

rod shaped (bacilli). They usually refract light and appear to be quivering due to Brownian movement. They are reported as few, moderate, or many. A large number of bacteria accompanied by a large number of WBCs indicates infection and inflammation of the urinary tract (cystitis, pyelonephritis) or genital tract (prostatitis, metritis, vaginitis, or balanitis).

Yeast bodies are often confused with RBCs or lipid droplets, but they do not dissolve in acetic acid, usually display characteristic budding, and may have double refractile walls (Figure 5-15). Yeast bodies usually are contaminants in urine samples, as yeast infections of the urinary tract are rare in domestic animals. Yeast infections of the external genitalia may cause yeast to be present in voided samples.

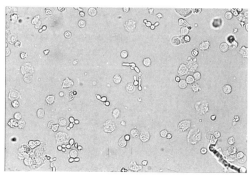

Figure 5-15. Yeast. (400X)

CASTS

Casts are formed in the lumen of the distal and collecting tubules of the kidney, where the concentration and acidity of urine are greatest. In the renal tubules, secreted protein precipitates in acidic conditions and forms casts shaped like the tubules in which they form. All casts are cylindric, with parallel sides. Cells in the area may also be incorporated into casts, imparting the morphologic features that allow them to be identified specifically. Casts dissolve while in alkaline urine, so cast identification and quantitation are best done in fresh samples that have not become alkaline with standing. Casts may also be disrupted with high-speed centrifugation and rough sample handling. A few hyaline casts or granular casts (0 to 1/HPF) may be seen in normal urine, but larger numbers of casts indicate a lesion in the renal tubules. The number of casts observed is not a reliable indicator of the severity of the urinary disease.

HYALINE CASTS. A few hyaline casts may be seen in urine from normal animals. These are clear, colorless, and highly refractile (Figures 5-16 and 5-17). They are difficult to see and can only be identified using dim light. They are cylindric, with parallel sides and usually rounded ends. Because these casts dissolve quickly in alkaline urine, they are rarely seen in the sediment of herbivores, which characteristically have alkaline urine. They are easier to identify in stained sediment and with phase-contrast microscopy than in unstained sediment. Hyaline casts indicate the mildest form of renal irritation. Their numbers are also increased with fever, poor renal perfusion, strenuous exercise, or general anesthesia. *Cylindroids* have the same significance as hyaline casts and resemble hyaline casts except that one end is tapered.

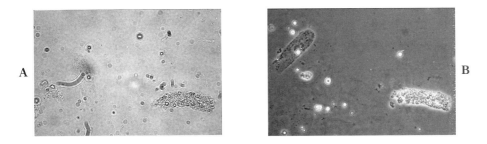

FIGURE 5-16. Hyaline and granular casts. **A,** Bright-field microscopy. **B,** Phase-contrast microscopy.

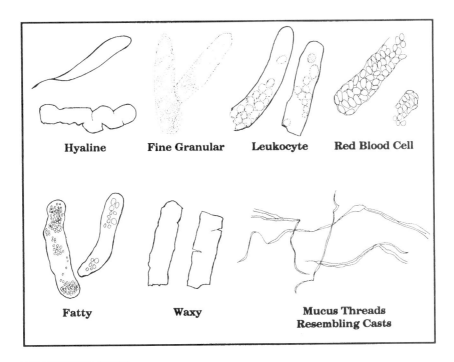

FIGURE 5-17. Various types of casts that may be found in urine.

GRANULAR CASTS. Granular casts are the most common type of cast seen in animals. These are simply hyaline casts containing granules (Figures 5-16, 5-17, and 5-18). The granules are from tubular epithelial cells and WBCs that became incorporated in the cast and then degenerated. Granular casts are seen in large numbers with acute nephritis and indicate more severe kidney damage than do hyaline casts.

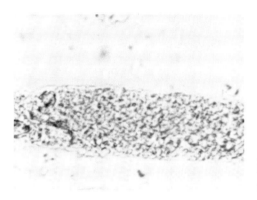

FIGURE 5-18.   Granular cast in canine urine. (500X)

EPITHELIAL CASTS.   Epithelial casts are comprised of epithelial cells from the renal tubules. Epithelial cells in casts are always of the renal epithelial type, as this is the only epithelial cell present at the site of cast formation. They are usually accompanied by granular casts. These casts are seen in acute nephritis or other conditions that cause degeneration of the renal tubular epithelium.

LEUKOCYTE CASTS.   Leukocyte casts contain WBCs (Figure 5-17). The presence of granular pus cells (WBCs) indicates inflammation in the renal tubules.

ERYTHROCYTE CASTS.   Erythrocyte casts are deep yellow to orange. The RBC membranes may or may not be visible (Figure 5-17). Erythrocyte casts indicate bleeding from the kidney.

WAXY CASTS.   Waxy casts resemble hyaline casts but are usually wider, with square ends rather than round ends and a dull, homogeneous, "waxy" appearance. They are more opaque than hyaline casts (Figures 5-17 and 5-19). They indicate chronic, severe degeneration of the renal tubules.

FATTY CASTS.   Fatty casts contain many small droplets of fat that appear as refractile bodies (Figure 5-17). They are frequently seen in cats with renal disease, as normal cats have fat in their renal parenchyma. They are occasionally seen in dogs with diabetes mellitus. Large numbers of fatty casts suggest degeneration of the renal tubules.

MUCUS THREADS.   Mucus threads are often confused with casts, but they do not have the well-delineated edges of casts. They more resemble a twisted ribbon than a cast (Figure 5-17). A large amount of mucus is normally present in

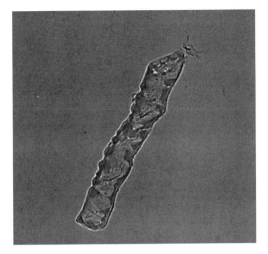

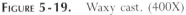
FIGURE 5-19. Waxy cast. (400X)

equine urine because horses have mucus glands in the renal pelvis and ureter. In other animals, mucus indicates urethral irritation or contamination of the sample with genital secretions.

SPERMATOZOA

Spermatozoa are occasionally seen in the urine sediment of intact male animals. They are easily recognized and have no clinical significance (Figures 5-10 and 5-20).

PARASITE OVA

Parasite ova may be seen in the urine sediment of animals with urinary parasites or because of fecal contamination at the time of collection of the urine sample. Parasites of the urinary tract include *Capillaria plica* (bladder worm of dogs and cats), *Dioctophyma renale* (kidney worm of dogs), and *Stephanurus dentatus* (kidney worm of pigs) (Figure 5-21).

FAT DROPLETS

In urine sediment, fat droplets are lightly green-tinged, highly refractile, spherical bodies of varying sizes (Figure 5-22). Because they vary in size, they

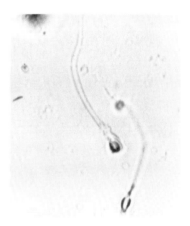

Figure 5-20. Spermatozoa in canine urine. (400X)

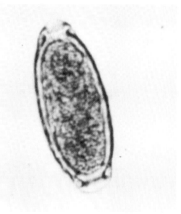

Figure 5-21. An egg of *Capillaria plica,* the bladderworm of dogs and cats. (400X)

can be distinguished from RBCs and yeast cells, which tend to be of uniform size. If a sediment smear is allowed to sit for a few moments before it is examined, fat droplets rise to a plane just beneath the coverslip, while other formed elements settle to the top of the slide. Any small, round structures found under the coverslip are usually fat globules. Uniformly sized, round structures found in a lower plane are usually RBCs. In sediment stained with Sudan III stain, fat droplets appear orange or red. Frequently, fat droplets from catheter lubricants or from oily surfaces of collecting vials and pipettes may contaminate urine. Fat in the urine (*lipuria*) is seen to some degree in most cats. Lipuria is also seen with obesity, diabetes mellitus, and hypothyroidism, and rarely after a high-fat meal.

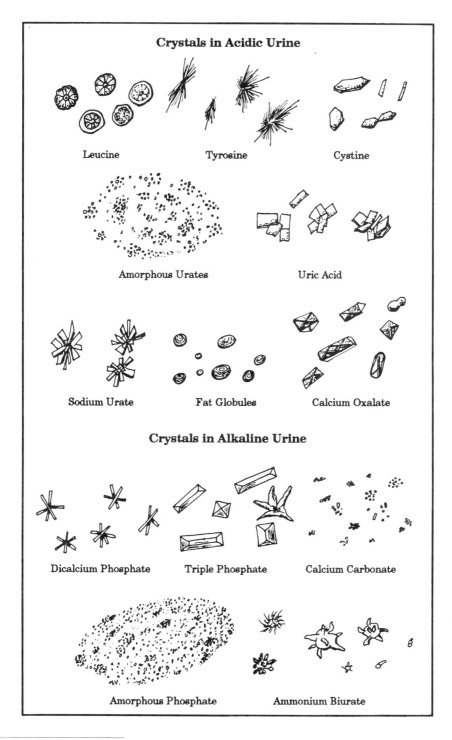

FIGURE 5-22. Various types of crystals that may be found in urine.

CRYSTALS

The presence of crystals in the urine is termed *crystalluria*. Crystalluria may or may not be of clinical significance. Certain crystals form as a consequence of their elements being secreted into the urine by normal renal activity. Other crystals form as a consequence of metabolic diseases. Crystal formation may lead to formation of urinary calculi. The type of crystals formed depends on the urine pH, concentration and temperature, and the solubility of the elements (Figure 5-22). If a urine sample is allowed to stand and cool before examination, the number of crystals in the sample increases because the materials that make up crystals are less soluble at lower temperatures. Refrigerated samples often have many more crystals than fresh samples. Sometimes crystals dissolve when a refrigerated sample is warmed to room temperature. Crystals are generally reported as occasional, moderate, or many.

TRIPLE PHOSPHATE.   Triple phosphate crystals are found in alkaline to slightly acidic urine. Triple phosphate crystals typically resemble coffin lids, though they may assume other shapes. Generally triple phosphate crystals are eight-sided prisms, with tapering sides and ends. Occasionally they may assume a fern-leaf shape, especially when the urine contains a high concentration of ammonia (Figures 5-22 and 5-23).

AMORPHOUS PHOSPHATE.   Amorphous phosphates are common in alkaline urine and appear as a granular precipitate (Figures 5-22 and 5-24).

CALCIUM CARBONATE.   Calcium carbonate crystals, commonly seen in the urine of horses, are round, with many lines radiating from their centers (Figures 5-22 and 5-25). They may also have a "dumbbell" shape.

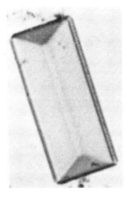

FIGURE 5-23.   Triple phosphate crystal in canine urine, resembling a coffin lid. (200X)

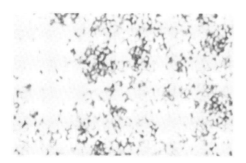

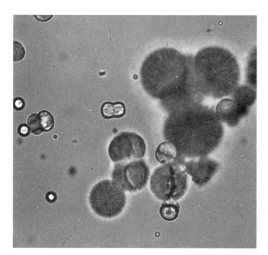

FIGURE 5-24. Amorphous phosphates in canine urine. (400X)

FIGURE 5-25. Calcium carbonate crystals in urine of a horse. (400X)

AMORPHOUS URATES.   Amorphous urates, which are seen in acidic urine, appear as a granular precipitate similar to amorphous phosphates, but amorphous phosphates are found in alkaline urine (Figure 5-22).

AMMONIUM BIURATE.   Ammonium biurate crystals are round, with long spicules (thorn apple shape) and a brownish color (Figures 5-22 and 5-26). Often the spicules fracture and the remaining crystal is brown, with fine radiating lines. They are most common in animals with liver disease, such as portacaval shunts.

CALCIUM OXALATE.   Calcium oxalate dihydrate crystals generally appear as small squares, containing an X across the crystal, resembling the back of an envelope (Figures 5-22 and 5-27). Calcium oxalate monohydrate crystals are very small and "dumbbell" shaped. Calcium dihydrate crystals are found in acidic and neutral urine and are commonly seen in small numbers in dogs and horses. The

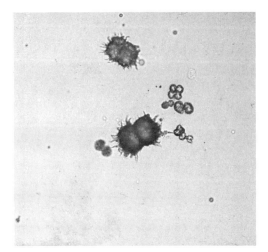

Figure 5-26. Ammonium biurate crystals in urine of a dog. (400X)

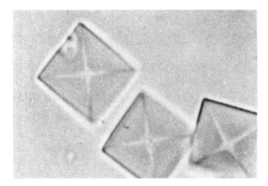

Figure 5-27. Calcium oxalate crystals, resembling a square envelope. (160X)

urine of animals poisoned with ethylene glycol (antifreeze) often contains large numbers of calcium oxalate crystals, especially calcium monohydrate crystals. Animals with oxalate urolithiasis may have large numbers of calcium oxalate crystals in their urine. Further, large numbers of oxalate crystals may indicate predisposition to oxalate urolithiasis.

Sulfonamide. Sulfonamide crystals may be seen in animals being treated with sulfonamides. They are less likely to be observed in alkaline urine, as these crystals are more soluble in alkaline urine. To prevent precipitation of these crystals in the renal tubules, it is advantageous to maintain alkaline urine and encourage the animal to drink as much as possible. Various sulfa drugs produce crystals that app⋯ typical for that drug.

LEUCINE, TYROSINE.   Animals with liver disease may have leucine and tyrosine crystals in their urine. Tyrosine crystals are dark and needle like (Figure 5-22). They are often found in small clusters.

CYSTINE.   Cystine crystals appear as six-sided (hexagonal), flat plates and can be associated with renal tubular dysfunction (Figures 5-22 and 5-28).

ARTIFACTS

Many artifacts may enter the urine sample during collection, transportation, or examination. It is important to be able to recognize these structures as irrelevant and not a normal part of the sediment. These contaminants can be a source of great confusion.

Air bubbles, oil droplets (usually due to lubricated catheters), starch granules (from surgical gloves), hair, fecal material, plant spores, dust, bacteria, and fungi may contaminate urine. Ova of intestinal parasites may be observed due to fecal contamination of the urine sample.

UROLITHIASIS

Uroliths are calculi (stones) composed of various minerals. They may be found anywhere in the urinary tract; their occurrence is termed *urolithiasis*. It is very important to determine the composition of these calculi, as their prevention and the prognosis depend on identification of their composition.

Mineral composition of uroliths may be determined to some degree with qualitative analysis, such as with the Oxford Stone Analysis Set for urinary calculi (Oxford Laboratories, Foster City, CA). A more accurate analysis of the mineral composition may be determined by submitting it intact to a reference laboratory for quantitative analysis (crystallography) (Urinary Stone Lab, Veterinary Medical Teaching Hospital, University of California, Davis, CA). Occasionally, a reasonable guess about the composition of a urolith may be made by its gross and radiographic appearance and the crystal types found in the sediment. Calculi may have a mixed composition, with a predominant crystal type.

TRIPLE PHOSPHATE.   In dogs and cats, the most common uroliths observed are triple phosphate uroliths. They are composed of salts of magnesium, ammonium, and calcium (the anions), and phosphate (the cation). These are generally radiopaque, hard, white or yellow, and powdery when crushed. They are common in alkaline urine. Alkaline urine often occurs in urinary tract infection in carnivores, especially with *Streptococcus* urinary tract infections.

Urate. Urate uroliths are composed of ammonium urate and are usually radiolucent, yellow, and brittle. These uroliths are seen mostly in Dalmatians, as this breed excretes much uric acid. They can sometimes be found in other dog breeds.

Cystine. Cystine uroliths are usually yellow, smooth, easily pulverized, and radiolucent.

Oxalate. Oxalate uroliths are composed of calcium oxalate and are radiopaque and hard. They do not crush easily and have sharp protrusions on their surface. They may severely traumatize the bladder.

Urolithiasis is a problem in castrated male ruminants. Lodging of calculi in the urethra obstructs the outflow of urine. It is a major problem in lambs and steers, particularly those fed high-concentrate rations. The most common calculi in these species are composed of calcium, magnesium, and ammonium carbonate, or calcium, magnesium, and ammonium phosphate.

Recommended Reading

1.   Osborne, Stevens: *Handbook of canine and feline urinalysis,* St Louis, 1981, Ralston Purina.

2.   *Modern urine chemistry,* Elkhart, IN, 1993, Miles Laboratories.

3.   Osborne, Finco, editors: *Canine and feline nephrology and urology,* 1995, Baltimore, Williams & Wilkins.

4.   Ling: *Lower urinary tract diseases of dogs and cats,* St Louis, 1995, Mosby.

INTERNAL PARASITES

C.M. Hendrix

This chapter discusses the roles that veterinary technicians play in assisting the veterinarian in diagnosing endoparasites (internal parasites) of domestic animals such as dogs, cats, cattle, horses, sheep, and poultry. Diagnosis of endoparasitism is one of the most frequently performed procedures in the veterinary clinical setting. As such, diagnoses must be performed accurately and in a timely manner so that the information may be related to the client and appropriate treatment initiated.

An accurate diagnosis of endoparasitism is based primarily upon the veterinarian's and the technician's awareness of parasites that are prevalent in the immediate geographic area or ecosystem. However, because of the mobility of clients during their lifetime, residence in or travel to another region should also be considered when endoparasitism is among several differential diagnoses.

Heavily parasitized animals often show clinical signs suggestive of the infected organ system. Depending on the system, these signs may include diarrhea or constipation, anorexia, vomiting, blood in the stool, or fat in the stool. Parasitized animals are frequently lethargic and display an unthrifty appearance characterized by weight loss or stunted growth, dull haircoat, dehydration, or anemia. The animal may also exhibit coughing or difficulty in breathing.

Internal parasites of domestic animals comprise several types of organisms that live internally in animals, feed on their tissues or body fluids, or compete directly for their food. These organisms range in size from too small to be seen with the naked eye (microscopic), to over a meter in length. Parasites also vary in their location within the host and in the means by which they are transmitted from one host to another. Because of these diverse variations, no single diagnostic test can identify all endoparasites.

The veterinary technician may be asked to perform a wide variety of diagnostic procedures to diagnose endoparasitism. These procedures usually detect the adult stages of a parasite or their eggs or larval stages in the animal's feces, urine, or blood. Mature parasites are seldom found because they are generally hidden within the body of the animal. The only way to detect their presence is by necropsy, or postmortem dissection. An assorted battery of diagnostic procedures may not be in common use in veterinary practices but are described in this chapter because they may be useful to veterinary technicians working in research or diagnostic laboratories.

This chapter includes illustrations and brief descriptions of some of the eggs, larvae, and adult parasites that may be diagnosed in common domesticated animals. Sometimes eggs of certain groups of parasites are quite similar; it may be difficult or impossible to differentiate individual species or genera based on their morphologic characteristics. Parasites with similar eggs are usually differentiated by fecal culture (procedure to be described later) and larval identification. This chapter does not provide descriptions of parasite larval cultures; those descriptions and methodologies are found in the reference texts listed at the end of this chapter.

The technician must remember that the diagnostic tests used to detect endoparasitism may be unreliable. An animal may be infected with endoparasites; however, if the infection is slight, no eggs or larvae may be observed in the specimens tested. If an inappropriate test is used, it is also possible that no parasites may be detected. Another common problem is trying to diagnose endoparasitism before the parasite completely develops. Many parasites can produce clinical disease before they become reproductively mature.

The time elapsed between initial infection with a parasite until the infection can be detected using common diagnostic procedures is called the *prepatent period*. The best example of this concept is trying to diagnose hookworm disease (*Ancylostoma caninum*) in a 1-week-old puppy by observation of eggs on fecal flotation. This is a waste of time because the minimum time for infection until adult hookworms are present in the bowel and begin to produce eggs (prepatent period) is 12 days. The astute veterinary practitioner uses not only fecal flotation results but also the puppy's history, clinical signs, and other laboratory tests (e.g., blood values) to arrive at a specific diagnosis of ancylostomiasis (infection with hookworms).

COMMON TYPES OF PARASITES

Complete coverage of the discipline of veterinary parasitology is beyond the scope of this textbook. Only the general types of parasites of domestic animals and their life cycle stages that may be recovered using commonly employed diagnostic procedures will be described. The reference textbooks listed at the end of this chapter can provide more detailed coverage of veterinary parasitology and specific parasites.

Internal parasites (endoparasites) live within an animal. These parasites derive their nutrition and protection at the expense of the infected animal, which is called the *host*. The various internal parasites have many different *life cycles*. Each parasite's life cycle is distinctive and is comprised of various developmental stages, which can occur all within the same host or separately within sequential hosts.

The host that harbors the adult, mature, or sexual stages of a parasite is called the *definitive host*. The dog is the definitive host for *Dirofilaria immitis;* adult male and female heartworms are found in the right ventricle and pulmonary arteries of the dog's heart. The host that harbors the larval, immature, or asexual stages of a parasite is called the *intermediate host*. The mosquito is the intermediate host for *D. immitis;* first, second, and third larval stages of *D. immitis* are found within the mosquito intermediate host.

The life cycle of most parasites has at least one stage at which it may be passed from one host to the next. Diagnostic procedures frequently detect this stage; thus, it is referred to as the *diagnostic stage*. The diagnostic stage of a parasite may leave the host through excreta, such as feces or urine, or it may be transmitted via the blood to its next host by an arthropod, such as a mosquito. The microfilarial stage is the diagnostic stage of *D. immitis;* the female mosquito takes in the microfilariae during a blood meal.

PROTOZOA (ONE-CELLED ORGANISMS)

Protozoa are unicellular or one-celled organisms, some of which may be parasitic in domestic animals. These protozoans can infect a variety of tissue sites within the definitive host. The most common sites for their detection are in blood samples (*blood protozoa* or *hemoprotozoa*) or within fecal samples (*intestinal protozoa*). The protozoan's life cycle may be very simple or it may be very complex.

Most hemoprotozoa seen in the United States are found in erythrocytes (red blood cells, RBCs) within a stained blood smear. Ticks usually serve as intermediate hosts and transmit the RBCs containing the hemoprotozoa from one animal to the next. *Babesia bigemina* is a tear-shaped or pear-shaped hemoprotozoan found within the RBCs of infected cattle. It is transmitted by *Boophilus annulatus,* a tick described in Chapter 7.

Trypanosomes are another group of hemoprotozoans occasionally found in the United States. Rather than being found within RBCs, trypanosomes are extracellular and "swim" within the blood. They are 3 to 10 times as long as a RBC is wide and are banana-shaped. They have a lateral undulating membrane and a thin, whip-like tail (flagellum) that is used for swimming. These parasites are also transmitted by blood-feeding arthropods (Reduviid bugs in Chapter 7).

Trematodes (flukes)

The trematodes (flukes) are flatworms with unsegmented, leaf-shaped bodies. In domestic animals in the United States, most adult flukes are found in the intestinal tract, the liver, or the lungs. In these sites, the hermaphroditic (having male *and* female sex organs) flukes lay eggs that are passed with the feces. The end portion of many fluke eggs has a small cap, lid, or door; this structure is called an *operculum* and is common among the flukes.

Within each fluke egg is a larval stage known as a *miracidium,* which hatches and exits the egg through the operculum. This stage penetrates the *first intermediate host,* which is usually a snail. Within the snail, the miracidium develops into a *sporocyst,* which then produces many tiny structures called *rediae.* Each redia may produce many *cercariae.* The cercaria exits the snail and may take one of three pathways to enter the definitive host: it may develop into a *metacercaria* and encyst upon vegetation, whereby it is ingested by the definitive host; it may be ingested by a *second intermediate host* and become encysted within that host, which is subsequently ingested by the definitive host; or it may directly penetrate the skin of the definitive host.

Flukes of veterinary importance include the liver flukes of cattle and sheep (*Fasciola hepatica, Fascioloides magna, Dicrocoelium dendriticum*) and the lung fluke of dogs and cats (*Paragonimus kellicotti*).

Cestodes (tapeworms)

Like trematodes, cestodes (tapeworms) are also flatworms. They differ, however, in that cestodes are ribbon-like and divided into a long chain of *proglottids* or segments connected like train cars behind a *scolex* or "head," by which the tapeworm attaches to the wall of the host's intestine. Most tapeworms release their proglottids one at a time or in short chains into the feces. Proglottids in the feces can be observed with the naked eye. A few tapeworms release eggs directly from the worm's uterus.

Tapeworm proglottids have muscles that enable them to move about. Pet owners often observe these tapeworms as "little white worms" crawling on the pet's feces, haircoat, or bedding. These fresh proglottids are said to resemble "cucumber seeds." When the proglottids dry out, they resemble uncooked grains of rice.

Tapeworm proglottids often contain eggs when they are passed into the feces. These eggs contain *hexacanth embryos,* which are embryos with an internal structure with six hooks.

These hexacanth embryos are ingested by an intermediate host, usually a mammalian host, such as a rabbit. The hexacanth embryo grows within the tissues of the intermediate host to a "bladder worm" stage, which is a fluid-filled larval stage. The definitive host becomes infected by ingesting the intermediate host containing the bladderworm larval stage. Examples of tapeworms that develop into the bladderworm stage in the intermediate host is the canine Taeniid tapeworm (*Taenia pisiformis*) and the coenurus tapeworm (*Multiceps multiceps*). In some tapeworms (*Echinococcus granulosus, E. multilocularis*), the larval stage within the vertebrate host is a *hydatid cyst.*

When the intermediate host is an arthropod, such as a flea or a grain mite, the hexacanth embryo develops into a microscopic larval stage known as a *cysticercoid.* The cysticercoid stage is tiny and contains a small fluid-filled space. The definitive host becomes infected by ingesting the intermediate host containing the cysticercoid larval stage. The cysticercoid stage develops in the fringed tapeworms of cattle (*Thysanosoma actinoides*) and the double-pored tapeworm of dogs and cats (*Dipylidium caninum*).

Nematodes (roundworms)

Nematodes are often referred to as roundworms and are the most important group of parasites in veterinary parasitology. They may be found in almost any tissue of domestic animals, including the intestines, skin, lungs, kidneys, urinary bladder, nervous tissue, and blood.

Nematodes as a group have diverse, complicated life cycles. Their eggs or larvae are most commonly recovered from the feces. The eggs of nematodes infecting the kidney or urinary bladder may be recovered from the urine.

Examples of intestinal nematodes include large roundworms (*Toxocara canis, Toxascaris leonina*), hookworms (*Ancylostoma caninum, Uncinaria stenocephala*), and whipworms (*Trichuris vulpis*). Urinary roundworms include canine kidney worms (*Dioctophyma renale*). Respiratory roundworms include the lungworms of cattle and sheep (*Dictyocaulus* species and *Muellerius capillaris*). Nematodes of the blood vasculature are a special group, of which the heartworm of dogs (*Dirofilaria immitis*) is an example. Adult female heartworms give birth to small, worm-like prelarval (embryonic) stages called *microfilariae.* The microfilariae are often observed in a peripheral blood smear and are approximately 310 μ long. These microfilariae can be transmitted to other animals by mosquitos.

Acanthocephalans (Thorny-Headed Worms)

Acanthocephalans (thorny-headed worms) are uncommon parasites with very complicated life cycles. On the cranial end of these helminths is a spiny proboscis, which is used to attach to the lining of the intestine wall. Thorny-headed worms do not have a true gut; they absorb nutrients through their body wall. Acanthocephalans are usually recovered at necropsy.

The most "famous" acanthocephalan is *Macracanthorhynchus hirudinaceus,* a parasite of pigs. This parasite has the dubious honor of possessing the longest scientific name among the parasites of domestic animals. *Oncicola canis* is the acanthocephalan of dogs.

COMMON ENDOPARASITES OF DOMESTIC ANIMALS

Following are descriptions of most of the common endoparasites in domestic animals in the United States. Information is given on the organ or organ system parasitized in the host, *prepatent period* (time from initial infection until the diagnostic stage can be recovered) where appropriate, description of the diagnostic stage (life cycle stage commonly used to make a diagnosis, such as eggs or larvae), and diagnostic stage most commonly identified.

Endoparasites of Dogs and Cats

Parasites of the Gastrointestinal Tract

Nematodes (Roundworms)

Spirocerca lupi, the esophageal worm, is a nematode that often forms nodules in the esophageal wall of dogs and cats. Occasionally it may be found in gastric nodules in cats. Adult worms reside deep within these nodules and expel their eggs through fistulous openings in the granuloma. Eggs are passed through the host animal's esophagus and out in the feces. The thick-shelled eggs are 30 to

37 μ by 11 to 15 μ and contain a larva when they are laid; these eggs have a unique "paper clip" shape. Figure 6-1 shows the characteristic ovum of *S. lupi*. Eggs can usually be observed on fecal flotation and can be recovered when vomitus has been subjected to a standard fecal flotation procedure. Radiographic or endoscopic examination may reveal characteristic granulomas within the esophagus or within the stomach. The prepatent period is 6 months.

Physaloptera species are stomach worms of dogs and cats. Although they are occasionally found in the lumen of the stomach or small intestine, *Physaloptera* species are usually firmly attached to the mucosal surface of the stomach, where they suck blood. At this site, it is possible to view these nematodes using an endoscope. Their diet consists of blood and tissue derived from the host's gastric mucosa. Their attachment sites continue to bleed after the parasite detaches. Vomiting, anorexia, and dark, tarry stools may be observed in affected animals.

The adults are creamy white, sometimes tightly coiled, and 1.3 to 4.8 cm long. They are often recovered in the pet's vomitus and can be confused with ascarids (roundworms). A quick way to differentiate the two parasites is to break open an adult specimen and (if that specimen happens to be female) examine the egg type microscopically. The eggs of *Physaloptera* species are small, smooth, thick-shelled, and embryonated when passed in the feces. Eggs are 30 to 34 μ by 49 to 59 μ and contain a larva when they are laid. Figure 6-2 shows the characteristic ovum of *Physaloptera* species. Eggs can usually be recovered on a standard fecal flotation, using solutions with a specific gravity above 1.25. The prepatent period is 56 to 83 days.

Aonchotheca putorii is commonly referred to as the gastric capillarid of cats. It was once known by a former name, *Capillaria putorii*. This capillarid

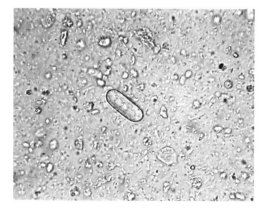

FIGURE 6-1. Characteristic ovum of *Spirocerca lupi*. The thick-shelled eggs contain larvae and measure 30 to 38 μ by 11 to 15 μ. Eggs can be usually observed on fecal flotation and can be recovered when vomitus has been subjected to a standard fecal flotation procedure.

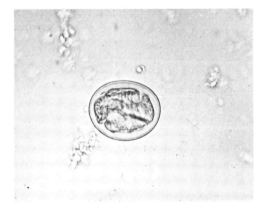

Figure 6-2. Characteristic ovum of *Physaloptera* species. The oval, thick-shelled eggs contain larvae and measure 49 to 58 μ by 30 to 34 μ. Eggs can be usually recovered on a standard fecal flotation, using solutions with a specific gravity above 1.25.

frequently parasitizes mustellids, such as mink, but it has also been reported in cats. These nematodes are rarely reported in North America. The eggs of *A. putorii* are easily confused with other trichinelloid nematodes (see the section following on feline whipworms). Their eggs are 53 to 70 μ by 20 to 30 μ and exhibit a net-like surface similar to that of the eggs of *Eucoleus aerophilus,* an upper respiratory capillarid. The eggs of *A. putorii* are dense, less delicate than those of *E. aerophilus,* and organized in a longitudinal formation. They have flattened sides and contain a one- or two-celled embryo that fills the egg.

Ollulanus tricuspis is "the feline trichostrongyle." This parasite is usually associated with vomiting in cats. It is most commonly identified by examining the cat's vomitus with a dissecting or compound microscope. Feline vomitus can also be examined using a standard fecal flotation procedure. The best flotation solution for identification is a modified Sheather's flotation solution. Adult female *O. tricuspis* are 0.8 to 1.0 mm long and have three major tail cusps (hence, the epithet *tricuspis*). Adult males are 0.7 to 0.8 mm long and have a copulatory bursa. The female worms are viviparous (bear live young). The infective third-stage larvae (500 by 22 μ) mature to adults in the cat's stomach. Free-living stages are not required for completion of the life cycle. Transmission occurs through ingestion of vomitus from infected cats.

Toxocara canis, T. cati, and *Toxascaris leonina* are the ascarids of dogs and cats. These roundworms are found in the small intestine of dogs and cats in most areas of the world. All young puppies and kittens presented to a veterinary clinic should be examined for these large, robust nematodes. Adult ascarids may vary from 3 to 18 cm in length and when passed are usually tightly coiled, much like a coiled bed spring. The eggs of *Toxocara* species are spherical, with a deeply pigmented center and a rough, pitted outer shell. Eggs of *T. canis* are

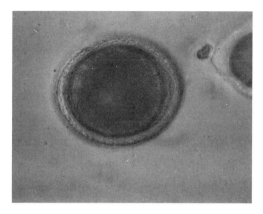

FIGURE 6-3. Characteristic ovum of *Toxocara* species. These eggs are spherical, with a deeply pigmented center and a rough, pitted outer shell. Eggs of *T. canis* are 75 to 90 µ in diameter.

75 to 90 µ in diameter (Figure 6-3), while those of *T. cati* are smaller, only 65 to 75 µ in diameter (Figure 6-4). The eggs of *Toxascaris leonina* are spherical to ovoid, with dimensions of 75 by 85 µ. These eggs have a smooth outer shell and a hyaline or "ground glass" central portion. Figure 6-5 shows the characteristic ovum of *Toxascaris leonina*. The prepatent period for *T. canis* is 21 to 35 days, while that of *T. leonina* is 74 days.

Ancylostoma caninum (canine hookworm), *A. tubaeforme* (feline hookworm), *A. braziliense* (canine and feline hookworm), and *Uncinaria stenocephala* (northern canine hookworm) are small intestinal nematodes. Hookworms are found throughout the world and are common in tropical and subtropical areas of North America. Hookworm infection, which can produce severe anemia in young kittens and puppies, can be a serious problem in kennels and catteries. The prepatent period depends on the species of hookworm and the route of infection.

Eggs of all hookworm species are oval or ellipsoid and thin-walled and contain 8 to 16 cells when passed in the pet's feces. Because these eggs larvate rapidly in the external environment (as early as 48 hours after feces are passed), fresh feces are needed for diagnosing hookworm infections. Eggs of *A. caninum* are 56 to 75 µ by 34 to 47 µ (Figures 6-6 and 6-8). Those of *A. tubaeforme* are 55 to 75 µ by 34.4 to 44.7 µ. Those of *A. braziliense* are 75 by 45 µ and those of *U. stenocephala*, 65 to 80 µ by 40 to 50 µ. These eggs can be usually recovered on a standard fecal flotation.

Strongyloides stercoralis and *S. tumiefaciens* are often referred to as "intestinal threadworms." These nematodes are unique in that only a parthenogenetic female (female that can lay eggs without copulation with a male) is parasitic in the host. Parasitic males do not exist. These females produce eggs, but in dogs

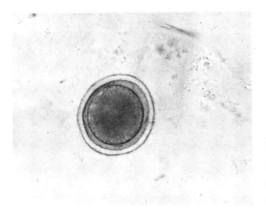

FIGURE **6-4.** Characteristic ovum of *Toxocara cati.* These eggs are smaller than those of *T. canis,* measuring only 65 to 75 μ in diameter.

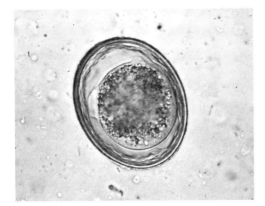

FIGURE **6-5.** Characteristic ovum of *Toxascaris leonina.* These eggs are spherical to ovoid, with dimensions of 75 by 85 μ. They have a smooth outer shell and a hyaline or "ground glass" central portion.

these eggs hatch in the intestine, releasing first-stage larvae. Figure 6-7 shows the parasitic adult females, eggs, and first-stage larvae of *Strongyloides* species. The larvae are 280 to 310 μ long and have a rhabditiform esophagus, with a club-shaped cranial corpus, a narrow median isthmus, and a caudal bulb. The prepatent period is 8 to 14 days.

Trichuris vulpis, the canine whipworm, and *T. campanula* and *T. serrata,* the feline whipworms, reside in the cecum and colon of their respective hosts. Canine whipworms are common, but feline whipworms are quite rare in North America and diagnosed only sporadically throughout the world. Whipworms derive their name from the fact that the adults have a thin, filamentous cranial end (the lash of the whip) and a thick caudal end (the handle of the whip). The egg of the whipworm is described as trichinelloid or trichuroid. It has a thick, yellow-brown, symmetric shell with polar plugs at both ends. The eggs are

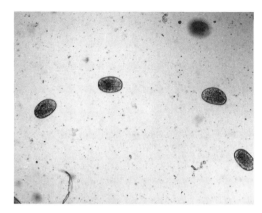

FIGURE 6-6. Characteristic hookworm ovum. The eggs of *Ancylostoma caninum* are 56 to 75 μ by 34 to 47 μ, those of *A. tubaeforme,* 55 to 75 μ by 34.4 to 44.7 μ, those of *A. braziliense,* 75 by 45 μ, and those of *U. stenocephala,* 65 to 80 μ by 40 to 50 μ.

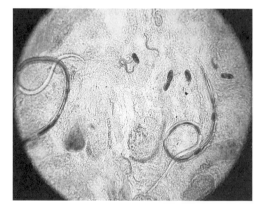

FIGURE 6-7. Parasitic adult females, eggs, and first-stage larvae of *Strongyloides* species. These larvae are 280 to 310 μ long and have a rhabditiform esophagus, with a club-shaped cranial corpus, a narrow median isthmus, and a caudal bulb.

unembryonated (not larvated) when laid. Eggs of *T. vulpis* are 70 to 89 μ by 37 to 40 μ. Figure 6-8 shows the characteristic egg of *T. vulpis.* The prepatent period for *T. vulpis* is 70 to 90 days.

The eggs of *T. campanula* and *T. serrata* may be easily confused with those of *Aonchotheca putorii, Eucoleus aerophilus,* and *Personema feliscati,* parasites of the feline stomach, respiratory tract, and urinary system, respectively. The eggs of *T. campanula* average 63 to 85 μ by 34 to 39 μ. When examining a cat's feces for feline trichurids, it is important to be aware of *pseudoparasites,* eggs of trichurids or capillarids that parasitize such hosts as mice, rabbits, or birds (an outdoor cat's prey). The eggs of these trichurids or capillarids may pass unaltered through the cat's gastrointestinal system, remaining intact and unembryonated.

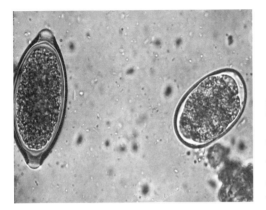

FIGURE 6-8. Characteristic ovum of *Trichuris vulpis*. Eggs of *T. vulpis* are 70 to 89 μ by 37 to 40 μ (*left*). On the *right* is the characteristic ovum of *A. caninum*, 56 to 75 μ by 34 to 47 μ.

Enterobius vermicularis is the human pinworm and *does not* parasitize dogs or cats! Nevertheless, the family pet is often falsely incriminated by family practitioners or pediatricians as a source of pinworm infection in young children. The veterinary technician should remember this rule: *Pinworms are parasites of omnivores (mice, rats, monkeys, people) and herbivores (rabbits, horses) but never carnivores (dogs, cats).*

CESTODES (TAPEWORMS)

Dipylidium caninum is often called the "double-pored" or "cucumber seed" tapeworm. This tapeworm is the most common tapeworm found in the small intestine of the dog and cat, owing to the fact that the dog or cat becomes infected by ingesting the flea intermediate host. Fleas often contain this parasite's infective cysticercoid stage. This tapeworm has motile, terminal, gravid proglottids, which are usually found on the feces (Figure 6-9), on the pet's haircoat, or in the bedding of the host. In the fresh state, these proglottids resemble cucumber seeds; hence the common name, the "cucumber seed" tapeworm. These terminal proglottids have a lateral pore located along the midpoint of each of their long edges; hence the second common name, the "double-pored" tapeworm.

If fresh proglottids are teased or broken open, they may reveal thousands of unique egg packets, each containing 20 to 30 hexacanth embryos. Figure 6-10 shows the unique egg packet of *D. caninum*. The proglottids of *D. caninum* often dry out in the external environment. As they lose moisture, they shrivel up and resemble uncooked grains of rice. If reconstituted with water, the dried proglottids usually assume their former cucumber-seed appearance. The prepatent period for *D. caninum* is 14 to 21 days.

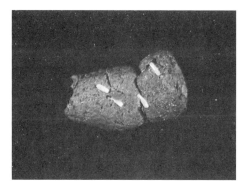

FIGURE 6-9. Characteristic motile, terminal, gravid proglottids of *Dipylidium caninum* on canine feces. In the fresh state, these proglottids resemble cucumber seeds; hence the common name, the "cucumber seed" tapeworm.

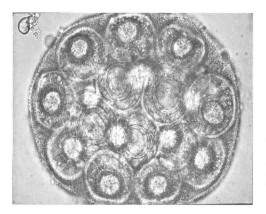

FIGURE 6-10. Characteristic egg packet of *Dipylidium caninum.* Each egg packet may contain up to 20 to 30 hexacanth embryos.

Taenia pisiformis, T. hydatigena, and *T. ovis* are the canine taeniids. As with *D. caninum, Taenia* tapeworms appear as motile, terminal, gravid proglottids on the feces, on the pet's haircoat, or in the bedding of the host. In the fresh state, these proglottids have a single lateral pore located along the midpoint of either of their long edges (as opposed to the "double-pored" tapeworm).

As with *D. caninum,* if these fresh proglottids are teased or broken open, they may reveal thousands of hexacanth embryos. The proglottids of *Taenia* species also dry out in the external environment and resemble uncooked grains of rice. If reconstituted with water, they too usually assume their former single-pored appearance. If gravid proglottids of *Taenia* species are recovered from a dog's or cat's feces, the proglottid should be torn open or macerated in a drop of saline solution on a glass slide to reveal the characteristic eggs under the compound microscope.

The eggs of taeniid tapeworms are slightly oval and are 43 to 53 μ by 43 to 49 μ in diameter (*T. pisiformis*), 36 to 39 μ by 31 to 35 μ in diameter (*T. hydatigena*) and 19 to 31 μ by 24 to 26 μ (*T. ovis*). Eggs of *Taenia* species contain a single *oncosphere* with three pairs of hooks. The oncosphere is often called a hexacanth embryo. Figure 6-11 shows the unique features of this taeniid tapeworm. The eggs are very similar to those of *Echinococcus* and *Multiceps* species.

Taenia taeniaeformis, or *Hydatigera taeniaeformis,* is called the "feline tapeworm" or the "feline taeniid." This tapeworm is observed infrequently in cats allowed to roam and prey upon house and field mice and rats. The egg of this tapeworm is 31 to 36 μ in diameter and contains a single oncosphere with three pairs of hooks. The oncosphere is often called a hexacanth embryo. As with the eggs of the canine taeniids, the eggs are very similar to those of *Echinococcus* species. Figure 6-11 shows the unique features of this taeniid tapeworm.

Multiceps multiceps and *M. serialis* are also tapeworms of the small intestine of canids. The eggs of *M. multiceps* are 29 to 37 μ in diameter, while those of *M. serialis* are elliptic and measure 31 to 34 μ by 29 to 30 μ. Both contain a single oncosphere with three pairs of hooks. As with the eggs of the canine and feline taeniids, the eggs of *Multiceps* species are very similar to those of *Echinococcus* species. Figure 6-11 shows the unique features of this taeniid tapeworm.

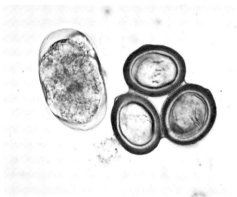

Figure 6-11. Characteristic ova of the taeniid tapeworms are slightly oval and 43 to 53 μ by 43 to 49 μ in diameter (*T. pisiformis*), 36 to 39 μ by 31 to 35 μ in diameter (*T. hydatigena*), and 19 to 31 μ by 24 to 26 μ (*T. ovis*). Eggs of *Taenia* species contain a single oncosphere with three pairs of hooks. The oncosphere is often called a hexacanth embryo. The eggs are quite similar to those of *Echinococcus* and *Multiceps* species. The dissimilar ovum is that of *A. caninum*, the hookworm.

Echinococcus granulosus and *E. multilocularis* are tapeworms associated with unilocular and multilocular hydatid disease. *Echinococcus granulosus* is the hydatid cyst tapeworm of dogs, while *E. multilocularis* is the hydatid cyst tapeworm of cats. These are important parasites because of their extreme zoonotic potential. The egg of *E. granulosus* is ovoid and 32 to 36 μ by 25 to 30 μ. It contains a single oncosphere with three pairs of hooks. The egg of *E. multilocularis* is ovoid and 30 to 40 μ. It contains a single oncosphere with three pairs of hooks. These eggs are very similar in appearance to those of *Taenia* and *Multiceps* species. Figure 6-11 shows the unique features of this taeniid tapeworm.

The adult *Echinococcus* is a tiny tapeworm, only 1.2 to 7.0 mm in length. The entire tapeworm only has three proglottids: immature, mature, and gravid. When passed, the tiny gravid proglottids are often overlooked by the client, the veterinary technician, and the veterinarian. Definitive diagnosis of *Echinococcus* infection is best achieved by identifying adult tapeworms taken from the host's intestinal tract. In the rare instances in which *Echinococcus* infection is suspected, antemortem diagnosis is accomplished by purging the dog or cat using arecoline hydrobromide PO at 3.5 mg/kg and collecting the feces. This procedure is usually only performed when this infection is strongly suspected. Entire worms or their proglottids may be collected from the final clear mucus. Because of the severe zoonotic potential, all evacuated material should be handled with caution. *Rubber gloves should be worn!* After the feces have been examined, they should be incinerated.

Spirometra species are often referred to as "zipper tapeworms" or sparganosis tapeworms. These tapeworms are often found in the small intestine of both the dog and cat. These tapeworms are often found in pets in Florida and along the Gulf Coast of North America. This tapeworm is a clinical oddity because it produces an operculated egg. Each proglottid of *Spirometra* species has a central spiral uterus and an associated uterine pore through which eggs are released. These tapeworms characteristically release eggs until they exhaust their uterine contents. Gravid segments are usually not discharged into the pet's feces.

The tapeworm is unique because while it is attached to the host's jejunum, the mature proglottids often separate along the longitudinal axis for a short distance. The tapeworm appears to "unzip." Hence its common name, the "zipper tapeworm." Spent "zipped" and "unzipped" proglottids often appear in the feces of the pet. Figure 6-12 shows the unique features of this pseudotapeworm.

The egg of *Spirometra* species resembles that of a fluke (digenetic trematode). The egg has a distinct operculum at one end of the pole of the shell. The

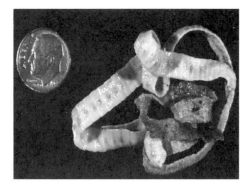

Figure 6-12. Spent proglottids of *Spirometra mansonoides,* the "zipper tapeworm." This tapeworm is unique because while it is attached to the host's jejunum, the mature proglottids often separate along the longitudinal axis for a short distance. The tapeworm appears to "unzip"; hence its common name, the "zipper tapeworm." Spent "zipped" and "unzipped" proglottids often appear in the feces of the pet.

eggs are oval and yellowish-brown. They average 60 by 36 μ, have an asymmetric appearance, and are rather pointed at one end. When the eggs rupture, a distinct operculum is visible. The eggs are unembryonated when passed in the feces. Figure 6-13 shows the unique features of the egg of this pseudotapeworm.

Diphyllobothrium species are often referred to as "broad fish tapeworms." This tapeworm can be 2 to 12 m in length; however, it probably does not attain this maximum length in dogs and cats. Each proglottid of this tapeworm has a central rosette-shaped uterus and an associated uterine pore through which eggs are released. These tapeworms continually release eggs until they exhaust their uterine contents. The terminal proglottids become senile rather than gravid and detach in chains rather than individually.

The egg of *Diphyllobothrium* species also resembles that of a fluke (digenetic trematode). The egg is oval and has a distinct operculum at one end of the shell. The eggs are light brown, averaging 67 to 71 μ by 40 to 51 μ. They tend to be rounded on one end. The operculum is present on the end opposite the rounded end. The eggs are unembryonated when passed in the feces.

Trematodes (Flukes)

Platynosomum fastosum is the "lizard poisoning fluke" of cats. The adult flukes inhabit the liver, gallbladder, bile ducts, and less commonly the small intestine.

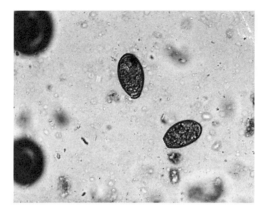

FIGURE 6-13. Characteristic ovum of *Spirometra mansonoides.* The egg of *Spirometra* species resembles that of a fluke (digenetic trematode). The egg has a distinct operculum at one end of the shell. The eggs are oval and yellowish-brown. They average 60 by 36 μ and have an asymmetric appearance. They tend to be rather pointed at one end.

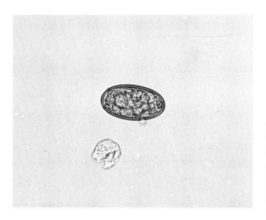

FIGURE 6-14. Characteristic ovum of *Platynosomum fastosum,* the "lizard poisoning fluke" of cats. The brownish, operculated eggs are 34 to 50 μ by 20 to 35 μ.

The brownish, operculated eggs are 34 to 50 μ by 20 to 35 μ. Figure 6-14 shows the features of the egg of *P. fastosum.*

Nanophyetus salmincola is the "salmon poisoning fluke" of dogs in the Pacific Northwest region of North America. The adult fluke inhabits the small intestine and serves as a vector for rickettsial agents, which produce "salmon poisoning" and "Elokomin fluke fever" in dogs. The eggs are unembryonated when laid and measure 52 to 82 μ by 32 to 56 μ. Figure 6-15 shows the features of the

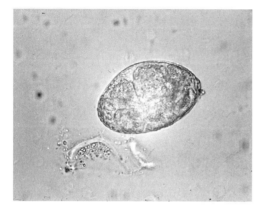

FIGURE 6-15. Characteristic ovum of *Nanophyetus salmincola*. The eggs are unembryonated when laid and measure 52 to 82 μ by 32 to 56 μ. They have an indistinct operculum and a small, blunt point at the end opposite the operculum.

egg of *N. salmincola*. They have an indistinct operculum and a small, blunt point at the end opposite the operculum.

Alaria species are intestinal flukes of dogs and cats and are found throughout the northern half of North America. Their ova are large, golden brown, and operculated. They are 98 to 134 μ by 62 to 68 μ. Figure 6-16 shows the features of the egg of *Alaria* species.

PROTOZOANS (UNICELLULAR ORGANISMS)

Isospora species (coccidians) are protozoan parasites of the small intestine of both dogs and cats. They produce a clinical syndrome known as coccidiosis, one of the most commonly diagnosed protozoan diseases in puppies and kittens. Coccidiosis is rarely a problem in mature animals. The *oocyst* is the diagnostic stage observed in a fecal flotation of fresh feces; it is unsporulated in fresh feces

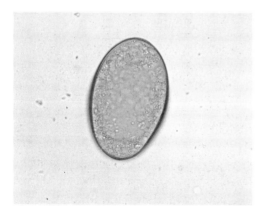

FIGURE 6-16. Characteristic ovum of *Alaria* species, the "intestinal flukes" of dogs and cats. They are found throughout the northern half of North America. The eggs are large, golden brown, and operculated. They measure 98 to 134 μ by 62 to 68 μ.

and varies in size and shape among the common *Isospora* species. Figure 6-17 shows an unsporulated oocyst and Figure 6-18 shows a sporulated oocyst of *Isospora* species.

The canine coccidians and their oocyst measurements are *Isospora canis*, 34 to 40 µ by 28 to 32 µ; *I. ohioensis*, 20 to 27 µ by 15 to 24 µ; and *I. wallacei*, 10 to 14 µ by 7.5 to 9 µ. The feline coccidians and their measurements are *Isospora felis*, 38 to 51 µ by 27 to 29 µ, and *I. rivolta*, 21 to 28 µ by 18 to 23 µ. The prepatent period varies among species but is usually 7 to 14 days.

Toxoplasma gondii is another intestinal coccidian of cats. Its oocysts are usually diagnosed using a standard fecal flotation. Oocysts of *T. gondii* are unsporulated in fresh feces and measure 10 by 12 µ. Several immunodiagnostic tests using whole blood or serum are available for diagnosis of *T. gondii* infection. The prepatent period is highly variable, ranging from 5 to 24 days, and depends on the route of infection.

Cryptosporidium is another coccidian parasite that parasitizes the small intestine of a wide variety of animals, including dogs and cats. The sporulated oocysts in the feces are oval to spherical and measure only 4 to 6 µ. Diagnosis is by a standard fecal flotation. The oocysts are extremely small and may be observed just under the coverslip, not in the same plane of focus as other oocysts and parasite ova. Examination of fresh fecal smears using special stains (modified acid-fast stain) is also helpful. Because people may become infected with *Cryptosporidium* species, feces suspected of harboring this protozoan should be handled with great care. Figure 6-19 shows the features of the oocysts of *Cryptosporidium* species.

Sarcocystis is another coccidian parasite found in the small intestine. Several species infect dogs and cats. Identification of an individual species can be quite

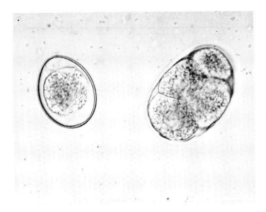

Figure 6-17. Unsporulated oocyst of *Isospora* species. Oocysts vary greatly in size. Also see Figure 6-18. The ovum on the *right* is that of *A. caninum.*

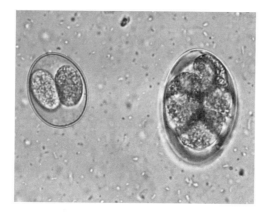

Figure 6-18. Sporulated oocyst of *Isospora* species. The canine coccidians and their measurements are *Isospora canis,* 34 to 40 µ by 28 to 32 µ; *I. ohioensis,* 20 to 27 µ by 15 to 24 µ; and *I. wallacei,* 10 to 14 µ by 7.5 to 9 µ. The feline coccidians and their measurements are *Isospora felis,* 38 to 51 µ by 27 to 29 µ, and *I. rivolta,* 21 to 28 µ by 18 to 23 µ. The ovum on the *right* is that of *A. caninum.*

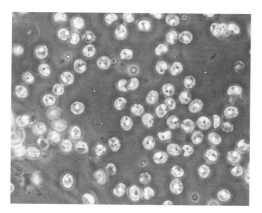

Figure 6-19. Oocysts of *Cryptosporidium* species.

difficult. The oocysts of *Sarcocystis* species are sporulated when passed in the feces. Each oocyst contains two sporocysts, each with four sporozoites. These individual oocysts measure 12 to 15 µ by 8 to 12 µ and may be recovered in a standard fecal flotation of fresh feces.

Giardia species are flagellated protozoans often recovered from the feces of dogs and cats with diarrhea, but they may also be recovered from animals with normal stools. This parasite occurs in two morphologic forms: a motile feeding stage (the *trophozoite*) and a resistant cyst stage. The motile stage is pear-shaped and dorsoventrally flattened, and contains four pairs of flagella. It measures 9 to 21 μ by 5 to 15 μ. Two nuclei and a prominent adhesive disc are present on the cranial portion of the cell, resembling a pair of eyes staring back at the observer. Figure 6-20 shows a motile trophozoite of *Giardia* species.

The mature cysts are oval and are 8 to 10 μ by 7 to 10 μ. They have a refractile wall and four nuclei. Immature cysts, which represent recently encysted motile forms, contain only two nuclei. Figure 6-21 shows cysts of *Giardia* species. In dogs, diarrhea may begin as early as 5 days after exposure to *Giardia,* with cysts first appearing in the feces at 1 week.

Diagnosis is by a standard fecal flotation. Zinc sulfate (specific gravity 1.18) is considered the best flotation medium for recovering cysts. Cysts are often distorted, with a semi-lunar appearance. The motile trophozoite can be occasionally found on a direct smear of fresh feces using isotonic saline. Lugol's iodine may be used to visualize the internal structures of cysts and trophozoites. Fecal immunodiagnostic tests are also commonly employed.

PARASITES OF THE CIRCULATORY SYSTEM

NEMATODES (ROUNDWORMS)

Dirofilaria immitis is often referred to as the canine heartworm; however, this nematode has also been known to parasitize cats and ferrets. Adult heartworms are found within the right ventricle, the pulmonary artery, and the fine branches of that artery. This parasite is often recovered in a variety of aberrant sites, such as the brain, the anterior chamber of the eye, and within subcutaneous sites. The prepatent period in dogs is approximately 6 months.

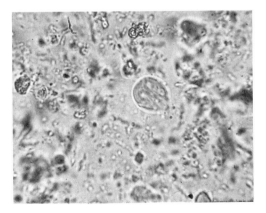

FIGURE 6-20. Motile trophozoite of *Giardia* species.

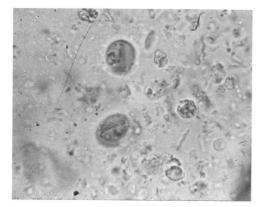

Figure 6-21. Cysts of *Giardia* species. The mature cysts are oval and measure 8 to 10 μ by 7 to 10 μ. They have a refractile wall and four nuclei. Immature cysts, which represent recently encysted motile forms, contain only two nuclei.

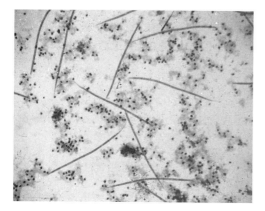

Figure 6-22. Microfilariae of *Dirofilaria immitis* from a peripheral blood sample subjected to the modified Knott's test. The microfilariae of *D. immitis* average 310 μ in length. In contrast, the microfilariae of *Dipetalonema reconditum* average 285 μ in length.

In microfilaremic dogs, diagnosis is by observing microfilariae in blood samples using one of several concentration techniques (modified Knott's test) or the commercially available filter techniques (Figures 6-22 and 6-23). For infected dogs with no circulating microfilariae, infection can also be diagnosed using commercially available immunodiagnostic tests.

It is important to remember that a subcutaneous filariid of dogs, *Dipetalonema reconditum,* also produces microfilariae in the peripheral blood. The microfilariae of this nonpathogenic nematode must be differentiated from those of *D. immitis* (Figures 6-22 and 6-23).

TREMATODES (FLUKES)

Heterobilharzia americana, the canine schistosome, is a blood fluke that parasitizes the mesenteric veins of the small and large intestines and portal veins of the

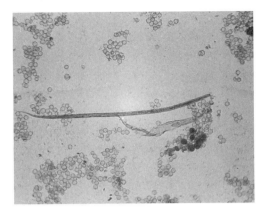

FIGURE 6-23. An individual microfilaria of *Dirofilaria immitis* from a peripheral blood sample subjected to the modified Knott's test. Note the tapered cranial end and straight tail. Microfilariae of *Dipetalonema reconditum* have a blunt (rounded) cranial end and may exhibit a shepherd's crook (hooked) tail.

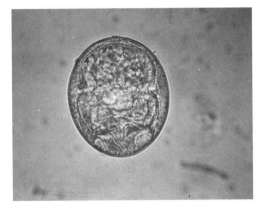

FIGURE 6-24. Characteristic thin-shelled ovum of *Heterobilharzia americana*. These ova are approximately 80 by 50 μ and contain a miracidium.

dog. This fluke is enzootic in the mud flats of the Mississippi delta and the coastal swampland of Louisiana. Although this fluke inhabits the vasculature, it manifests its presence by bloody diarrhea. Infected dogs also exhibit emaciation and anorexia. Diagnosis is by identification of the thin-shelled egg, about 80 by 50 μ, which contains a *miracidium*. Figure 6-24 shows the morphologic features of the egg of *Heterobilharzia americana*. The prepatent period is approximately 84 days.

PROTOZOANS (UNICELLULAR ORGANISMS)

Babesia canis is an intracellular parasite found within the erythrocytes of dogs. It is also referred to as a *piroplasm* (pear-shaped body). Diagnosis is by observing basophilic, pear-shaped trophozoites in RBCs on stained blood smears. Figure 6-25 shows the trophzoites of *B. canis* within canine RBCs.

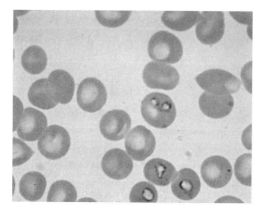

FIGURE 6-25. Basophilic, pear-shaped trophozoites of *Babesia canis* within canine RBCs in a stained blood smear.

Cytauxzoon felis is another intracellular parasite that has been sporadically reported in the RBCs of cats in sites (Missouri, Arkansas, Georgia, Texas) throughout the United States. It also produces piroplasms; however, these bodies have been described as shaped like a "bejeweled ring" and are referred to as the ring form in stained blood smears. Cytauxzoonosis is a rapidly fatal disease, and its prognosis is poor.

PARASITES OF THE RESPIRATORY SYSTEM

PENTASTOMIDS (TONGUEWORMS)

Pentastomids (tongueworms) resemble helminths but are actually an arthropod. *Linguatula serrata* is the "canine pentastome" or the "canine tongueworm." Pentastomes are usually parasites of snakes and reptiles, but this tongueworm parasitizes the nasal and respiratory passages of dogs. It resembles a helminth but is a type of arthropod (it has a mite-like larval stage). Figure 6-26 shows the unique appearance of the adult *L. serrata*. The pentastome eggs measure 70 by 90 µ (Figure 6-27). On the inside of the egg, one can see the mite-like larval stage with jointed claws.

NEMATODES (ROUNDWORMS)

Aelurostrongylus abstrusus is the feline lungworm. The adults live in the terminal respiratory bronchioles and alveolar ducts, where they form small egg nests or nodules. The eggs of this parasite are forced into the lung tissue, where they hatch to form characteristic first-stage larvae, approximately 360 µ long. Each larva has a tail with an S-shaped bend and a dorsal spine (Figure 6-28). Characteristic larvae on fecal flotation or the Baermann technique can determine

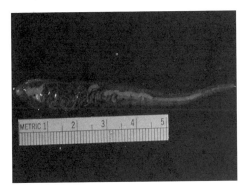

FIGURE 6-26. Adult female *Linguatula serrata,* the "canine pentastome" or "canine tongueworm." This parasite of the nasal and respiratory passages of dogs resembles a helminth, but it is actually a type of arthropod (it has a mite-like larval stage).

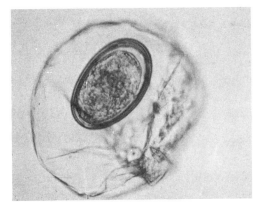

FIGURE 6-27. Characteristic ovum of *Linguatula serrata.* The pentastome eggs measure 70 by 90 μ. In the interior of many pentastome eggs, one may observe a mite-like larval stage with jointed claws.

their presence. It is also possible to recover the larvae on tracheal washing (Figure 6-29). The prepatent period is approximately 30 days.

Filaroides osleri, F. hirthi, and *F. milksi,* the canine "lungworms," are found in the trachea, the lung parenchyma, and the bronchioles, respectively. The larva is 232 to 266 μ in length and has a short, S-shaped tail. *Filaroides* species are unique among the nematodes in that their first-stage larvae are immediately infective for the canine definitive host. No period of development is required outside the host. Diagnosis is by finding these characteristic larvae on fecal flotation or by using the Baermann technique. Figure 6-30 shows the unique infective larvae of *F. osleri.* Nodules of *F. osleri* are usually found at the bifurcation of the trachea, where they can be observed via endoscopic examination. The prepatent period for *F. osleri* is approximately 10 weeks.

Eucoleus aerophilus (Capillaria aerophila) is a capillarid nematode found in the trachea and bronchi of both dogs and cats. The prepatent period is approximately

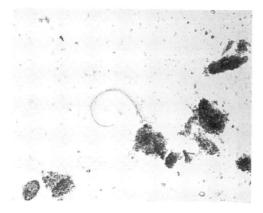

Figure 6-28. Characteristic first-stage larva of *Aelurostrongylus abstrusus,* the "feline lungworm." The larva is approximately 360 μ long and has a tail with an S-shaped bend and a dorsal spine. Diagnosis is accomplished by finding these characteristic larvae on fecal flotation or by using the Baermann technique.

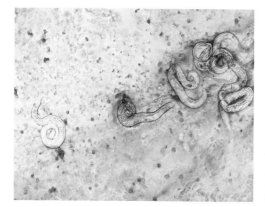

Figure 6-29. Numerous first-stage larvae of *Aelurostrongylus abstrusus,* recovered on tracheal washing.

40 days. In standard fecal flotations, eggs of *Eucoleus* species are often confused with those of *Trichuris* (whipworms). Eggs of *E. aerophilus* are smaller than whipworm eggs (59 to 80 μ by 30 to 40 μ), more broadly barrel-shaped, and lighter in color. The egg also has a rough outer surface with a netted appearance.

Eucoleus böehmi is found in the nasal cavity and frontal sinuses of dogs. Its eggs are smaller and have a smoother outer surface than those of *E. aerophilus.* Its shell has a pitted appearance. This parasite can be detected using a standard fecal flotation.

TREMATODES (FLUKES)

Paragonimus kellicotti is the "lung fluke" of dogs. Adult hermaphroditic flukes occur in cystic spaces within the lung parenchyma of both dogs and cats. These cystic spaces connect to the terminal bronchioles. The eggs are found in sputum

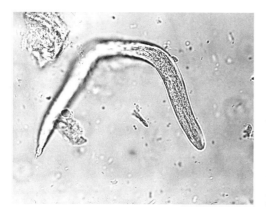

FIGURE 6-30. Characteristic, infective first-stage larva of *Filaroides osleri,* a canine "lungworm." The larva is 232 to 266 μ in length and has a short, S-shaped tail.

or feces. They are yellowish brown with an operculum and measure 75 to 118 μ by 42 to 67 μ. Figure 6-31 shows the operculated ovum of *P. kellicotti.* Fluke eggs are usually recovered using fecal sedimentation techniques; however, the eggs of *P. kellicotti* can be recovered using standard fecal flotation solutions. The eggs of *P. kellicotti* can also be recovered in the sputum via tracheal washing. The adult flukes within the cystic spaces of the lung parenchyma can also be observed using thoracic radiography. This fluke's prepatent period is 30 to 36 days.

PARASITES OF THE UROGENITAL SYSTEM

NEMATODES (ROUNDWORMS)

Dioctophyma renale is the "giant kidney worm" of dogs. This largest of parasitic nematodes frequently infects the right kidney of dogs and gradually ingests the renal parenchyma, leaving only the capsule of the kidney. Eggs may be recovered by centrifugation and examination of the urine sediment. They are characteristically barrel-shaped, bipolar, and yellow brown. The egg shell has a pitted appearance. Eggs measure 71 to 84 μ by 46 to 52 μ. Figure 6-32 shows the characteristic ovum of *D. renale. D. renale* may also occur freely within the peritoneal cavity. When it is in this location, eggs are not passed to the external environment. The prepatent period is approximately 18 weeks.

Capillaria plica and *C. feliscati* are nematodes of the urinary bladder of dogs and cats, respectively. Their eggs may be found in urine or in feces contaminated with urine. Eggs are clear to yellow in color, measure 63 to 68 μ by 24 to 27 μ, and have flattened bipolar end plugs. Their outer surface is roughened. These eggs may be confused with those of the respiratory and gastric capillarids and with those of the whipworms.

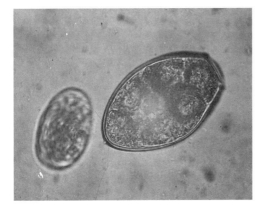

FIGURE **6-31.** Characteristic ovum of *Paragonimus kellicotti*, the "lung fluke" of dogs recovered using a standard fecal flotation. The eggs may be found in either sputum or feces but are often recovered on fecal flotation. The yellowish-brown, operculated eggs measure 75 to 118 μ by 42 to 67 μ. The egg on the *left* is that of *A. caninum*.

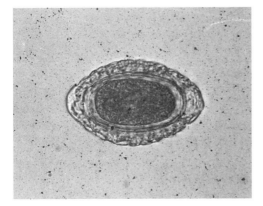

FIGURE **6-32.** Characteristic ovum of *Dioctophyma renale* recovered from urine sediment. These eggs are characteristically barrel-shaped, bipolar, and yellow brown. The egg shell has a pitted appearance. Eggs measure 71 to 84 μ by 46 to 52 μ.

PARASITES OF THE EYE AND ADNEXA

NEMATODES (ROUNDWORMS)

Thelazia californensis is the "eyeworm" of dogs and cats. Adult parasites can be recovered from the conjunctival sac and lacrimal duct. Examination of the lacrimal secretions may reveal eggs or first-stage larvae.

As mentioned previously, *Dirofilaria immitis* can be recovered from a variety of aberrant sites, such as the anterior chamber of the eye.

ENDOPARASITES OF CATTLE AND OTHER RUMINANTS

PARASITES OF THE GASTROINTESTINAL TRACT

NEMATODES (ROUNDWORMS)

The "bovine trichstrongyles" comprise several genera of nematodes within the abomasum and small and large intestine of cattle and other ruminants. Genera that produce "trichostrongyle-type eggs" are *Bunostomum, Cooperia, Chabertia, Haemonchus, Oesophagostomum, Ostertagia,* and *Trichostrongylus.* These seven genera (and there are others) produce oval, thin-shelled eggs. They contain four or more cells and are 70 to 120 µ long. Some of these ova can be identified to their respective genus; however, identification is usually quite difficult because mixed infections are quite common.

Upon identification of the characteristic eggs, the veterinary technician should record the finding as "trichostrongyle-type egg." They *should not* be recorded as individual genus names. Identification to genus and species is usually performed by fecal culture and larval identification. Figure 6-33 shows representative examples of "trichostrongyle-type" eggs.

Nematodirus species and *Marshallagia* species are also "bovine trichostrongyles"; however, their eggs are much larger than those of the genera mentioned previously. Their eggs are the largest in the trichostrongyle family. Figure 6-34 shows the large eggs of *Nematodirus* species. In a standard fecal flotation, the eggs of *Nematodirus* species are large (150 to 230 µ by 80 to 100 µ) and have tapering ends and 4 to 8 cells. The eggs of *Marshallagia* species are also large (160 to 200 µ by 75 to 100 µ) have parallel sides and rounded ends, and contain 16 to 32 cells.

Strongyloides papillosus is often referred to as the "intestinal threadworm." These nematodes are unique in that only a parthenogenetic female (female that lays eggs without copulating with a male) is parasitic in the host. Parasitic males do not exist. These females produce larvated eggs measuring 40 to 60 µ by 20 to 25 µ. Eggs are usually recovered in flotation of fresh feces. The prepatent period is 5 to 7 days (see Figure 6-7 for the parasitic adult females, eggs, and first-stage larvae of *Strongyloides* species).

Trichuris ovis is commonly called the "whipworm," infecting the cecum and colon of ruminants. The section on nematode parasites of the gastointestinal tract of dogs and cats contains details on the gross morphology of adult whipworms. The egg of the whipworm is described as trichinelloid or trichuroid. It has a thick, yellow-brown, symmetric shell with plugs at both ends. The eggs are unembryonated (not larvated) when laid. Eggs of bovine whipworms measure 50 to 60 µ by 21 to 25 µ.

CESTODES (TAPEWORMS)

Moniezia species are tapeworms found in the small intestine of cattle, sheep, and goats. These tapeworms produce eggs with a characteristic square or triangular shape. Two species are common, *Moniezia benedini* in cattle and *M. expansa* in cattle, sheep, and goats. The eggs of both species can be easily differentiated using standard fecal flotation procedures. Figure 6-35 shows

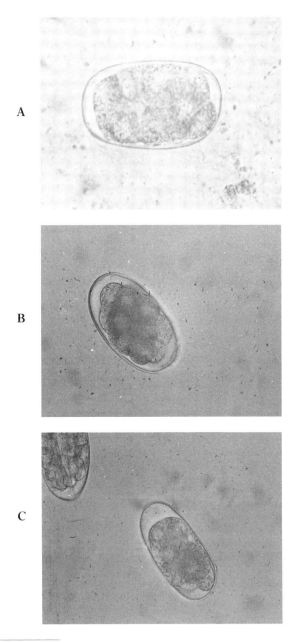

Figure 6-33. **A** to **C,** Characteristic "trichostrongyle-type" ova of the bovine trichostrongyles. These oval, thin-shelled eggs contain four or more cells. They measure 70 to 120 μ in length. Some of these ova can be identified by their respective genus; however, identification is usually quite difficult because mixed infections are quite common.

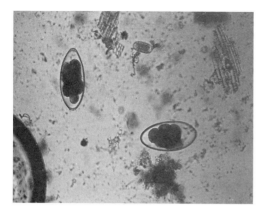

FIGURE 6-34.   Characteristic large ova of *Nematodirus* species. In standard fecal flotation, the eggs of *Nematodirus* species are larger than those of other bovine trichostrongyles (150 to 230 μ by 80 to 100 μ), have tapering ends, and four to eight cells.

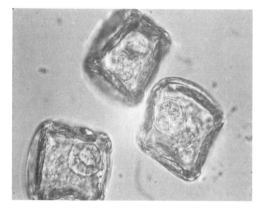

FIGURE 6-35.   Characteristic ova of *Moniezia* species. The eggs of *M. expansa* are triangular or pyramidal and 56 to 67 μ in diameter. The eggs of *M. benedini* are square or cuboidal and approximately 75 μ in diameter.

representative eggs of *Moniezia* species. The eggs of *M. expansa* are triangular or pyramidal and 56 to 67 μ in diameter. The eggs of *M. benedini* are square or cuboidal and approximately 75 μ in diameter. The prepatent period for these tapeworms is approximately 40 days.

 Thysanosoma actinoides is the "fringed tapeworm," found in the bile ducts, pancreatic ducts, and small intestine of ruminants. Eggs of this tapeworm occur in packets of 6 to 12 eggs, with individual eggs measuring 19 by 27 μ.

TREMATODES (FLUKES)

"Rumen flukes" are comprised of two genera, *Paramphistomum* and *Cotylophoron*. These adult flukes reside in the rumen and reticulum of cattle, sheep, goats, and many other ruminants. The eggs of *Paramphistomum* measure 114 to 176 μ by 73 to 100 μ, while the eggs of *Cotylophoron* measure 125 to 135 μ by 61 to 68 μ. The prepatent period of *Paramphistomum* species is 80 to 95 days.

Fasciola hepatica is the "liver fluke" of cattle, sheep, and other ruminants. The hermaphroditic adult flukes are found in the bile ducts of the liver. The eggs measure 140 by 100 μ and are yellowish-brown, oval, and operculated. Figure 6-36 shows a representative egg of *F. hepatica*. The prepatent period for *F. hepatica* is approximately 56 days.

Dicrocoelium dendriticum is the "lancet fluke" of sheep, goats, and oxen. These tiny flukes reside within the fine branches of the bile ducts. The brown eggs have an indistinct operculum and measure 36 to 45 μ by 20 to 30 μ.

Eggs of the above mentioned trematodes may be recovered from feces using fecal sedimentation or a commercially available fluke egg recovery test.

PROTOZOANS (UNICELLULAR ORGANISMS)

Ruminants serve as host to many species of *Eimeria*. It is often difficult to identify individual species of coccidia because their oocysts are so similar in size and shape. The two most common species of coccidia in cattle, *E. bovis* and *E. zurnii,* can be differentiated on a standard fecal flotation. Oocysts of *E. bovis* are oval, have a micropyle, and measure 20 by 28 μ, while those of *E. zurnii* are spherical, lack the micropyle, and measure 15 to 22 μ by 13 to 18 μ. When oocysts are recovered on fecal flotation, the observation is usually noted as "coccidia."

Cryptosporidium is another coccidian parasite that parasitizes the small intestine of a wide variety of animals, including cattle, sheep, and goats. The sporulated oocysts in the feces are colorless and transparent and measure only 5.0 to 4.5 μ. Diagnosis is by standard fecal flotation and stained fecal smears.

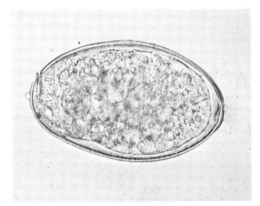

FIGURE 6-36. Characteristic operculated ovum of *Fasciola hepatica,* the "liver fluke" of cattle, sheep, and other ruminants. The eggs measure 140 by 100 μ and are yellowish-brown and oval.

Because people may become infected with *Cryptosporidium* species, feces suspected of harboring this protozoan should be handled with great care (see Figure 6-19 for features of the oocysts of *Cryptosporidium* species).

PARASITES OF THE CIRCULATORY SYSTEM

NEMATODES (ROUNDWORMS)

Elaeophora schneideri, the "arterial worm," is found in the common carotid arteries of sheep in the western and southwestern United States. Microfilariae are 270 μ in length by 17 μ in thickness, bluntly rounded cranially, and tapering caudally. They are found in the skin, usually in the capillaries of the forehead and face. Filarial dermatitis is seen on the face, poll region, and feet of sheep.

Diagnosis is by observation of characteristic lesions and identification of microfilariae in the skin. The most satisfactory means of diagnosis is to macerate a piece of skin in warm saline and examine the material for microfilariae after about 2 hours. In sheep, microfilariae are rare and may not be found in the skin of infected animals. Postmortem examination may be necessary to confirm the diagnosis. The prepatent period is 18 weeks or longer.

PROTOZOANS (UNICELLULAR ORGANISMS)

Babesia bigemina is an intracellular parasite found within the RBCs of cattle. This parasite is a large piroplasm, 4 to 5 μ in length by about 2 μ wide. It is characteristically pear-shaped and occurs in pairs, forming an acute angle within the erythrocyte. The intermediate host for this protozoan parasite is the tick, *Boophilus annulatus.*

PARASITES OF THE RESPIRATORY SYSTEM

NEMATODES (ROUNDWORMS)

Dictyocaulus species are lungworms of cattle (*D. viviparus*), sheep, and goats (*D. filaria*). Adults are found in the bronchi. The prepatent period varies with the species but is approximately 28 days. Eggs are usually coughed up and swallowed and hatch in the intestine, producing larvae that may be recovered in the feces.

Larvae of *D. filaria* have brownish food granules in their intestinal cells, a blunt tail, and a cranial cuticular knob. They are 550 to 580 μ in length. Larvae of *D. viviparus* also have brownish food granules in their intestinal cells but have a straight tail. They lack the cranial cuticular knob. They are 300 to 360 μ in length. Figure 6-37 shows representative eggs and larvae of *D. viviparus.*

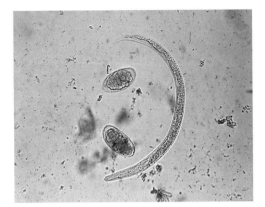

Figure 6-37. Representative eggs and larvae of *Dictyocaulus* species, cattle "lungworms."

Muellerius capillaris is often called the "hair lungworm." Adults are found within the bronchioles, mostly in nodules in the lung parenchyma of sheep and goats. The eggs develop in the lungs of the definitive host and the first-stage larvae are coughed up, swallowed, and passed out with the feces. They are 230 to 300 µ long. The larval tail has an undulating tip and a dorsal spine. Figure 6-38 shows representative eggs and larvae of *M. capillaris.*

Protostrongylus species adults occur in the small bronchioles of sheep and goats. Again, the eggs develop in the lungs of the definitive host and the first-stage larvae are coughed up, swallowed, and passed out with the feces. These larvae are 250 to 320 µ long. This nematode's larval tail has an undulating tip but lacks the dorsal spine.

The Baermann technique is used to diagnose lungworm infection in ruminants.

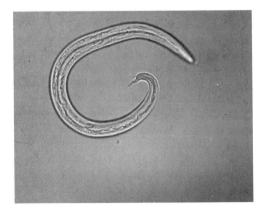

Figure 6-38. First-stage larva of *Muellerius capillaris,* the "hair lungworm" of sheep and goats. First-stage larvae are 230 to 300 µ long. The larval tail has an undulating tip and a dorsal spine.

PARASITES OF THE EYE AND ADNEXA

NEMATODES (ROUNDWORMS)

Thelazia rhodesii and *T. gulosa* are the "eyeworm" of cattle, sheep, and goats. Adult parasites can be recovered from the conjunctival sac and lacrimal duct. Examination of the lacrimal secretions may reveal eggs or first-stage larvae. Figure 6-39 shows adult *Thelazia* in the conjunctival sac of a cow.

PARASITES OF THE ABDOMINAL CAVITY

Setaria cervi is the "abdominal worm" of cattle. Adults are found free within the peritoneal cavity. The sheathed microfilariae are approximately 250 by 7 μ. Diagnosis is by demonstration of microfilariae in blood smears.

ENDOPARASITES OF HORSES

PARASITES OF THE GASTROINTESTINAL TRACT

ARTHROPODS (LARVAL FLIES)

These parasites are odd in that their adult form is an ectoparasite and their larval form is an endoparasite.

Larval *Gasterophilus* species or "horse bots" parasitize the stomach of horses. Because these stages are larval or immature stages of nonparasitic adult flies, no demonstrable egg stage can be recovered from horse feces. It is via the feces that the third larval stage exits the gastrointestinal tract; therefore, this stage may be recovered from the feces. The brown larvae are up to 20 mm in length and have dense spines on the cranial border of each segment. A pair of distinct mouth hooks is found on the cranial end of the first segment and a spiracular

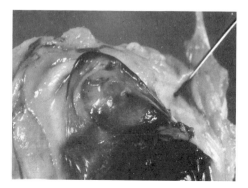

FIGURE **6-39.**   Adult *Thelazia* species, the "eyeworm," in the conjunctival sac of a cow.

plate on the caudal end. The veterinary technician should be able to grossly identify horse bots as *Gasterophilus* species.

Nematodes (roundworms)

Habronema species and *Draschia megastoma* are nematodes found in the stomach of horses. *Habronema microstoma* and *H. muscae* occur on the stomach mucosa, just beneath a thick layer of mucus; *D. megastoma* is often associated with large, thickened fibrous nodules within the stomach mucosa. Larvae of both may parasitize skin lesions, causing a condition known as "summer sores" (see Chapter 7 for a description of this condition and the larvae). The prepatent period is approximately 60 days. Larvated eggs or larvae may be recovered on a standard fecal flotation. The eggs of both genera are elongated and thin walled and measure 40 to 50 μ by 10 to 12 μ.

Trichostrongylus axei is another nematode that may infect the stomach of horses. They are unusual in that they can also infect cattle and sheep. Their eggs are classified as "strongyle-type" eggs (see discussion following).

Parascaris equorum is often called the "equine ascarid" or "equine roundworm." It is found in the small intestine of horses, particularly young foals. The prepatent period is 75 to 80 days. Eggs recovered from the feces of young horses are oval and brown. The shell is thickened, with a finely granular surface. The eggs measure 90 to 100 μ in diameter. The center of the egg contains one or two cells. Figure 6-40 shows an egg of *P. equorum.* Eggs can be easily recovered on standard fecal flotation.

Strongyles are nematodes that parasitize the large intestine of horses and are typically divided into two types: large strongyles and small strongyles. The small strongyles are comprised of several genera that vary in pathogenicity. The

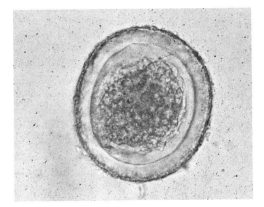

Figure 6-40. Characteristic ovum of *Parascaris equorum,* the "equine ascarid" or the "equine roundworm." The shell is thickened, with a finely granular surface. The eggs measure 90 to 100 μ in diameter. The center of the egg contains one or two cells.

large strongyles are the most pathogenic of the strongyles. *Strongylus vulgaris, S. edentatus,* and *S. equinus* comprise the large strongyles. Figure 6-41 shows a typical strongyle-type ovum produced by both small and large strongyles.

Regardless of whether these endoparasites are a small strongyle or a large strongyle, their eggs are virtually identical. Identification to the species level is accomplished by fecal culture and identification of larvae. Strongyle eggs are most often observed in a standard fecal flotation. They contain an 8- to 16-cell morula and measure approximately 70 to 90 μ by 40 to 50 μ. When these characteristic eggs are found on fecal flotation, the observation is recorded as "strongyle-type" ova, rather than as a particular species of strongyles.

Strongyloides westeri is often referred to as the "intestinal threadworm" of horses. These nematodes are unique in that only a parthenogenetic female (one that can lay eggs without copulating with a male) is parasitic in the host. Parasitic males do not exist. These females produce larvated eggs measuring 40 to 52 μ by 32 to 40 μ. Eggs are usually recovered on flotation of fresh feces. The prepatent period is 5 to 7 days (see Figure 6-7 for the parasitic adult females, eggs, and first-stage larvae of *Strongyloides* species).

Oxyuris equi is the "pinworm" of horses. The adult worms are found in the cecum, colon, and rectum. Adult worms are often observed protruding from the horse's anus. The adult female worms attach their eggs to the anus with a gelatinous, sticky material that produces anal pruritus in infected horses. Eggs can also be recovered from the feces. The eggs are 90 by 40 μ, with a smooth, thick shell. They are operculated and slightly flattened on one side. The eggs may be larvated. Figure 6-42 shows the egg of *Oxyuris equi*. The prepatent period is approximately 4 to 5 months. Diagnosis is by finding the characteristic eggs on microscopic examination of cellophane tape impressions or by scraping the surface of the anus.

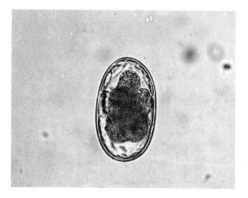

FIGURE **6-41.** "Strongyle-type ovum" of horses. These eggs contain an 8- to 16-cell morula and measure approximately 70 to 90 μ by 40 to 50 μ. When these characteristic eggs are found on fecal flotation, the observation is recorded as "strongyle-type" ova, rather than as a particular species of strongyle.

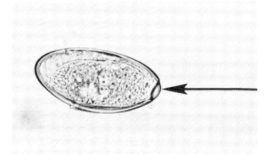

Figure 6-42. Characteristic ovum of *Oxyuris equi,* the "pinworm" of horses. The eggs are 90 by 40 μ, with a smooth, thick shell. They are operculated and slightly flattened on one side. The eggs may be larvated.

Cestodes (tapeworms)

Anoplocephala perfoliata, A. magna, and *Paranoplocephala mamillana* are the "equine tapeworms." *Anoplocephala perfoliata* is found in the small and large intestine and cecum. *A. magna* is found in the small intestine and occasionally the stomach. *P. mamillana* is also found in the small intestine and occasionally the stomach. The eggs of *A. perfoliata* are thick walled, with one or more flattened sides, and measure 65 to 80 μ in diameter. Those of *A. magna* are similar but slightly smaller, measuring 50 to 60 μ. The eggs of *P. mamillana* are oval and thin walled, measuring 51 by 37 μ. Eggs of all three species have a three-layered egg shell, with the innermost lining being called the *pyriform (pear-shaped) apparatus.* The hexacanth embryo can be visualized just inside the pyriform apparatus. Eggs of all equine tapeworms can be recovered using a standard fecal flotation. The prepatent period of all three species ranges from 28 to 42 days.

Protozoans (unicellular organisms)

Eimeria leuckarti is a coccidian found in the small intestine of horses. This protozoan demonstrates unique oocysts that are quite large (80 to 87 μ by 55 to 60 μ), with a thick wall, a distinct micropyle, and a dark brown color. These oocysts can be recovered on fecal flotation and are the largest coccidian oocysts. They are frequently observed on histopathologic examination. The prepatent period ranges from 15 to 33 days.

Parasites of the circulatory system

Protozoans (unicellular organisms)

Babesia equi and *B. caballi* are intracellular parasites found within the RBCs of horses. They are also referred to as the "equine piroplasms." Diagnosis is by observing basophilic, pear-shaped trophozoites in RBCs on stained blood smears. Trophozoites of *B. equi* may be round, amoeboid, or pyriform (pear-shaped). Four organisms may be joined, giving the effect of a Maltese cross. Individual organisms are 2 to 3 μ long. Trophozoites of *B. caballi* are pyriform, round, or oval and 2 to 4 μ long. They occur characteristically in pairs at acute angles to each other.

PARASITES OF THE RESPIRATORY SYSTEM

NEMATODES (ROUNDWORMS)

Dictyocaulus arnfieldi, the "equine lungworm," is found in the bronchi and bronchioles of horses, mules, and donkeys. Its eggs are ellipsoid and embryonated, measuring approximately 80 to 100 μ by 50 to 60 μ. Eggs can be recovered on fecal flotation of fresh (less than 24 hours old) feces. Larvae hatch from the eggs within a few hours after feces are passed. The prepatent period for the equine lungworm is 42 to 56 days.

PARASITES OF THE EYE AND ADNEXA

Thelazia lacrymalis is the "eyeworm" of horses throughout the world. Adult parasites can be recovered from the conjunctival sac and lacrimal duct. Examination of the lacrimal secretions may reveal eggs or first-stage larvae.

The unsheathed microfilariae of *Onchocerca cervicalis* have been incriminated as causing periodic ophthalmia and blindness in horses. These may be detected by ophthalmic examination.

PARASITES OF THE ABDOMINAL CAVITY

Setaria equina is the "abdominal worm" of horses. Adults are found free within the peritoneal cavity. The sheathed microfilariae are 240 to 256 μ long. Diagnosis is by demonstration of microfilariae in blood smears.

ENDOPARASITES OF SWINE

PARASITES OF THE GASTROINTESTINAL TRACT

NEMATODES (ROUNDWORMS)

Ascarops strongylina and *Physocephalus sexalatus* are the "thick stomach worms" of the porcine stomach. Both of these nematodes produce thick-walled, larvated eggs that can be recovered on fecal flotation. The eggs of both species are quite similar. The eggs of *A. strongylina* are 34 to 39 μ by 20 μ and have thick shells surrounded by a thin membrane that produces an irregular outline. The eggs of

P. sexalatus are 34 to 39 µ by 15 to 17 µ. The prepatent period for both species is approximately 42 days.

Hyostrongylus rubidus is referred to as the "red stomach worm" of swine. The eggs are "trichostrongyle type," that is, they are oval, thin-shelled eggs. They contain four or more cells and measure 71 to 78 µ by 35 to 42 µ. These eggs can be recovered on fecal flotation. As with bovine trichostrongyles, definitive diagnosis can only be made by fecal culture and larval identification. The prepatent period is approximately 20 days.

Ascaris suum, the "swine ascarid" or the "large intestinal roundworm," is the largest nematode found within the small intestine of pigs. The eggs can be recovered on standard fecal flotation. They are oval and golden brown, with a thick albuminous shell bearing prominent projections. These eggs measure 70 to 89 µ by 37 to 40 µ. Figure 6-43 shows the egg of *A. suum.*

Strongyloides ransomi, the "intestinal threadworm" of pigs, is unique in that only a parthenogenetic female is parasitic in the host. Parasitic males do not exist. These females produce larvated eggs measuring 45 to 55 µ by 26 to 35 µ. Eggs are usually recovered in flotation of fresh feces. The prepatent period is 3 to 7 days (Figure 6-7 shows the parasitic adult females, eggs, and first-stage larvae of *Strongyloides* species).

Oesophagostomum dentatum, the "nodular worm of swine," is found in the large intestine of swine. The prepatent period is 50 days. Their eggs are "trichostrongyle type," that is, they are oval, thin-shelled eggs. They contain 4 to 16 cells and measure 40 by 70 µ. These eggs can be recovered on a standard fecal flotation. As with bovine trichostrongyles, definitive diagnosis can only be made by fecal culture and larval identification.

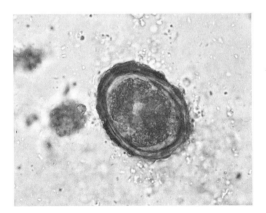

FIGURE 6-43. Characteristic ovum of *Ascaris suum*, the "swine ascarid" or the "large intestinal roundworm" of pigs. The eggs are oval and golden brown, with a thick, albuminous shell bearing prominent projections. They measure 70 to 89 µ by 37 to 40 µ.

Trichuris suis is commonly called the "whipworm," infecting the cecum and colon of swine. (See the section on nematode parasites of the gastointestinal tract of dogs and cats for details on gross morphology of adult worms.) The egg of the whipworm is described as trichinelloid or trichuroid. It has a thick, brown, barrel-shaped shell with plugs at both ends. The eggs are unembryonated (not larvated) when laid. Eggs of porcine whipworms measure 50 to 60 μ by 21 to 25 μ. The prepatent period is 42 to 49 days.

ACANTHOCEPHALANS (THORNY-HEADED WORMS)

Macracanthorhynchus hirudinaceus is the "thorny-headed worm" of the small intestine of swine; it is called "thorny-headed" because of its spiny proboscis, which it embeds as an anchor into the small intestinal mucosa of the host. The eggs have a triple-layered shell, are oval, and measure 67 to 100 μ by 40 to 65 μ. Figure 6-44 shows the eggs of *M. hirudinaceus*. The eggs can be recovered on a standard fecal flotation. The prepatent period is 60 to 90 days.

PROTOZOANS (UNICELLULAR ORGANISMS)

Balantidium coli is the "ciliated protozoan" found in the large intestine of swine. Although it is commonly observed during microscopic examination of fresh diarrheic feces, it is generally considered to be nonpathogenic. Two morphologic stages can be found in feces: the "cyst" stage and the motile "trophozoite" stage. Both stages may vary in size. This is a large protozoan parasite. The trophozoites may be 150 by 120 μ, with a sausage- to kidney-shaped macronucleus. It is covered with numerous rows of cilia and moves about the microscopic field with lively motility. The cyst is spherical to ovoid and 40 to 60 μ in diameter, with a slight greenish-yellow color. Both of these stages may be easily recognized by microscopic examination of the intestinal contents or fresh, diarrheic feces. Figure 6-45 shows the trophozoite stage of *B. coli* recovered on fecal flotation. Figure 6-46 shows *B. coli* in histopathologic section.

Cryptosporidium is another coccidian parasite that parasitizes the small intestine of a wide variety of animals, including swine. The sporulated oocysts in the feces are colorless and transparent and measure only 4.5 to 5.0 μ. Diagnosis is by standard fecal flotation and stained fecal smears. Because people may become infected with *Cryptosporidium* species, feces suspected of harboring this protozoan should be handled with great care. See Figure 6-19 for features of the oocysts of *Cryptosporidium* species.

Isospora suis is the coccidian that parasitizes the small intestine of swine, especially young piglets. Oocysts are usually found on flotation of fresh feces. They are subspherical, lack a micropyle, and measure 18 to 21 μ. Postmortem

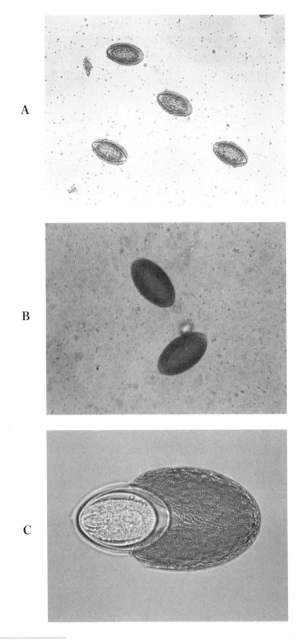

Figure 6-44. **A** to **C,** Ova of *Macracanthorhynchus hirudinaceus,* the "thorny-headed worm" of the small intestine of swine. The eggs have a triple-layered shell, are oval, and measure 67 to 100 μ by 40 to 65 μ.

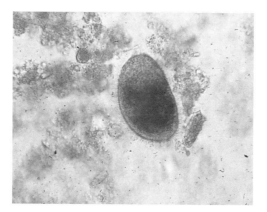

FIGURE 6-45. Trophozoite stage of *Balantidium coli,* the "ciliated protozoan" found in the large intestine of swine. The trophozoites may be 150 by 120 μ, with a sausage- to kidney-shaped macronucleus. They are covered with numerous rows of cilia and move about the microscopic field with lively motility. The cyst is spherical to ovoid and 40 to 60 μ in diameter, with a slight greenish-yellow color.

diagnosis in piglets exhibiting clinical signs, but not shedding oocysts, can be achieved by direct smear of the jejunum stained with Diff-Quik. Diagnosis is by observation of the banana-shaped merozoites. The prepatent period is 4 to 8 days. Figure 6-47 shows features of the oocysts of *Isospora suis.*

PARASITES OF THE RESPIRATORY SYSTEM

NEMATODES (ROUNDWORMS)

Metastrongylus apri, the "swine lungworm," is found within the bronchi and bronchioles of pigs. The oval, thick-walled eggs measure 60 by 40 μ and contain larvae. Eggs can be recovered on fecal flotation using a flotation medium with a specific gravity above 1.25 or by using the fecal sedimentation technique. The prepatent period is approximately 24 days.

PARASITES OF THE URINARY SYSTEM

NEMATODES (ROUNDWORMS)

Stephanurus dentatus, the "swine kidney worm," is found in the kidney, ureters, and perirenal tissues of pigs. Their eggs are "strongyle-type," that is they are oval, thin-shelled eggs, containing 4 to 16 cells, and measuring 90 to 120 μ by

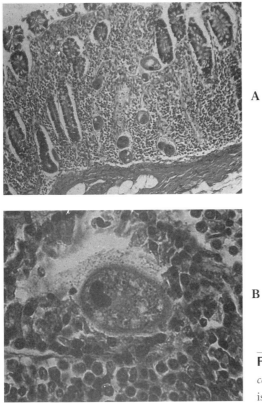

A

B

Figure 6-46. A and B, *Balantidium coli* in a histopathologic section. This is a very large protozoan parasite.

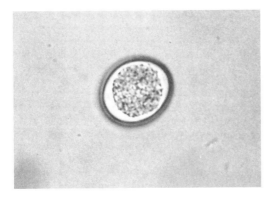

Figure 6-47. Oocyst of *Isospora suis*.

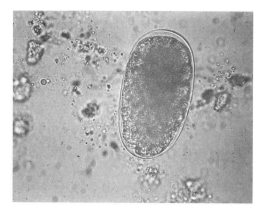

FIGURE 6-48. Egg of *Stephanurus dentatus,* the "swine kidney worm." These eggs are "strongle type," that is, they are oval, thin-shelled eggs, containing 4 to 16 cells and measuring 90 to 120 µ by 43 to 70 µ. Eggs can be recovered from the urine using urine sedimentation.

43 to 70 µ. Eggs can be recovered from the urine using urine sedimentation. Figure 6-48 shows the features of the eggs of *Stephanurus dentatus.* The prepatent period is extremely long, approximately 9 to 24 months.

DIAGNOSIS OF ALIMENTARY PARASITISM

Parasites can infect the oral cavity, esophagus, stomach, small and large intestines, and other internal organs of animals. Detection of these parasites involves collection and microscopic examination of feces. Diagnosis is usually by finding life cycle stages of the parasite within the feces. These stages include eggs, oocysts, larvae, segments (tapeworms), and adult organisms. The following procedures can be performed by veterinary technicians to detect parasitic infections.

COLLECTION OF FECAL SAMPLES

Fecal samples collected for routine examination should be as fresh as possible. Specimens that cannot be examined within a few hours of excretion should be refrigerated or mixed with equal parts of 10% formalin. The need for fresh feces stems from the fact that eggs, oocysts, and other life cycle stages may be altered by development, making diagnosis extremely difficult.

SMALL ANIMAL FECAL SAMPLES

Several methods are used for collecting feces from companion animals. A fecal sample can be collected by the owner immediately after the animal has defecated. The feces may be stored in any type of container, such as a Zip-Loc bag or a clean, small jar. Veterinary hospitals may dispense containers to their clients for this purpose. In either case, only a small amount of feces (1 teaspoon) is required for proper examination. All specimens should be properly identified with the owner's name, animal's name, and species of animal.

Fecal samples can also be collected directly from the animal at the veterinary hospital, using a gloved finger or fecal loop. If a glove is used, the feces can remain in the glove, with the glove turned inside out, tied and labeled. Samples collected with a fecal loop should be used for direct examination only, as the amount collected is relatively small.

LARGE ANIMAL FECAL SAMPLES

Fecal specimens collected from livestock can either be obtained directly from an individual animal's rectum, or from a number of animals to comprise a pooled sample. Samples collected directly from an individual animal using a gloved hand can remain in the glove, with the glove turned inside out, tied, and labeled.

Pooled samples are collected from a number of animals housed together and then commingled in a single container. These samples are used to get an idea of the degree of infection within the group. Pooled samples can be collected in any type of container, as long as it is clean and can be tightly sealed. These samples should be labeled with the species, pen or group number, owner, and time of collection.

EXAMINATION OF FECAL SAMPLES

Several precautions should be taken during fecal examination:

- *Handle fecal samples with care.* The feces may contain parasites, bacteria, or viruses that are zoonotic (i.e., hazardous to people). Appropriate clothing and gloves should be worn. If gloves are not worn, hands should be frequently washed with soap and water. No food or drink should be allowed in the examination area.
- *Clean the laboratory area thoroughly after the examinations are completed.* Spilled materials create a hazardous area in which to work and could pose a serious threat to one's health.

- *Maintain good records.* Records should contain the date, owner's name, and any parasites found in the sample. If the sample is negative, it should be recorded as such.

GROSS EXAMINATION OF FECES

Several characteristics of the feces should also be recorded and reported to the veterinarian. They are as follows:

- *Consistency.* Fresh feces should be somewhat formed, depending on the species of animal. Diarrhea or constipation could be the result of a parasitic infection.
- *Color.* Fecal color can be affected by the food an animal eats. Also malabsorption or a parasitic infection may alter the color of feces.
- *Blood.* Blood can impart a dark reddish-brown color to feces or it can appear as bright red streaks in the feces. In either case, blood can indicate a severe parasitic infection or other serious intestinal diseases. Blood in the feces is an important clinical finding and should be brought to the attention of the veterinarian. Digested blood has a dark, tarry appearance.
- *Mucus.* Mucus in the feces can be a result of digestive disorders or a parasitic infection. In either case, its presence should be reported to the veterinarian.
- *Parasites.* Adult parasites or tapeworm segments can be found in the feces. Adult roundworms resemble strings of spaghetti, whereas tapeworm segments look more like pieces of rice. Tapeworm segments can be identified by microscopic examination. The segments of two common tapeworms infecting dogs and cats are shown in Figure 6-49. Figure 6-50 shows the segments found in livestock feces.

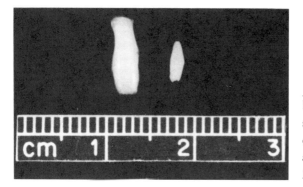

FIGURE 6-49. Mature segments of the most common tapeworms of dogs and cats. *Left, Taenia. Right, Dipylidium.*

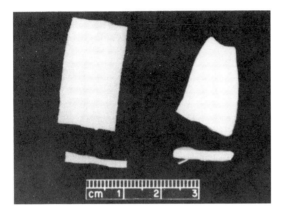

Figure 6-50. Chains and individually mature segments of tapeworms of cattle, *Moniezia* (*left*) and horses, *Anoplocephala* (*right*).

Occasionally, a client may submit a dried tapeworm segment. To identify the tapeworm species, the dried segments must be soaked in saline for 1 to 4 hours. Once the segments are rehydrated, they can be identified by size, shape, and the eggs contained within.

Segments of some tapeworm species do not contain eggs, and some segments may have expelled their eggs before the examination was conducted. In either case, a tapeworm segment can be identified as such by finding small mineral deposits (*calcareous bodies*) within the segment (Figure 6-51). This is done by crushing the tapeworm-like segment between two glass slides and examining the material with a microscope.

Microscopic examination of feces

Microscopic examination of feces is the most reliable method to detect parasitic infections. A microscope with 4X, 10X, and 40X objectives is required for proper examination of a fecal specimen (see Chapter 1). A mechanical stage is helpful. A micrometer is also useful but not required (Procedure 6-1).

Fecal specimens should be routinely examined with the 10X objective. The examination should begin at one corner of the slide and end at the opposite corner moving over the slide in a systematic pattern (Figure 6-52). The microscope should be continually focused with the fine-tuning knob during the examination. The initial plane of focus should be that of air bubbles, as most eggs are found in this plane. Any material found during the initial scan, including parasite eggs, can be more closely examined using the more powerful objectives.

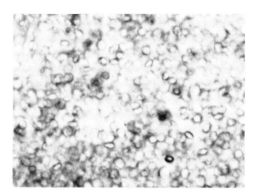

FIGURE 6-51. Microscopic calcium deposits (calcareous bodies) in tapeworm tissue.

PROCEDURE 6-1. Examination of tapeworm segments

Materials: Thumb forceps
Dissection needles (hypodermic needles work well)
Microscope slides and coverslips
Saline
Wooden applicator sticks

1. Remove the segment from the feces with thumb forceps and place in a drop of saline on a slide.
2. Using the dissection needles, pull the segment into several small pieces. Crush the pieces with a wooden applicator stick.
3. Remove the large pieces. Add more saline, if needed, and place a coverslip on the slide.
4. Examine the slide with the microscope (described later) for tapeworm eggs.

CALIBRATING THE MICROSCOPE. The size of the various stages of many parasites is often important for correct identification. Some examples are *Trichuris* vs. *Capillaria* eggs and *Dipetalonema* vs. *Dirofilaria* microfilariae. Accurate measurements are easily obtained by using a calibrated eyepiece on the microscope. Calibration must be performed on every microscope to be used. Each objective (lens) of the microscope must be individually calibrated.

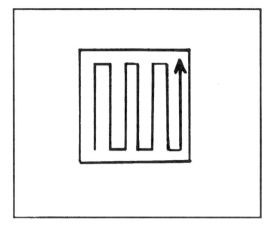

FIGURE 6-52. Diagram of a scheme of movement of the microscopic field to thoroughly examine the area under the coverslip.

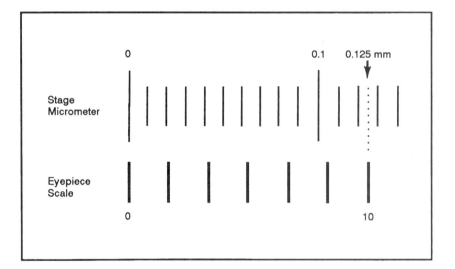

FIGURE 6-53. Stage micrometer and eyepiece scale used to calibrate a microscope.

The *stage micrometer* is a microscope slide etched with a 2-mm line marked in 0.01-mm (10-μ) divisions (Figure 6-53). Note that 1 micron (μ) equals 0.001 mm.

The *eyepiece scale* is a glass disc that fits into and remains in one of the microscope eyepieces. This disc is etched with 30 hash marks spaced at equal intervals (Figure 6-53). The number of hash marks on the disc may vary with different manufacturers, but the calibration procedure is the same for all.

The stage micrometer is used to determine the distance in microns between the hash marks on the eyepiece scale for each objective lens of the microscope being calibrated. This information is recorded and labelled on the microscope for future reference.

To begin the calibration procedure, start on low power (10X) and focus on the 2-mm line of the stage micrometer. Note that 2 mm equals 2000 μ. Rotate the eyepiece so that the hash-mark scale is horizontal and parallel to the stage micrometer scale (Figure 6-53). Align the zero ("0") point on both scales.

Determine the point on the stage micrometer aligned with the "10" hash mark on the eyepiece scale. In Figure 6-53, this point is at 0.125 mm on the stage micrometer.

Multiply this number by 100. In our example, 0.125 × 100 = 12.5 μ. This means that at this power (10X), the distance between each hash mark on the eyepiece scale is 12.5 μ.

Repeat these steps at each magnification (10X, 40X, 100X). Record the information on a label and attach it to the calibrated microscope. For example,

OBJECTIVE	DISTANCE BETWEEN HASH MARKS (μ)
10X	12.5
40X	2.5
100X	1.0

To measure an object, such as a parasite egg, place one end of the egg on the zero mark and count the number of divisions to the other end of the egg. Multiply the number of divisions counted by the calibration factor for the objective being used.

For example, a trichostrongyle egg is 24 divisions long and 13.5 divisions wide when measured with the 40X objective. The calibration factor for the 40X objective in our hypothetical microscope is 2.5. Therefore the egg is 24 × 2.5 = 60 μ long and 13.5 × 2.5 = 33.75 μ wide.

To measure microfilariae, align the head with the zero mark and count the number of divisions to the very end of the tail. To measure round parasite eggs, measure through the middle of the egg. For more accurate measurements, use the higher objective (40X instead of 10X).

EXAMINING DIRECT SMEARS.   A direct smear of feces is used to rapidly estimate an animal's parasite burden. This procedure is also used to detect some of the motile protozoa found in feces.

Advantages of direct smears include short preparation time and minimal equipment required to run the procedure. Disadvantages include the small amount of feces examined, which may not be enough to detect a low parasite burden, and the amount of fecal debris on the slide, which could be confused with parasitic material.

A fecal sample for a direct smear preparation can be obtained from an animal using a fecal loop or a rectal thermometer (after measuring the animal's temperature). Either way, only a very small amount of feces is needed (Procedure 6-2).

CONCENTRATION METHODS FOR FECAL EXAMINATION

The following methods are used to concentrate parasitic material in feces. A concentration technique makes it possible to examine a large amount of feces in a relatively short time. Also, a low parasite burden can easily be identified. Two types of procedures are most often used in veterinary hospitals: *flotation* and *sedimentation*.

FLOTATION SOLUTIONS.   Fecal flotation methods are based on the *specific gravity* of parasitic material and fecal debris. *Specific gravity* refers to the weight of an object as compared with the weight of an equal volume of water. The specific

---

PROCEDURE 6-2.   Direct smear procedure

Materials: Microscope slide and coverslip
            Applicator stick or toothpick
            Optional: Lugol's iodine or new methylene blue

1. Place a drop of saline or water on the microscope slide with an equal amount of feces. A drop of stain may be added at this time.
2. Thoroughly mix the feces and saline or water with the applicator stick to form a homogeneous emulsion.
3. Make a smear on the slide. Be sure the smear is thin enough to see newspaper print through it.
4. Remove any large pieces of feces. Add more saline or water if needed and apply a coverslip.
5. Examine the smear using the 10X objective for parasite eggs and larvae or the 40X objective for motile protozoal organisms.

gravity of most parasite eggs is between 1.100 and 1.200 g/ml, while the specific gravity of water is 1.000 (Procedure 6-3).

To allow for flotation of parasite eggs, oocysts, and other life cycle stages, the flotation solution must have a higher specific gravity than that of the parasitic material. Several salt and sugar solutions work well for flotation. Most have a specific gravity of 1.200 to 1.250. In this range, heavy fecal debris sinks

---

PROCEDURE 6-3.   Preparation of flotation solutions

SUGAR SOLUTION (SHEATHER'S SOLUTION)
1. Pour 355 ml of warm water into a beaker. Add a stir bar and place on a hot plate. Heat the water on high, but not to the boiling point.
2. Slowly add 1 lb of granulated sugar to the water, stirring constantly. Allow the sugar to dissolve completely before removing from the heat source.
3. Add 6 ml of 40% formalin or liquid phenol after the solution has completely cooled.
4. Check the specific gravity of the solution with a hydrometer (Figure 6-54) before using. (Hydrometers are available from scientific supply houses.)
5. If the specific gravity is below the desired range, heat the solution and add more sugar.
6. If the specific gravity is above the desired range, add water and stir.

SODIUM NITRATE SOLUTION
1. Add about 315 g of sodium nitrate to 1 L of water while stirring. Heating is not necessary, but it hastens the dissolution process.
2. Check the specific gravity and adjust as needed.

ZINC SULFATE SOLUTION
1. Add about 386 g of zinc sulfate to 1 L of water while stirring. Heating is not necessary, but it hastens the dissolution process.
2. Check the specific gravity and adjust as needed.

SATURATED SODIUM CHLORIDE SOLUTION
1. Add table salt to water until the salt no longer dissolves but tends to settle to the bottom of the container. The specific gravity of this solution cannot go any higher than 1.200.

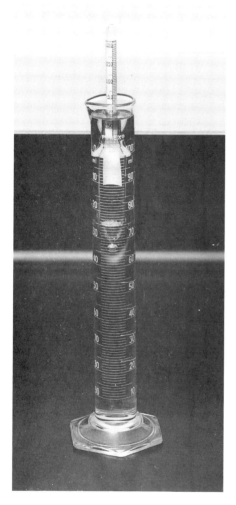

Figure 6-54. Measuring the specific gravity of a flotation solution with a hydrometer.

to the bottom of the container, while parasitic material rises to the top of the solution.

   Sodium nitrate solution is the most common fecal flotation solution used in veterinary hospitals today. This solution is efficient for floating parasite eggs, oocysts, and larvae. It can be purchased with commercial diagnostic test kits or in individual aliquots. The major disadvantage of using sodium nitrate is the expense. Sodium nitrate also forms crystals and distorts eggs if allowed to sit longer than 20 minutes.

   Another solution commonly used for flotation is *sugar solution*. Sugar solution is inexpensive and does not crystallize or distort eggs. Sugar solution can be made anywhere and has a long shelf life. Although it is sticky to work with, spilled sugar solution can be cleaned up with warm, soapy water.

Zinc sulfate solution is more commonly used in diagnostic laboratories. Zinc sulfate floats protozoal organisms with the least amount of distortion. It is generally used in combination with one of the previously mentioned solutions.

The least desirable solution used is saturated *sodium chloride* solution. This solution corrodes laboratory equipment, forms crystals, and severely distorts parasite eggs. Saturated sodium chloride solution is also a poor flotation medium, as the maximum specific gravity obtainable is 1.200, allowing heavier eggs to remain submerged.

As there are a number of choices in flotation solutions, so there are a number of choices in flotation techniques (Procedure 6-4).

STANDARD FECAL FLOTATION.   The standard or simple fecal flotation is one of the most common flotation techniques used in veterinary hospitals. This technique uses a test tube or vial, in which feces and flotation solution are mixed. A coverslip or microscope slide is placed on top of the test tube and the unit is allowed to sit undisturbed. Any parasite eggs in the feces float to the top and stick to the underside of the coverslip or microscope slide. The coverslip or slide is then removed and microscopically examined for parasitic material.

Although the standard flotation technique is easy to perform, it is less efficient at floating parasitic material than the centrifugal technique, described later in this chapter.

Commercial flotation kits use the same principle as the standard flotation technique. These kits contain a vial with a filter; some also include prepared flotation solution. Examples of commercial flotation kits include Fecalyzer (EVSCO Pharmaceuticals, Buena, NJ), Ovassay (Synbiotics, San Diego, CA), and Ovatector (BGS Medical Products, Venice, FL) (Figure 6-55). These kits are easy to use, but they are expensive. Some practices reduce the expense by washing and reusing the vials and filters.

CENTRIFUGAL FLOTATION.   Centrifugal flotation for parasite eggs, oocysts, and other parasitic material is the most efficient method available. It requires less time to perform than the standard flotation method. The only drawback to this procedure is that it requires a centrifuge with a horizontal (nonfixed) rotor that can hold 15-ml centrifuge tubes (see Chapter 1). If such a centrifuge is available, centrifugal flotation is preferred, as it is easy to perform and samples can be run individually or in batches.

PROCEDURE 6-4.   Standard flotation procedure

Materials: Flotation solution
           Shell vial or test tube and test tube rack
           Waxed paper cups
           Cheesecloth cut into 6 × 6-inch squares
           Wooden tongue depressor
           Microscope slides and coverslips

1. Take about 2 g (1/2 tsp) of feces and place it in the cup. Add 20 ml of flotation solution. Using a tongue depressor, mix the feces and flotation solution until no large fecal pieces remain.
2. Wrap cheesecloth around the lip of the cup, while bending the cup to form a spout. Pour the mixture through the cheesecloth, into a vial. Fill the vial so that a meniscus is formed (Figure 6-56). If there is not enough fluid in the cup, fill the vial with as much mixture as is available and then fill the remainder with flotation solution.
3. Gently place a coverslip on top of the vial.
4. Allow the unit to remain undisturbed for 10 to 20 minutes (sugar solution requires a longer waiting time than does sodium nitrate). If the preparation is not allowed to sit this long, some eggs will not have time to float to the surface. If allowed to sit for more than an hour, some eggs might become waterlogged and sink, or the eggs may become distorted.
5. Carefully remove the coverslip by picking it straight up and placing it on a microscope slide, with the wet side adjacent to the slide.
6. Examine the area of the slide under the coverslip, as described earlier in this chapter, using the 10X objective. Record any parasitic material found in the sample.

If you are testing multiple samples, a numbering system helps keep the samples in order. Assign a number to the patient and the corresponding centrifuge tube. This minimizes the chances of error (Procedure 6-5).

FECAL SEDIMENTATION

Fecal sedimentation concentrates parasite eggs, oocysts, and other parasitic material by allowing them to settle to the bottom of a tube of liquid, usually water. A disadvantage of this technique is the amount of fecal debris that mixes

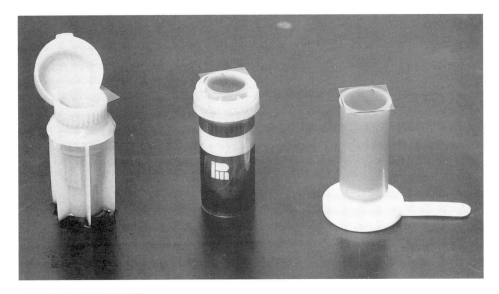

FIGURE 6-55. Three examples of commercial fecal flotation kits. From *left* to *right*, Fecalyzer (EVSCO Pharmaceuticals, Buena, NJ), Ovassay (Synbiotics, San Diego, CA), and Ovatector (BGS Medical Products, Venice, FL).

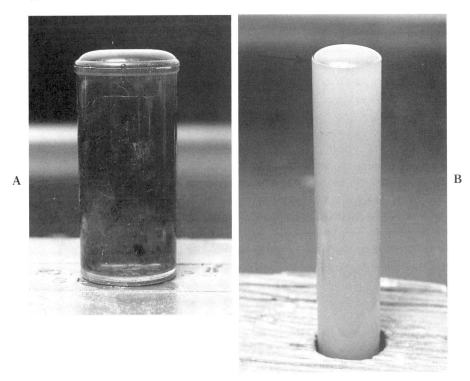

FIGURE 6-56. **A,** Vial filled with flotation solution, showing appearance of the meniscus. **B,** Test tube filled with flotation solution, showing appearance of the meniscus.

PROCEDURE 6-5.   Centrifugal flotation procedure

Materials: Same as for standard flotation, but omits the vials
15-ml centrifuge tube
Microscope slides and coverslips

1. Prepare the fecal mixture as described in the standard flotation procedure.
2. Strain the mixture through cheesecloth into the 15-ml centrifuge tube. Fill the tube to the top. (If using a fixed-rotor centrifuge, the tube should be filled half way and a coverslip should not be used.) Apply a coverslip to the top of the tube. Always balance the centrifuge with a 15-ml tube filled with flotation solution and a coverslip placed on top. Be sure all tubes are marked for identification after centrifugation.
3. Centrifuge the tubes for 3 to 5 minutes at 1300 to 1500 rpm (400 to 650 gravities).
4. Remove the coverslip, or use a wire loop or glass rod to remove the top part of fluid in the tube and place on a microscope slide. Microscopically examine the sample, using the 10X objective as previously described.

---

with the parasitic material, which makes microscopic examination somewhat difficult.

This procedure is used to detect heavy eggs that would not float in flotation solution, or eggs that would become distorted by the flotation solution. Parasite eggs considered too heavy for flotation are trematode (fluke) eggs. Although some flotation solutions can be adjusted to a specific gravity of 1.300 to float these eggs, such solutions are not routinely used because distortion can occur (Procedure 6-6).

QUANTITATIVE FECAL EXAMINATION

Quantitative procedures are used to determine the number of eggs or oocysts present in each gram of feces. These procedures are used as a rough indication of the number of parasites present within a host. Their usefulness is limited, however, by the fact that the various parasite species produce different numbers of eggs. Also egg production by the parasites may be sporadic, and the number of eggs may not correlate with the number of parasites present. The last item is the most significant disadvantage because, in most cases, clinical signs of disease are caused by immature parasites that have not yet begun producing eggs or larvae.

Several quantitative procedures can be performed in veterinary hospitals. These include the Stoll egg count technique, the modified Wisconsin double centrifugation technique, and the McMaster technique. These procedures are fairly easy to perform; each requires its own equipment. Two quantitative techniques are described in Procedures 6-7 and 6-8. Other quantitative procedures may be found in the reference books listed at the end of this chapter.

EXAMINATION OF FECES FOR PROTOZOA AND COCCIDIA

PROTOZOAL TROPHOZOITES.   All of the previously described procedures can be used to detect protozoal cysts. However, some protozoans do not form cysts and pass out of the host in trophozoite form. *Trophozoites* are one-celled, motile organisms that lack the rigid wall of a cyst, making flotation without distortion or death of the trophozoite impossible. Therefore the direct smear technique, using saline and a stain, is the procedure of choice when examining a fecal sample for protozoal organisms.

In a direct smear, trophozoites can be recognized by their movement. *Balantidium coli* is bean-shaped and covered with cilia. It moves in a slow, tumbling fashion. *Giardia* is pear shaped and has five to eight flagella. It moves with a jerky motion. Trichomonads are long, slender organisms with a single flagellum attached to the dorsal surface, forming a sail-like structure that ripples as the organism glides through debris. Amoebas move with a flowing motion, extending a part of the body (*pseudopod*) and moving the rest of the body after it.

Stains can also be used to recognize certain structural characteristics of trophozoites and cysts. Lugol's iodine and new methylene blue are common stains used with the direct smear procedure. These stains do not preserve the slide but do facilitate examination of the specimen, making identification easier (Procedure 6-9).

PROCEDURE 6-6. Fecal sedimentation procedure

Materials: Waxed paper cups
Cheesecloth cut in 6 × 6-inch squares
Wooden tongue depressors
Centrifuge and 15-ml tubes
Pasteur pipettes with bulbs
Microscope slides and coverslips

1. Mix about 2 g of feces with tap water in a waxed paper cup. Strain the mixture through cheesecloth into a centrifuge tube (as described for the centrifugation procedure), filling the tube half full.
2. Balance the centrifuge with tubes filled with equal amounts of water. Centrifuge for 3 to 5 minutes at 1300 to 1500 rpm. If a centrifuge is unavailable, allow the tube to sit undisturbed for 20 to 30 minutes.
3. Slowly pour the liquid off the top without disturbing the sediment layer (including the fine, silty material) on the bottom.
4. Using a pipette, transfer a small amount of the fine sediment to a microscope slide. Also transfer a small amount of sediment to a different slide. Apply a coverslip to the drops of sediment and examine microscopically. Lugol's iodine may be mixed with the drop of sediment before a coverslip is applied; this facilitates identification of protozoal cysts or trophozoites.

If a protozoal parasite cannot be identified on direct smears, fecal smears containing protozoal trophozoites can be dried, stained with Diff-Quik, Wright's, or Giemsa stain, and sent to a diagnostic laboratory. There are many other procedures used for staining and preserving protozoal trophozoites. Most of these procedures are used in diagnostic laboratories and will not be explained here.

COCCIDIA. Several coccidial parasites require special staining techniques for identification. Two procedures will be discussed in this chapter.

The *acid-fast staining technique* is used to identify *Cryptosporidium* in the feces. *Cryptosporidium* is a parasite of the gastrointestinal tract of many animals, including people. The oocysts are 2 to 8 μ in diameter and are almost undetectable in flotation solution to the inexperienced eye. Acid-fast staining can aid detection of the oocysts in a fecal smear (Procedure 6-10).

PROCEDURE 6-7.   Wisconsin double centrifugation technique

1. Weigh out a fecal sample (5 g for cattle, 2 g for horses or swine).
2. Place 12 ml of water in a small cup and add the feces to it.
3. Stir well with a wooden tongue depressor and mash the material until it is completely broken up.
4. Pour the mixture through an ordinary tea strainer into another cup, stirring the material while pouring.
5. Press the remaining material with the tongue depressor until nearly dry.
6. Squirt 2 to 3 ml of water into the small cup just emptied and rinse down the sides. Pour this rinsing fluid through the material in the strainer.
7. Press the material in the strainer until dry again and discard.
8. Stir the mixture in the second cup and immediately pour it into a 15-ml centrifuge tube.
9. Centrifuge the tube at 1500 rpm for 10 minutes.
10. Decant the fluid from the tube, being careful not to pour off the fine material on the surface of the sediment.
11. Fill the tube half full of sugar solution (specific gravity 1.27) and mix the sediment and sugar solution with a wooden applicator stick, being careful to scrape the sides and bottom of the tube while mixing.
12. Finish filling the tube with sugar solution and place in the centrifuge.
13. With a pipette, add sugar solution to the tube until it is full enough to place a coverslip on top. There should not be an air bubble under the coverslip nor should the material overflow so that it runs down the sides of the tube.
14. Centrifuge at 1500 rpm for 10 minutes.
15. Remove the coverslip by lifting straight upward and place it on a microscope slide. If done properly, there should be a good thickness of material under the coverslip.
16. Using the 10X objective, scan the entire slide, counting all parasite eggs.

For cattle:

Total number = eggs/5 g of feces; total number × 91 = eggs/lb of feces

For horses and swine:

Total number = eggs/2 g of feces; total number × 227 = eggs/lb of feces

---

Procedure 6-8. Modified Wisconsin technique

1. Weigh out 5 g of feces.
2. Mix the feces thoroughly with 45 ml of water in a small cup.
3. Withdraw 1 ml of suspended mixture and place into a 15-ml centrifuge cup.
4. Fill the tube with sugar solution (specific gravity 1.27) and place a coverslip on the tube.
5. Centrifuge the tube at 1200 rpm for 5 minutes.
6. Remove the coverslip and place on a microscope slide. Scan the slide, counting all parasite eggs or oocysts seen.
7. Multiply the number of eggs or oocysts counted by 10 to determine the eggs per gram (epg) of feces.

Procedure 6-9. Preparation of Lugol's iodine

Before preparing this solution, the technician should remove all jewelry, as this solution permanently stains precious metals.

1. Dissolve 10 g of potassium iodide in 100 ml of distilled water in a glass beaker.
2. Add 5 g of powdered iodine crystals to the solution and stir until all of the iodine has dissolved. This produces a 5% Lugol's iodine solution (therapeutic strength). This solution should be stored in an amber bottle, away from light.
3. For staining, this 5% Lugol's solution must be diluted by adding 1 part 5% Lugol's solution to 5 parts distilled water. This staining solution must be remade every 3 weeks because it deteriorates.

The second procedure uses Diff-Quik stain for identification of *Isospora*. *Isospora* is a coccidian found in the gastrointestinal tract (especially the jejunum) of many animals, but it is of most concern in pigs. This parasite can cause the death of many piglets before any oocysts are found in the feces using conventional flotation methods. Therefore an intestinal mucosal scraping must

Procedure 6-10. Acid-fast staining technique

Materials: Glass pipette
Microscope slide
Timer
Hot plate or Bunsen burner
Carbol fuchsin stain[a]
Acid alcohol[b]
New methylene blue stain[c]

1. Make a thin (paper thin) smear of feces using a glass pipette and allow to air dry.
2. Fix the smear by heating on a hot plate at a setting of 1.5 for 2 to 3 minutes or by passing the slide through a Bunsen burner flame, specimen side up.
3. Flood the slide with carbol fuchsin stain and heat the slide until the stain steams.
4. Remove the slide from the heat and let it sit for 5 minutes. Rinse with tap water.
5. Decolorize by adding acid alcohol for 10 to 20 seconds, then rinse with tap water. Repeat this step until the film on the slide appears light pink.
6. Add new methylene blue stain for 20 to 30 seconds. Rinse with tap water.
7. Blot dry with a paper towel and examine microscopically using the oil-immersion objective.
8. Oocysts appear as bright fluorescent red objects, while bacteria and yeasts stain blue.

[a]*Carbol fuchsin stain:*

Basic fuchsin	0.3 g
95% ethanol	10 ml
Liquefied phenol	5 ml
Distilled water	95 ml

Dissolve the basic fuchsin in ethanol. Mix the phenol with distilled water and then add this to the ethanol. Mix and let stand for several days. Filter before using.

[b]*Acid alcohol:*

95% ethanol	97 ml
Concentrated hydrochloric acid	3 ml

[c]*Methylene blue stain:*

Methylene blue chloride	0.3 g
Distilled water	100 ml

be stained and examined for other diagnostic stages (schizonts, merozoites) of this parasite. This procedure involves scraping the mucosa of the jejunum and smearing the scrapings onto microscope slides. After the slides are air dried, they are stained with Diff-Quik and examined with the oil-immersion objective.

For accurate results with either of these procedures, several samples should be examined. If such examination is not possible, feces or intestines may be sent to a diagnostic laboratory. Collection and shipping of parasitic specimens are described later in this chapter.

FECAL CULTURE

Fecal cultures involve rearing infective larvae of strongyles, trichostrongyles, or hookworms for identification. Several techniques are available for this purpose.

The first procedure uses a covered glass jar that has been rinsed with 0.1% sodium carbonate solution. Sodium carbonate solution is used to inhibit mold growth while allowing the parasite eggs to develop. Formed feces are placed in the jar, which is then stored at room temperature in a dark area for 7 to 10 days. The contents of the jar should be kept moist but not soggy. If no water droplets are seen condensing on the inside of the jar, add a few drops of water or sodium carbonate. Vermiculite or sand should be added to bovine feces or feces that contain a lot of water.

Larvae can be found in the condensation droplets in the culture jar. The larvae can be collected by rinsing the jar with a small amount of water, collecting the rinsings, and concentrating the larvae by centrifugation. The larvae found in the sediment after centrifugation can be placed on a microscope slide and examined after coverslip application. The slide is then briefly heated with a match to "relax" or straighten the larvae and curtail their movement.

When examining for larvae, numbers of larvae do not necessarily correlate with numbers of eggs present in the feces. Development from egg to larva may take longer with some species than with others, and some parasite species may produce more eggs than others. For example, *Hemonchus contortus* and *Strongyloides papillosus* are found in greater numbers and their eggs develop faster than those of *Trichostrongylus* and *Cooperia*.

Culture of canine feces for *Strongyloides stercoralis* filariform larvae uses the same technique described previously. Most *filariform larvae* appear within 24 to 48 hours. *Rhabditiform larvae* may be evident first. If this occurs, allow the sample to stand for no less than 96 hours so the larvae can mate and produce filariform larvae.

Another method uses a covered Petri dish and filter paper. Feces are placed in the middle of a piece of moistened filter paper, which is then placed in the Petri dish. The Petri dish is covered and placed in a dark area at room temperature for 7 to 10 days. The dish is rinsed and the rinsings are collected as previously described. Technicians who wish to do a fecal culture and identify larvae should refer to the chapters on larval identification in the reference by Georgi, listed at the end of this chapter.

SAMPLE COLLECTION AT NECROPSY

Necropsy (postmortem examination) is an important method of diagnosing many diseases, including parasitism (see Chapter 10). The types of lesions produced by immature parasites, any adult parasites found in the body cavity and tissues, and histopathologic examination of infected tissues are used in diagnosis. Veterinary technicians are responsible for the samples collected, making sure they are contained, preserved, labeled, and shipped properly.

Two methods can be used to recover parasites from the digestive tract at necropsy: the *decanting method* and the *sieving method* (Procedures 6-11 and 6-12). With either method, it is important to separate the different parts of the digestive tract and work with the contents of each individually.

Parasites recovered from the digestive tract can be preserved in 70% alcohol or 10% neutral buffered formalin for later identification. Occasionally, "bladder worms" or "cysticerci" may be found attached to the viscera of domestic animals. A "bladder worm" is a fluid-filled, balloon-like structure that is actually a larval tapeworm. These should be handled with care, as the fluid within the bladder can be allergenic and may also be zoonotic. To identify the parasites recovered, consult the references listed at the end of this chapter. If in-hospital diagnosis is not possible, the samples can be preserved as previously described and sent to a diagnostic laboratory for identification.

SHIPPING PARASITOLOGIC SPECIMENS

Any parasitologic specimen shipped to a diagnostic laboratory should be preserved with alcohol or formalin, unless otherwise directed by laboratory personnel. Specimens should be packaged in a leak-proof container and sealed with Parafilm or tape. If specimen containers are found leaking, the shipment

PROCEDURE 6-11.   Decanting method

Materials: Buckets (large enough to hold the contents of each
            part of the digestive tract and an equal volume of water)
            Knives
            Metal spatulas
            Stirring spoons or paddles
            Dissecting pans
            Dissecting microscope or magnifying glass
            Thumb forceps

1. Open each section of the digestive tract and pour its contents into a
   bucket. Using a spatula, scrape the interior lining of the organ into the
   bucket or examine the scrapings separately.
2. Add an equal amount of water to the contents of each bucket and mix
   thoroughly.
3. Allow the contents to sit undisturbed for about 45 minutes.
4. Carefully pour off the liquid, leaving the sediment in the bottom of the
   bucket. Add an equal amount of water and repeat the above procedure
   until the water over the sediment becomes clear.
5. Pour off the clear water, then transfer the sediment to a dissecting pan.
6. Using a dissecting microscope or magnifying glass, examine a number of
   small samples of the sediment. Any parasites found should gently be
   removed with thumb forceps and preserved (discussed later in this
   chapter).

will not be delivered. Feces can be sent fresh or mixed at a ratio of 1:3 with
10% formalin. Whole parasites or segments can be preserved in alcohol or
formalin and placed in a leak-proof container (clean small jar, medicine vial,
clot tube).

All specimen containers should be labeled as to the site from which the
specimen was obtained, the owner's name, the animal's species, name, or
identification number, and the referring veterinarian (including telephone
number and address). The labeled specimen container should be placed in a
shockproof shipping container to prevent breakage during shipping. Styrofoam
containers filled with shredded newspaper work well for shipping parasitologic
specimens.

PROCEDURE 6-12. Sieving method

Materials: Same as for decanting method
Testing sieves (#18 and #45, Sargent-Welch Scientific)

1. Place the contents of each section of digestive tract and the scrapings in a bucket and mix with water, as previously described.
2. Pour the mixture through the #18 sieve and then through the #45 sieve. Wash the sieves' contents with water.
3. Examine the solid material in the sieves, as described for the sediment in the decanting method.

A cover letter should be included with the specimen and should contain a brief history of the animal, findings upon necropsy, and the reason for submitting the samples to the laboratory (e.g., fecal examination, special staining, species identification). Without this background information, the diagnostic laboratory is unlikely to provide accurate results.

MISCELLANEOUS PROCEDURES FOR DETECTION OF ENDOPARASITES

CELLOPHANE TAPE TECHNIQUE. The cellophane tape technique is used to detect the equine pinworm, *Oxyuris equi* (Procedure 6-13). Pinworms are nematodes found in horses, rodents, and people. They live in the colon and, as adults, migrate out the rectum to lay eggs on the skin around the anus. The eggs are contained within a sticky substance and fall off as the substance hardens or as the animal scratches. For this reason, pinworm eggs are usually not seen in a routine fecal examination (Figure 6-42).

BAERMANN TECHNIQUE. The Baermann technique is used to recover nematode larvae from feces, tissues, or soil. This technique uses warm water to stimulate larvae to move about. As the larvae do so, they sink to the bottom of the funnel for collection and identification (Procedure 6-14).

Procedure 6-13. Cellophane tape technique

Materials: Transparent cellophane tape (e.g., Scotch)
          Tongue depressor
          Microscope slide

1. Wrap the cellophane tape in a loop around the tongue depressor, with the sticky side out.
2. Press the tape to the skin around the horse's anus. Stand to the side of the horse and not directly behind it.
3. Place a drop of water on the slide. Remove the tape from the tongue depressor and place it, sticky side down, on top of the water.
4. Examine the slide for pinworm eggs (see Figure 6-42).

Procedure 6-14. Baermann technique

Materials: Baermann apparatus
          Cheesecloth or gauze square about twice the diameter of the funnel
          Microscope slides and coverslips

1. Spread the cheesecloth out on the support screen in the Baermann apparatus. Take 5 to 15 g of fecal, soil, or tissue sample and place it on the cheesecloth. Fold any excess cheesecloth over the top of the sample. Be sure the sample is covered by the warm water or saline; add more if necessary.
2. Allow the apparatus to remain undisturbed overnight.
3. Hold a microscope slide under the cut-off pipette and open the pinch clamp only long enough to allow a large drop to fall on the slide. Apply a coverslip to the slide and examine it microscopically for larvae. Repeat by examining several slides before concluding the sample is negative.

This technique is performed with a Baermann apparatus (Figure 6-57). The apparatus consists of a ring stand and ring holder, a glass funnel with a piece of rubber tubing on the end, a clamp, and a wire net or cheesecloth. With the apparatus set up as shown in Figure 6-57, the sample is placed on the wire screen or cheesecloth, and warm water is added to barely cover the sample. All air bubbles are allowed to flow from the tube of the funnel by releasing the clamp. The apparatus is allowed to sit undisturbed for 12 to 24 hours.

A drop of fluid from the bottom of the funnel is removed (usually the first drop) and placed on a microscope slide. If any larvae are found swimming on the slide, heat the slide with a match to render them immobile.

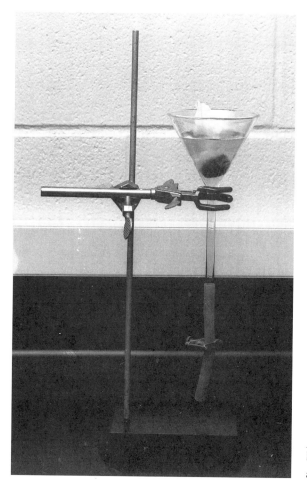

FIGURE 6-57. Baermann apparatus.

Larvae recovered from fresh large animal feces are almost always those of lungworms. Larvae from *Strongyloides stercoralis* can be found in *fresh* canine feces. If the feces are not fresh, all sorts of parasitic and nonparasitic larvae and adults may be seen. For more detailed information on the descriptions of larvae, consult the reference by Bowman.

DIAGNOSIS OF BLOOD PARASITISM

Dirofilaria immitis, the canine heartworm, is the most important parasite of the vascular system in domestic animals in the United States. For this reason, in-hospital blood examinations are commonly performed to detect heartworms.

The following procedures can be performed by veterinary technicians to identify *Dirofilaria immitis.* As mentioned earlier, a clean environment and proper handling of samples are vital to quality control in any laboratory. Any sample handled improperly may result in inaccurate results.

COLLECTION OF BLOOD SAMPLES

Sterile equipment and alcohol are required for collecting a blood sample from an animal. Blood may be collected using a syringe and needle or a Vacutainer (Becton-Dickinson, Rutherford, NJ). If blood is collected with a syringe and needle, the inside of the syringe should be coated with an anticoagulant, such as heparin. If a Vacutainer is used, an EDTA (lavender top) tube is used. Unless serum is required, as with some of the immunodiagnostic test kits, a clot tube (red top) should be used. All samples should be labeled with the owner's name, animal's name, and date of collection.

Microfilariae are more numerous in the blood stream at certain times of the day. To increase the probability of collecting microfilariae, blood should be collected in the afternoon, as the microfilariae of *Dirofilaria immitis* are most numerous in the circulating blood at this time.

EXAMINATION OF THE BLOOD

General observations of the blood should be noted. For example, a blood sample that appears watery may be due to anemia. Clinical pathology tests on the blood can also aid in diagnosis of parasitism. Heartworm microfilariae may be seen during the differential WBC count. A high eosinophil count may also indicate parasitism (Procedure 6-15).

DIRECT EXAMINATION.   Direct examination of the blood for microfilariae is the simplest procedure to perform. This procedure detects movement of microfilariae and other parasites among the red blood cells. As with direct examination of feces, direct examination of blood requires only a small sample. However, unless parasites are present in large numbers, they may be missed. For this reason, the direct smear is *not* a good diagnostic technique for diagnosing microfilariae.

Microfilariae of primary interest are those of *Dirofilaria immitis,* the canine heartworm, and *Dipetalonema reconditum,* a subcutaneous parasite of dogs. Differentiation between the two is extremely important, as treatment for heartworms is expensive, somewhat stressful, and involves use of arsenical compounds.

In a direct blood smear, microfilariae of *Dirofilaria* coil and uncoil, while those of *Dipetalonema* glide smoothly across the slide. However, this is not always the case. Also, the number of *Dirofilaria* microfilariae in a sample is greater than that of *Dipetalonema.* Again, this is not always the case. Direct examination of the blood is only used to determine the presence of microfilariae, not the type. For this, a concentration technique, which "relaxes" and stains microfilariae, is used. These procedures will be discussed later in this chapter.

Trypanosomes are another type of parasite found in the blood. These protozoa occur in tropical areas and occasionally in the United States. Trypanosomes can be seen swimming among the cells of a diluted blood smear (single cell thickness) but are more easily identified in stained smears.

PROCEDURE 6-15.   Direct examination of blood

Materials: Blood collection equipment
            Microscope slides and coverslips

1. Immediately after collecting the blood sample, place a single drop of blood onto the microscope slide and add a coverslip.
2. Examine the slide using the 10X microscope objective. Watch for localized areas of movement among the red blood cells, which may indicate the presence of parasites.

Microfilariae can also be found in large animals. *Setaria* is a long, white nematode found in the serous membranes of cattle and horses. Adults are most often seen during abdominal surgery, and microfilariae are found during differential WBC count.

THIN BLOOD SMEAR

The thin blood smear is prepared and stained in exactly the same way as a blood smear for a differential WBC count (Procedure 6-16). When doing a differential WBC count on an animal, the veterinary technician should note any parasitic organisms seen. Occasionally, microfilariae may be found. Because of their size, microfilariae are usually found along the feathered edge. Because differentiation of the microfilariae is not possible in a thin blood smear, other procedures must be performed for identification. Trypanosomes, protozoans, and rickettsiae may also be found among or within cells. As with the direct smear procedure, a small blood sample is used and mild parasitic infections may be missed.

THICK BLOOD SMEAR

A thick blood smear examines a slightly greater volume of blood than does a thin blood smear. Again, microfilariae may be seen, but they cannot be easily differentiated using this method (Procedure 6-17).

PROCEDURE 6-16.   Thin blood smear

Materials: Microscope slides
Blood smear stain (Diff-Quik, Wright's, Giemsa)

1. Place a glass slide on a flat surface. Add a drop of blood near one end of the slide.
2. Place the end of a second slide near the middle of the first slide at a 45-degree angle (Figure 6-58). Holding the second slide at that angle, gently pull the slide backward, into the drop of blood. Allow the blood to spread across the edge of the second slide.
3. Holding the first slide firmly, smoothly push the second slide across and off the end of the first slide. This should form a thin smear on the first slide, with a nice feathered edge.
4. Allow the slide to air dry, and stain. After staining, the slide can be examined using the oil-immersion objective.

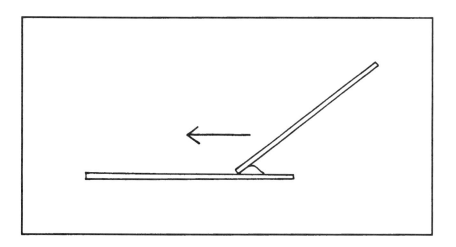

FIGURE 6-58. As viewed from the side, the correct angle and direction of movement for preparation of a thin blood smear.

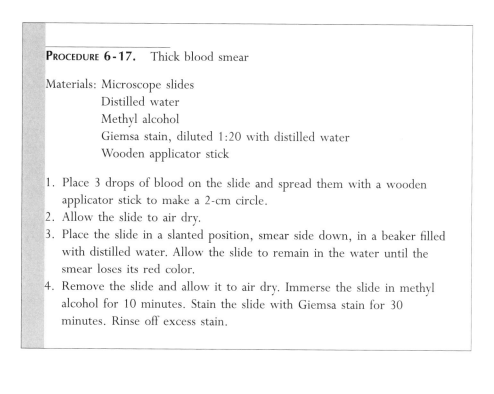

PROCEDURE 6-17. Thick blood smear

Materials: Microscope slides
Distilled water
Methyl alcohol
Giemsa stain, diluted 1:20 with distilled water
Wooden applicator stick

1. Place 3 drops of blood on the slide and spread them with a wooden applicator stick to make a 2-cm circle.
2. Allow the slide to air dry.
3. Place the slide in a slanted position, smear side down, in a beaker filled with distilled water. Allow the slide to remain in the water until the smear loses its red color.
4. Remove the slide and allow it to air dry. Immerse the slide in methyl alcohol for 10 minutes. Stain the slide with Giemsa stain for 30 minutes. Rinse off excess stain.

BUFFY COAT METHOD

The buffy coat method is a concentration technique used on a small volume of blood. When blood is placed in a microhematocrit tube and centrifuged, for determining the packed cell volume (PCV), it separates into three layers: plasma, WBC layer (buffy coat) and RBC layer (Figure 6-59). Microfilariae can be found on the surface of the buffy coat layer (Figure 6-60). This technique is quick and can be done in conjunction with a PCV and total protein evaluation. However, differentiation of microfilariae is not possible (Procedure 6-18).

The following concentration techniques can be used for differentiating *Dirofilaria immitis* from *Dipetalonema reconditum.*

MODIFIED KNOTT'S TECHNIQUE

The modified Knott's technique is a simple procedure that allows differentiation of microfilariae (Procedure 6-19). This technique concentrates, "relaxes," and stains microfilariae, while lysing red blood cells to make the microfilariae more visible.

Figures 6-61 and 6-62 and Table 6-1 for differentiating microfilariae show the characteristics that can be used when identifying microfilariae. Always examine as many microfilariae as possible, as mixed infections can occur. The most accurate method for differentiation is measuring the length and width of the body. However, with some practice, general characteristics of the microfilariae can be used for identification if a means of measuring microfilariae is not available.

FILTER TECHNIQUE

Filter techniques are the most common method used in veterinary practices for detection of microfilariae in the blood. Several diagnostic kits are available for

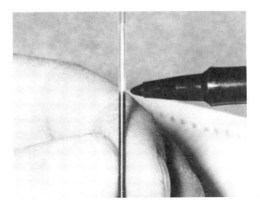

FIGURE 6-59. Buffy coat in a hematocrit tube.

PROCEDURE 6-18.   Buffy coat method

Materials: Microhematocrit tubes and sealer
Microhematocrit centrifuge
Small file or glass cutter
Microscope slides and coverslips
Saline
Methylene blue stain (diluted 1:1000 with distilled water)

1. Fill the microhematocrit tube with blood, and seal.
2. Centrifuge for 3 minutes.
3. Read the PCV, if desired, then find the buffy coat layer between the red blood cells and plasma (Figure 6-59).
4. Using a file, scratch the tube at the level of the buffy coat. Carefully snap the tube and save the part of the tube containing the buffy coat and plasma. Gently tap the tube onto a slide, ejecting the buffy coat layer with a small amount of plasma. Save the rest of the plasma for a total protein determination, if desired.
5. Add a drop of saline and a drop of stain to the buffy coat. Apply a coverslip and examine for microfilariae (Figure 6-60).

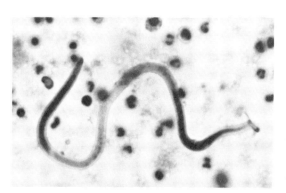

FIGURE 6-60.   Microfilaria in a buffy coat smear from canine blood.

this procedure, including Di-Fil Test Kit (EVSCO, Buena, NJ) and Filarassay*F Heartworm Diagnostic Test Kit (Pitman-Moore, Mundelein, IL). These kits come complete with filters, lysing solution, stain, and directions for use.

Procedure 6-19   Modified Knott's technique

Materials: 15-ml centrifuge tube
         Centrifuge
         2% formalin (2 ml of 40% formalin diluted with 98 ml of
         distilled water)
         Methylene blue stain (diluted 1:1000 with distilled water)
         Pasteur pipettes and bulbs

1. Mix 1 ml of blood with 9 ml of 2% formalin in a centrifuge tube.
2. Centrifuge the tube at 1300 to 1500 rpm for 5 minutes.
3. Pour off the liquid supernatant, leaving the sediment at the bottom of the tube.
4. Add 2 to 3 drops of stain to the sediment. Using a pipette, mix the sediment with the stain.
5. Place a drop of this mixture onto a glass slide. Apply a coverslip and examine for microfilariae using the 10X objective.

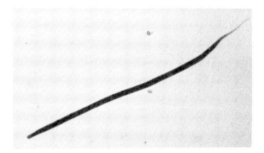

Figure 6-61.   Microfilaria of *Dirofilaria immitis,* found using the modified Knott's technique. Note the straight tail and tapering cranial end of the microfilaria.

Most kits require 1 ml of whole blood to test for heartworms. The blood is mixed with 9 parts of lysing solution and passed through a filter. The filter is rinsed, removed, and placed on a slide. A drop of stain is added and a coverslip applied, then the filter is microscopically examined for microfilariae (Figure 6-63). Differentiation of microfilariae is possible but difficult using the filter technique. If microfilariae are present, it is best to perform other diagnostic procedures for identification purposes.

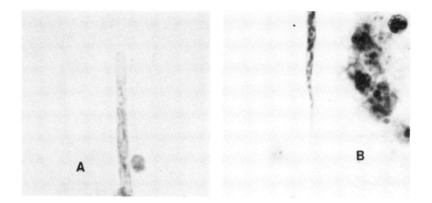

FIGURE **6-62.** Cranial **(A)** and caudal **(B)** ends of a *Dipetalonema reconditum* microfilaria.

TABLE **6-1.** Differentiation of microfilariae using the modified Knott's technique

	DIROFILARIA IMMITIS	*DIPETALONEMA RECONDITUM*
Body length	>310 μ	<290 μ
Mid-body width	>6 μ	<6 μ
Head	Tapered	Blunt
Tail	Straight	Hooked

ENZYME-LINKED IMMUNOSORBENT ASSAY

Enzyme-linked immunosorbent assay (ELISA) kits do not directly detect microfilariae but instead test the host's response to the parasites. These types of tests can be used for differentiating *Dirofilaria immitis* from *Dipetalonema,* and they can be used to identify an occult heartworm infection. An *occult infection* is one in which only one sex of adult worms is present, and no microfilariae are produced. Also, when an animal is treated with drugs that kill circulating microfilariae or render the adults unable to reproduce, again there are no circulating microfilariae.

Some ELISA kits detect the host's antibody response to the adult heartworms, while others detect the host's antibody response to the microfilariae (see Chapter 9). The most reliable ELISA kits test for the presence of

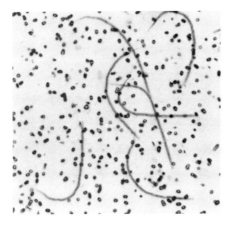

FIGURE 6-63.   Microfilariae in canine blood on a filter. The small, irregular structures are the holes in the filter paper, and the small circular objects are RBCs.

Dirofilaria antigen in the host's blood. Dirochek (Synbiotics, San Diego, CA) and Cite Heartworm Test Kit (IDEXX, Portland, ME) are two such diagnostic kits. These two procedures rely on a color change to indicate a positive response. As with any procedure, ELISA immunodiagnostic tests should be performed exactly according to the manufacturer's directions and in a clean environment to avoid contamination.

MISCELLANEOUS TESTS

Another type of heartworm diagnostic test kit (Heartworm Identification Test: ImmunoVet, Tampa, FL) works on the same principle as the Knott's and filter techniques, except the microfilariae remain alive. This test relies on the movement of the microfilariae, which can be unreliable at times.

Other tests use special stains to bring out certain characteristics of the microfilariae. These procedures are too cumbersome to be useful in private practice and are usually done in diagnostic laboratories.

RECOMMENDED READING

Bowman: *Georgi's parasitology for veterinarians,* ed 6, Philadelphia, 1995, WB Saunders.

Colville: *Diagnostic parasitology for veterinary technicians,* St Louis, 1991, Mosby.

Sloss, et al: *Veterinary clinical parasitology,* ed 6, Ames, Iowa, 1994, Iowa State University Press.

Eᴠᴛᴇʀɴᴀʟ Pᴀʀᴀsɪᴛᴇs

C.M. Hendrix

If a parasite resides on the surface of its host, it is termed an *ectoparasite*. The vast majority of ectoparasites are either insects (fleas, lice, flies) or arachnids (ticks, mites). A few nematodes have immature stages that occur in the skin or subcutaneous tissues.

This chapter is designed to aid the veterinary technician in diagnosis of ectoparasitism in dogs, cats, cattle, sheep, goats, horses, and swine. To diagnose an ectoparasitic infestation, the technician must be able to collect the ectoparasite and then identify the organism involved. This chapter explains procedures commonly used to collect ectoparasites from the host and describes those parasites so that a correct diagnosis can be made.

While a complete review of the biology of ectoparasites is beyond the scope of this chapter, a brief review of the life cycles of the major groups of ectoparasites is included.

COLLECTION OF SAMPLES

Sᴋɪɴ sᴄʀᴀᴘɪɴɢs

Skin scraping is one of the most common diagnostic procedures used in evaluating animals with dermatologic problems. Equipment needed includes an electric clipper with #40 blade, a scalpel or spatula, mineral oil in a small dropper bottle, and a compound microscope. Typical lesions or sites likely to harbor the particular parasite should be scraped (e.g., ear margins for *Sarcoptes scabiei* variety *canis*).

The scraping is performed with a #10 scalpel blade, used with or without a handle. A 165-mm stainless-steel spatula (Sargent-Welsh Scientific, Detroit, MI) is preferred by some clinicians. The scalpel blade should be held between the thumb and forefinger (Figure 7-1). Before the skin is scraped, the blade is dipped in a drop of mineral oil on the slide, or a drop of mineral oil may be placed on the skin.

During the scraping process, the blade must be held perpendicular to the skin. Holding it at another angle may result in an accidental incision. The average area scraped should be about 6 to 8 cm^2.

The depth of the scraping varies with the typical location of the parasite in question. When scraping for mites that live in tunnels (e.g., *Sarcoptes* species) or in hair follicles (e.g., *Demodex* species), the skin should be scraped until a small amount of capillary blood oozes from the scraped area. Clipping the area with a #40 blade before scraping enables better visualization of the lesion and removes excess hair that impedes proper scraping and interferes with collection of epidermal debris. For surface-dwelling mites (e.g., *Cheyletiella* or *Chorioptes* species), the skin is scraped superficially to collect loose scales and crusts. Clipping before scraping is not necessary when infestation with surface dwellers is suspected.

All scraped debris on the forward surface of the blade is then spread in a drop of mineral oil on the slide. A glass coverslip is placed on the material, and the slide is ready for microscopic examination using the 4X (scanning) objective. The slide should be examined systematically in rows so the entire area under the coverslip is evaluated. Low light intensity and high contrast increase visualization of translucent mites and eggs. If necessary, the slide may be evaluated using the 10X (low-power) objective.

Demonstration of the characteristic mite or egg is frequently diagnostic for most diseases. In certain circumstances, however, more than just identification

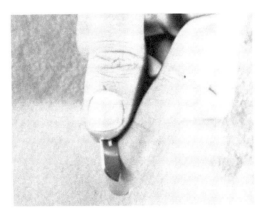

FIGURE 7-1. A scalpel blade can be safely held between the thumb and forefinger for skin scrapings.

of the parasite is necessary. For example, determination of live : dead ratios and observation of immature larval and nymphal stages of demodectic mites are important in determining a patient's prognosis. A decrease in the number of live mites and eggs during treatment is an excellent prognostic indicator.

CELLOPHANE TAPE PREPARATION

When attempting to demonstrate lice or mites that live primarily on the surface of the skin (e.g., *Cheyletiella*), a cellophane tape preparation may be used instead of a skin scraping. Clear cellophane tape (Scotch Transparent Tape, 3M, Minneapolis, MN) is applied to the skin to pick up epidermal debris. A ribbon of mineral oil is placed on a glass slide, and the adhesive surface of the tape is then placed on the mineral oil. Additional mineral oil and a coverslip may be placed on the tape to prevent the tape from wrinkling, but this is not necessary. The slide is then examined microscopically for parasites.

PARASITE IDENTIFICATION

When arthropods or helminths cannot be grossly identified, the intact specimen should be collected in a sealed container containing 10% formalin or ethyl alcohol and submitted to an arthropodologist / parasitologist for identification. A complete history should accompany the specimen. Do not fragment or squash the specimen, as this could distort morphologic features necessary for proper identification. Forensic identification of parasites is quite difficult.

TERMINOLOGY

Ectoparasites usually live on or in, or feed upon skin surfaces. Ectoparasites *infest* the skin or external surfaces of animals and produce an *infestation* on the animal. This is in contrast to internal parasites, or endoparasites, which *infect* the internal organs of domestic animals and produce an *infection* within that animal. In diagnostic parasitology, these terms should always be used in the proper context.

Life cycle describes the development of a parasite through its various life stages. Every parasite's life cycle has a definitive host and may have one or more intermediate hosts. The *definitive host* harbors the adult, sexual, or mature stages of a parasite. The *intermediate host* harbors the juvenile, asexual, or immature stages of a parasite.

Many of the ectoparasites in this chapter belong to the phylum Arthropoda or, more simply, "arthropods." All adult arthropods have jointed legs. Later on in this chapter, we will discuss ectoparasites that reside within the skin; these ectoparasites are not arthropods but rather belong to the phylum Nematoda, or more simply, the "roundworms."

CLASSIFICATION SYSTEM

In beginning biology, students must learn the classification scheme perfected by Linnaeus, an early biologist. Every living organism on this planet can be classified using the following classification scheme: kingdom, phylum, class, order, family, genus, and species. Students often remember this scheme with this simple mnemonic device, "King Philip came over for good spaghetti," where each letter in the sentence corresponds to the first letter in the Linnaean classification scheme.

Each classification scheme works like this. Every living thing is known by a scientific name that is made up of two components: the *genus* and the *specific epithet*. The dog's scientific name is *Canis familiaris,* where *Canis* is the *genus* and *familiaris* is the specific epithet or *species*. Similar species are grouped together into the same *genus*. Similar genera (plural of genus) are grouped together into the same *family*. Similar families are grouped together into the same *order*. Similar orders are grouped together into the same *class*. Similar classes are grouped together into the same *phylum*. Similar phyla are grouped together into the same *kingdom*. Therefore, the dog's classification scheme is as follows:

Kingdom: Animalia
> Phylum: Chordata
>> Subphylum: Vertebrata
>>> Class: Mammalia
>>>> Order: Carnivora
>>>>> Family: Canidae
>>>>>> Genus: *Canis*
>>>>>>> Species: *familiaris*

Every living thing on earth has its own distinct classification scheme.

PHYLUM: ARTHROPODA

Class: insecta

The first part of this chapter discusses the orders belonging to the class Insecta and the families belonging to the class Acarina and how these ectoparasites are relevant to veterinary practice. The following orders of Insecta are described:

- Order: Hymenoptera (ants, bees, wasps)
- Order: Hemiptera (true bugs)
- Order: Mallophaga (chewing or biting lice)
- Order: Anoplura (sucking lice)
- Order: Diptera (two-winged flies)
- Order: Siphonaptera (fleas)

Order: hymenoptera (ants, bees, wasps)

Fire ants are indigenous to the southeastern United States and can bite and sting almost any domestic animal. "Downer cows" and young newborn animals are particularly at risk to the perils of fire ants.

Bees, wasps, and hornets can sting domestic animals, particularly curious dogs and cats. When stung, the animals may show an extremely swollen nose or face.

Africanized honey bees ("killer bees") have now crossed the Mexico/United States border. Almost any domestic animal (and people) could stumble on a hive of these bees, angering the inhabitants. Death often results from thousands of killer bee stings.

Diagnosis.   If you suspect that ants, bees, wasps, or hornets may be causing problems, collect the intact hymenopteran in a sealed container containing 10% formalin or ethyl alcohol and submit it to an entomologist for identification.

Order: hemiptera (true bugs)

Two groups of hemipterans are of veterinary importance: Reduviid bugs (kissing bugs) and bed bugs. Reduviid bugs (kissing bugs) are periodic parasites, making frequent visits to the host to obtain a blood meal. Kissing bugs serve as intermediate hosts for *Trypanosoma cruzi*, a protozoan parasite that can produce a rare disease in people and dogs called Chagas' disease. This disease is also called South American trypanosomiasis and rarely occurs in the United States.

Kissing bugs take blood meals from an infected host and transmit the parasite as they defecate.

Bed bugs are dorsoventrally flattened, wingless hemipterans that often infest homes. They are periodic parasites, making frequent visits to the host to obtain a blood meal. Although bed bugs are human parasites, they may also be found in rabbit colonies, poultry houses, and pigeon colonies.

DIAGNOSIS. If you suspect that Reduviid bugs or bed bugs may be causing problems, collect the intact hemipteran in 10% formalin or ethyl alcohol and submit it to an entomologist for identification.

ORDERS: MALLOPHAGA (CHEWING OR BITING LICE) AND ANOPLURA (SUCKING LICE)

Lice are some of the most prolific ectoparasites of domestic animals. There are two orders of lice: the Mallophaga (chewing or biting lice) and Anoplura (sucking lice). Lice are dorsoventrally flattened, wingless insects. They have three body divisions: the head, with its mouthparts and antennae; the thorax, with its three pairs of legs and no wings; and the abdomen, the portion that bears the reproductive organs. These body divisions and their relationship to each other are important in diagnostic veterinary parasitology.

Members of the order Mallophaga or chewing/biting lice are smaller than sucking lice. They are usually yellow and have a large, rounded head. The mouthparts are mandibulate and are adapted for chewing or biting. Characteristically, the head of every chewing louse is wider than the widest portion of the thorax. On the thorax are three pairs of legs, which may be adapted for clasping or for moving rapidly among feathers or hairs. Chewing/biting lice may parasitize birds, dogs, cats, cattle, sheep, goats, and horses. Figure 7-2 shows assorted chewing lice of goats and fowl.

Members of the order Anoplura or sucking lice are larger than chewing lice. These lice are red to gray; their color usually depends on the amount of blood that has been ingested from the host. In contrast to the "big-headed" Mallophagans, Anoplurans have a head that is more narrow than the widest part of the thorax. Their mouthparts are of the piercing type and are adapted for sucking. Their pincer-like claws are adapted for clinging to the host's hairs. Although they are found on many species of domestic animals, sucking lice do not parasitize birds or cats. Figure 7-3 shows assorted sucking lice of sheep, swine, monkeys, and dogs.

Anoplurans and Mallophagans have the same type of life cycle. This life cycle has only three developmental stages.

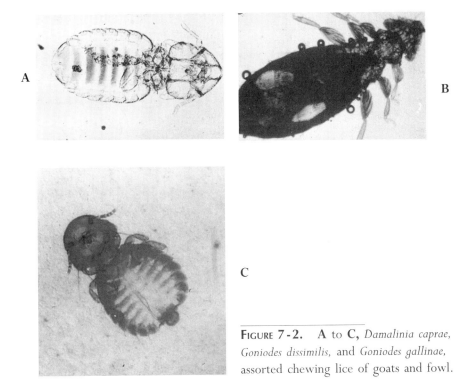

FIGURE 7-2.   **A** to **C,** *Damalinia caprae,*
Goniodes dissimilis, and *Goniodes gallinae,*
assorted chewing lice of goats and fowl.

The *egg stage* is also called a "nit." The nit is tiny, approximately 0.5 to 1.0 mm in length. It is oval, white, and usually found cemented to the hair or feather shaft. Figure 7-4 shows a gravid female sucking louse and an associated nit collected from a dog. Nits hatch about 5 to 14 days after being laid by the adult female louse.

The *nymphal stage* is similar in appearance to the adult. However, it is smaller and lacks functioning reproductive organs and genital openings. There are three nymphal stages, each progressively larger than its predecessor. The nymphal stage lasts from 2 to 3 weeks.

The *adult stage* is similar in appearance to the nymphal stage but larger. It has functional reproductive organs. Male and female lice copulate, the female lays eggs, and the life cycle begins again. It takes 3 to 4 weeks to complete the cycle. Nymphal and adult stages live no longer than 7 days if removed from the host. Eggs hatch within 2 to 3 weeks during warm weather but seldom hatch off the host.

Lice are usually transmitted by direct contact, but all life stages may be transmitted by fomites (inanimate objects such as blankets, brushes, and other

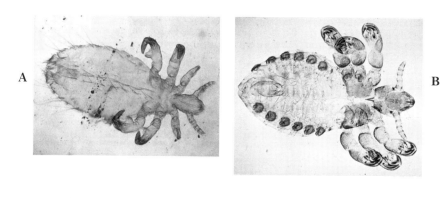

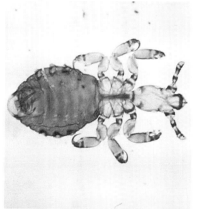

FIGURE 7-3. **A** to **C,** *Solenopotes capillatus, Haematopinus suis, Pedicinus obtusus,* and *Linognathus setosus,* assorted sucking lice of sheep, swine, monkeys, and dogs.

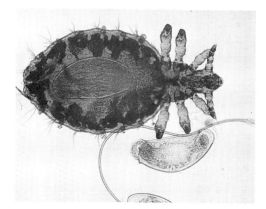

FIGURE 7-4. *Linognathus setosus,* a gravid female sucking louse and associated nit collected from a dog.

grooming equipment). Lice are easily transmitted among young, old, and malnourished animals. Veterinarians are often at a quandary to understand why certain animals in a flock or herd are heavily infested, while others have only a few lice.

Infestation by lice (whether Mallophagan or Anopluran) is referred to as *pediculosis*. Sucking lice can ingest blood to such a degree that they produce severe anemia; fatalities can occur, especially in young animals. The packed cell volume can drop as much as 10% to 20%. There may be as many as a million lice on severely infested animals. Infested animals become more susceptible to other diseases and parasites and may succumb to stresses not ordinarily pathologic to uninfested animals. When animals are poorly fed and kept in overcrowded conditions, they often become severely infested with lice and quickly become anemic and unthrifty.

DIAGNOSIS.   Careful examination of the haircoat or feathers of infested animals easily reveals lice and their accompanying nits. Hair clippings also serve as a good source for lice. Infestation of animals with a thick haircoat may be easily overlooked. A hand-held magnifying lens or Optivisor (binocular headband magnifier) may aid observation of adult/nymphal lice crawling through or clinging to hair or feathers, or tiny nits cemented to individual hairs.

Any lice and/or their nits observed may be collected with thumb forceps and placed in a drop of mineral oil on a glass microscope slide. A coverslip should be placed over the specimen and the slide examined using the 4X or 10X objective.

Identification of louse to genus and specific epithet is quite difficult. It is better to identify the specimen as being Anopluran (sucking) vs. Mallophagan (chewing or biting). Remember that the head of every chewing louse is wider than the widest portion of its thorax, while the sucking louse has a head that is more narrow than the widest part of the thorax.

ORDER: DIPTERA (TWO-WINGED FLIES)

This is a very large, complex order of insects. As adults, most members have one pair of wings (two wings); hence the ordinal name, Diptera (*Di-*, meaning two, and *-ptera*, meaning wing). Its members vary greatly in size, food source preference, and developmental stage that parasitizes the animal or produces lesions.

Dipterans produce two very contrasting pathologic scenarios. As adults, they may intermittently feed on vertebrate blood, saliva, tears, and mucus. As larvae, they may develop in the subcutaneous tissues. Dipterans that make frequent visits to the vertebrate host to intermittently feed on blood are referred to as *periodic parasites*. When dipteran larvae develop in the tissue or organs of vertebrate hosts, they produce a condition known as *myiasis*.

As periodic parasites, blood-feeding dipterans can be classified as to which sex feeds on vertebrate blood and as to food preference. In certain dipteran groups only the females feed on vertebrate blood; these female flies require vertebrate blood for laying their eggs. In this group are the biting gnats (*Simulium, Lutzomyia, Culicoides*), the mosquitoes (*Anopheles, Aedes, Culex*), the horse flies (*Tabanus*), and the deer flies (*Chrysops*).

In the second group of blood-feeding dipterans, both male and female flies require a vertebrate blood meal. These species include the stable fly *Stomoxys calcitrans,* the horn fly *Haematobia irritans,* and the sheep ked *Melophagus ovinus.*

Musca autumnalis (face fly) feeds on mucus, tears, and saliva of large animals, particularly cattle.

In the first dipteran group of periodic parasites, only the female dipterans feed on vertebrate blood. The tiniest members of this group are the biting gnats, *Simulium, Lutzomyia,* and *Culicoides.*

SIMULIUM (BLACK FLY)

Members of the genus *Simulium* are commonly called "black flies," although their coloration may vary from gray to yellow. They are also called "buffalo gnats" because their thorax is humped over the head, giving the appearance of a buffalo's hump (Figure 7-5). These are tiny flies, ranging from 1 to 6 mm in length. They have broad, unspotted wings with very prominent veins along the cranial margins of the wings. These tiny flies have serrated, scissor-like mouthparts that inflict very painful bites.

Because the females lay their eggs in well-aerated water, these flies are often found in the vicinity of swiftly flowing streams. They move in great swarms, inflicting painful bites and sucking the host's blood. These flies may keep cattle from grazing or cause them to stampede. The animal's ears, neck, head, and abdomen are favorite feeding sites. These flies also feed on poultry and can serve as an intermediate host for the protozoan parasite *Leukocytozoon.*

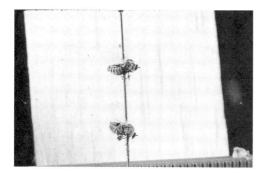

Figure 7-5. *Simulium* species, black flies. These tiny flies range in size from 1 to 6 mm in length.

DIAGNOSIS.   Black flies are most often collected in the field and are not found on animals presented to a veterinary clinic. They are identified by their small size, humped back, and strong venation in the cranial region of the wings. Identification of black flies is probably best left to an entomologist.

LUTZOMYIA *(NEW WORLD SAND FLY)*

Members of the genus *Lutzomyia* are commonly referred to as New World sand flies. They are tiny, moth-like flies, rarely over 5 mm in length. A key feature for their identification is that their body is covered with fine hairs. They tend to be active only at night and are weak fliers. These tiny flies transmit the protozoan parasite *Leishmania*.

DIAGNOSIS.   Like black flies, sand flies are most often collected in the field and are not found on animals presented to a veterinary clinic. They are identified by their small size and hairy wings and body. Identification of sand flies is probably best left to an entomologist.

CULICOIDES *(NO-SEE-UM)*

Culicoides gnats are also commonly known as "no-see-ums," "punkies," or even "sand flies." They are tiny gnats (1 to 3 mm in length) and quite similar in appearance to black flies. They inflict painful bites and suck the blood of their hosts. They are active at dusk and dawn, especially during the winter months. These gnats tend to feed on the dorsal or ventral areas of the host; the feeding site depends on the species of biting gnat.

Horses often become allergic to the bites of *Culicoides* gnats, scratching and rubbing bitten areas, causing alopecia, excoriations, and thickening of the skin. This condition has several names, including "Queensland itch," "sweat itch," and "sweet itch." Because it is often seen during the warmer months of the year, it is also referred to as "summer dermatitis." These flies also serve as the intermediate host for *Onchocerca cervicalis*, a nematode whose microfilariae are found in the skin of horses. These flies also transmit the blue-tongue virus of sheep.

DIAGNOSIS.   In contrast to the clear, heavily veined wings of black flies, the wings of *Culicoides* species are mottled. Identification of *Culicoides* species is probably best left to an entomologist.

ANOPHELES, AEDES, CULEX *(MOSQUITO)*

Although they are tiny, fragile dipterans, mosquitoes are some of the most voracious blood feeders on domestic animals and people (Figure 7-6).

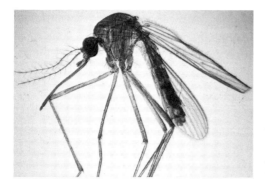

FIGURE 7-6. *Culex* species, one genus among several genera of mosquitoes.

Mosquitoes can plague livestock and in swarms have been known to keep cattle from grazing or to cause them to stampede. The feeding of large numbers of swarming mosquitoes can cause significant anemia in domestic animals. Large numbers of mosquitoes can be produced from eggs laid in relatively small bodies of water. Although they are known for spreading malaria (*Plasmodium* species), yellow fever, and elephantiasis among people, mosquitoes are probably best known in veterinary medicine as the intermediate host for the canine heartworm, *Dirofilaria immitis.*

DIAGNOSIS. Adult mosquitoes have wings and body parts covered by tiny, leaf-shaped scales. Identification of adult and larval *Anopheles, Aedes,* and *Culex* species is probably best left to an entomologist.

CHRYSOPS, TABANUS (DEER FLY, HORSE FLY)

Chrysops species (deer flies) and *Tabanus* species (horse flies) are large (up to 3.5 cm in length), heavy-bodied, robust dipterans with powerful wings. These flies also have very large eyes. Horse flies and deer flies are the largest flies in the dipteran group in which only the females feed on vertebrate blood. Figure 7-7 shows *Tabanus,* the largest blood-feeding dipteran. Horse flies are larger than deer flies. Deer flies have a dark band passing from the cranial to the caudal margin of the wings.

Adult flies lay eggs in the vicinity of open water. Larval stages of these flies are found in aquatic to semi-aquatic environments, often buried deep in mud at the bottom of lakes and ponds. Adults are seen in summer and are very fond of sunlight. Female flies feed in the vicinity of open water and have reciprocating, scissor-like mouthparts; they use these sharp, blade-like mouthparts to lacerate tissues and lap up the oozing vertebrate blood. These flies feed primarily on

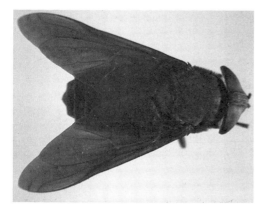

FIGURE 7-7. *Tabanus* species, the largest blood-feeding dipteran. This tabanid is approximately 2.5 cm in length.

large animals, such as cattle and horses. Preferred feeding sites include the underside of the abdomen around the navel, the legs, or the neck and withers.

Horse flies and deer flies feed a number of times at multiple feeding sites before they stop feeding. When disturbed by the animal's swatting tail or by the panniculus reflex (skin twitching), the flies leave the host, but the blood continues to ooze from the open wound. These fly bites are very painful. Affected cattle and horses become restless. These flies may act as mechanical transmitters of anthrax, anaplasmosis, and the virus of equine infectious anemia.

DIAGNOSIS. These flies are most easily recognized by their large, robust size and lacerating, scissor-like mouthparts. Species identification of intact adult and larval horse and deer flies is probably best left to an entomologist.

In the second group of blood-feeding dipterans, both male and female adult flies require a vertebrate blood meal. These species include the stable fly *Stomoxys calcitrans,* the horn fly *Haematobia irritans,* and the wingless ked *Melophagus ovinus.*

STOMOXYS CALCITRANS (STABLE FLY)

The stable fly, *Stomoxys calcitrans,* is often called the biting housefly. It is approximately the size of *Musca domestica,* the housefly. Rather than a sponging type of mouthpart, the stable fly has a bayonet-like proboscis that protrudes forward from the head (Figure 7-8). These flies are found worldwide. In the United States, they are found in the central and southeastern states, where cattle are raised. Both male and female flies are avid blood feeders, feeding on any domestic animal. They usually attack the legs and ventral abdomen and may also bite the ears. These flies also feed on the tips of the ears of dogs with pointed ears, especially the German Shepherd.

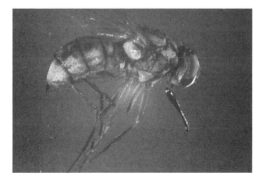

Figure 7-8. *Stomoxys calcitrans,* the stable fly. Note the bayonet-like proboscis that protrudes forward from the head. The stable fly is approximatley the same size as a housefly.

This fly feeds on both horses and cattle, with horses the preferred host. The fly usually lands on the host with its head pointed upward. It is a sedentary fly, not moving on the host. The flies inflict painful bites that puncture the skin and bleed freely. Stable flies stay on the host for short periods, during which they obtain the blood meals. This is an outdoor fly; however, in the late fall and during rainy weather, it may enter barns.

Stable flies are mechanical vectors of anthrax in cattle and equine infectious anemia. They are the intermediate host for *Habronema muscae,* a nematode found in the stomach of horses. When large numbers of stable flies attack dairy cattle, milk production can fall. Beef cattle may refuse to graze in the daytime when they are attacked by large numbers of flies; as a result, these cattle do not gain the usual amount of weight.

Diagnosis. The veterinary technician can easily identify the stable fly by its size (approximately the same size as a housefly) and its bayonet-like proboscis that protrudes forward from the head.

Haematobia irritans (Horn Fly)

Haematobia irritans is often called the horn fly. This dark-colored fly is approximately 3 to 6 mm in length, half the size of *Stomoxys calcitrans,* the biting housefly. Like the stable fly, the horn fly has a bayonet-like proboscis that protrudes forward from the head. These flies are found almost exclusively on cattle throughout North America.

When the air temperature is below 70° F, horn flies cluster around the base of the horns; hence the name horn fly. In warmer climates, thousands of flies often cluster on the host's shoulders, backs, and side; these areas are least disturbed by tail switching. On hot, sunny days, horn flies congregate on the ventral abdomen.

Adult horn flies spend most of their life on cattle and leave the host only to deposit their eggs in fresh cow manure. Using their tiny bayonet mouthparts, they feed frequently, sucking blood and other fluids, and cause considerable irritation. Females flies are more aggressive than males. Harassment by the flies and loss of blood often reduces weight gains and milk production in cattle. Horn flies probably cause greater losses in cattle in the United States than any other blood-sucking fly. Adult horn flies also cause focal midline dermatitis on the ventral abdomen of horses. These flies also serve as the intermediate host for *Stephanofilaria stilesi,* a filarial parasite that produces ventral, plaque-like lesions on the ventral abdomen of cattle.

DIAGNOSIS.   The veterinary technician can easily identify the horn fly by its dark color and its size (approximately half the size of a stable fly). Like the stable fly, the horn fly's bayonet-like proboscis protrudes forward from the head.

MELOPHAGUS OVINUS *(SHEEP KED)*

Melophagus ovinus is often called the sheep ked. Members of the order Diptera usually have one pair of wings (two wings). Keds are an exception to that rule; they are *wingless dipterans.* Keds are hairy, leathery, and 4 to 7 mm in length. The head is short and broad. The thorax is brown and the abdomen broad and grayish-brown. The legs are strong and armed with stout claws (Figure 7-9). Some say that keds have a "louse-like" appearance.

Keds are permanent ectoparasites of sheep and goats. Their pupal stages are often found attached to the wool or hair of the host. Keds are avid blood feeders. Heavy infestations can reduce the condition of the host considerably and even cause anemia. Their bites cause pruritus over much of the host's body; infested sheep often bite, scratch, and rub themselves, damaging the wool. Ked feces often stain the wool and do not wash out readily. Keds are most

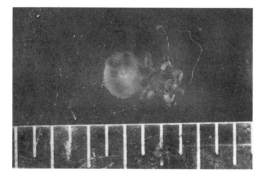

FIGURE 7-9.   *Melophagus ovinus,* the sheep ked. Keds are hairy, leathery, and 4 to 7 mm in length. The head is short and broad. The thorax is brown, and the abdomen broad and grayish-brown. The legs are strong and armed with stout claws.

numerous in the cold temperatures of the fall and winter months. Their numbers decline as temperatures warm in the spring and summer months.

DIAGNOSIS.   Close inspection of the wool and underlying skin reveals infestation by these wingless dipterans, with their unique appearance.

MUSCA AUTUMNALIS (FACE FLY)

The final periodic parasite among the dipteran flies is one that is not a blood feeder but instead feeds on mucus, tears, and saliva of large animals, particularly cattle. Face flies, *Musca autumnalis,* are so named because they gather around the eyes and muzzle of livestock, particularly cattle. They may also be found on the withers, neck, brisket, and sides. Face flies feed mostly on saliva, tears, and mucus. They are usually not considered blood feeders because their mouthparts are not piercing or bayonet-like. Instead, their mouthparts are adapted for sponging up saliva, tears, and mucus (Figure 7-10). They follow blood-feeding flies, disturb them during their feeding process, and then lap up the blood and body fluids that accumulate on the host's skin. Face flies are found on animals outdoors; they usually do not follow animals into barns.

Face flies produce considerable annoyance to the host. The irritation around the host's eyes stimulates the flow of tears, which attracts even more flies. This harassment ultimately interferes with the host's productivity. Face flies may be involved in the transmission of *Moraxella bovis,* a bacterium associated with infectious keratoconjunctivitis or pinkeye in cattle.

DIAGNOSIS.   Face flies are morphologically similar to the housefly, *Musca domestica.* These two species can be differentiated through minor differences in

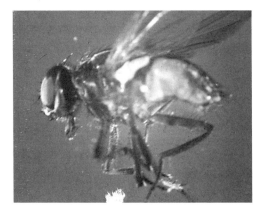

FIGURE 7-10.   *Musca autumnalis,* the face fly. Its mouthparts are adapted for sponging up saliva, tears, and mucus.

eye position and color of the abdomen. The veterinary technician should probably not attempt to speciate this fly; speciation requires the skills of a trained entomologist. Remember this rule of thumb: if the fly is found around the face of cattle or horses, it is probably a face fly.

MYIASIS-PRODUCING FLIES

With regard to their roles as ectoparasites, larval dipterans may develop in the subcutaneous tissues of many domestic animals. When dipteran larvae develop in the tissue or organs of vertebrate hosts, they produce a condition known as *myiasis.* Based on the degree of host dependence, there are two types of myiases. In *facultative myiasis,* the fly larvae are usually *free-living.* Under certain circumstances, these "normally free-living" larvae can adapt to a parasitic dependence on a host. In *obligatory myiasis,* the fly larvae are *completely parasitic,* that is, they are completely dependent on the host to develop through the life cycle. In other words, without the host, the obligatory parasites die.

FACULTATIVE MYIASIS-PRODUCING FLIES

MUSCA DOMESTICA (HOUSE FLY), CALLIPHORA, PHAENICIA, LUCILIA, PHORMIA (BLOW FLY, BOTTLE FLY), AND SARCOPHAGA (FLESH FLY). Dipteran larvae that produce facultative myiasis include the housefly *Musca domestica,* the blow flies or bottle flies *Calliphora, Phaenicia, Lucilia,* and *Phormia* species, and the flesh fly *Sarcophaga.* Larval stages of these flies are usually associated with skin wounds contaminated with bacteria or with a matted haircoat contaminated with feces.

Under normal conditions, adult flies of these genera lay their eggs in decaying animal carcasses or in feces. In facultative myiasis, the adult flies are attracted to an animal's moist wound, skin lesion, or soiled haircoat. These sites provide the adult fly with a moist medium on which it feeds. As adult female flies feed in these sites, they lay eggs. These eggs hatch, producing larvae (maggots) that move independently about the wound surface, ingesting dead cells, exudate, secretions, and debris, but not live tissue. This condition is known as "fly strike" or "strike." These larvae irritate, injure, and kill successive layers of skin and produce exudates.

Maggots can tunnel through the thinned epidermis into the subcutis. This process produces tissue cavities in the skin that measure up to several centimeters in diameter. Unless the process is halted by appropriate therapy, the infested animal may die from shock, intoxication, histolysis, or infection. A peculiar, distinct, pungent odor permeates the infested tissue and the affected animal. Advanced lesions may contain thousands of maggots. It is important to remember that as adults, these flies can be pestiferous flies in a veterinary clinical setting. These flies are "vomit drop" feeders and fly from feces to food, spreading bacteria on their feet and their disgorged stomach contents.

DIAGNOSIS. A tentative diagnosis of maggot infestation in any domestic animal can easily be made by a veterinary technician, as maggots can be observed in an existing wound or among the soiled, matted haircoat. When facultative myiasis has been diagnosed, the veterinarian must rule out the possibility of obligatory myiasis caused by *Cochliomyia hominivorax*.

OBLIGATORY MYIASIS-PRODUCING FLIES

COCHLIOMYIA HOMINIVORAX (PRIMARY SCREWWORM). In obligatory myiasis, the dipteran larvae lead a parasitic existence. Only one fly in North America, *Cochliomyia hominivorax,* is a primary invader of fresh, uncontaminated skin wounds of domestic animals. These larvae must not be confused with the larvae of the facultative myiasis-producing flies described previously. *Cochliomyia hominivorax* is often referred to as the "screwworm fly." Economically it is the most important fly that attacks livestock in the southwestern and southern United States.

Adult female flies are attracted to fresh skin wounds on any warm-blooded animal, where they lay batches of 15 to 500 eggs in a shingle-like pattern at the edge of wounds. Several thousand eggs are laid by the female during her lifetime. The eggs are cream-colored and elongated. They hatch within 24 hours. Larvae enter the wound, where they feed for 4 to 7 days before developing into third-stage (fully grown) larvae. They can be as long as 1.5 cm in length. At this stage they resemble a wood screw; hence the name "screwworm." When fully grown, the larvae drop to the ground and pupate for about a week, after which the adult flies emerge. The adult male and female fly breed only once during their lifetime, a fact that is used to control these flies biologically.

DIAGNOSIS. Adult flies are shiny and greenish-blue, with a reddish orange head and eyes, and are 8 to 15 mm long. Larvae are often identified by their wood screw shape and by the deeply pigmented tracheal tubes on the dorsal aspect of the caudal ends. Because of the obligatory nature of the screwworm with regard to breeding in the fresh wounds of any warm-blooded animal, the veterinarian must report any screwworm infestations to both state and federal authorities. *Cochliomyia hominivorax* has been eradicated from the United States but occasionally surreptitiously enters the country in imported animals.

Cuterebra (wolf, warble)

Larvae of the genus *Cuterebra* infest the skin of rabbits, squirrels, mice, rats, chipmunks, and occasionally dogs and cats. There is a large discrepancy concerning the descriptions of larval *Cuterebra*. Most of the specimens recovered in a veterinary setting are second- or third-stage larvae. Second-stage larvae are grub-like, 5 to 10 mm long, and cream to grayish white. They are often sparsely covered with tiny, black, tooth-like spines. Third-stage larvae are large, robust, coal-black, and heavily spined. Larval stages are usually found in swollen, cyst-like subcutaneous sites, with a fistula or pore communicating to the outside environment. The larval *Cuterebra* breathes through this pore.

Eggs are laid by adult flies near the entrance to rodent burrows. Pets usually contract this parasite while investigating or hunting rodent prey. As a result, the most commonly affected sites in dogs and cats are the subcutaneous tissues of the neck and face. Most cases occur during the late summer and early fall. Among the myiasis-producing flies, this dipteran larva is known for its aberrant or erratic migrations, having been found in a variety of extracutaneous sites, the cranial vault, the eye, and the pharyngeal regions. Clinical signs vary with the site of infection/infestation. Larvae are often discovered in subcutaneous sites during physical examination. They are usually removed surgically by enlarging the breathing pore and removing the larva with thumb forceps. Great care must be taken not to crush the larva during extraction, as anaphylaxis might result.

Diagnosis. Cuterebrosis is diagnosed by observing the characteristic swollen, cyst-like subcutaneous lesion, with a fistula or central pore communicating to the outside environment. Second- or third-stage larvae are usually removed from this lesion.

Hypoderma (ox warble, cattle grub)

Two larval stages of *Hypoderma* flies infect cattle: *Hypoderma lineatum* and *H. bovis*. *Hypoderma lineatum* is found in southern United States; both species are found in northern United States and in Canada. The adult flies are heavy and resemble honey bees; the adults are often called "heel flies."

The life cycle is almost a year in length. Adult flies are bothersome to cattle because they approach cattle to lay eggs. Animals often become apprehensive and disturbed and attempt to escape the fly by running away, an action that is called "gadding." The eggs are about 1 mm long and attached to hairs on the legs of cattle. *Hypoderma lineatum* deposits a row of six or more eggs on an individual hair shaft, while *H. bovis* lays its eggs singly. The larvae hatch in about 4 days and crawl down the hair shaft to the skin, through which they penetrate. They wander through the subcutaneous connective tissue in the leg, migrating to the esophagus (*H. lineatum*) or the region of the spinal canal and epidural fat (*H. bovis*), until they reach the subcutaneous tissues of the back. Here the larvae create breathing holes in the skin of the dorsum, through which they later exit and fall to the ground to pupate. The adult flies emerge from the pupae.

Diagnosis. Adults are bee-like and covered with yellow to orange hairs. Mature larvae are 25 to 30 mm long, cream to dark brown, and covered with small spines. Lesions consist of large, cyst-like swellings on the back, with a central breathing pore. As with *Cuterebra* species, great care must be taken not to crush the larva during extraction, as anaphylaxis might result.

Order: siphonaptera (fleas)

Of all the ectoparasites discussed thus far, the flea is perhaps the most economically important insect to the veterinarian; treating flea infestations can be a veterinary practice builder. Because of the extreme popularity of dogs and cats and the prolific nature of the flea (hence its ability to return after populations are exterminated on the animal and in the animal's environment), special attention should be paid to detecting the various life cycle stages of fleas both on the pet and in the pet's environment.

Fleas are siphonapterans, small (4 to 5 mm in length), laterally compressed, wingless insects with powerful hind legs that are used for jumping. Figure 7-11 shows the life stages of *Ctenocephalides felis,* the cat flea. Adult fleas have piercing-sucking (siphon-like) mouthparts that are used to suck the blood

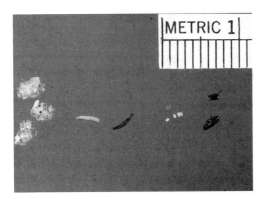

Figure 7-11. Life stages of *Ctenocephalides felis,* the cat flea. *Left* to *right,* pupae, larvae, eggs, adult male and female.

of their host. Figure 7-12 shows the morphologic details of the adult female and male *Ctenocephalides felis,* the cat flea. Over 2000 species of fleas have been identified throughout the world. Adult fleas are always parasitic, feeding on both mammals and birds. Dogs and cats are host to comparatively few species of fleas.

Ctenocephalides felis, the cat flea, is the most common flea found on dogs and cats. The dog flea, *Ctenocephalides canis,* is uncommon and occurs far less frequently on dogs than does the cat flea.

Echidnophaga gallinacea is also known as the stick-tight flea of poultry (Figure 7-13). A common flea of chickens and guinea fowl, it also feeds on dogs and cats. This flea has unique feeding habits. The female flea inserts its mouthparts into the skin of the host and remains attached at that site. On first

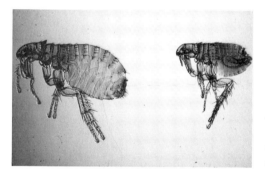

Figure 7-12.   Morphologic details of the adult female and male *Ctenocephalides felis,* the cat flea.

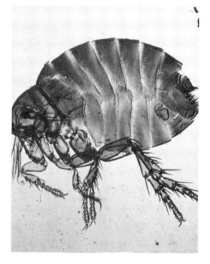

Figure 7-13.   Adult *Echidnophaga gallinacea,* the stick tight flea of poultry.

observation, one might think that these specimens resemble attached ticks; however, they are indeed fleas.

Fleas are not commonly found on horses or ruminants. In barns where feral cats abound and where excessive bedding is used, fleas have been found on calves in very large numbers and can produce significant anemia. *Pulex irritans,* the human flea, has been recovered from dogs and cats, especially in the southeastern United States.

While the adult flea is the stage most commonly encountered, the veterinary technician may also be presented with flea eggs, larval fleas, or flea droppings from the pet's environment. Flea eggs and larvae are commonly found in the owner's bedclothes, the pet's bedding, travel carriers, dog houses, or clinic cages. Flea eggs resemble tiny pearls; they are non-sticky, 0.5 mm long, white, oval, and rounded at both ends (Figure 7-14). Flea larvae resemble tiny fly maggots. They are 2 to 5 mm long, white (after feeding they become brown) and sparsely covered with hairs (Figure 7-15). Flea larvae spin a sticky, silky cocoon that often becomes covered with environmental debris. This is the pupal stage (Figure 7-16).

DIAGNOSIS. Because adult fleas spend most of their time on the host, flea infestation is usually obvious. However, in animals with flea-allergy dermatitis, fleas may be so few on the pet as to make diagnosis of flea infestation quite difficult.

Definitive diagnosis of flea infestation requires demonstration of the adult fleas and/or their droppings (flea dirt, flea feces, flea frass) (Figure 7-17). Adult fleas defecate large quantities of partially digested blood, commonly called "flea dirt." These feces are reddish-black and can appear as fine pepper-like specks, comma-shaped columns, or long coils.

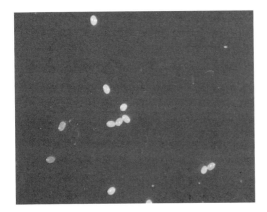

FIGURE 7-14. Eggs of *Ctenocephalides felis,* the cat flea.

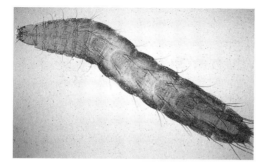

FIGURE 7-15. Larva of *Ctenocephalides felis,* the cat flea.

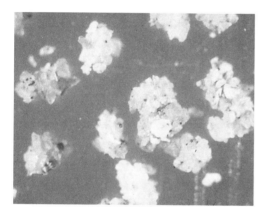

FIGURE 7-16. Sand-covered pupae of *Ctenocephalides felis,* the cat flea.

Adult fleas are usually encountered on the animal but may also be collected in the pet's environment. When recovered from the pet, the larger fleas with an orange to light brown abdomen are females; the smaller, darker specimens are males.

One can easily collect fleas by spraying the pet with an insecticide. In a few minutes, dead fleas drop off the animals. Alternatively, fleas may be collected using a fine-toothed flea comb, available at any veterinary supply store or pet store.

"Flea dirt" can be used to diagnose current or recent flea infestation. To collect a sample of flea dirt, just comb the pet with a flea comb and place the collected samples on a white paper towel moistened with water. Rubbing the flea dirt with a fingertip causes the flea dirt to dissolve, producing a characteristic blood-red or rust-red color.

CONTROL. Flea control is important because fleas not only cause discomfort and irritation to the pet, but they also serve as intermediate hosts to certain

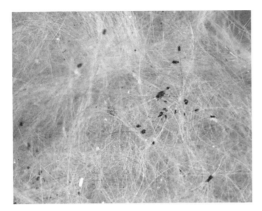

Figure 7-17. Flea dirt, flea feces, or flea frass of *Ctenocephalides felis*, the cat flea.

helminth parasites. Fleas serve as intermediate host for *Dipylidium caninum,* the double-pored tapeworm of dogs and cats, and as intermediate host for *Dipetalonema reconditum,* a filarial parasite that resides in the subcutaneous tissues of dogs. Some types of fleas can also transmit disease, such as bubonic plague and endemic typhus, to people.

CLASS: ACARINA (MITES AND TICKS)

Mites and ticks of veterinary importance are members of the class Acarina.

MITES OF VETERINARY IMPORTANCE

The first group of parasitic mites can be classified together as "sarcoptiform" mites. Sarcoptiform mites have several key characteristics or features in common. These mites can produce severe dermatologic problems in a variety of domestic animals. This dermatitis is usually accompanied by a severe pruritus. Sarcoptiform mites are small, barely visible to the naked eye, and approximately the size of a grain of salt. Their bodies have a round to oval shape. Sarcoptiform mites have legs with pedicels or stalks at the tip. The pedicels may be long or short. If the pedicel is long, it may be straight (unjointed) or jointed. At the tip of each pedicel, there may be a tiny sucker. Veterinarians and veterinary technicians should use the description of the pedicel (long or short, jointed or unjointed) to identify these sarcoptiform mites.

Sarcoptiform mites can be divided into two basic families: Sarcoptidae, which burrow or tunnel within the epidermis, and Psoroptidae, which reside on the surface of the skin or within the external ear canal. The Sarcoptidae includes *Sarcoptes, Notoedres,* and *Cnemidocoptes* species, while the Psoroptidae includes *Psoroptes, Chorioptes,* and *Otodectes* species.

FAMILY: SARCOPTIDAE

Sarcoptic mites burrow or tunnel within the epidermis of the infested definitive host. The entire 4-stage life cycle is spent on the host. Male and female mites breed on the skin surface. Female mites penetrate the keratinized layers of the skin and burrow or tunnel through the epidermis. Over a 10- to 15-day period, the female deposits 40 to 50 eggs within the tunnel. Following egg deposition, the female dies. Larvae emerge from the eggs in 3 to 10 days and exit the tunnel to wander on the skin surface. These larvae molt to the nymphal stage within minute pockets in the epidermis. Nymphs become sexually active adults in 12 to 17 days and the life cycle begins again.

SARCOPTES SCABIEI (SCABIES MITES). The disease caused by *Sarcoptes scabiei* is called scabies or sarcoptic acariasis. This condition is considered extremely pruritic.

Certain varieties of mites infest specific hosts. For example, *Sarcoptes scabiei* variety *canis* infests only dogs, and *Sarcoptes scabiei* variety *suis* infests only pigs. Almost every domestic species has its own distinct variety of this mite.

Scabies in dogs is caused by *Sarcoptes scabiei* variety *canis,* which produces an erythematous, papular rash. Scaling, crusting, and excoriation are common. The ears, lateral elbows, and ventral abdomen are most likely to harbor mites. The host's entire body, however, may be infested. These mites are spread by direct contact and can affect all dogs in a household or kennel. Scabies is extremely contagious. Also, the dog owner can become infested with this mite, but the infestation in people is self-limiting. The mites burrow into human skin, producing a papule-like lesion, but they do not establish a full-blown infestation in people. This mite is considered to cause a *zoonosis,* that is, a disease that can be transmitted from animals to people. Some dogs may be asymptomatic carriers of this mite. *Sarcoptes scabiei* variety *felis,* which causes scabies in cats, is an extremely rare mite.

Among large animals, pigs are most commonly affected by scabies. Lesions caused by *Sarcoptes scabiei* variety *suis* include small, red papules, alopecia, and crusts, most commonly on the trunk and ears. Scabies in cattle (*Sarcoptes scabiei* variety *bovis*) is rare. The main infested areas are the head, neck, and shoulders. Scabies in horses (*Sarcoptes scabiei* variety *equi*) is even more rare. The main infested area is the neck. *Sarcoptes scabiei* variety *ovis* does not infest the fleece of sheep and goats; rather, the face is the main area affected.

DIAGNOSIS. Areas with an erythematous, papular rash and crust should be scraped, especially the areas most associated with sarcoptic infestation (ears, lateral elbows, and ventral abdomen of dogs). Repeated scrapings may be necessary to detect mites. Adult sarcoptic mites are oval and 200 to 400 μ in diameter, with eight legs. The key morphologic feature used to identify this species is *the long, unjointed pedicel with sucker on the end of some of the legs* (Figure 7-18). The anus is located on the caudal end of the body. The eggs of *Sarcoptes* mites are oval (Figure 7-19).

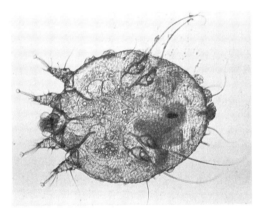

FIGURE 7-18. Adult *Sarcoptes scabiei* mite. Note the long, unjointed pedicels (stalks), with suckers on the ends.

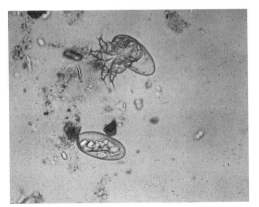

FIGURE 7-19. Oval eggs of *Sarcoptes scabiei.* Note the emergence of a six-legged larval mite.

NOTOEDRES CATI (FELINE SCABIES MITE). *Notoedres cati* infests mainly cats; but on occasion it can parasitize rabbits. This sarcoptiform mite is found chiefly on the ears, back of the neck, face, feet, and in extreme cases on the entire body. The life cycle is like that of *Sarcoptes scabiei,* with the mite burrowing or tunneling in the superficial layers of the epidermis. The characteristic lesion of notoedric acariasis is a yellowing crust in the region of the ears, face, or neck.

DIAGNOSIS. Notoedric mites are easier to demonstrate in cats than sarcoptic mites in dogs. Likely infestation sites should be scraped. Like *Sarcoptes* species, *Notoedres* mites have *a long, unjointed pedicel with sucker on the end of some of the legs.* Adult notoedric mites are similar to sarcoptic mites but are smaller, with a dorsal anus. The eggs of notoedric mites are oval.

CNEMIDOCOPTES PILAE (SCALEY LEG MITE OF BUDGERIGARS). *Cnemidocoptes pilae* causes scaley leg in budgerigars or parakeets. This mite tunnels in the superficial layers of the epidermis of the pads and shanks of the feet. In severe cases the beak and cere may also be affected. The mite characteristically produces a yellow to gray-white mass that resembles a honeycomb. This condition can be quite disfiguring to the parakeet. The parasites pierce the skin underlying the scales, causing an inflammation with exudate that hardens on the surface and displaces the scales superficially. This process causes the thickened, scaly nature of the skin. A related species, *Cnemidocoptes mutans,* produces scaly leg in chickens and turkeys.

DIAGNOSIS. Infested sites should be scraped. Great care should be taken in handling infested birds, as parakeets are quite fragile. The eight-legged, globular mites are about 500 µ in diameter. Adult female mites have very short legs and no suckers on the end of their legs (Figure 7-20). Adult males have longer legs and *a long, unjointed pedicel with suckers on the end of some of the legs.*

FAMILY: PSOROPTIDAE

Members of the family Psoroptidae reside on the surface of the skin or within the external ear canal. The entire five-stage life cycle (egg, larva, protonymph, deutonymph or pubescent female, adult ovigerous female) is spent on the host. Adult male and female mites breed on the skin surface. The female produces 14 to 24 elliptic, opaque, shiny white eggs that hatch within 1 to 3 days. The six-legged nymphs are small, oval, soft, and grayish-brown. The eight-legged nymphs are slightly larger than larvae. Larval and nymphal stages may last 7 to 10 days. The life cycle is completed in 10 to 18 days. Under favorable

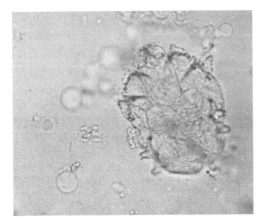

Figure 7-20. Adult female *Cnemidocoptes pilae* mite. The adult male has longer legs and a long, unjointed pedicel with suckers on the end of some of the legs.

conditions, psoroptic mites can live off the host for 2 to 3 weeks or longer. Under optimum conditions, mite eggs may remain viable for 2 to 4 weeks.

***Psoroptes cuniculi* (ear canker mite of rabbits).** *Psoroptes cuniculi* occurs most commonly in the external ear canal of rabbits but has also been found in horses, goats, and sheep. These mites live on the surface of the skin and feed on the rabbit host by puncturing the epidermis to obtain tissue fluids. Within the external ear canal of the infested host are the characteristic dried crusts of coagulated serum. The rabbit's ears appear to be packed with dried corn flakes. Affected animals shake their head and scratch their ears. Lesions sometimes occur on the head and legs. Severely infested animals may become debilitated. Loss of equilibrium may occur, with head tilt.

Diagnosis. The mites within the crusty debris inside the ear can be easily isolated. The brownish-white female is large, up to 750 µ long. The mites exhibit characteristic *long, jointed pedicels with suckers on the ends of some of the legs* (Figures 7-21 and 7-22). The anus is in a terminal slit.

***Psoroptes* species (scab mite of large animals).** *Psoroptes ovis, P. bovis,* and *P. equi* are the scab mites of large animals, residing on sheep, cattle, and horses, respectively. These mites are very host specific and reside within the thick-haired or long-wooled areas of the animal. They are surface dwellers and feed by puncturing the epidermis to feed on lymphatic fluid. Serum exudes through the puncture site. After the serum coagulates and forms a crust, wool is lost. The feeding site is extremely pruritic and the animal excoriates itself, producing further wool loss. The mites then migrate to adjacent undamaged

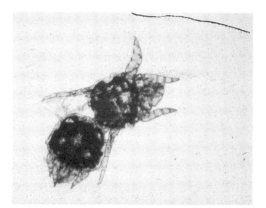

FIGURE 7-21. Adult *Psoroptes cuniculi* mites.

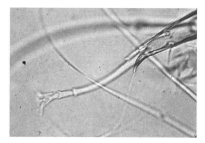

FIGURE 7-22. Detail of the long, jointed pedicel on the leg of *Psoroptes cuniculi.*

skin. As the mites proliferate, tags of wool are pulled out and the fleece becomes matted. Finally, patches of skin are exposed and the skin becomes parchment-like, thickened, and cracked. The skin may bleed easily. Infested sheep constantly rub against fences, posts, farm equipment, and anything else that might serve as a scratching post. The disease is spread by direct contact or infested premises.

Psoroptes bovis in cattle produces lesions on the withers, neck, and rump. These consist of papules, crusts, and wrinkled, thickened skin. *Psoroptes equi* in horses is rare and affects the base of the mane and the tail.

Because of the intense pruritus and the highly contagious nature of the infestation, the occurrence of *Psoroptes* species in large animals should be reported to state and federal authorities, as well as the United States Department of Agriculture.

DIAGNOSIS. These mites are host specific. Adults are up to 600 μ in length. Psoroptic mites exhibit characteristic *long, jointed pedicels with suckers on the ends of some of the legs.*

CHORIOPTES SPECIES (FOOT AND TAIL MITE, ITCHY LEG MITE). *Chorioptes equi, C. bovis, C. caprae,* and *C. ovis* are the foot and tail mites of large animals, residing on horses, cattle, goats, and sheep, respectively. These mites are found on the skin surface on the distal (lower) part of the hind legs but may spread to the flank and shoulder area. On cattle, they are frequently found in the tail region, especially in the area of the escutcheon. These mites do not spread rapidly or extensively. They puncture the skin, causing serum to exude. Thin crusts of coagulated serum form on the skin surface. The skin eventually wrinkles and thickens although pruritus is not severe.

Infested horses stamp, bite, and kick, especially at night. Mites typically infest the pasterns, especially those of the hind legs.

DIAGNOSIS. The characteristic mites can be identified from skin scrapings of infested areas. Chorioptic mites have *short, unjointed pedicels, with suckers on the ends of some of the legs* (Figure 7-23). The female mites are about 400 μ long.

OTODECTES CYNOTIS (EAR MITE). Ear mites, *Otodectes cynotis,* are a common cause of otitis externa in dogs and cats. Although they occur primarily in the external ear canal, ear mites may be found on any area of the body. A common infestation site is the tail and head region. As dogs and cats curl up to sleep, their head (and ears) are often in close proximity to the base of the tail. These mites are spread by direct contact and are highly transmissible both among and between the canine and feline species.

Ear mites are found within the external ear canal, where they feed on epidermal debris and produce intense irritation. Infection is usually bilateral. The host responds to the mite infestation by shaking its head and scratching its

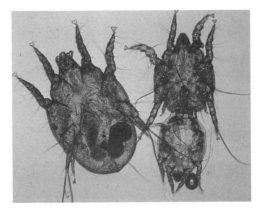

FIGURE 7-23. Female and male *Chorioptes* species. Note this mite's short, unjointed pedicels.

ears. Severe infestations may cause otitis media, with head tilt, circling, and convulsions. Auricular hematomas may develop.

DIAGNOSIS. Mites are usually identified by using an otoscope; through an otoscope the mites appear as white, motile objects. The brown exudate collected by swabbing the ear may be placed in mineral oil on a glass slide and the mites observed with a low-power microscopic objective. These mites are fairly large, approximately 400 µ; they can also be easily seen with a magnifying glass or even the unaided eye. The mites exhibit characteristic *short, unjointed pedicels, with suckers on the ends of some of the legs* (Figures 7-24 and 7-25). The anus is terminal.

MISCELLANEOUS MITES
This group of parasitic mites can be grouped together because they are not sarcoptiform mites. They can, however, produce severe dermatologic problems in a variety of domestic animals. These mites lack pedicels or stalks on their legs that are so important in identifying sarcoptiform mites.

DEMODEX SPECIES. Mites of the genus *Demodex* reside in the hair follicles and sebaceous glands of people and most domestic animals. In many species, they are considered normal, nonpathogenic fauna of the skin. These mites are host specific and are not transmissible from one host species to another. The clinical disease, caused by an increased number of these mites, is called *demodicosis.*

Demodex mites resemble "eight-legged alligators." They are elongated mites with short, stubby legs. Adult and nymphal stages have eight legs, while the larvae have six. Adult *Demodex* mites are approximately 250 µ long (Figure 7-26). The eggs are spindle-shaped or tapered at each end (Figure 7-27).

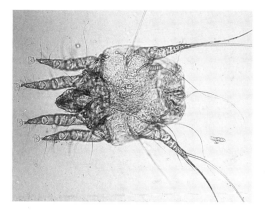

FIGURE 7-24. Adult female *Otodectes cynotis* mite.

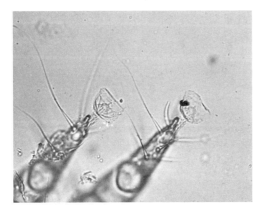

Figure 7-25. Detail of the leg of *Otodectes,* with a short, unjointed pedicel.

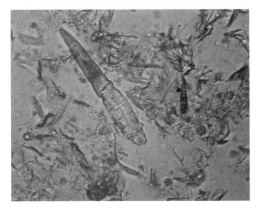

Figure 7-26. Adult *Demodex canis* mite.

There are five stages in the life cycle of *Demodex* species: egg, larva, protonymph, deutonymph, and adult. The developmental periods of these various life cycle stages are not well known.

Of all the domestic animals infested with *Demodex* species, the dog is the most commonly and most seriously infested. Small numbers of these mites are considered part of the normal skin flora of all dogs. In dogs with immunodeficiencies, however, these mites proliferate and cause skin disease.

Demodicosis occurs in two forms in dogs: localized demodicosis and generalized demodicosis. The predominant clinical sign of the localized form is patchy alopecia, especially of the muzzle, face, and forelimbs. It is thought that the mites are acquired during intimate contact when the puppy nurses the dam. As a result of that close contact, localized demodicosis often develops in the region of the face. Generalized demodicosis is characterized by diffuse alopecia, erythema, and secondary bacterial contamination over the entire body surface

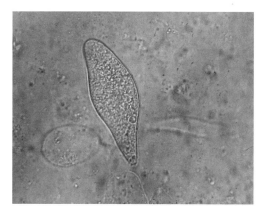

Figure 7-27. Egg of *Demodex canis.* Eggs are spindle-shaped or tapered at each end.

of the dog. An inherited defect in the dog's immune system is thought to be an important factor in development of generalized demodicosis.

Cats are infested by two species of demodectic mites: *Demodex cati* and an unnamed species. *Demodex cati* is an elongated mite, quite similar to *D. canis.* The unnamed species has a broad, blunted abdomen, as compared with the elongated one of *D. cati.* The presence of either species on the skin of cats is rare. In localized feline demodicosis, there are patchy areas of alopecia, erythema, and occasionally crusting on the head (especially around the eyes), ears, and neck. In generalized feline demodicosis, the alopecia, erythema, and crusting usually involve the entire body. Demodicosis has also been associated with ceruminous otitis externa.

Demodectic mites reside in the hair follicles of other species of domestic animals but rarely produce clinical disease. Cattle and goats are most commonly infested but then only rarely.

In cattle, *Demodex bovis* causes large nodules (abscesses) on the shoulders, trunk, and lateral aspects of the neck. In goats, *Demodex caprae* occurs in small papular or nodular lesions on the shoulders, trunk, and lateral aspect of the neck. In sheep, *Demodex ovis* rarely causes pustules and crusting around the coronet, nose, ear tips, and periorbital areas. In pigs, *Demodex phylloides* rarely produces pustules and nodules on the face, abdomen, and ventral neck. In horses, *Demodex equi* occurs around the face and eyes and rarely produces clinical disease.

DIAGNOSIS. Skin areas with altered pigmentation, obstructed hair follicles, erythema, or alopecia should always be scraped. In localized demodicosis, the areas most commonly affected are the forelegs, perioral region, and periorbital regions. In generalized demodicosis, the entire body may be affected; however, the face and feet usually are the most severely involved. In dogs, areas of apparently normal skin should also be scraped to determine if the disease is generalized. The areas should be clipped and a fold of skin gently squeezed to express any mites from the hair follicles. Scraping should be continued until capillary blood oozing is observed because these mites live deep in the hair follicles and sebaceous glands (Figure 7-28).

Nodular lesions in large animals should be incised with a scalpel and the caseous material within smeared on a slide with mineral oil, covered with a coverslip, and examined microscopically for mites.

The mites on the slide should be counted and the live : dead ratio determined. Note the presence of any larval or nymphal stages or eggs. During therapy for *Demodex* species, a decrease in the number of eggs and live mites is a good prognostic indicator.

***CHEYLETIELLA* SPECIES (WALKING DANDRUFF).** Mites of the genus *Cheyletiella* are surface-dwelling (non-burrowing), residing in the keratin layer of the skin and in the haircoat of the definitive host, which may be a dog, cat, or rabbit. These mites ingest keratin debris and tissue fluids. *Cheyletiella* mites are sometimes referred to as "walking dandruff" because the mites resemble large, mobile flakes of dandruff. Cheylettid mites have distinct key morphologic features. They are large (386 by 266 μ) and visible to the naked eye. Using the compound microscope, one can easily see their most characteristic key morphologic feature, their enormous hook-like accessory mouthparts (palpi). These palpi assist the mite in attaching to the host as it feeds on tissue fluids. The mite also has "comb-like" structures at the tip of each leg. Members of the

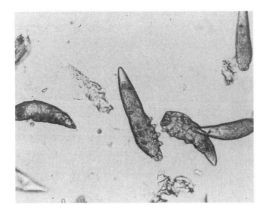

FIGURE 7-28. A deep skin scraping produces numerous mites of *Demodex canis.*

genus are also known for their characteristic body shape resembling a shield, a bell pepper, an oak acorn, or a western horse saddle when viewed from above (Figure 7-29). Eggs are 235 to 245 μ long and 115 to 135 μ wide (smaller than louse nits) and supported by cocoon-like structures bound to the host's hair shaft by strands of fibers. Two or three eggs may be bound together on one hair shaft.

DIAGNOSIS. The key feature of *Cheyletiella* infestation is often the moving white "dandruff" flakes along the dorsal midline and head of the host. A hand-held magnifying lens or Optivisor (binocular headband magnifier) are often used to view questionable flakes or hairs; these are perhaps the quickest methods of diagnosing cheyletiellosis. A fine-toothed flea comb may be used to collect mites; combing dandruff-like debris onto black paper often facilitates visualization of these highly mobile mites. Using clear cellophane tape to entrap mites collected from the haircoat often simplifies viewing with the compound microscope.

***TROMBICULA* SPECIES (CHIGGER).** The chigger (*Trombicula* species) is yellow to red, six-legged, and 200 to 400 μ in diameter. The larval stage is the only developmental stage that parasitizes people, domestic animals, and wild animals. The larvae are most common in the late summer and early fall and are transmitted by direct contact with the ground or with foliage in fields or heavy underbrush. Nymphal and adult chiggers are nonparasitic and are free living in nature.

Chigger larvae *do not burrow into the skin* as commonly believed nor do they feed primarily on host blood. Their food consists of the serous components of tissues. Chiggers attach firmly to the host and inject a digestive fluid that

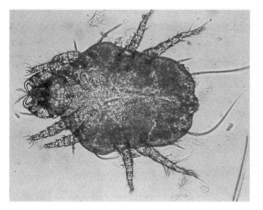

FIGURE 7-29. Adult *Cheyletiella* mite.

liquefies host cells. The host's skin becomes hardened and a tube called a stylostome forms at the chigger's attachment site. Chiggers suck up the liquefied host tissues. When the mite has finished feeding, it loosens its grip and falls to the ground. The injected digestive fluid causes the attachment site to itch intensely. Cutaneous lesions tend to be restricted to areas of the body that come in contact with the ground, such as the limbs, interdigital areas, and ventrum, as well as the head and ears.

The most common chigger mite affecting animals and people is *Trombicula alfreddugesi* (the North American chigger). Lesions consist of an erythematous, often pruritic papular rash on the ventrum, face, feet, and legs.

Diagnosis. Chigger infestation (trombiculosis) is diagnosed by an orange, crusting dermatosis, a history of exposure (roaming the outdoors), and identification or the typical six-legged larvae in skin scrapings or on collection from the host. The larvae remain attached to the skin only for several hours. Consequently, trombiculosis may be difficult to diagnose, as the pruritus persists after the larvae have dropped.

Pneumonyssoides (pneumonyssus) caninum (nasal mite of dogs). *Pneumonyssoides (Pneumonyssus) caninum* is a rare mite that lives in the nasal passages and associated sinuses of dogs. Nasal mites are generally considered to be nonpathogenic; however, reddening of the nasal mucosa, sneezing, head shaking and rubbing the nose often accompany infestation. Fainting, labored breathing, asthma-like attacks, and orbital disease have been associated with this mite. Sinusitis caused by these mites may lead to disorders of the central nervous system. Owners may observe these mites exiting the animal's nostrils.

The life cycle is unknown, but it apparently takes place entirely within the host. Adult males, adult females, and larvae have been identified, but no nymphal stages have been observed. Transmission probably occurs via direct contact with an infested animal.

Diagnosis. The mites are oval and pale yellow. They measure 1 to 1.5 mm by 0.6 to 0.9 mm. They have a smooth cuticle, with very few hairs. The larvae have six legs and the adults have eight legs. All legs are located on the cranial half of the body.

Ornithonyssus sylviarum (northern mite of poultry) and *Dermanyssus gallinae* (red mite of poultry). These two mites parasite poultry, but they differ in the sites they tend to infest. *Ornithonyssus sylviarum* is a 1-mm, elongated to oval mite usually found on birds but may also be found in their nests or houses. They feed intermittently on the birds, producing irritation, weight loss, decreased egg production, anemia, and even death. These mites have been known to bite people.

Dermanyssus gallinae is another 1-mm, elongated to oval, whitish, grayish or black mite that feeds on birds. This mite has a distinct red color when it has recently fed on its host's blood. *Dermanyssus gallinae* lays its eggs in cracks and crevices in the walls of poultry houses. Nymphs and adults are periodic parasites, hiding in the crevices of the poultry houses and making frequent visits to the host to feed. Because of their blood feeding activity, they may produce significant anemia and much irritation to the host. Infested birds are listless and egg production may drop. Loss of blood may result in death. These mites also occur in birds' nests in the eaves of houses or in air conditioners. The mites can migrate into homes and infest people.

DIAGNOSIS.   *Ornithonyssus sylviarum* is usually found on the avian host, while *Dermanyssus gallinae* is a periodic parasite, usually found in the host's environment. Specimens should be cleared in lactophenol and the anal plates examined with a compound microscope. The anus of *O. sylviarum* is on the cranial half of the anal plate, while the anus of *D. gallinae* is on the caudal half.

TICKS OF VETERINARY IMPORTANCE

Ticks are small to medium-sized acarines with dorsoventrally compressed, leathery bodies. The tick's head, the *capitulum,* has cutting organs called *chelicerae,* a penetrating, anchor-like sucking organ, the *hypostome,* and four accessory appendages, two *chelicerae* and two *pedipalps,* that act as sensors and supports when the tick fastens to the host's body. The tick's body may be partially or entirely covered by a hard, chitinous plate, the *scutum.* Mouthparts may be concealed under the tick's body or may extend from the cranial border. Most ticks are inornate, that is, they are reddish or mahogany, without markings. Some species are ornate, that is, they have distinctive white patterns on the dark scutum background. Adult ticks are eight-legged, with claws on the ends of the legs.

Ticks are important parasites because of their voracious blood feeding activity. They are also important because they can transmit many parasitic, bacterial, viral, and other diseases, such as borreliosis (Lyme disease), among animals and from animals to people. These pathogenic organisms may be transmitted passively or the tick may serve as an obligatory intermediate host.

Ticks are also important because the salivary secretions of some female ticks are toxic and can produce a syndrome known as "tick paralysis" in people and animals. Tick species commonly associated with tick paralysis are *Dermacentor andersoni* (the Rocky Mountain spotted fever tick), *D. occidentalis* (the Pacific Coast tick), *Ixodes holocyclis* (the paralysis tick of Australia), and *D. variabilis* (the wood tick).

Ticks of veterinary importance can be divided into two families: the Argasid or soft ticks and the Ixodid or hard ticks. Argasid ticks lack a scutum, or hard, chitinous plate. The mouthparts of the adults cannot be seen when viewed from the dorsal aspect. Ixodid ticks have a hard, chitinous scutum that covers all of the male tick's dorsum and about a third or less of the female's dorsum. Depending on the degree of engorgement, male ticks are much smaller than female ticks.

Two species of Argasid ticks are important: *Otobius megnini* (the spinose ear tick) and *Argas persicus* (the fowl tick). There are thirteen economically important tick species in the Ixodid family. These include *Rhipicephalus sanguineus, Ixodes scapularis, Dermacentor* species, and *Amblyomma* species. Of these species, only *R. sanguineus* infests buildings; the remaining ticks attack their hosts outdoors.

Specific identification of ticks is difficult and should be performed by a veterinary parasitologist or a trained arthropodologist. Ticks are usually identified by the shape and length of the capitulum, the shape and color of the body, and the shape and markings on the scutum. Male and unengorged female ticks are easier to identify than engorged females. It is most difficult to determine the species of larval or nymphal ticks. Common species can be identified by their size, shape, color, body markings, host, and location on the host.

There are four major stages in the life cycle of ticks: egg, larva, nymph, and adult. Following engorgement on the host, female ticks drop off the host and seek protected places, such as within cracks and crevices or under leaves and branches to lay their eggs (Figure 7-30). The six-legged larvae, or *seed ticks,* hatch from the eggs and feed on a host (Figure 7-31). The larva molts to the eight-legged nymphal stage, which resembles the adult stage but lacks the functioning reproductive organs of the adult stage. After one or two blood meals, the nymph matures and molts to the adult stage. During the larval, nymphal, and adult stages, ticks may infest one to three or even many different host species. This ability to feed on several hosts during the life cycle plays an important role in the transmission of disease pathogens among hosts. Any infestation of domestic animals by mites or ticks is referred to as *acariasis.*

Most ticks do not tolerate direct sunlight, dryness, or excessive rainfall. They can survive as long as 2 to 3 years without a blood meal, but females

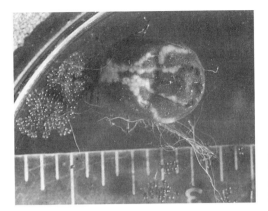

Figure 7-30. Adult female *Dermacentor variabilis* tick laying hundreds of eggs.

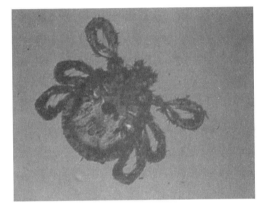

Figure 7-31. Six-legged larval *Rhipicephalus sanguineus.*

require blood before egg fertilization and deposition. Tick activity is restricted during the cold winter months.

Argasid (soft) ticks

***Otobius megnini* (spinose ear tick).** *Otobius megnini,* the spinose ear tick, is an unusual soft tick in that only the larval and nymphal stages are parasitic. The adult stages are not parasitic but are free living, found in the environment of the definitive host, usually in dry, protected places, in cracks and crevices, under logs, and on fence posts. The larval and nymphal stages feed on horses, cattle, sheep, goats, and dogs. These ticks usually are associated with the semi-arid or arid areas of the southwestern United States. With widespread interstate movement of animals, this soft tick may occur throughout North

America. As with most soft ticks, the mouthparts may not be visible when viewed from the dorsal aspect (Figure 7-32). The nymphal stage is widest in the middle, almost violin-shaped. It is covered with tiny, backward-projecting spines; hence the name "spinose." Larvae and nymphs are usually found within the ears of the definitive host; hence the name "ear tick."

Spinose ear ticks are extremely irritating to the definitive host. They often occur in large numbers, deep within the external ear canal. These ticks imbibe large amounts of host blood; however, because they are soft ticks, they do not enlarge with feeding. Large numbers may produce ulceration deep within the ear. The ears become highly sensitive and the animals may shake their head. The pinnae may become excoriated by the animal's shaking and rubbing its head.

DIAGNOSIS. The ticks may be visualized in the ear with an otoscope. Any waxy exudate should be examined for larval and nymphal spinose ear ticks.

ARGAS PERSICUS (FOWL TICK). *Argas persicus,* the fowl tick, is a soft tick of chickens, turkeys, and wild birds. These ticks are periodic parasites, hiding in cracks and crevices during the day and becoming active during the night, when they feed intermittently on the avian host. The adults are 7 mm long and 5 mm wide. In the unengorged state, they are reddish brown. Following engorgement, they are slate blue. These ticks are flat and leathery, and the tegument is covered with tiny bumps. As soft ticks, they lack a scutum. The mouthparts are not visible when the adult tick is viewed from the dorsal aspect.

Heavily infested birds may develop anemia. These ticks are worrisome to birds, particularly at night. Egg production by hens may decrease or cease.

DIAGNOSIS. All stages of this tick may be collected from birds, but they are usually found in cracks, crevices, and contaminated bedding in poultry houses.

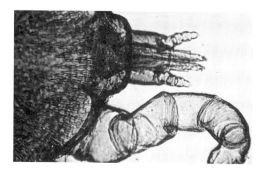

FIGURE 7-32. *Otobius megnini,* the spinose ear tick, is an unusual soft tick in that only the larval and nymphal stages are parasitic. These mouthparts may not be visible when viewed from the dorsal aspect.

IXODID (HARD) TICKS

RHIPICEPHALUS SANGUINEUS (BROWN DOG TICK). *Rhipicephalus sanguineus,* the brown dog tick, is an unusual hard tick in that it may invade both kennel and household environments. This tick is widely distributed throughout North America. It has an inornate, uniformly reddish-brown scutum, and it feeds almost exclusively on dogs. *Rhipicephalus sanguineus* also has a distinguishing morphologic feature. Its basis capitulum has prominent lateral extensions that give this structure a decidedly hexagonal appearance (Figure 7-33). The engorged female is often slate gray in color. In southern climates, the tick is found outdoors, but in northern climates it becomes a serious household pest, breeding indoors.

The bites of this tick can be very irritating to dogs. Severe infestations can cause heavy blood loss. This tick is also an intermediate host for *Babesia canis,* the agent that causes piroplasmosis in dogs.

DIAGNOSIS. This tick can be identified by its inornate brown color and characteristic lateral projections of the basis capitulum. These ticks are unique in that they can be found in indoor or kennel environments.

DERMACENTOR VARIABILIS (AMERICAN DOG TICK, WOOD TICK). *Dermacentor variabilis,* the American dog tick or wood tick, is found primarily in the eastern two thirds of the United States; however, with increased mobility of American households, the tick may occur throughout the country. Unlike *R. sanguineus,* this tick only

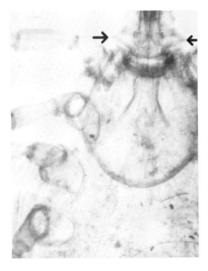

FIGURE 7-33. Lateral expansion of the basis capitulum (base of the head) (*arrows*) of an adult *Rhipicephalus sanguineus.* This key morphologic feature is used to identify this parasite, which can breed in the host's environment.

inhabits grassy, scrub brush areas, especially roadsides and pathways. This three-host tick initially feeds on small mammals and rodents; however, dogs (and people) can serve as hosts for this ubiquitous tick. This tick is a seasonal annoyance to people and domestic animals. It can serve as a vector of Rocky Mountain spotted fever, tularemia, and other diseases, and may also produce tick paralysis in animals and people. This tick has a dark brown, ornate scutum, with white striping. Unfed adults are approximately 6 mm long, while adult engorged females are about 12 mm long and blue-gray in color (Figure 7-34).

DIAGNOSIS. This tick can be identified by its morphologic features. It has a rectangular base of the capitulum and characteristic white markings on the dorsal shield.

AMBLYOMMA AMERICANUM (LONE STAR TICK). *Amblyomma americanum,* the Lone Star tick, gets its common name from a characteristic white spot on the apex of its scutum. The spot is more conspicuous on male ticks than on female ticks. This tick is distributed throughout the southern United States but is also found in the Midwest and on the Atlantic coast.

This three-host tick is found most often in the spring and summer months, parasitizing the head, belly, and flanks of wild and domestic animal hosts. It also feeds on people and is said to have a painful bite. It can produce anemia and has been incriminated as a vector of tularemia and Rocky Mountain spotted fever.

DIAGNOSIS. *Amblyomma americanum* is easily identified by a characteristic white spot on the apex of the scutum.

AMBLYOMMA MACULATUM (GULF COAST TICK). *Amblyomma maculatum,* the Gulf Coast tick, is a three-host tick found in the ears of cattle, horses, sheep, dogs,

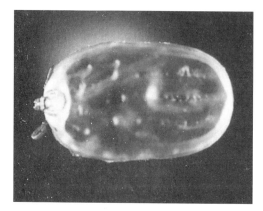

FIGURE 7-34. Adult female *Dermacentor variabilis.* Unfed adults are approximately 6 mm long, while engorged adult females are about 12 mm long and a blue-gray color.

and people. It occurs in areas of high humidity on the Atlantic and Gulf coasts. It produces severe bites and painful swellings and is also associated with tick paralysis. This tick has silvery markings on its scutum. Larval and nymphal stages occur on ground birds throughout the year. The number of adult ticks on cattle decreases during the winter and spring and increases in the summer and fall. When the ear canals of cattle and horses are infested, the pinna may droop and become deformed.

DIAGNOSIS. *Amblyomma maculatum* is easily identified by the silvery markings on its scutum (Figure 7-35).

BOOPHILUS ANNULATUS (TEXAS CATTLE FEVER TICK). *Boophilus annulatus* is often called the Texas cattle fever tick or the North American tick. This one-host tick has historical significance in that it is the first arthropod shown to serve as an intermediate host for a protozoan parasite, *Babesia bigemina* of cattle, a milestone in veterinary parasitology. This tick has been completely eradicated from the United States; however, any *Boophilus* infestation should be reported to the proper regulatory agencies. The tick should be identified by a specialist and control methods applied. *Boophilus annulatus* frequently enters the United States from Mexico.

The engorged female is 10 to 12 mm in length and the male 3 to 4 mm. The mouthparts are very short and there are no festoons on the caudal aspect of the abdomen.

Because this is a one-host tick, larvae, nymphs, and adult ticks may be found on the same animal. They do not have to leave the host to complete the life cycle. Animals with heavy infestations are restless and irritated. In an attempt to rid themselves of ticks, they rub, lick, bite, and scratch themselves.

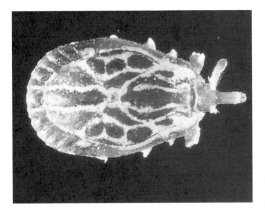

FIGURE 7-35. Ornate adult male *Amblyomma maculatum.*

Irritated areas may become raw and secondarily infected. Heavily infested cattle may become anemic.

Diagnosis. Suspect ticks from an enzootic area or from animals originating from the Texas-Mexico border should be submitted to a laboratory recommended by regulatory agencies.

PHYLUM NEMATODA (ROUNDWORMS)

CLASS SECERNENTEA

The next part of this chapter discusses the superfamilies belonging to the class Secernentea and how these skin-dwelling parasites are relevant to veterinary practice. The following superfamilies are described:

SUPERFAMILY: RHABDITOIDEA

PELODERA STRONGYLOIDES *(FREE-LIVING SAPROPHYTIC NEMATODE)*

Pelodera strongyloides is a free-living saprophytic nematode that normally lives in moist soil. These are facultative parasites. They are normally free-living; however, under certain circumstances, they can invade mammalian skin and develop to a parasitic existence. Male and female adult *P. strongyloides* nematodes are found in soil mixed with moist organic debris, such as straw. The females produce eggs that hatch into first-stage larvae. These larvae invade the superficial layers of damaged or scarified skin, producing mild dermatitis. The skin may become reddened, denuded, and covered with a crusty material. Occasionally a pustular dermatitis develops. Because dogs become infested by lying on contaminated soil, these lesions are usually observed on the ventrum or medial (inner) surface of the limbs. Larvae of *P. strongyloides* can also be recovered from the skin of cattle recumbent on soil containing these larvae.

Diagnosis. These larvae (and possibly adults) can be identified in superficial skin scrapings. Larvae of *P. strongyloides* are 596 to 600 μ long. These larvae must be differentiated from the microfilariae of the canine heartworm, *Dirofilaria immitis,* the microfilariae of *Dipetalonema reconditum,* and the first-stage larvae of *Dracunculus insignis.*

Superfamily: spiruroidea (spirurid nematodes)

Habronema *and* draschia *species*

Adult *Habronema* nematodes are found on the stomach mucosa of horses, under a thick layer of mucus. Adult *Draschia* species produce large, fibrous nodules in the equine stomach wall; the nematodes reside within the nodules. The adults do not parasitize the skin; however, their larval stages can be deposited by flies (*Musca domestica, Stomoxys calcitrans*) into skin wounds on horses. Here the larvae produce a condition known as "cutaneous habronemiasis," "cutaneous draschiasis," or "summer sores."

The lesions vary in size and have an uneven surface consisting of a soft, reddish-brown material covering a mass of firmer granulations. These lesions are seen on body parts most susceptible to trauma, such as the legs, withers, male genitalia, and medial canthus of the eye. Infested wounds tend to increase in size and do not respond to ordinary treatment until the following winter, when they spontaneously heal.

Diagnosis.   Diagnosis of cutaneous habronemiasis is based on clinical signs and skin biopsies, which may reveal cross or longitudinal sections of these aberrant *Habronema* or *Draschia* larvae.

Superfamily: filarioidea (filarial nematodes)

Onchocerca cervicalis

Microfilariae of *Onchocerca cervicalis,* the filarial parasite of horses, produce recurrent dermatitis and periodic ophthalmia. The adults live in the ligamentum nuchae. Females produce microfilariae that migrate to the dermis via connective tissue. This parasite is spread by the biting midge, *Culicoides* species. The midge feeds on a horse's blood and ingests the microfilariae, which develop to the infective third stage within the fly. When the fly bites another horse, larvae are injected into the connective tissue and develop to adults during migration to the ligamentum nuchae.

The characteristic signs of cutaneous onchocerciasis include patchy alopecia, scaling on the head, neck, shoulders, and ventral midline, and sometimes intense pruritus.

Many infected horses are asymptomatic. Microfilariae of *Onchocerca* concentrate in certain areas, with the ventral midline the most common area of concentration. Because over 90% of normal hosts are probably infected with *O.*

cervicalis, detection of microfilariae in the skin of the ventral midline is not diagnostic for cutaneous onchocerciasis. However, the presence of microfilariae in diseased skin in highly indicative of, though not diagnostic of, cutaneous onchocerciasis.

Diagnosis.   *Onchocerca* microfilariae may be demonstrated by the following procedure. After clipping the skin site and performing a surgical scrub, a 6-mm punch biopsy is used to obtain a skin sample (see Skin Biopsy, Chapter 12). With a single-edged razor blade or scalpel blade, half of the tissue is minced in a small amount of preservative-free physiologic saline on a glass slide and allowed to stand for 5 to 10 minutes. Drying of the specimen is prevented by placing the slide in a covered chamber with a small amount of saline. The slide is then examined with a low-power (10X) objective. Because the translucent microfilariae are difficult to observe, low-intensity light and high contrast (achieved by lowering the condenser) are essential. Live microfilariae are identified by their vigorous swimming activity at the edge of the tissue. *Onchocerca cervicalis* microfilariae are slender and 207 to 140 µ long. The other half of the biopsy should be submitted for routine histopathologic examination.

STEPHANOFILARIA STILESI

Stephanofilaria stilesi is a small nematode found in the skin of ruminants, such as cattle, goats, and buffalo, and of wild mammals. It commonly causes dermatitis along the ventral midline of cattle in the United States. The infective larvae are transmitted by the bites of horn flies, *Haematobia irritans.* The skin lesions are thought to be caused by both adult and microfilarial stages.

The lesions caused by *S. stilesi* are located near the umbilicus and consist of small, red papules initially. Later, the lesions develop into large pruritic areas (up to 25 cm) of alopecia, with thick, moist crusts.

Diagnosis.   The adults (less than 6 mm long) and microfilariae may be found in deep skin scrapings after the crusts have been removed from the lesions.

DIPETALONEMA RECONDITUM *(SUBCUTANEOUS FILARIAL PARASITE OF DOGS)*

Adult *Dipetalonema reconditum* is a nonpathogenic parasite that resides in the subcutaneous tissues of the dog. It may also be found within a body cavity. Occasional subcutaneous abscesses and ulcerated areas have been associated with this parasite. The intermediate host for this parasite is the flea, *Ctenocephalides felis.* Because this parasite is found in enzootic areas where

Dirofilaria immitis is present, it is necessary to differentiate the microfilariae of these two filarial parasites (see Chapter 6).

DIAGNOSIS. Adults of *D. reconditum* are rarely recovered from their subcutaneous sites. Microfilariae may be rarely recovered in deep skin scrapings that draw blood. When subjected to the modified Knott's procedure, the microfilariae of *D. reconditum* average about 285 µ in length, with a button-hook tail and a blunt (broom handle-shaped) cranial end. They must be differentiated from microfilariae of *D. immitis,* first-stage larvae of *Pelodera strongyloides,* and first-stage larvae of *Dracunculus insignis.*

DIROFILARIA IMMITIS *(CANINE HEARTWORM)*

Dirofilaria immitis, the canine heartworm, normally resides in the right ventricle and pulmonary arteries of its definitive host, the dog. Adult heartworms can also occur aberrantly and may be found in a variety of extravascular sites, including cystic spaces in the subcutaneous sites (Figure 7-36). When adult heartworms are found aberrantly, they are usually single, immature, isolated worms. Any female heartworms found within the cyst will not have been fertilized by a male heartworm. Therefore, such females are not gravid and do not produce microfilariae.

Adult female heartworms in the right ventricle and pulmonary arteries can produce microfilariae after mating with adult males. These microfilariae may be occasionally recovered in deep skin scrapings that draw blood.

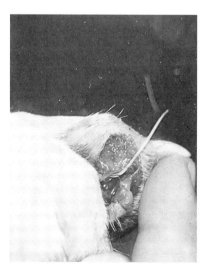

FIGURE 7-36. Aberrant adult *Dirofilaria immitis* heartworm in a subcutaneous interdigital cyst in a dog.

DIAGNOSIS.   Aberrant adult *D. immitis* heartworms within cystic spaces in the skin can be removed surgically. When subjected to the modified Knott's procedure, the microfilariae of *D. immitis* are 310 to 320 μ long, with a straight tail and tapering cranial end. They must be differentiated from the microfilariae of *D. reconditum,* first-stage larvae of *Pelodera strongyloides,* and first-stage larvae of *Dracunculus insignis.*

SUPERFAMILY: DRACUNCULOIDEA

DRACUNCULUS INSIGNIS *(GUINEA WORM)*

Dracunculus insignis, the Guinea worm, is a nematode found in the skin of dogs. The adult female nematode resides subcutaneously and produces a draining, ulcerous lesion in the skin, usually on the dog's limb. The cranial end of the female worm extends from this ulcer. When the female worm within the lesion comes in contact with water, its uterus prolapses through the worm's cranial end and ruptures, releasing a mass of first-stage larvae into the water. These larvae are 500 to 750 μ long and have a unique, long tail (Figure 7-37). The larvae are ingested by tiny crustaceans in the water; within the crustaceans, the larvae develop to the infective third stage. Dogs become infected with *D. insignis* by drinking water containing the infected crustaceans.

DIAGNOSIS.   If *D. insignis* infection is suspected, the ulcer with its associated worm should be dipped in cool water. The cool water is a stimulus for the female worm to expel her larvae. The water containing expelled larvae should be centrifuged and the sediment examined for the characteristic first-stage larvae. Larvae of *D. insignis* must be differentiated from the microfilariae of

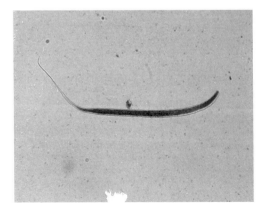

FIGURE 7-37.   Unique first-stage larva of *Dracunculus insignis.* These larvae are 500 μ to 750 μ long and have a characteristic long tail.

Dirofilaria immitis, microfilariae of *Dipetalonema reconditum,* and first-stage larvae of *Pelodera strongyloides.* Once identified, the adult female worm can be removed surgically.

PHYLUM ANNELIDA (SEGMENTED WORMS)

CLASS HIRUDINEA (LEECHES)

- Order: Gnathobdellida

HIRUDO MEDICINALIS (MEDICINAL LEECH)

Leeches are annelids; they are not considered to be true helminths but are often described as parasitic worms. As ectoparasites of people, domestic animals, and wild animals, leeches are members of the phylum Annelida and the class Hirudinea. Leeches can have a pathologic or beneficial role in veterinary medicine.

The term *hirudiniasis* is derived from the classic Linnaean nomenclature and is defined as invasion of the nose, mouth, pharynx, or larynx by leeches, or the attachment of leeches to the skin. Leeches are voracious blood feeders; depending on the number that attach to the host, the host may become anemic and may die from blood loss. Leeches have recently gained favor as postsurgical tools in reconstructive and microvascular surgery. *Hirudo medicinalis,* the medicinal leech, has been used in reconstructive and microvascular surgery in people; such use in veterinary medicine is forthcoming.

DIAGNOSIS. Leeches are segmented worms with slender, leaf-shaped bodies devoid of bristles. A typical leech has two suckers, a large and adhesive caudal sucker and a smaller cranial one that surrounds the mouth. Most leeches are found in fresh water and a few in salt water; some are terrestrial varieties.

RECOMMENDED READING

Bowman: *Georgi's parasitology for veterinarians,* ed 6, Philadelphia, 1995, WB Saunders.

Colville: *Diagnostic parasitology for veterinary technicians,* St Louis, 1991, Mosby.

Sloss, et al: *Veterinary clinical parasitology,* ed 6, Ames, Iowa, 1994, Iowa State University Press.

FUNCTION TESTS

B.F. Feldman and R.R. de Gopegui

Function tests are a challenge in that they provoke organs to demonstrate their operational integrity. Because they probe actual function, such tests may discover abnormalities latent or even disguised in other clinical data.

Because organs integrate a variety of stimuli and responses to those stimuli, exploring their function can mean exploring a chain of events. This has two implications. First, a single test may be employed to examine different links in this chain. Second, these links must be known to identify any that have failed when a test result is abnormal.

Most function tests involve direct observation of a traceable substance in the body. The fate of this substance in the normal animal must be known before alterations are interpreted. It is also essential to know the values deemed normal by your particular laboratory. If these data are unavailable, normal control samples should accompany each test procedure or the data obtained may be worse than useless.

There are four main types of function tests: gastrointestinal, hepatic, renal, and endocrine. Pulmonary function tests are also important but are performed in specialized hospitals only.

TESTS OF GASTROINTESTINAL FUNCTION

The principal functions of the gastrointestinal (GI) tract are assimilation of nutrients (digestion and/or absorption) and excretion of waste products. Most nutrients are ingested in a form that is either too complex or insoluble for absorption. Within the GI tract these substances are solubilized and degraded enzymatically to simple molecules that can be absorbed across the mucosal epithelium.

Gastrointestinal diseases are common in veterinary practice. Specific diagnosis is essential, especially when the disease is chronic. Therefore function tests are very useful in guiding treatment. Sometimes GI function tests are described as equivalent to exploratory laparotomy.

Malassimilation can be classified by pathophysiologic process into maldigestive or malabsorptive forms. *Maldigestion* results from altered gastric secretion and lack of, or decreased amounts of, digestive enzymes, usually secreted by the pancreas, and less often, by the intestinal mucosa. *Malabsorption* is most often caused by an acquired disease of the small intestinal wall or by bacterial overgrowth syndromes. Before clinical signs of maldigestion are seen, about 90% of the pancreas must be either nonfunctional or destroyed.[1,11,32] The small intestine of a dog can function well with up to 85% loss, but greater than 50% loss may result in "short bowel syndrome" that cannot be compensated for by adaptive mechanisms.[18,21]

Laboratory tests may evaluate gastric hydrochloric acid secretion, but most of them are directed to detect malassimilation and its origin. These tests are based on examination of feces for fecal dietary nutrients and fecal enzyme activities and serum for concentrations of orally administered substrates or metabolites and specific tests for endogenous substances.

MAXIMAL GASTRIC ACID SECRETION

This test may be indicated in patients with gastroduodenal ulcer or gastric mucosal atrophy. The maximal gastric acid output may be assessed by histamine-induced secretion or pentagastrin-induced secretion. The patient must be fasted and anesthetized to accomplish these tests. Gastric intubation with the patient in left lateral recumbency is also required before stimulant administration (Procedure 8-1).

FECAL EXAMINATION

Do not ignore your senses. First insights into GI function come from simple fecal examinations. In this case, the functional challenge is provided by the patient's diet; no clinical intervention is needed. Grossly, stools may reveal excess fat (*steatorrhea*). They may be bulky, pale, and malodorous, especially with severe pancreatic insufficiency.

PROCEDURE 8-1. Protocol for pentagastrin-stimulated gastric secretion[16]

1. Fast the animal for 24 hours before anesthesia.
2. Anesthesize and place the dog in left lateral recumbency.
3. Insert a monogastric tube, instill water (60 ml), and aspirate gastric contents. Collect two samples of gastric juice 30 minutes later to assess unstimulated gastric secretion.
4. Inject pentagastrin IM at 6 µg/kg.
5. Collect four samples of gastric juice every 15 minutes over 1 hour and calculate the acid output (mmol/kg/hour).

Normal hydrochloric acid peak output in dogs is 1.86 to 3.64 mmol/kg/hour at 30 minutes after pentagastrin administration and 1.65 to 3.42 mmol/kg/hour at 45 minutes after pentagastrin administration.

MICROSCOPIC EXAMINATION

Microscopic examination explores abnormalities or reveals them when the stool appears normal. Procedure 8-2 lists a protocol for microscopic examination. It is also useful, for comparison, to perform these tests on a normal animal given the same diet as the patient. Remember, these tests are qualitative. At best, they point you in the right direction. Fecal fat, starch, and muscle tests vary with dietary content and intestinal motility. It is wise to repeat them.

Of the nutrients, absorption of fat is the least physiologically efficient; the entire small intestine is required. Steatorrhea, then, is a forerunner and accompaniment of nearly all malabsorption syndromes. Steatorrhea of *neutral fats* (undigested/nonsplit) is revealed by treating the stool with Sudan III or IV stains. Large oil globules stain red-orange. Up to two or three such globules normally are found per high-power field (40X objective). Larger numbers suggest pancreatic lipase deficiency.

Digested fats (free fatty acids/split fats) do not color with Sudan stains unless acidification and heat melt them into neutral droplets that stain as described previously. Again, more than two or three droplets per high-power field indicate malfunction, particularly intestinal malassimilation. Fecal protease activity should be present in such cases (see Fecal Protease Test).

Lugol's iodine demonstrates starch granules in feces (*amylorrhea*): these stain blue-black, with a turquoise fringe. Persistent amylorrhea indicates pancreatic

PROCEDURE 8-2. Protocol for microscopic examination of feces

FECAL NEUTRAL FAT
Add 2 drops of water to a stool sample on a glass slide and mix. Add 2
drops of 95% ethanol with several drops of saturated Sudan III or IV stain
in 95% ethanol. Mix, apply coverslip, and examine for more than a few
red-orange droplets.

FECAL FREE FATTY ACIDS
Add several drops of glacial acetic acid to a stool sample on a glass slide
and mix. Add several drops of Sudan III or IV stain, mix, apply coverslip,
and heat gently over a Bunsen burner until it just bubbles. Air cool and
repeat two to three times. Examine for more than a few red-orange
droplets.

FECAL STARCH AND MUSCLE FIBER
Mix a stool sample with several drops of Lugol's iodine on a glass slide,
apply a coverslip, and examine for blunt, striated muscle fibers or
blue-black starch granules. Muscle fiber may also be seen in unstained
smears.

amylase deficiency, but it is a relatively insensitive test for pancreatic
malfunction.

Also seek *creatorrhea* (fecal muscle fibers) in a patient eating a meat-based
diet. A fresh fecal smear is stained with Lugol's, methylene blue, or Wright's
stain and examined under high power. Undigested fibers have blunt ends and
prominent cross striations. The presence of two to three striated muscle fibers
per high-power field is supportive of maldigestion. They are products of
deficient protein digestion (usually pancreatic), one form of protein-losing
gastroenteropathy. However, the results tend to be excessively variable and
insensitive because most carnivorous pets usually eat cooked meat.

FECAL WEIGHT
Fecal weight is one of the simplest (but most unesthetic) ways to differentiate
disorders of maldigestion, malabsorption, colitis, and nonsteatorrheic small
intestine disease. Knowing the weight of feces and the period of collection
allows one to calculate a 24-hour fecal weight (Procedure 8-3).

PROCEDURE 8-3.   Protocol for the fecal weight test in dogs

1. Feed a commercial canned meat-based dog food at 50 g/kg body weight once daily for 2 to 3 days.
2. Collect and weigh all feces passed in each subsequent 24-hour period.
3. Divide the resultant fecal weight by the weight of the dog in kilograms.

Results: Feces from dogs with maldigestion or malabsorption are three to four times heavier than the feces of normal dogs or of those with nonsteatorrheic diarrheal disease.

FECAL PROTEASE TEST

A quick, inexpensive estimate of pancreatic protease function is made by observing the effect of a fecal suspension on gelatin (Procedure 8-4). The substrate is provided in a test tube of gelatin (tube test). Digestion of the gelatin implies fecal (and presumably intestinal) protease activity. As you might suspect, the test's convenience is offset by inaccuracy.

What does a negative (no protease activity) test mean? It can mean true pancreatic insufficiency, but normal animals often have negative tests because of the normal daily flux in fecal protease concentrations. Do not be misled. False negatives also arise from trypsin inhibitors or exhaustion of proteases during digestion. Remember that the old x-ray film digestion test is, quite simply, inaccurate. Always run simultaneous controls. Repeat negative tests at least three times before lending them credence.

For correct interpretation of these results, fresh feces must be used. If not quickly analyzed, the sample should be frozen.

Also beware of positive tests; the protease activity revealed may be only bacterial. This is pronounced when the client is tardy in submitting feces collected 1 to 2 days earlier. Serial fecal dilutions exceeding 1:100 in the tube test reduce the influence of these bacterial proteases. That is, protease activity at fecal dilutions exceeding 1:100 is appropriate and nonbacterial in origin.

FECAL OCCULT BLOOD

Blood loss into the gut is another cause of protein-losing gastroenteropathy. Dramatic bleeding is evident as black feces (*melena*) or frank fecal blood (*hematochezia*). Less obvious, subtle bleeding is a significant sign of GI ulcers, neoplasia, or parasitism. Chronic, low-level bleeding may lead to iron-deficiency anemia.

Procedure 8-4.   Protocol for the fecal protease test

Tube test
1. Dilute 1 part feces with 9 parts 5% sodium bicarbonate.
2. Add 1 ml of the above mixture to 2 ml of melted 7.5% gelatin at 37°C.
3. Incubate at 37° C for 1 hour, or at room temperature for 2.5 hours.
4. Refrigerate for 20 minutes.
5. If the mixture fails to form a gel, the test is positive. Confirm positive tests by diluting feces up to 1:100. Negative results at these dilutions indicate fecal protease deficiency.

Run two control samples
1. Diluent only (negative control).
2. Normal feces (positive control).

Useful reagents to detect insidious bleeding include orthotoluidine (Occult-est: Ames) and benzidine (Hemoccult: SmithKline Beecham). Impregnated strips or tablets are oxidized to a colored product by hemoglobin peroxidase activity in the feces. Both reagents are so sensitive that they respond to dietary hemoglobin and myoglobin; therefore, the patient's diet must be meat-free for 3 days before the test. We recommend a cottage cheese and rice diet, 50% of each, before testing. This precaution is less pertinent in herbivores, but check that their diet has not been supplemented with meat and bone meal.

Guaiac test.   The guaiac test is the preferred test for occult fecal blood because it is less affected by diet (Procedure 8-5). It is less sensitive but still detects fecal blood volumes as small as 5 to 20 ml. Dietary restriction is still advised. Guaiac may also be used to test for blood in urine and gastric juice. Note that many gum guaiac preparations vary in sensitivity. Alcohol solutions of guaiac, as well as 3% hydrogen peroxide solutions, are unstable. Check these with known positive controls. False negatives are also caused by excessive reducing compounds in the medium (as with vitamin C supplementation); this is a problem when seeking blood in canine urine because dogs overproduce vitamin C and dump the excess vitamin into the urine.

Total fecal fat.   Practitioners anxious to confirm steatorrhea may consider a test of total fecal fat. The test is quite sensitive but unesthetic. Preferably a diet

---

PROCEDURE 8-5. Protocol for the guaiac fecal occult blood test

1. Smear feces sparingly on a piece of filter paper. Also smear a positive control sample (0.05 ml of venous blood in 50 ml of water) on another paper.
2. Add 2 drops each of glacial acetic acid, gum guaiac solution (20 g in 100 ml 95% ethanol), and 3% hydrogen peroxide (fresh!) to each sample.
3. Observe for color change and rapidity of color change.
   Trace: faint green-blue in 1 minute
   1+: light blue appearing slowly
   2+: clear blue appearing fairly fast
   3+: deep blue almost immediately
   4+: deep blue immediately
4. The control should give a 1+ reaction.

---

of known fat content is fed for a few days, then all feces are collected for 24 to 72 hours. The bulky or watery feces that often typify suspect patients heighten this challenge.

All feces are mixed thoroughly (a clean coffee can and agitator are handy) and an aliquot is removed for fat analysis. Neutral fats and free fatty acids can be differentiated if desired. Normal fat excretion is less than 6 g/24 hours (2% to 5% of dietary intake). The test is predictably expensive and nullified if fecal collection is less than accurate.

FECAL PROTEOLYTIC ACTIVITY. Because the BT-PABA test and trypsin-like immunoreactivity (TLI) tests are not well developed for feline species, an assay for fecal proteolytic activity should be used for evaluation of exocrine pancreatic insufficiency in cats and other species.

Fecal proteolytic activity can be determined colorimetrically using an azocasein or azoalbumin substrate, or a radial enzyme diffusion method.[22,38]

SERUM TESTS

FAT/LIPID ABSORPTION
Lipid absorption relies on bile, pancreatic lipase, and a healthy intestinal mucosa. Associated lesions cause steatorrhea and prevent the normal hyperlipemia

that follows a fatty meal. Lipemia, as judged by plasma turbidity, is then a gauge of GI function.

The patient is fasted for 12 hours and a baseline blood sample is drawn and centrifuged. Should you encounter fasting lipemia (in diabetes mellitus, starvation, feline steatitis, hypothyroidism, hyperadrenocorticism, liver/biliary disease, familial hyperlipemia of Schnauzers, white muscle disease of sheep, or hyperlipemia of ponies, among others), the test must be abandoned. If the plasma is clear, proceed by giving corn oil (3 ml/kg) or peanut oil (2 ml/kg) PO. Draw more blood samples at hourly intervals for 4 hours. This plasma should be cloudy. Clear follow-up samples indicate disturbed absorptive function, but where? Some argue that this test is no more than the simple discovery of steatorrhea.

However, a variation in approach to the test can better define the lesion. The test is repeated on another day but the oil is preincubated at room temperature for 20 minutes with pancreatic enzymes. If the postchallenge plasma is now cloudy, pancreatic enzyme deficiency is implied. If it is clear, inadequate bile production or intestinal malassimilation must be considered.

The fat absorption test may yield false negatives (no fat absorption) with delayed gastric emptying (fat induces this), gastric inactivation of added pancreatic enzymes, or enteritis.

Slight lipemia before oil administration indicates increased concentrations of very low lipoproteins (mainly triglycerides and cholesterol). The enzyme lipoprotein lipase usually clears plasma of triglycerides; the activity of this enzyme is enhanced by insulin, thyroid hormones, glucagon, and heparin. Determination of triglyceride concentrations of slightly lipemic plasma may reveal increased triglyceride concentration; this could be attributed to disease of hepatic, pancreatic, renal or endocrine origin. Slight postprandial lipemia may also be seen in some canine patients with malabsorptive syndromes.

MONOSACCHARIDE ABSORPTION TESTS

These tests more specifically probe intestinal function. Again, the agent is given PO, and blood concentrations are the yardstick of absorption.

D-XYLOSE ABSORPTION.   D-xylose is a 5-carbon sugar absorbed passively in the jejunum and excreted rapidly by the kidneys. Because xylose absorption is simple and the agent is not metabolized, its fate can be readily traced. Xylose absorption is inefficient and often affected by some intestinal diseases. Nonetheless, the test is relatively insensitive because control values are variable.

The test is performed as described in Procedure 8-6 in dogs and horses. Interference from rumen flora precludes use of the oral test in cattle and sheep; the alternative injection of monosaccharides into the abomasum is difficult enough to make its use rare.

Abnormal xylose absorption indicates intestinal malassimilation, specifically malabsorption. Note, however, that only slight differences separate normal and abnormal ranges; diseased animals can have normal results. Animals with lymphangiectasia still can have normal results as the lymphatics do not participate in xylose absorption. The rate of xylose absorption depends only on the amount given, the size of the absorptive area, intestinal blood circulation, and gastric emptying. The latter may be delayed by cold or hypertonic solutions, pain, apprehension, or feeding. Fasting or radiographs to confirm an empty stomach are required. Vomiting, of course, falsely lowers blood values, as does ascites (xylose enters pooled fluids). Bacteria have the ability to metabolize xylose; therefore, bacterial overgrowth can be monitored by this test. If bacterial overgrowth is suspected (intestinal stasis, pancreatic enzyme deficiency), repeat the test after 24 hours' use of oral tetracycline. Finally, renal disease falsely elevates blood xylose concentrations.

The fate of D-xylose has also been followed in dogs by collecting a 5-hour urine sample after a 25-g oral dose and determining the total xylose excreted. This method is more laborious but requires only one xylose assay.

Cats were thought to have plasma concentrations and kinetics similar to dogs.[23] Other studies found xylose uptake to be variable in cats and plasma concentration did not increase to the levels found in dogs.[12,13] Peak plasma concentration of xylose in normal cats ranged between 12 and 42 mg/dl when a dosage of 500 mg/kg body weight was used.[17]

False-negative results can be caused by delayed gastric emptying, abnormal intestinal motility, reduced intestinal blood flow, bacterial overgrowth, and sequestration of xylose in ascitic fluid. False-positive results may be caused by decreased glomerular filtration rate; hence, it is important to make sure that the patient is fully hydrated and not azotemic at the time of testing.

Of the oral dose of xylose, 18% is excreted through the kidneys within 5 hours.

GLUCOSE ABSORPTION. This test offers both advantages and drawbacks. Glucose is cheap, readily available, and easily assayed. However, the test is not very sensitive; the intestine has a large, active absorptive reserve for glucose and only extensive lesions are detected. Most crucial, the test is not specific. Glucose, as a major energy currency, is involved in intricate biochemical

Procedures 8-6. Protocol for the monosaccharide absorption test in dogs and horses

Oral xylose absorption in dogs

1. Fast the patient for 16 hours.
2. Collect a heparinized blood sample for baseline xylose measurement.
3. Give 5% xylose solution at 500 mg/kg via stomach tube.
4. Draw heparinized blood samples at 30, 60, 90, 120, 180, and 240 minutes after xylose administration and submit for xylose determination.[23]
5. Plot a blood xylose concentration vs. time curve. A peak of less than 45 mg/dl between 30 and 90 minutes is abnormal. Peak values of 45 to 50 mg/dl are possibly abnormal. A peak above 50 mg/dl is probably normal.

Oral glucose absorption in dogs

1. Fast the patient for 16 hours.
2. Collect a blood sample in a sodium fluoride tube for baseline glucose determination.
3. Give glucose PO at 1 g/kg.
4. Collect blood at 30-minute intervals to 180 minutes using sodium fluoride as the anticoagulant and submit for glucose determination.
5. Animals with intestinal malabsorption fail to develop a serum glucose concentration of 160 mg/dl by 60 minutes. The baseline serum glucose concentration should be attained by 120 to 180 minutes.

Glucose and xylose absorption in horses

1. Fast the patient for 12 to 18 hours.
2. Withhold water for the first 2 hours of the test.
3. Collect baseline blood samples (heparinized for xylose, sodium fluoride for glucose).
4. Give xylose at 0.5 g/kg as a 10% aqueous solution or anhydrous glucose at 1 g/kg as a 20% aqueous solution via stomach tube.
5. Collect blood at 30-minute intervals for 4 to 5 hours. Centrifuge and keep plasma at 0° C (32° F) until analyzed.
6. Maximum blood xylose level of 20.6 ± 4.8 mg/dl is expected at 60 minutes. The preadministration blood glucose concentration should be doubled by 120 minutes.
7. Do not run tests simultaneously, as they cause mutual interference.

reactions that can distort test results. Indeed, the same test is sometimes used to explore endocrine disorders (diabetes mellitus or hyperinsulinism). Always interpret glucose absorption results realizing that hepatic or pancreatic disease can interfere.

Increased endogenous epinephrine enhances enterocytic glucose absorption as well as glycogen liberation from liver, muscles, and erythrocytes. It inhibits glucose absorption by erythrocytes. Increased cortisol (endogenous or exogenous) enhances enterocytic glucose absorption.

The glucose absorption test is seldom performed in small animals; results are inconsistent in dogs with consistent xylose tests. The test may also cause diarrhea. Despite problems, glucose absorption is often the test of choice in equine practice because of its economy and simplicity. The main indication is weight loss without anorexia.

The glucose absorption test is described in Procedure 8-6. Glucose absorption is decreased by rumen flora, bacterial overgrowth, vomiting, and delayed gastric emptying. Note that the fasting recommended to normalize gastric function, if prolonged to 36 hours, actually decreases glucose absorption in normal horses.

In normal dogs the blood sugar level is less than 120 mg/dl and reaches 160 mg/dl during the test. It then returns to normal by the end of the second hour. In patients with diabetes mellitus or exocrine pancreatic insufficiency, the fasting blood sugar level is usually more than 120 mg/dl. It reaches 180 mg/dl during the test and will not return to normal during the test period.

DISACCHARIDE DIGESTION AND ABSORPTION TEST

Intestinal brush border disaccharidase cleaves ingested sugars into glucose and other monosaccharides for absorption. Lack of disaccharidase causes malabsorption, such as lactose intolerance in people. To explore this in monogastric (nonruminant) animals, the suspect sugar (usually lactose, maltose, or sucrose) is given PO and its progress monitored via blood glucose determinations. Such tests are rarely performed. There are little data on normal animals, and the test is fraught with the previously mentioned difficulties associated with the glucose absorption test.

STARCH TOLERANCE TEST

Food is withheld for 12 hours and a blood sample is taken; then starch is administered via stomach tube at 3 g/kg. The starch is prepared by mixing each 3-g starch aliquot with 1.5 ml of warm water. Subsequent blood samples are taken at 30-minute intervals for 150 minutes. The serum glucose in normal dogs should increase to 125 to 130 mg/dl within an hour. Dogs with malassimilation have a flatter absorption curve than normal. If the results of the xylose and this starch tolerance test are combined, the two tests may be able to distinguish between exocrine pancreatic insufficiency and malabsorption.

BT-PABA TEST

BT-PABA test was the best tool to check pancreatic function before the trypsin-like immunoreactivity test became available. N-benzoyl-L-tyrosyl-p-aminobenzoic acid (BT-PABA; Bentiromide: Adria Labs) is a chymotrypsin-labile peptide that, when given PO, is split by this pancreatic protease into a p-aminobenzoic acid (PABA) free moiety. This is absorbed rapidly into the blood, conjugated in the liver, and excreted in urine. The success of this chain of reactions is evaluated by measuring plasma or urinary PABA concentrations (Procedure 8-7). Note that several organs participate. Abnormal results may reflect pancreatic enzyme insufficiency, intestinal malassimilation, or renal disease. A subsequent or simultaneous xylose absorption test helps identify the dysfunctioning organ.

The test has proven useful in diagnosis of exocrine pancreatic insufficiency in dogs.[2,35,39] Affected dogs excrete less than 15% of the orally administered BT-PABA in 6 hours, while normal dogs excrete more than 70%. Dogs that are experimentally pancreatectomized excrete less than 5%. Dogs that excrete greater than 20% in urine within 6 hours may not require pancreatic enzyme replacement.

The large variations apparent in response of the BT-PABA test in normal cats limit the clinical usefulness of the test in cats with malassimilation.[33]

Actually, protease deficiency is the least likely pancreatic failure; when detected, lipase and amylase deficiencies usually accompany it. BT-PABA results correlate well with measurements of intestinal enzyme activity and 24-hour fecal fat tests. This accuracy is altered by previous use of chloramphenicol, sulfonamides, or diuretics.

COMBINED BT-PABA AND XYLOSE TEST

This test is used so that both digestion and absorption can be evaluated simultaneously (Procedure 8-8).

SERUM FOLATE AND COBALAMIN

Serum concentrations of folate and cobalamin may be assessed by radioimmunoassay (RIA). Both concentrations tend to be decreased in malabsorption. Folate is absorbed in proximal intestine, whereas cobalamin is absorbed in the

---

PROCEDURE 8-7. Protocol for the PABA test

1. Fast the patient for 18 hours.
2. Give PABA at 0.25 ml (16.7 mg)/kg (Bentiromide: Adria Labs) via stomach tube, followed by 25 to 100 ml of water.
3. Collect all urine produced in the subsequent 6 hours via catheter, or collect blood samples before the test and at 30-minute intervals for 2 hours after PABA is given. Centrifuge the blood and remove the plasma.
4. Submit an aliquot of urine to determine total PABA excreted, or submit all plasma samples for PABA measurement.
5. Normal 6-hour urinary PABA excretion is greater than 70% of the administered dose. Patients excreting less than 15% require enzyme replacement therapy. Intermediate results suggest partial pancreatic insufficiency or intestinal malassimilation.
6. Normal canine plasma PABA concentrations:
   Before test: 39.5 ± 15 µg/dl
   30 minutes: 500.5 ± 15.1 µg/dl
   60 minutes: 670.4 ± 140.6 µg/dl
   90 minutes: 636.4 ± 124.6 µg/dl
   120 minutes: 560.7 ± 116.6 µg/dl
   A 60-minute plasma PABA concentration of less than 125 µg/dl indicates the need for enzyme therapy. A 60-minute plasma PABA less than the 120-minute value, or in the range of 150 to 350 µg/dl, suggests intestinal malassimilation as the primary problem.

---

ileum. Bacterial overgrowth may also alter these concentrations; folate synthesis is increased in bacterial overgrowth, while some bacteria may decrease the cobalamin availability. Reference intervals in dogs are 3.7 to 8.8 µg/L for folate and 200 to 490 ng/L for cobalamin in serum.[31]

NITROSONAPHTHOL TEST

The nitrosonaphthol test is used to determine bacterial overgrowth. The small intestine bacteria degrade tyrosine to parahydroxyphenylacetic acid that is excreted in urine. The reaction of the urine parahydroxyphenylacetic acid with 1-nitroso-2-naphthol is denoted by a color change of the urine to orange. False-positive results may appear in liver disease (Procedure 8-9).

PROCEDURE 8-8. Protocol for the combined BT-PABA and xylose test

1. Prepare a solution of 100 ml containing 1 g of BT-PABA and 10 g of D-xylose. This solution can be frozen and used at a dosage of 5 ml/kg body weight.
2. Fast the patient overnight and then give the oral dose via stomach tube.
3. Collect blood in heparin tubes at 0, 30, 60, 90, 120, 180, and 240 minutes after administration and analyze for PABA and xylose concentrations.
4. The peak plasma concentration of PABA is at least 400 μg/dl in normal dogs.

PROCEDURE 8-9. Protocol for the nitrosonaphthol test for gastrointestinal bacterial overgrowth[4]

1. Place 1 ml of 2.6-N nitric acid in a test tube.
2. Add 1 drop of 2.5% sodium nitrite and add 0.1 ml of 0.1% 1-nitroso-2-naphthol (diluted in ethanol).
3. Mix and add 5 drops of urine.
4. Mix again and look for color change to orange. The test is positive if color change appears within 2 to 5 minutes.

ADMINISTRATION OF [51]CR-EDTA

Intestinal permeability may be assessed, after intragastric administration of [51]crethylendiaminotetraacetic acid (^{51}Cr EDTA), by quantitation of 24-hour urinary excretion. This test requires counting radioactive ^{51}Cr EDTA in a γ counter. Intestinal permeability is increased in dogs with gluten-sensitive enteropathy, small intestinal bacterial overgrowth, and giardiasis.[15]

CELLOBIOSE/MANNITOL TEST

The cellobiose/mannitol test has been proposed to assess the intestinal permeability in gluten-sensitive enteropathy in Irish Setter dogs. Intestinal absorption of mannitol is reduced with villus atrophy, while cellobiose permeability (passive absorption) is increased with jejunal damage. Therefore in gluten-sensitive enteropathy, the cellobiose/mannitol (C/M) ratio is increased (Procedure 8-10).

TRYPSIN-LIKE IMMUNOREACTIVITY

This is the most convenient and accurate test of pancreatic digestive function. Most of the pancreatic secretions enter the pancreatic duct, but small amounts leak from the basolateral aspect of the acinar cells into the blood. The serum content of the enzyme trypsinogen is derived only from the pancreas. This unique characteristic of trypsinogen prompted development of a radioimmunoassay technique for detecting the minute amount of serum trypsinogen or trypsin-like immunoreactivity (TLI) using antibodies to trypsin. These antibodies are species specific. TLI provides a sensitive and specific test for diagnosis of exocrine pancreatic insufficiency in dogs.[37] Assays for TLI have not been well developed for feline species.

Dogs with exocrine pancreatic insufficiency have a serum TLI of less than 2.5 µg/L. Normal dogs have a range of 5 to 35 µg/L. Dogs with other causes of malassimilation may have normal serum TLI. Dogs with chronic pancreatitis may have normal TLI values or between 2.5 and 5 µg/L.

Serum TLI decreases in parallel with functional pancreatic mass. The inflammation associated with acute and probably chronic pancreatitis may

---

PROCEDURE 8-10.   Protocol for the cellobiose/mannitol test for gastrointestinal permeability[14]

1. Fast the animal for 15 hours.
2. Obtain a urine sample.
3. Prepare an isotonic solution of cellobiose (5 g) and mannitol (2 g) in 100 ml water; administer by gastric intubation. Leave the animal fasted but with free access to water.
4. Collect urine samples for 6 hours.
5. Determine urine concentrations of cellobiose and mannitol by spectrophotometry.
6. Determine the percentage recovery of mannitol and cellobiose and calculate the cellobiose/mannitol ratio.
7. The C/M ratio for normal dogs is 0.05.

enhance leakage of trypsinogen and trypsin from the pancreas and increase TLI. Also, decreased glomerular filtration rate increases TLI (trypsinogen is a small molecule that easily passes into the glomerular filtrate). Serum TLI is an important indicator of functional pancreatic mass. It is most informative if coupled with BT-PABA and fecal fat results to characterize and diagnose malassimilation.

Serum TLI increases after eating (especially proteins), but values remain within reference intervals. Therefore food should be withheld for at least 3 hours and preferably 12 hours before taking a blood sample. The blood is coagulated at room temperature, and the serum stored at $-20°$ C until assay. The recommended radioimmunoassay kit is the Gamma-Vet Canine TLI (Immunodiagnostic Systems, Tyne & Wear, England).

TESTS OF LIVER FUNCTION

The liver's metabolic and transport functions are numerous. It plays a key role in conjugation and excretion of exogenous compounds, such as bilirubin and bile acids, as well as numerous exogenous drugs. Production of various proteins, metabolism of carbohydrates and lipids, and conversion of ammonia to urea are also important metabolic functions, making it an essential organ for maintenance of life. Malfunctions in these pathways result in predictable clinical signs of jaundice, hypoalbuminemia, problems with hemostasis, hypoglycemia, hyperlipoproteinemia, and hepatoencephalopathy.

DYE EXCRETION

Among the liver's many functions is excretion of certain wastes and foreign substances. This function can be exploited to test the liver's health.

BSP CLEARANCE.   Sulfobromophthalein (BSP) is an organic dye. While an excellent test, the usefulness of BSP clearance is limited by the availability of the dye. Injected intravenously, BSP is retrieved by the liver, conjugated and excreted in the bile by a pathway shared by bilirubin. Its disappearance from the plasma then depends on hepatic blood flow and bile flow as well as hepatocellular integrity. This disappearance is assayed as a half-life or percent dye retention (Procedure 8-11).

BSP clearance is a sensitive hepatic function test, especially useful for detecting chronic lesions or portosystemic shunts with no leakage of liver enzymes. Coagulation defects and mysterious anemias may sometimes be

PROCEDURE 8-11. Protocol for BSP clearance

DOGS AND CATS

1. Fast the patient for 12 hours. Also withdraw all medication for this period.
2. Inject BSP IV at 5 mg/kg. (*Caution:* Perivascular BSP causes major sloughing! Also, old solutions of BSP can crystallize and cause anaphylaxis.)
3. Collect a 5-ml blood sample from the opposite cephalic vein 30 minutes after BSP injection. Centrifuge and avoid hemolysis.
4. Submit plasma for BSP determination and calculate the percentage of retention at 30 minutes.
5. Normal is less than 5% retention at 30 minutes.

CATTLE AND HORSES (**1000** LB OR MORE)

1. Collect an initial blood sample.
2. Inject 20 ml of 0.5% BSP (or 1 g of BSP) IV.
3. Collect blood samples from the opposite jugular vein at 2- to 3-minute intervals between 5 and 15 minutes postinjection (record the times).
4. Centrifuge the samples, avoid hemolysis, and submit for BSP analysis.
5. Plot the clearance curve and calculate the half-life.
6. Normal half-life is 2.5 to 4 minutes.

SHEEP AND GOATS

1. Half-life or percent retention may be determined.
2. For percent retention, inject BSP IV at 5 mg/kg and collect blood samples from the opposite jugular vein 10 minutes later. Centrifuge the sample and submit plasma for BSP analysis. Calculate percent retention at 10 minutes.
3. For half-life determination, collect an initial blood sample, inject BSP IV at 5 mg/kg, and collect two to three blood samples from the opposite jugular vein within 7 minutes of injection (record the times). Submit plasma for BSP analysis and half-life determination.
4. Normal percent retention (sheep) is 6% ± 2% at 10 minutes. Normal half-life for sheep and goats is about 2 ± 0.3 minutes.

SWINE

1. Determine percent retention as for sheep and goats. Give BSP IV at 6 mg/kg.
2. Normal percent retention at 10 minutes is 3% to 4% for a 100-kg pig, and 1.4% ± 0.9% for a 30-kg pig.

explained by BSP test results. In horses, the test is handy in differentiating jaundice of hepatic disease from that of simple anorexia and hepatoencephalopathy from wobbler syndrome. Specific indications in ruminants include fascioliasis, liver abscesses, ketosis, and photosensitization. BSP clearance can aid diagnosis of aflatoxicosis in swine.

Hepatic lesions delay BSP excretion. Delays due to hepatocellular injury indicate a loss of at least 55% of the liver's functional mass. The magnitude of delay is poorly correlated to both the extent of hepatic lesions, when mild, and the clinical signs of liver dysfunction.

Delayed BSP clearance can be erroneous. Slowed BSP excretion results from perivascular dye injection (painful!), poor hepatic perfusion (shock, heart failure, dehydration), and fever. Ascites also interferes with BSP clearance, as the dye lingers in pooled fluids. Certain inborn defects of BSP metabolism occur without liver disease, notably in some Southdown and Corriedale sheep. Obesity prolongs BSP retention because the amount of BSP per unit of body mass is relatively increased. Finally, remember that bilirubin competes with BSP for excretion by the liver. For this reason, do not perform the BSP test in animals with hyperbilirubinemia of 3 mg/dl or more. The results will tell you no more than the already apparent jaundice.

Two conditions may disguise liver disease by speeding BSP clearance. Because albumin carries BSP in the plasma, hypoalbuminemia (nephrotic syndrome, protein-losing gastroenteropathies, extreme liver disease) speeds clearance by increasing hepatic access to the free dye. Phenobarbital use also hastens BSP clearance.

BSP clearance has no correlation with the extent of fatty infiltration of the liver.

INDOCYANINE GREEN CLEARANCE.   Indocyanine green (ICG) is an organic dye similar to BSP. Introduced to human medicine because of occasional reactions to BSP, it is used to estimate hepatic blood flow. ICG clearance is now being used by veterinarians instead of BSP because BSP is no longer available for clinical use.

Preinjection plasma is required to prepare a blank and a standard solution. This test can be used in both fed and fasted animals, but the latter are preferred. An IV dosage of 0.8 to 1.1 mg/kg body weight is recommended for horses, while 1 mg/kg body weight is recommended for dogs and 1.5 mg/kg body weight for cats. Usually five to six plasma samples are collected between 0, 5, 10, 15, and 30 minutes postinjection. ICG concentration is measured photometrically at 805 nm and the half-life is determined. Normal ICG clearances are as follows: dogs, 8.4 ± 2.3 minutes; horses (fed), 3.5 ± 0.67 minutes; horses (fasted), 1.6 ± 0.57 minutes. Normal 30-minute retention is $< 14.7 \pm 5\%$ in dogs and $\leq 7.3 \pm 2.9\%$ in cats.[8]

Delayed ICG clearance has been reported in a variety of disorders, such as hyperbilirubinemia, hypoproteinemia, decreased hepatic blood flow, hepatic necrosis, and extrahepatic bile duct obstruction.[19]

AMMONIA TOLERANCE

The liver's enzyme constituents include those involved in the urea cycle. Liver disease may impair ammonia detoxification, leading to hepatoencephalopathy. Random blood ammonia measurements may be normal in these patients, but challenge with overwhelming exogenous ammonia loads may reveal liver dysfunction. Rectal administration is more reliable because some dogs regurgitate ammonium chloride solution when it is given orally. However, oral administration of ammonium chloride may be accomplished with dry powder in gelatin capsules (Procedure 8-12).

The ammonia tolerance test is used to detect abnormal portal blood flow, particularly congenital portovascular anomalies.[30] In affected animals, plasma liver enzyme levels are often normal. The test's chief limitation is in the handling of blood samples. You must consult your particular laboratory for sample handling recommendations. In general, the blood must be centrifuged immediately and the serum placed on ice and analyzed within 1 to 3 hours of collection or frozen at $-20°$ C. Whole blood cannot be tested, as its ammonia content increases with storage. Although the test can dramatically elevate the blood ammonia level, it does not cause or worsen neurologic signs. Occasional vomiting is the only problem.

PROTHROMBIN TIME

Prothrombin is a vitamin K-dependent coagulation protein (factor) made by the liver. Activated by tissue thromboplastin and calcium, it initiates a coagulation cascade involving liver coagulation factors I, II, V, VII, and X. A prolonged prothrombin time (PT), the time from activation to clotting, indicates coagulation factor insufficiency and possible liver necrosis, cirrhosis, or poor bile secretion (bile is vital for vitamin K absorption). The PT factors are shorter lived than albumin; the PT may be prolonged in acute liver disease. Unfortunately, the test is insensitive. Only extensive lesions are detected because of the liver's large reserve capacity for PT factor synthesis.

The PT is often a mere prebiopsy screening test. If the PT is prolonged, vitamin K_1 therapy may help locate the problem. Long PTs shortened by

Procedure 8-12.   Protocol for the ammonia tolerance test

1. Consult your regional diagnostic laboratory about blood specimen handling.
2. Fast the patient for 12 hours and give enemas to clear the lower bowel of feces. Obtain a baseline blood sample.
3. For rectal administration, give ammonium chloride at 0.1 g/kg as a 5% solution infused 20 to 30 cm into the rectum. For oral administration, give 0.1 mg/kg (maximum of 3 g) dissolved in 20 to 50 ml of water via stomach tube.
4. Collect a second blood sample 30 minutes after administration and another at 60 minutes postadministration. The blood should be kept on ice until it is analyzed (within 3 hours).
5. Blood ammonia levels:

	Before ammonia loading	After ammonia loading
Normal	80 ± 36 µg/dl	156 ± 71 µg/dl
Abnormal	236 ± 116 µg/dl	1049 ± 256 µg/dl

6. Rectal ammonia tolerance results increase only minimally in normal blood (less than 2.5 times the baseline). Increases greater than 2.5 times the baseline value indicate hepatic failure or portosystemic shunting.

Note: Always consult your diagnostic laboratory for their reference intervals ("normal values").

subcutaneous but not oral K_1 use suggest obstructive/biliary difficulties. No reduction of the PT with K_1 administration by either route suggests diffuse hepatic disease. If the PT is reduced after subcutaneous injection of K_1 but remains 4 or more seconds longer than in controls, suspect advanced liver disease. This warrants a guarded prognosis (Procedure 8-13). The PT test must be done carefully and in duplicate. Always run a normal homologous plasma sample as a control and dilute the thromboplastin reagent until the control PT is 7 to 10 seconds.

BILE ACID CONCENTRATIONS

Bile acids are synthesized by hepatocytes from cholesterol and are conjugated with glycine or taurine. Conjugated bile acids are secreted across the canalicular

PROCEDURE 8-13. Protocol for determining prothrombin time

1. Obtain a blood sample in a sodium citrate tube.
2. Centrifuge at 3000 rpm for 10 minutes, then remove plasma.

AUTOMATED
1. Add 0.1 ml of plasma to cuvettes.
2. Activate the coagulyzer.
3. If the PT is greater than or equal to 60 seconds, the test must be repeated manually.

MANUAL
1. Add 0.1 ml of plasma to a test tube in a 37° C (98.6° F) water bath and wait 1 minute.
2. Forcibly blow 0.2 ml of commercial thromboplastin-calcium chloride (warmed to 37° C) into the plasma tube. Start timing simultaneously.
3. Keep the tube in the 37° C bath and shake gently.
4. Stop timing when a visible clot just begins to form.
5. Run homologous controls simultaneously to obtain normal values.

membrane and reach the small intestine via the biliary system. Any process that impairs the hepatocellular, biliary, or portal enterohepatic circulation of bile acids results in elevated serum bile acid (SBA) levels. The great advantage of SBA determinations as a liver function test is that they evaluate the major anatomic component of the hepatobiliary system, and they are very stable *in vitro* (Procedure 8-14).

Increased fasting SBA levels were observed in patients with extrahepatic biliary obstruction, cholangiohepatic-portosystemic shunt, biliary cirrhosis, and hepatic lipidosis. Postprandial values are more valuable in portosystemic vascular abnormalities or acquired shunts. Fasting bile acid levels may be greater than postprandial levels in spontaneous gallbladder contraction, slow intestinal transit, altered response to cholecystokinin, and altered gastrointestinal flora. Low bile acid levels may appear in hepatobiliary disease if diarrhea and steatorrhea are present.[8]

Additional comparative studies are still needed to evaluate this test in comparison with other established tests in determining or diagnosing hepatopathy in each animal species.

Procedure 8-14. Protocol for determination of serum bile acid concentrations

1. Obtain blood samples from dogs after fasting for 12 hours and again 2 hours after eating (see fat/lipid absorption).
2. Separate serum from blood cells within 1 hour and store at −20° C.
3. Determine bile acid concentration by radioimmunoassay or an enzymatic colorimetric procedure. The latter has also been validated for equine serum.

Enzymatic method

This measures all nonsulfated conjugated and unconjugated 3-alphahydroxy bile acids.

1. To each of two test tubes, add 0.2 ml of serum and 0.2 ml of 200-mM sodium pyruvate.
2. To one tube add 0.5 ml of the 3-alpha-hydroxysteroid dehydrogenase reaction mixture (prepared as described in #6, or from the kit, Enzabil [Nyegaard & Co., Oslo, Norway]).
3. To the other tube add 0.5 ml of the reference reaction mixture (prepared or from the kit). This mixture has the same constituents as the reaction mixture described above, except it has no 3-alpha-hydroxysteroid dehydrogenase.
4. Incubate the tubes at 37° C (water bath) for 10 minutes. Add 0.1 ml of 1.33-M phosphoric acid solution to each tube after incubation and mix thoroughly.
5. The final volume in each tube is 1 ml. Read the light absorbance at 540 nm to determine the difference between the reaction tube and the reference tube.
6. A standard solution is prepared from sodium taurocholate (400 µmol/L), pooled serum (species specific), and various buffers.[7]
7. Bile acid concentration equals:

$$\frac{\text{Sample Concentration} \times \text{Standard Concentration}}{\text{Standard Concentration}}$$

Radioimmunoassay method

The conjugated bile acid, solid-phase radioimmunoassay kit (Conjugated Bile Acids Solid-Phase Radioimmunoassay Kit: Becton-Dickinson Immunodiagnostics, Orangeburg, NJ) consists of assay tubes coated with rabbit antiserum against conjugated bile acids, a bile acid tracer that contains iodoglycocholic acid dissolved in buffers, and sodium taurocholate standards (0, 0.4, 2.0, 6.0, 15, and 50 µmol/L) in buffer solutions.

PROCEDURE **8-14.**—*continued*

1. Mix 25 μl of serum or standard with 1 ml of bile acid tracer solution in the assay tube and incubate the tubes for 1 hour in a 37° C water bath to allow antigen-antibody interaction.
2. Aspirate the solution from each tube and rinse the tubes with 1 ml of sterile distilled water. Determine the radioactivity remaining in the tubes with an automatic gamma scintillation counter calibrated for ^{125}I measurement.
3. Calculate the conjugated bile acid concentration (μmol/L) of each sample from the standard curve.[29]

RESULTS

Normal fasting concentrations:

Dogs	≤ 5.0 μmol/L
Cats	≤ 2.0 μmol/L
Horses	5.9 ± 2.7 μmol/L

Normal values 2 hours after feeding:

Dogs	≤ 15.5 μmol/L
Cats	≤ 10.0 μmol/L
Horses	5.9 ± 2.7 μmol/L

Equine bile acid concentrations do not change after feeding; only an insignificant increase is observed.

Note: In horses, an increase of 17 times greater than the baseline value is expected in cholestasis. An increase greater than ten-fold above the baseline value was observed in hepatocellular necrosis.

Fasting concentrations in dogs and cats >15 μmol/L are suggestive of disease.

Postprandial levels >25 μmol/L in dogs and >20 μmol/L in cats are suggestive of disease.

CAFFEINE CLEARANCE

This is a specific assay of hepatic microsomal function. Demethylation of caffeine depends only on the specific P448 microsomal system of healthy hepatocytes; therefore, it accurately reflects aberrations in hepatocellular function. This test is now used in human medicine; few experimental studies have been performed in canine species.[5,28]

Caffeine sodium benzoate is dissolved in 2 ml of sterile water (50:50 wt/wt) and 7 mg of caffeine/kg body weight are then injected IV. Plasma samples are collected from 15 to 480 minutes, and the caffeine concentration (µg/ml) is measured by automated enzyme immunoassay. Plasma caffeine clearance and half-life are calculated.

Normal half-life values in dogs are 6 ± 0.6 hours and clearance is 1.7 ± 0.1 ml/min/kg. Elimination of caffeine is prolonged in hepatic insufficiency, with a clearance of 0.8 ± 0.1 ml/min/kg.

Delta bilirubin concentration

Delta bilirubin has been identified as a fourth, firmly bound bilirubin fraction of total bilirubin. It is composed of a portion covalently bound to albumin and a portion that is nonenzymatically derived from albumin and monoconjugated bilirubin. Small amounts of delta bilirubin have been detected in healthy people and human patients with physiologic jaundice and hemolysis. Its concentration is increased (less than 50% of total bilirubin levels) in patients with a variety of hepatobiliary diseases.

Unlike conjugated bilirubin, delta bilirubin is not filtered by the glomeruli; hence, its clearance seems to be linked to that of albumin. Because of its slow clearance from serum, delta bilirubin is thought to cause persistence of jaundice following resolution of active hepatobiliary disease in people.

Delta bilirubin concentrations, when present over time in people, are prognostic of clinical outcome in numerous pathologic conditions, including but not limited to conjugated hyperbilirubinemia. In people with large fluctuations in total bilirubin and conjugated bilirubin values, fluctuations of both absolute and percentage delta bilirubin concentration mirror the patient's clinical status and thus seem to be more sensitive than hepatic enzyme measurements or liver function tests in assessing the prognosis. The differing patterns of delta bilirubin concentrations over time might be useful in distinguishing patients with irreversible liver damage from those with sufficient hepatic regenerative capacity.

The Kodak Ektachem multilayer dry film method measures total bilirubin by the classic diazo reaction and unconjugated and conjugated bilirubin by the difference in their spectral properties. Delta bilirubin is then calculated by the equation:

$$\text{Delta Bilirubin} = \text{Total Bilirubin} - (\text{Unconjugated Bilirubin} + \text{Conjugated Bilirubin})$$

Total bilirubin, unconjugated bilirubin, and conjugated bilirubin values are determined with the Kodak Ektachem unit. The Kodak method is sensitive and superior for determination of bilirubin fractions. The observed delta bilirubin concentration range in one study in healthy horses was 3 to 6 μmol/L, and the concentration range in sick horses was 0 to 36 μmol/L.[20]

TESTS OF KIDNEY FUNCTION

To compare the kidney with a filter is tempting but naive. Blood coursing through the kidney is not just cleansed but is *changed*. Ion concentrations are regulated, and influential messengers, such as renin, erythropoietin, and activated vitamin D, are added. Hence, monitoring kidney function may be critical.

SODIUM SULFANILATE AND PSP CLEARANCE

These two tests have been used, with success, in the past. Because they are no longer commonly used, however, many veterinarians have not heard of them. They are useful and easily performed and have been included here for completeness.

Kidney filtration is evaluated by injecting inert traceable substances that are excreted in the urine. Sodium sulfanilate is removed only by glomerular filtration in dogs (Procedure 8-15); its disappearance from the plasma is an index of glomerular filtration. The test can detect unilateral nephrectomy, as well as diminished renal function in dogs before azotemia develops. The half-life of sodium sulfanilate is prolonged up to five times in horses with glomerulonephritis. Although the test is also performed in cats, the mode of sodium sulfanilate excretion is not confirmed in this species.

Phenolsulfonphthalein (PSP) is an organic dye excreted by the renal tubules. Nonetheless, its clearance is accepted as a measure of renal blood flow, as this usually limits its efflux more than tubular secretion rates. PSP clearance (Procedure 8-15) is decreased only when more than two thirds of the nephrons are nonfunctional, or when renal perfusion is compromised.

Both of these tests have been largely abandoned in favor of endogenous creatinine clearance.

ENDOGENOUS CREATININE CLEARANCE

Creatinine is derived from degraded muscle or dietary creatinine. It is always present in the blood. Because creatinine appears in the glomerular filtrate with negligible tubular secretion, it is a natural tracer of glomerular filtration. Fortunately, its short-term blood concentrations are stable enough to satisfy the clearance formula used for steady infusion studies of inulin and p-aminohippuric acid, the renal function standards.

Procedure 8-15. Protocol for sodium sulfanilate and PSP clearance

Sodium sulfanilate clearance in dogs, cats, and horses

1. Inject sodium sulfanilate IV at 20 mg/kg (10 mg/kg for horses).
2. Obtain heparinized blood samples at 30, 60, and 90 minutes postinjection. Submit for sodium sulfanilate analysis.
3. Plot the disappearance curve and determine half-life.
4. Dogs: normal half-life is 66 ± 11 minutes; cats: normal half-life is 45.1 ± 7 minutes; horses: normal half-life is 39.5 ± 4 minutes.

PSP urinary test

1. Empty the bladder.
2. Give 6 mg of PSP IV, regardless of patient size.
3. Insert a urinary catheter 10 minutes later.
4. Empty the bladder 15 minutes after PSP injection and rinse with sterile saline until 20 minutes after PSP injection. Save the urine sample and the rinse.
5. Submit an aliquot of the bladder rinse for PSP analysis and determine the percent of total PSP dose excreted.
6. Normal PSP clearance is 43.8 ± 11.1%. Any value less than 30% is abnormal.

PSP plasma test in dogs and cats

1. Give PSP IV at 5 mg/kg.
2. Obtain 3.0-ml blood samples in EDTA at 15, 25, and 35 minutes after PSP injection. Submit for PSP determination.
3. Plot the disappearance curve and determine half-life.
4. Normal half-life is 18 to 24 minutes.

The test is relatively simple (Procedure 8-16). You need only a measure of blood creatinine and an accurate, timed urine collection. Be precise. Sloppy bladder catheterization and sampling ruin the results, especially with the briefer methods. The bladder must be rinsed before and after the test, saving the after-rinses with the urine for creatinine analysis. Clearance is calculated by dividing urinary creatinine excretion (urine creatinine concentration times urine volume) by plasma creatinine concentration. The estimate, if imperfect, is quite practical.

PROCEDURE 8-16. Protocol for endogenous creatinine clearance

1. Obtain a blood sample for creatinine analysis.
2. Catheterize the bladder and rinse the bladder several times with sterile saline. Discard the rinse. Empty the bladder.
3. Begin timing immediately and collect all urine for a 20-minute or 24-hour period (the latter is more precise).
4. At the end of this period (20 minutes or 24 hours), empty the bladder. Measure the total urine volume collected. Rinse the bladder thoroughly with sterile saline. Empty the bladder and save the rinses. Submit an aliquot of urine rinse saline for creatinine analysis:
5. Calculate creatinine clearance with the equation:

$$\text{Creatinine Clearance} = \frac{Uv \times Uc}{Pc}$$

6. Normal clearance in dogs is 2.8 ± 0.96 ml/min/kg.

Uv = urine volume; Uc = urine creatinine concentration; Pc = plasma creatine concentration

---

MODIFIED WATER-DEPRIVATION TEST, VASOPRESSIN RESPONSE

With polyuria/polydipsia, the initial impulse is to blame the kidney. That is too simple. Diuresis and subsequent polydipsia may mean failing nephrons, or kidney function disrupted by hyperadrenocorticism (Cushing's disease), diabetes mellitus, or nephrogenic diabetes insipidus. Or the kidneys may be normal but not receiving the signal to concentrate urine, as in neurogenic diabetes insipidus. Finally, the diuresis may be a totally appropriate renal compensation for pathologic water intake (psychogenic polydipsia).

Some background on the control of urine concentration is essential. Vasopressin or antidiuretic hormone (ADH), from the neurohypophysis, signals the kidneys to retain water. Targeted on the renal collecting duct, it increases the duct's permeability to water. Water in the urine passes out of the collecting duct and into the hypertonic renal medulla, concentrating the urine that remains behind in the collecting duct. If the system fails (inappropriate diuresis), either the neuroendocrine pathway that releases ADH in response to hypovolemia/plasma hyperosmolarity has been interrupted, or the nephrons are unable to respond.

Water-deprivation test.   We examine this system by watching the response to endogenous or exogenous ADH. The trick is to safely dehydrate the patient until there is a definite stimulus for endogenous ADH release (usually at about 5% body weight loss). That endpoint varies. When denied water, patients dehydrate at different rates and must be monitored for weight loss, clinical signs of dehydration, and increased urine osmolarity or specific gravity. At the endpoint, the kidney should be under strictest endocrine orders to concentrate urine. Continued diuresis and dilute urine indicate lack of endogenous ADH or unresponsive nephrons. In dogs with kidney failure, this unresponsiveness precedes azotemia.

Contraindications to this test include dehydration and azotemia. Dehydrated patients risk hypovolemia and shock. They should already have maximal ADH release; if they could concentrate urine, they would. The test then is useless and dangerous, especially in animals with diabetes insipidus or neurogenic diabetes insipidus. Azotemia already attests to kidney dysfunction. Again, the test reveals nothing new and adds a prerenal component to the azotemia.

Vasopressin response.   When patients have these signs or a previous water-deprivation test has failed, a vasopressin response test is indicated. This is simply a challenge with exogenous ADH; it focuses on the kidney's ability to respond. Urine osmolarity or specific gravity is the index of function. Normal kidneys should concentrate urine with this technique, despite the patient's free access to water. Vasopressin must be handled carefully, as it is a labile drug and settles out in oil suspensions. Test failures may result from use of old or poorly mixed solutions. Also, IM vasopressin injection causes pain. Because of vasopressin's vasomotor activity, its use is theoretically contraindicated in pregnancy. However, we have observed no ill effects from its use.

Note that in both tests, even normal kidneys may be unable to concentrate urine to normal extremes. Diuresis quickly washes solutes from the renal medulla, weakening the osmotic gradient that draws water from the collecting ducts. Gradual water deprivation over 3 to 5 days before use of the water deprivation test is recommended to renew renal solutes. This also lets you preview the impact of dehydration on the animal. Some argue, however, that this technique is not superior and simply increases the costs of hospitalization. They prefer a rapid test, at least initially.

MODIFIED WATER-DEPRIVATION TEST. Both of these tests may be combined in a single protocol that may differentiate several causes of polyuria/polydipsia (Procedure 8-17). The modified water-deprivation test is specifically contraindicated in patients with known renal disease, uremia due to prerenal or primary renal disorder, or suspected or obvious dehydration.

URINE PROTEIN/CREATININE RATIO

Quantitative assessment of renal proteinuria is of diagnostic significance in renal disease. In the absence of inflammatory cells in the urine, proteinuria indicates glomerular disease. For accurate determination of proteinuria, a 24-hour urinary protein value should be determined. This is a tedious task and errors are common. A mathematical method that compares the urine protein concentration to the urine creatinine concentrations in a single urine sample is more accurate and comprehensive. This urine protein to creatinine (P/C) ratio is based on the concept that the tubular concentration of urine increases both the urinary protein and creatinine concentrations equally.

This method has been validated for canine species. Usually 5 to 10 ml of urine are collected between 10 AM and 2 PM, preferably by cystocentesis. The urine sample should be kept at 4° C or stored at −20° C. The sample is centrifuged and the supernatant is used. The protein concentration for each sample can be determined by the trichloroacetic acid-ponceau S method (mg/dl) or by using commercial kits for microprotein determination (Microprotein Rapid Stat Diagnostic Kit: Lancer Division of Sherwood Medical, St. Louis, MO).[10] The creatinine concentration can be determined in mg/dl by the alkaline picric method, or by the semiautomated chemistry method (CKDA: American Monitor Corp., Indianapolis, IN).[3]

The urine P/C ratio for healthy dogs should be less than 1. A urine P/C ratio greater than 1 may indicate nephrotic syndrome. A P/C ratio greater than 10 indicates severe glomerulonephritis.[6,36]

TESTS OF GLOMERULAR FUNCTION (GLOMERULAR FILTRATION RATE)

Glomerular function may also be assessed by clearance of radioactive isotopes, such as ^{125}I-iothalamate, ^{131}I-iodohippurate, ^{14}C-inulin, ^{3}H-tetraethylammonium, and [99M]Tc-diethylenetriaminepentaacetic acid. The complexity of these methods has limited their usefulness and they are rarely used outside research institutions.[24]

FRACTIONAL CLEARANCE OF ELECTROLYTES

Fractional clearance (FC) of sodium, potassium, phosphorus, and chloride is increased with renal parenchymal damage. These tests allow differentiation

PROCEDURE 8-17.   Protocol for the modified water-deprivation test in dogs

PREPARATION

1. 72 hours before the test, limit water intake to 120 ml/kg/day in small portions.
2. 48 hours before the test, limit water intake to 90 ml/kg/day.
3. 24 hours before the test, limit water intake to 60 to 80 ml/kg/day.

WATER DEPRIVATION

Before the test:

1. Withdraw food and all water.
2. Empty the bladder completely.
3. Determine the exact body weight.
4. Check the urine osmolality/specific gravity.
5. Obtain a BUN determination to check for azotemia.
6. Check hydration and CNS status.

During the test:

1. Completely empty the bladder and determine the exact body weight every 30 to 60 minutes.
2. Check the urine specific gravity and osmolality at each interval.
3. Check hydration and CNS status at each interval.
4. Recheck the BUN and serum osmolality values.
5. Weigh the patient at each interval.

After the test:

If the dog is clinically dehydrated, appears ill, or has lost about 5% of its body weight:

1. Obtain a blood sample for determination of the vasopressin concentration.
2. Empty the bladder.
3. Collect a final urine sample and check specific gravity and osmolality.

VASOPRESSIN RESPONSE

1. Give 2 to 5 pressor units of aqueous vasopressin IM.
2. Continue withholding food and water.
3. Monitor the patient as follows:
   - Empty the bladder every 30 minutes for 1 to 2 hours maximum.
   - Check urine osmolality ± specific gravity.
   - Check BUN.
   - Check hydration and CNS status.
   - Weigh patient.

PROCEDURE 8-17.—*continued*

AFTER TESTING

1. Introduce small amounts of water (10 to 20 ml/kg) every 30 minutes for 2 hours.
2. Monitor the patient for vomiting, hydration, and CNS status.
3. If the patient is well 2 hours after the test, provide water *ad lib.*

TEST RESULTS

Normal:
1. Urine specific gravity $\geq$1.048.
2. Urine osmolality $\geq$1700 mOsm/kg.
3. Exogenous ADH does not further concentrate the urine after water deprivation.

Psychogenic polydipsia:
1. Urine osmolality is below normal. It can be similar to or above that of serum.
2. Urine specific gravity is 1.015 to 1.020.
3. Exogenous ADH does not further concentrate urine.

Nephrogenic diabetes insipidus:
1. Urine osmolarity does not exceed that of plasma (290 to 310 mOsm).
2. Urine specific gravity is 1.010 to 1.012.
3. Exogenous ADH does not further concentrate urine.
4. The animal dehydrates rapidly.

Neurogenic diabetes insipidus:
1. Urine osmolarity does not exceed 300 mOsm.
2. Urine specific gravity is 1.010 to 1.012.
3. Exogenous ADH causes a 50% to 500% increase in urine concentration (specific gravity 1.020 to 1.030).
4. The animal dehydrates rapidly.

Partial diabetes insipidus:
1. Urine osmolarity is 300 to 1000 mOsm.
2. Exogenous ADH does not further concentrate urine.
3. The animal dehydrates slowly.

Hyperadrenocorticism (Cushing's disease):
1. Urine osmolarity is 300 to 1000 mOsm.
2. Exogenous ADH concentrates urine slightly.
3. The animal dehydrates slowly.

between prerenal problems and renal failure because in prerenal problems, normal results may be expected. Normal results are[9]:

- Dogs: Sodium <1; potassium <20; chloride <1; phosphorus <39
- Cats: Sodium <1; potassium <24; chloride <1.3; phosphorus <73

Fractional clearance may be caluclated using the following equation, where U is the electrolyte concentration in urine and P is the electrolyte concentration in plasma:

$$FC_{electrolyte} = \frac{U_{electrolyte} \times P_{creatinine}}{U_{creatinine} \times P_{electrolyte} \times 100}$$

TESTS OF ADRENOCORTICAL FUNCTION

THE ADRENAL AXIS

Adrenocortical function tests are relatively common. Adrenal dysfunction is increasingly common, too often because of misuse of corticosteroids.

The adrenal axis starts with the hypothalamus. Stimuli originating in the brain, as from stress, cause the hypothalamus to secrete corticotropin-releasing factor (CRF). Under the influence of CRF, the adenohypophysis secretes adrenocorticotrophic hormone (ACTH), the hormone that stimulates adreno-cortical growth and secretion, particularly of glucocorticoid-synthesizing tissue. Cortisol is the major hormone released in domestic mammals. It, in turn, feeds back to inhibit both CRF and ACTH release, completing a balanced system.

True or mimicked hyperfunction of the system is a common complaint. Brain or pituitary tumors leading to secondary bilateral adrenal hyperplasia, idiopathic adrenal hyperplasia, or neoplasia (one or both glands) may all cause excessive endogenous cortisol release and hyperadrenocorticism (Cushing's disease). Overenthusiastic glucocorticoid therapy is the most common exogenous cause of cortisol excess.

Because exogenous, like endogenous, glucocorticoids inhibit adrenotrophic hormones, iatrogenic hyperadrenocorticism is accompanied by the paradox of atrophied adrenal glands. Sudden withdrawal of exogenous glucocorticoids can lead to adrenal hypofunction. However, hypoadrenocorticism (Addison's disease), by definition, includes mineralocorticoid deficiency, which does not occur in iatrogenic disease caused by rapid withdrawal of glucocorticoids. Addison's disease may result from overuse of lysodren (for adrenal hyperplasia) or from idiopathic causes.

Screening tests for hyperadrenocorticism must be carefully interpreted because many dogs with nonadrenal disease (such as diabetes mellitus, liver disease, or renal disease) may have false-positive results.

URINE CORTISOL/CREATININE RATIO

Urine cortisol/creatinine ratio is not a specific test to diagnose hyperadrenocorticism. It, however, helps rule out hyperadrenocorticism. Abnormal results may appear in dogs with hyperadrenocorticism or other diseases, such as diabetes, pyometra, liver failure, or hypercalcemia[26] (Procedure 8-18).

ACTH RESPONSE

Animals with suspected hypoadrenocorticism (Addison's disease) or hyperadrenocorticism (Cushing's disease) can be evaluated with an ACTH response test (Procedure 8-19). The rationale assumes that the adrenal glands will respond to exogenous ACTH stimulation by glucocorticoid release in proportion to the glands' size and development. Hyperplastic adrenal glands have exaggerated responses, while hypoplastic adrenal glands show diminished responses. The test, then, can detect these abnormalities but not reveal their ultimate cause.

The ACTH response test is just a screening test. There is one potential problem: adrenal glands that are hyperactive from neoplasia may be insensitive to ACTH. Nonetheless, current figures indicate that the test is 84% accurate in diagnosing adrenocortical hyperfunction.

In the past, the adrenal glucocorticoid response to ACTH was monitored indirectly by following eosinophil counts. This proved inaccurate, as eosinophils

---

PROCEDURE 8-18. Protocol for urine cortisol/creatinine ratio

1. Obtain a urine sample, attempting to avoid stress.
2. Determine cortisol and creatinine concentrations in μmol/L.
3. Normal canine ratio is less than 1.35×10^{-5}.
   - With spontaneous hyperadrenocorticism, the ratio is between 2×10^{-5} and 210×10^{-5}.
   - With polyuria-polydipsia, the ratio is between 0.8×10^{-5} and 15×10^{-5}.

Procedure 8-19.   Protocol for the ACTH response test

Dogs

1. Collect a plasma sample for cortisol determination before and 1 hour after IM injection of 0.25 mg (25 units) of cosyntropin (Cortrosyn: Organon).

   or

   Collect a plasma sample for cortisol determination before and 2 hours after IM injection of ACTH gel (Cortigel: Savage) at 1 unit/lb. Separate and freeze the plasma samples immediately.
2. Results (vary with laboratory and method of cortisol measure):

Adrenal condition	Pretest cortisol level[a]	Posttest cortisol level[a]
Normal	1-8 µg/dl	8-15 µg/dl
Hyperadrenal[b]	2.5-10.8 µg/dl	11.7-35.7 µg/dl (>15 µg/dl)
Hypoadrenal	0.1-3.5 µg/dl	0.1-6.0 µg/dl[c]

Horses

1. Collect plasma for a baseline cortisol determination (handle as above).
2. Administer 1 unit of ACTH gel/kg and collect plasma samples for cortisol determinations 2, 4, and 8 hours later.
3. Results:
   - Normal: Double or triple baseline value in 4 to 8 hours.
   - Hyperadrenal: four-fold or greater increase from baseline value in 4 to 8 hours.

[a] Competitive protein-binding determination.
[b] Some hyperfunctioning tumors may not respond to ACTH, causing false negatives.
[c] Note that 50% of dogs with Addison's disease have posttest cortisol levels lower than pretest levels.

are usually not numerous in peripheral blood. The method was largely abandoned in favor of plasma cortisol determinations. Note that sporadic measurements of plasma cortisol without some test challenge are diagnostically unreliable, as normal and abnormal ranges overlap. Remember, use of prednisone and prednisolone can interfere with plasma cortisol measurements.

DEXAMETHASONE SUPPRESSION

Dexamethasone suppression tests evaluate the adrenal glands differently, using the adrenal feedback loops. The low-dosage test confirms or replaces the ACTH response test for hyperadrenocorticism (Cushing's disease). The high-dosage test goes further, differentiating pituitary from adrenal causes of hyperadreno-corticism (Procedure 8-20).

PROCEDURE 8-20. Protocol for dexamethasone suppression tests in dogs

LOW DOSAGE

1. Obtain a blood sample for baseline plasma cortisol determination at 8 AM. (Some clinicians also do a 2- or 3-hour test as well.)
2. Immediately give dexamethasone IV at 0.01 mg/kg.
3. At 4 PM (see comment in Step 1 above), obtain postinjection plasma sample for cortisol determination.
4. Results:

ADRENAL CONDITION	PRETEST CORTISOL LEVEL	POSTTEST CORTISOL LEVEL
Normal	1.1-8.0 µg/dl	0.1-0.9 µg/dl (<1.4)
Hyperadrenal	2.5-10.8 µg/dl	1.8-5.2 µg/dl (>1.4)

HIGH DOSAGE

1. Use the same protocol as above, except the dexamethasone dosage is 0.1 mg/kg.
2. Results:
   - Pituitary-dependent hyperadrenocorticism: Normal values as above
   - Adrenal-dependent hyperadrenocorticism: As for hyperadrenal values above

Note: Successful suppression is defined as a 50% decrease in the plasma cortisol concentration from the baseline value. In 15% of dogs with pituitary-dependent hyperadrenocorticism, the plasma cortisol level is not suppressed by 50%. About 20% of dogs with adrenal-dependent hyperadrenocorticism have suppression of the plasma cortisol level by less than 50%, but all values remain above these considered adequate for suppression (greater than 1.5 µg/dl).

Dexamethasone, a potent glucocorticoid, suppresses ACTH release from the normal pituitary gland, resulting in a drop in plasma cortisol concentration. Hyperadrenocorticism of any etiology is usually resistant to suppression from small dexamethasone doses, as a diseased pituitary gland is abnormally insensitive to the drug and continues elaborating excessive ACTH (although 35% of dogs with pituitary-dependent hyperadrenocorticism have a 4-hour post-dexamethasone cortisol level at the baseline concentration.) Neoplastic adrenal glands are autonomously secreting cortisol, independent of endogenous ACTH control. The excessive cortisol production suppresses secretion of ACTH by the normal pituitary gland through negative-feedback inhibition. Small doses of dexamethasone do not affect plasma cortisol measurements. However, such doses may complicate test results and can only differentiate normal animals from those with hyperadrenocorticism.

With larger dexamethasone doses, more differences appear. The sensitivity of a diseased pituitary gland to dexamethasone is incomplete; large dexamethasone doses overcome it and the abnormally high plasma ACTH and cortisol concentrations fall. Abnormal adrenal glands, however, continue to autonomously secrete cortisol. Thus plasma cortisol concentrations unresponsive to all dexamethasone doses are probably caused by primary adrenal gland disease. Suppression by large but not small doses suggests pituitary gland disease. The test has 73% accuracy in differentiating pituitary from adrenal causes.

A protocol for combined high-dosage dexamethasone test and ACTH response test is described in Procedure 8-21. Although combined protocol is a step saver, possibly ambiguous results necessitate more tests and expense. The ACTH response segment of the test is particularly prone to error. Because dexamethasone alters the adrenal responsiveness to ACTH (enhances or inhibits, depending on the duration of activity), the timing of the test is crucial. Normal standards must be newly established for any changes in protocol.

ENDOGENOUS ACTH CONCENTRATIONS

Although not strictly a function test, assay of plasma ACTH concentrations may be a helpful diagnostic aid for hypo- and hyperadrenocorticism. Normal plasma ACTH concentrations range from 20 to 100 pg/ml, averaging 46 pg/ml. Animals with functioning adrenocortical tumors have extremely low concentrations (less than 20 pg/ml) from the negative-feedback effect, as do animals with pituitary-dependent hypoadrenocorticism. Those with pituitary-dependent hyperadrenocorticism have variable but often high concentrations (29 to 340 pg/ml; usually greater than 40 pg/ml), responsible for secondary adrenal hyperfunction. Dogs with primary hypoadrenocorticism have ACTH concen-

---

PROCEDURE 8-21. Protocol for combined dexamethasone suppression and ACTH response tests in dogs

1. Obtain a baseline blood sample for cortisol determination, centrifuge, remove the serum, and freeze immediately (handle all samples this way).
2. Give dexamethasone IV at 0.1 mg/kg.
3. Obtain a second blood sample in 3 to 4 hours.
4. Give ACTH (Cortigel:Savage) (timing crucial!) IM at 2.2 units/kg to a maximum of 40 units and collect a third blood sample 2 hours later. Alternatively, you may use 0.25 mg of cosyntropin (Cortrosyn:Organon) IV and obtain a third blood sample 1 hour later.
5. Submit serum samples for cortisol analyses.
6. Results (normal values vary with the laboratory):

	BASELINE **CORTISOL LEVEL**	**POSTDEXAMETHASONE** **CORTISOL LEVEL**	**POSTACTH** **CORTISOL LEVEL**
Normal	0.5-4.0 µg/dl	<1.5 µg/dl	8-15 µg/dl
Pituitary-dependent hyperadrenocorticism	Normal to increased	>50% suppression	>20% suppression
Adrenocortical tumor	Normal to increased	<30% suppression	Variable

7. Wait 48 hours before repeating the test.

---

trations over 50 pg/ml.[26] Many laboratories across the nation now offer the assay; the price is no longer prohibitive.

TESTS OF THYROID FUNCTION

Thyroid hormones have pervasive effects, influencing the metabolic rate, growth, and differentiation of all body cells. Because the clinical signs of thyroid malfunction are numerous and confusing, function tests are valuable.

The thyroid glands are governed like the adrenal cortices. Thyrotropin-releasing factor (TRF) from the hypothalamus encourages the anterior pituitary to release thyrotropin or thyroid stimulating hormone (TSH). TSH enhances thyroid growth, function, and thyroxine release. Thyroxine is really comprised of two kinds of hormones, T_3 and T_4, varying in their extent of iodination. T_4 is also converted to more active T_3 in tissues. Thyroxine completes the regulatory cycle by inhibiting TRF and TSH release.

Thyroid disease is manifested primarily as hypofunction in dogs, horses, ruminants, and swine, and hyperfunction in cats. The cause may be dietary iodine deficiency or excess, or goitrogens, most common in large animals. Primary glandular disease (neoplasia, autoimmune disease, idiopathic atrophy) or pituitary/hypothalamic disease (secondary and tertiary thyroid disease, respectively) may also be responsible. In food animals, diagnosis is based on clinical signs (abortion, stillbirths, alopecia, and goiter in fetuses and neonates), serum thyroxine concentrations, serum protein-bound iodine concentrations, and pasture iodine analyses. Feeds may be examined for goitrogenic plants (brassicas) or excess calcium, which decreases iodine uptake.

TSH RESPONSE

This test is used on small animals (except in cats with hyperthyroidism) and horses and provides the most reliable diagnostic separation of patients with normal vs. abnormal thyroid function (Procedure 8-22). The major problem with this test is availability of low-cost TSH.

Baseline thyroxine concentrations are used diagnostically but normal values vary dramatically. Their diagnostic inadequacy mirrors that of plasma cortisol determinations. Exogenous TSH challenge may sort out borderline cases and separate real hypothyroid patients from those with other illness or drug-depressed thyroxine concentrations and may also pinpoint the site of the lesions.

The test is usually used to explore canine hypothyroidism. After TSH is injected, thyroid response (usually serum T_4 levels; the most reliable index) is followed. An increase in the serum T_4 level occurs in normal animals. Primarily exhausted or insensitive thyroids do not respond to exogenous TSH. Indeed, endogenous TSH concentrations are already high from failing thyroxine inhibition. Therefore there is no increased serum T_4 level in these animals. With pituitary or brain disease, however, the thyroid glands remain responsive. Such lesions result in too little endogenous thyrotropin. Although an increase in the serum T_4 level is expected in animals with pituitary or brain lesions, 2 to 3 days of TSH challenge may be necessary before increased serum T_4 levels are seen. The extra TSH is required to overcome chronic glandular atrophy, similar to "priming the pump."

Procedure 8-22.   Protocol for the TSH response test

Dogs and Cats

1. Collect a blood sample for a baseline serum T_4 determination.
2. Administer TSH IV at 5 units/10 kg (dogs) or at 1 unit/kg (cats).
3. Collect a second blood sample 4 to 6 hours later for a serum T_4 determination.
4. Results:
    - Euthyroid patients: second serum T_4 level is increased above baseline (consult your laboratory for reference intervals).
    - Primary hypothyroidism: Little or no increase in the second serum T_4 level above baseline; the baseline serum T_4 level is normal or low.
    - Secondary or tertiary hypothyroidism: Second serum T_4 level is greater than baseline, and the baseline value is low. This response may require 2 to 3 days' "priming" with 5 to 10 units of TSH given SC or IM daily to overcome thyroid atrophy.

Horses

1. Collect a blood sample for a serum T_4 determination.
2. Give 20 units of TSH IM.
3. Collect a second blood sample 12 hours postinjection for another serum T_4 determination.
4. Results: An increase of greater than two times the baseline value indicates normal gland function.*

---

*Always weigh the significance of an increased serum T_4 value together with the absolute value of the baseline concentration. For example, pre- and postinjection serum T_4 values of 0.2 μg/dl and 0.4 μg/dl, respectively, represent a doubling of the T_4 serum level, but both values are very low; the patient could still have primary hypothyroidism.

Hypothyroidism's insidious onset is rarely recognized. If it is suspected, be aware that animals with early primary hypothyroidism may have some slight TSH responsiveness. Glucocorticoids seem to inhibit both TSH and thyroxine secretion, so euthyroidism with only low serum T_3 levels often accompanies Cushing's disease or vigorous glucocorticoid therapy. Fortunately, the TSH and ACTH response tests may be performed simultaneously. In such animals, the glands remain responsive to TSH but the absolute values of pre- and postchallenge serum T_4 are low or low resting with normal post-TSH values.

Feline hyperthyroidism is usually due to functional thyroid adenomas. Oddly, with exogenous TSH challenge, there is little or no increase in the serum T_4 level, as in canine primary hypothyroidism. This suggests that either the neoplasm functions independently of the trophic hormone or is already manufacturing and leaking thyroxine at maximum capacity. A lack of TSH responsiveness, appropriate clinical manifestations, and high baseline plasma thyroxine concentrations all attest to feline hyperthyroidism.

In horses, iodine-deficiency hypothyroidism is rare because iodized salt usually is offered free choice or in feeds. Overzealous iodine supplementation with kelp meal or vitamin-mineral mixes, however, provokes hypothyroidism and goiter. Excessive use of iodine inhibits thyroid function. When assessing thyroid function in horses, remember that normal serum T_4 values are 1 to 3 μg/dl. This is lower than in other species. Hypothyroidism should only be suspected with serum T_4 concentrations of less than 0.5 μg/dl.

Rare tumors of the pars intermedia of the pituitary, compressing the anterior pituitary, may cause secondary hypothyroidism in older horses. Because pituitary damage induces a plethora of signs, the TSH response test may be especially helpful. On the horizon for thyroid testing is the plasma TSH and TRH assay, like the ACTH assay for adrenal function. A radioimmunoassay for TSH is available for people, but the antiglobulin has doubtful specificity for animal TSH. Already popular are nuclear medicine studies of thyroid function involving radioactive tracers. However, these are rather expensive and laborious.

TRH RESPONSE

This test is used on small animals and provides a reliable diagnostic separation of patients with normal vs. abnormal thyroid function. FT_4 is the fraction of thyroxine that is not bound to protein. FT_4 levels are less influenced by nonthyroidal diseases or drugs than total T_4 (TT_4) concentrations. Exogenous TRH challenge may sort out borderline cases and separate real hypothyroid and hyperthyroid patients from those with other illness or drug-depressed thyroxine concentrations. The test is usually used to explore canine hypothyroidism when TSH is not available. Baseline serum TT_4 and FT_4 concentrations are determined. Four hours after 100 μg or 200 μg (total dose) of TRH is injected intravenously, thyroid response (serum TT_4 and FT_4 levels) is followed. An increase of the serum TT_4 (1.7 times) and FT_4 (1.9 times) concentrations, compared with baseline concentrations, occurs in normal animals. Evaluation of FT_4 levels allows a clearer distinction between euthyroid and hypothyroid dogs when TT_4 results are equivocal.[34]

TRH response may be used to diagnose mild-to-moderate feline hyperthyroidism. Baseline serum TT_4 and FT_4 concentrations are determined. Four hours after TRH is injected intravenously at 100 µg/kg, serum TT_4 and FT_4 levels are determined. An increase of the serum TT_4 less than 50%, compared with baseline concentrations, occurs in hyperthyroid cats. Increases between 50% and 60% are borderline, and increases over 60% rule out hyperthyroidism.[27]

TESTS OF GLUCOSE HOMEOSTASIS

The remaining endocrine function tests focus on maintenance of blood glucose levels. This is crucial, as brain cells, among others, must constantly be supplied with glucose as fuel. Accordingly, glucose metabolism is very closely regulated. Glucagon, thyroxine, growth hormone, epinephrine, and glucocorticoids are all agents favoring hyperglycemia. They boost blood glucose levels by encouraging glycogenolysis, gluconeogenesis, and/or lipolysis, while discouraging glucose entry into cells. Insulin is the sole hypoglycemic hormone. Promoting glucose flux into its target cells, it also triggers anabolism, a process that converts glucose to other substances. This regulatory effect prevents blood glucose concentration from exceeding the renal threshold, with the consequent spilling of glucose into the urine.

Regulation of blood glucose levels is complex. The pancreatic islets respond directly to blood glucose concentrations and release insulin (from the beta cells) or glucagon (from the alpha cells) as needed. Glucagon release also directly stimulates insulin release. Epinephrine is under direct sympathetic neural control; hyperglycemia is one aspect of the classic "flight or fight" state. The other hormones mentioned respond to hypothalamic/pituitary command. At any one time, most of these agents are shifting the blood glucose concentration up or down.

Because only insulin lowers blood glucose concentrations, aberrations of insulin action have the most obvious clinical effects. Hypofunction (diabetes mellitus) or hyperfunction (hyperinsulinism) can occur.

GLUCOSE TOLERANCE
Glucose tolerance tests directly challenge the pancreas with a glucose load and measure insulin's effect via blood or urine glucose concentrations. If adequate insulin is released and its target cells have healthy receptors, the artificially elevated blood glucose drops to normal within roughly 2 hours, and no glucose appears in the urine. Prolonged hyperglycemia and glucosuria are consistent

with diabetes mellitus. Profound hypoglycemia after challenge may indicate a glucose-responsive, hyperactive beta-cell tumor of the pancreas.

The oral glucose tolerance test has been described earlier in this chapter as a test of intestinal absorption. Because test results are affected by abnormal intestinal function (enteritis, hypermotility, etc.) and excitement (as from gastric intubation), an IV glucose tolerance test is preferred. The IV test is the only practical option for ruminants.

With the IV glucose tolerance test (Procedure 8-23), a challenge glucose load is injected after a 12- to 24-hour fast (except in ruminants). Blood glucose is subsequently checked and its progress mapped as a tolerance curve. Results

---

PROCEDURE 8-23. Protocol for the intravenous glucose tolerance test

1. Check the animal's diet. If it is low in carbohydrates, feed a high-carbohydrate diet (100 to 200 g/day for dogs) for 3 days before the test.
2. Fast the animal for 12 to 24 hours or long enough to lower the blood glucose level to 70 mg/dl in patients with suspected hyperinsulinism (do not fast ruminants). *Fasting is very dangerous in dogs with insulinoma!*
3. Obtain a preinjection blood sample in a sodium fluoride tube for a baseline blood glucose determination.
4. Begin timing the trial as you infuse a sterile 50% glucose solution IV at 0.5 g/kg. Complete the infusion in exactly 30 seconds for small animals and within 2 to 3 minutes for large animals.
5. Obtain blood samples at 5, 15, 25, 35, 45, 60, 90, and 120 minutes after glucose infusion, using sodium fluoride as an anticoagulant, and submit all blood samples for glucose assay.
6. Plot glucose values on a semilog graph and determine the serum glucose half-life or turnover rate.
7. Results (values in species other than dogs and cats may be comparable):
   - Dogs: The postinfusion blood glucose level should fall to baseline by 90 minutes. The normal half-life of glucose is 25 ± 8 min and the normal turnover time is 2.76 ± 0.91%/min. A turnover time of 2.0%/min indicates diabetes mellitus, and >2.0%/min but <2.5%/min indicates an insulin-secreting tumor (see text).
   - Cats: The postinfusion blood glucose level should fall to baseline by 120 to 180 minutes.

are standardized as disappearance half-live or glucose turnover rates (turnover rate = 0.693/half-life × 100).

Decreased glucose tolerance (increased half-life, decreased turnover rate) occurs in diabetes mellitus and less consistently in hyperthyroidism, hyperadrenocorticism, hyperpituitarism, and severe liver disease. Increased glucose tolerance (decreased half-life, increased turnover rate) is observed with hypothyroidism, hypoadrenocorticism, hypopituitarism, and hyperinsulinism. However, results can be erroneous. Normal animals on low-carbohydrate diets may manifest "diabetic curves." Hence, we recommend 2 to 3 days of high-carbohydrate meals before testing. The IV glucose tolerance test results are so variable in normal horses, depending on diet and fasting, that they are not very useful.

Frankly, glucose tolerance tests are usually unnecessary. Persistent hyperglycemia and glucosuria, frequently with a history of polyuria, polydipsia, polyphagia, and weight loss, are sufficient to diagnose diabetes mellitus. The test may be of value in detecting hyperinsulinism, as most beta-cell tumors of the pancreas are not rapidly responsive to glucose. They may even cause diabetic glucose tolerance curves because insulin-antagonist hormones are released due to the initial hypoglycemia. Glucose tolerance test results are also affected by patient stress and chemical restraint. Serum glucose measurements themselves may be erroneously low if blood samples are not anticoagulated and are allowed to sit at room temperature. However, the test is still used.

The best use for the glucose tolerance test is in animals with borderline hyperglycemia without glucosuria. However, this test is not cost effective for the owner and may not result in significant therapeutic change. This dilemma is most often seen in cats in which high renal thresholds for glucose and stress-induced hyperglycemia are common and misleading.

Extra information may be obtained from the IV glucose tolerance test if immunoreactive insulin concentrations are followed simultaneously. This protocol may differentiate diabetes mellitus due to absolute lack of insulin from that due to target-cell insensitivity.

INSULIN TOLERANCE

This test also probes the causes of diabetes mellitus. Specifically, it checks the responsiveness of target cells to challenge with 0.1 unit (or more) of crystalline zinc insulin/kg SC or IM. Serum glucose levels are measured in blood samples obtained before insulin injection (fasting-blood glucose) and every 30 minutes after injection, for 3 hours. If the serum glucose level fails to drop to 50% of the fasting concentration within 30 minutes of insulin injection (insulin resistance), the insulin receptors are unresponsive or insulin action is being severely antagonized. The latter occurs in hyperadrenocorticism, the primary indication for the test in horses. Insulin resistance profoundly influences prognostic and therapeutic decisions.

If the insulin-induced hypoglycemia persists for 2 hours (hypoglycemia unresponsiveness), suspect hyperinsulinism, hypopituitarism, or hypoadreno-corticism. Because the test may cause this hypoglycemia, with possible weakness and convulsions, always have a glucose solution on hand for rapid IV administration.

GLUCAGON TOLERANCE

The main indications for this test are repeated normal or borderline results with the amended insulin:glucose ratio test (see discussion following) or lack of an insulin assay. The glucagon tolerance test gives us another assessment of hyperinsulinism. Glucagon stimulates the pancreatic beta cells directly and indirectly to increase the blood insulin level. In normal animals, glucagon injection (0.03 mg/kg IV up to a total of 1 mg in dogs and 0.5 mg in cats) transiently elevates the blood glucose level to greater than 135 mg/dl. In normal animals, this concentration returns to fasting concentrations. If the animal has a pancreatic beta-cell tumor, the serum glucose level peak is lower than normal and is followed within 1 hour by hypoglycemia (serum glucose less than 60 mg/dl), as excessive insulin is secreted by the stimulated neoplasm.

To perform the test, the patient is fasted until the serum glucose level dips below 90 mg/dl (usually less than 10 hours). Glucagon is injected and sodium fluoride-anticoagulated blood samples are obtained before glucagon injection and 1, 3, 5, 15, 30, 45, 60, and 120 minutes after injection to monitor the glucose response. Unfortunately, the test is insensitive and may cause hypogly-cemia convulsions up to 4 hours later. Patients must be fed immediately after the test and observed for hours.

AMENDED INSULIN : GLUCOSE RATIO

You can better assess the cause of hyperinsulinism by taking simultaneous measurements of serum glucose and insulin levels. Hypoglycemia normally inhibits insulin secretion. Pancreatic beta-cell tumors, hyperactive and unre-sponsive to glucose, secrete an abundance of insulin inappropriate to the prevailing blood glucose concentration. Although fasting serum insulin concen-trations are often normal in hyperinsulinism, ratios of insulin to glucose concentrations are usually aberrant.

The absolute ratio of insulin to glucose can be amended to increase diagnostic accuracy. The amended insulin:glucose ratio (AIGR) subtracts 30 from the serum glucose concentration (Procedure 8-24). At a serum glucose level of 30 mg/dl or less, insulin is normally undetectable, so this discriminant puts the zero of both the glucose and insulin scale at the same physiologic place. Because abnormally high insulin concentrations are more obvious at low serum glucose concentrations, the AIGR is most valuable in animals with a hypoglycemia of less than 60 mg/dl. However, the test is not totally dependable. Repeat the procedure or try other tests if the results are unconvincing.

PROCEDURE 8-24. Protocol for amended insulin : glucose ratio determination

1. Feed the patient a normal meal at 8 AM, then begin fast.
2. Obtain a blood sample in a sodium fluoride tube every 2 to 3 hours for blood glucose assays. Save any samples with blood glucose values less than 60 mg/dl* for the immunoreactive insulin assay (usually occurs within 6 to 10 hours). Stop the test. If an immediate blood glucose assay is unavailable, obtain blood samples for 8 hours and then stop the test. Instruct the laboratory to measure the serum insulin concentration on the sample with the lowest blood glucose value. If the blood glucose value does not fall below 60 mg/dl in 8 to 10 hours, feed the patient at 5 PM, 8:30 PM and 12 PM and repeat the test by beginning fasting at midnight and obtaining blood samples from 8 AM to 5 PM the next day (if necessary).
3. Feed the patient several small meals over the next 2 hours after testing to avoid postprandial reactive hypoglycemia.
4. Compute the AIGR:

$$AIGR = \frac{\text{Plasma Insulin Level (U/ml)} \times 100}{\text{Plasma Glucose Level (mg/dl)} - 30}$$

5. *Results:* A normal AIGR for dogs is 8.2 to 25.6.[†] Some authors suggest any ratio less than 30 is normal. If the animal is insulinopenic (insulin concentration less than 6 U/ml), it probably does not have a pancreatic beta-cell tumor, regardless of the AIGR.

---

*Patients with hyperinsulinism usually do not exhibit clinical signs at this level of hypoglycemia.
[†]Varies with the laboratory.

Miscellaneous tests of insulin release

When results of a glucagon response test or AIGR are equivocal, glucose, leucine, tolbutamide, or calcium challenges may be tried. These substances, like glucagon, may provoke a hyperinsulinemic response from pancreatic islet-cell tumors, resulting in decreased serum glucose levels. However, tumors vary in their sensitivity to these agents and false negatives (no response) can occur. These tests are also dangerous, as they can precipitate severe, prolonged hypoglycemia.

References

1. Anderson: Pancreatitis in dogs, *Vet Clin North Am* 2:79-97, 1972.

2. Batt, et al: A new test for the diagnosis of exocrine pancreatic insufficiency in the dog, *J Small Anim Pract* 20: 185-192, 1979.

3. Bonsnes and Taussky: On the colorimetric determination of creatinine by the Jaffe reaction, *J Biol Chem* 158:581-591, 1945.

4. Burrows and Merritt: Assessment of gastrointestinal function. In Anderson, editor: *Veterinary gastroenterology,* ed 2, Philadelphia, 1992, Lea & Febiger, pp 16-42.

5. Callery, et al: Hepatic insufficiency after portacaval shunting is prevented by prior intraportal pancreatic islet autotransplantation, *Surgery* 106:257-266, 1989.

6. Center, et al: 24-hour urine protein/creatinine ratio in dogs with protein-losing nephropathies, *JAVMA* 187:820-824, 1985.

7. Center, et al: Direct spectrophotometric determination of serum bile acid in dogs and cats, *Am J Vet Res* 45:2043-2050, 1984.

8. Center: Pathophysiology, laboratory diagnosis, and diseases of the liver. In Ettinger and Feldman, editors: *Textbook of veterinary internal medicine,* ed 4, Philadelphia, 1995, WB Saunders, pp 1261-1312.

9. Di Bartola: Clinical approach and laboratory evaluation of renal disease. In Ettinger and Feldman, editors: *Textbook of veterinary internal medicine,* ed 4, Philadelphia, 1995, WB Saunders, pp 1706-1719.

10. DiBartola, et al: Urinary protein excretion and immunopathologic findings in dogs with glomerular disease, *JAVMA* 177:73-77, 1980.

11. DiMagno, et al: Relations between pancreatic enzyme outputs and malabsorption of severe pancreatic insufficiency, *N Engl J Med* 288: 813-815, 1973.

12. Edwards and Russell: Probable vitamin K–deficient bleeding in two cats with malabsorption syndrome secondary to lymphocytic-plasmacytic enteritis, *J Vet Int Med* 1:97-101, 1987.

13. Emm, et al: The rate of D-xylose absorption in normal cats, *Aust Vet J* 60:30-32, 1983.

14. Hall and Batt: Differential sugar absorption for the assessment of canine intestinal permeability: the cellobiose/mannitol test in gluten-sensitive enteropathy of Irish setters, *Res Vet Sci* 51:83-87, 1991.

15. Hall and Batt: Enhanced intestinal permeability to ^{51}Cr-labeled EDTA in dogs with small intestinal disease, *J Am Vet Med Assoc* 196:91-95, 1990.

16. Happé and de Bruijne: Pentagastrin-stimulated gastric secretion in the dog (orogastric aspiration technique), *Res Vet Sci* 33:232-239, 1982.

17. Hawkins, et al: Digestion of bentiromide and absorption of xylose in healthy cats and absorption in cats with infiltrative intestinal disease, *Am J Vet Res* 47:567-569, 1986.

18. Joy and Patterson: Short bowel syndrome following surgical correction of double intussusception in a dog, *Can Vet J* 19:254-259, 1978.

19. Kaneko: *Clinical biochemistry of domestic animals,* ed 4, New York, 1989, Academic Press, p 380.

20. Lumsden, et al: Contribution of delta bilirubin to the interpretation of hyperbilirubinemia in the horse—a pilot study, *Can Vet J* 32:169-172, 1991.

21. Macby, et al: The short bowel revisited, *Surgery* 79:1-2, 1976.

22. McGowan and Wills: The diagnostic value of fecal trypsin estimation in chronic pancreatic disease, *J Clin Pathol* 15:62-68, 1962.

23. Merritt and Duely: Phloroglucinol microassay for plasma xylose in dogs and horses, *Am J Vet Res* 44:2184-2185, 1983.

24. Moe and Heiene: Estimation of glomerular filtration rate in dogs with [99M]Tc-DTPA and iohexol, *Res Vet Sci* 58:138-143, 1995.

25. Morris, et al: Diarrhoea and increased intestinal permeability in laboratory Beagles associated with proximal small intestinal bacterial overgrowth, *Lab Anim* 28:313-319, 1994.

26. Nelson, et al: Endocrine, metabolic, and lipid disorders. In Willard, Tvedten, and Turnwald, editors: *Small animal clinical diagnosis by laboratory methods,* ed 2, Philadelphia, 1994, WB Saunders, pp 147-178.

27. Peterson: Hyperthyroid diseases. In Ettinger and Feldman, editors: *Textbook of veterinary internal medicine,* ed 4, Philadelphia, 1995, WB Saunders, pp 1466-1487.

28. Renner, et al: Caffeine: a model compound for measuring liver function, *Hepatology* 4:38-46, 1984.

29. Rodbard, et al: Rapid calculation of radioimmunoassay results, *J Lab Clin Med* 74:770-781, 1969.

30. Rothuizen: Rectal ammonia tolerance test in the evaluation of portal circulation in dogs with liver disease, *Res Vet Sci* 33:22-25, 1982.

31. Rutgers, et al: Small intestinal bacterial overgrowth in dogs with chronic intestinal disease, *J Am Vet Med Assoc* 206:187-193, 1995.

32. Saunders and Wormsley: Pancreatic extracts in the treatment of pancreatic exocrine insufficiency, *Gut* 16:157-162, 1975.

33.   Sherding, et al: Bentiromide : xylose test in healthy cats, *Am J Vet Res* 43:2272-2273, 1982.

34.   Sparkes, et al: Assessment of dose and time responses to TRH and thyrotropin in healthy dogs, *J Small Anim Pract* 36:245-251, 1995.

35.   Strombeck and Harrold: Evaluation of 60-minute blood p-aminobenzoic acid concentration in pancreatic function testing of dogs, *JAVMA* 180:419-421, 1982.

36.   White, et al: Use of protein-to-creatinine ratio in a single urine specimen for quantitative estimation of canine proteinuria, *JAVMA* 185:882-885, 1984.

37.   Williams and Batt: Diagnosis of canine exocrine pancreatic insufficiency by the assay of serum trypsin-like immunoreactivity, *J Small Anim Pract* 24:583-588, 1983.

38.   Williams, et al: Fecal proteolytic activity in clinically normal cats and in a cat with exocrine pancreatic insufficiency, *JAVMA* 197:210-212, 1990.

39.   Zimmer and Todd: Further evaluation of bentiromide in the diagnosis of canine exocrine pancreatic insufficiency, *Cornell Vet* 75:426-440, 1985.

IMMUNOLOGY AND SEROLOGY

E. Hill

It has long been known that animals in the recovery phase of an infectious disease are resistant to reinfection. *Immunity* (from the Latin *immunis,* meaning safe) was the word used to describe this state of heightened resistance.

The goal of the body's immune response is to combat the effects of foreign substances on vital bodily processes. To accomplish this, the body must be able to recognize minute differences among foreign substances and between foreign substances and itself. After a substance is recognized as foreign, there must be a means of responding to it physiologically, thus eliminating or limiting any harmful effects of the agent. To facilitate a future immune response to an encounter with the same agent, memory components for the foreign material are required.

Occasionally, the immune system malfunctions, resulting in such disorders as allergy, immunodeficiency, neoplasia, or auto-immune disease.

This chapter reviews the basic principles of immunity and the immune response and the practical applications of immunology that have been developed, including vaccination and immunodiagnostic procedures.

THE IMMUNE RESPONSE

Vertebrate species have two major internal defense systems: the *innate* or *non-specific immune system* and the *acquired* or *specific immune system.* Foreign bodies, such as bacteria, viruses, and fungi, first encounter barriers of the innate immune system. These include the skin; physical and biochemical components in the nasopharynx, gut, lungs, and genitourinary tract; and the body's inflammatory response. The body also has populations of commensal bacteria that compete with invading pathogens.

Another major function of the innate system is *phagocytosis,* a nonspecific response. Phagocytic cells (the chief phagocyte is the macrophage) ingest and destroy inert particles, viruses, bacteria, and cellular debris. Macrophages are found throughout the body. In the blood they are called monocytes. From the blood they migrate to various tissues and organs and are then called macrophages or other specialized names. They locate in connective tissue, liver, brain, lung, spleen, bone marrow, and lymph nodes and together comprise the mononuclear phagocytic system.

If foreign bodies evade the innate immune system, they then encounter the acquired immune system, which is more sophisticated. The acquired immune system has the ability to respond specifically to foreign substances. These substances, or *antigens,* can be bacterial, viral, fungal, or altered endogenous cells of the host's body. Their presence initiates humoral and cellular responses that neutralize, detoxify, and eliminate these foreign materials from the host.

Lymphocytes and their progeny are the cell types largely responsible for the acquired immune system. This line of defense is not, however, divorced from the innate immune system. It is now clear that macrophages process antigens and present them to antigen-committed lymphocytes. That is, they act as antigen-presenting cells.

Lymphoid stem cells develop first in the yolk sac and then in the fetal liver (Figure 9-1). The bone marrow assumes this responsibility near parturition and serves as the source of these cells throughout postnatal life. The lymphoid stem cells are destined to further mature in one of two places: the bone marrow or the thymus. B-lymphocytes mature in the bone marrow, while T-lymphocytes mature in the thymus.

The acquired immune system is divided into two components: the *humoral immune system* and the *cell-mediated immune system.*

THE HUMORAL IMMUNE SYSTEM

Lymphocytes that mature in the bone marrow (B-cells) are concerned chiefly with production and secretion of immunoglobulin (Ig) molecules, which are also known as *antibodies.* Many clones of B-cells differentiate, each of which is programmed to respond to a specific antigen. Their maturation process consists of three stages: the lymphoblast, the prolymphocyte, and the mature lymphocyte. The mature cells leave the bone marrow to seed secondary lymphoid organs, chiefly the spleen and lymph nodes.

When an antigen enters the body and encounters its mature antigen-committed B-cell (one that will specifically bind with that invading antigen), the antigen and B-cell interact. The B-cell processes the antigen and couples it

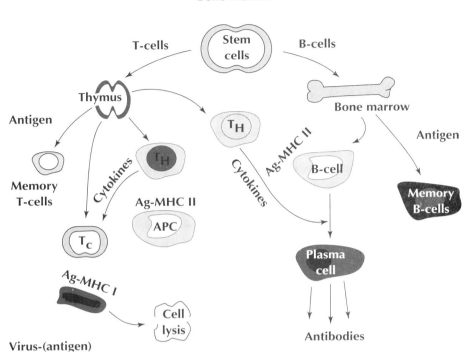

FIGURE 9-1. Pathways of lymphoid cells in the immune response. Stem cells in the bone marrow give rise to T- and B-lymphocytes. Lymphocytes mature in the thymus and bone marrow. Memory and effector cells differentiate and proliferate upon interaction with antigens. T_H, T-helper lymphocytes. T_C, T-cytotoxic lymphocyte. *APC,* antigen-presenting cell.

with an MHC II molecule (major histocompatibility complex) from its (B-cell) surface. A T-helper lymphocyte then binds with the antigen/MHC II complex and releases cytokines. One of its cytokines "helps" B-cells proliferate and differentiate into antibody-secreting plasma cells. The B-cells may also differentiate into memory B-cells, which respond faster to a second exposure of antigen (Figure 9-1). MHC I and MHC II molecules are involved in interactions between T- and B-lymphocytes, between T-lymphocytes and antigen-presenting cells, and between T-lymphocytes and antigen-infected cells (Figure 9-1).

Antibodies (immunoglobulins) are proteins consisting of two distinct functional portions. One portion of the antibody molecule, the variable portion, is specific for the antigen. The other portion of the antibody molecule, the constant portion, is the same in all antibodies of the same class. When an antigen is encountered by an appropriate antibody, the antibody binds to the antigen to form a complex.

Immunoglobulins (Ig) are divided into distinct classes, each with unique biologic properties. The most abundant of these classes is IgG, the major immunoglobulin in serum. It plays the major role in humoral immunity.

IgM, the largest antibody, is the first antibody to appear in response to exposure to an antigen. Its concentration rapidly declines, followed by an increase in IgG concentration, which is also specific for the same antigen. Functions of IgG and IgM include bacterial toxin neutralization, activation of complement, and phagocytic enhancement.

IgA prevents attachment of pathogens to mucosal surfaces and is important in protection of the respiratory, intestinal, and urogenital tracts. High levels of IgE are found in allergic and parasitized individuals. IgD is a B-lymphocyte surface antigen receptor in some species.

CELL-MEDIATED IMMUNITY

Lymphoid stem cells that mature in the thymus develop into *T-cell lymphocytes*. Like that of B-cells, their maturation process consists of three morphologically distinct stages: lymphoblast, prolymphocyte, and lymphocyte. As these cells mature, they develop receptors to specific antigens and become "immunocompetent or antigen-committed" T-lymphocytes. Then, after contact with a specific antigen, the cells proliferate and differentiate into either *memory cells* or *effector cells* against that antigen.

Memory cells recognize antigens to which they have previously been exposed. On a subsequent encounter, they elicit a more rapid immune response.

There are different types of T-effector cells, such as helper T-cells (CD4+) and cytotoxic T-cells (CD8+). CD4+ and CD8+ refer to surface molecules, or markers, found on helper T (T_H) and cytotoxic T (T_C) lymphocytes, respectively. These terms are noteworthy because it is the T_H (CD4+) lymphocytes for which HIV (human immunodeficiency virus), the AIDS virus, has a special affinity. T-helpers, in addition to their function in humoral immunity, affect the actions of other cells, such as cytotoxic T-lymphocytes.

An antigen may be picked up by an antigen-presenting cell (APC), such as a macrophage, which then processes it and brings it to its surface in association with its MHC II molecule. A T-helper cell can then link with the antigen and

MHC II and release cytokines. Cytokines affect the actions of cytotoxic T-lymphocytes. A cytotoxic T-lymphocyte attaches to an infected cell that has processed antigen and an MHC I molecule on its surface. For example, this may be a virus-infected cell. Cytokines cause a cytotoxic lymphocyte to ultimately lyse a body cell that is infected with an endogenous organism, like the virus (Figure 9-1).

IMMUNIZATION

Animals become actively resistant to disease by having the disease and developing antibodies, or by being vaccinated or immunized, in which case they also develop their own antibodies. They become passively resistant by receiving maternal antibodies in the colostrum, or by receiving preformed antibodies by injection.

Vaccine is produced by injecting a suspension of microorganisms into an animal for the purpose of eliciting an antibody response but not causing the disease. The microorganisms may be either attenuated (weakened but still alive) or inactivated (killed). Attenuated vaccines normally cause a longer-lasting, more potent immune response. Inactivated vaccines are generally safer and have no ability to cause disease. After some time and when the antibody titer (serum level) is high enough, the injected animal's serum is collected and processed. An adjuvant may be added to the vaccine to enhance the normal immune response. Some adjuvants do this by simply slowing the rate of antigen elimination from the body so the antigen is present longer to stimulate antibody production.

Vaccines may be given subcutaneously or intramuscularly, depending on the vaccine. Other vaccines can be aerosolized and given intranasally. Some vaccines can be put in the feed or drinking water. Fish can be vaccinated by putting the vaccine into their water.

PASSIVE IMMUNITY

Establishing passive immunity requires use of antibodies that have been produced in a donor animal. A *donor animal* is vaccinated with a pathogen. When its serum antibodies reach a high concentration, the animal is bled and the globulin portion containing the antibodies is separated and purified. The protection that an animal receives from an injection of this immune globulin is short lived but immediate.

DISORDERS OF THE IMMUNE SYSTEM

Some immune responses have an adverse effect on the host animal. Among *hypersensitivity reactions* are *allergies; anaphylactic shock,* a severe reaction that may occur within seconds after an antigen enters the circulation; *autoimmune hemolytic anemia,* a condition causing destruction of red blood cells by the host itself; *glomerulonephritis,* caused by deposition of antibody-antigen complexes in the kidney; and *contact hypersensitivity reactions,* such as reactions to contact with poison ivy.

In addition to the hypersensitivity reactions just described, the immune system may also show *deficiencies.* There may be a deficiency in phagocytes or in immunoglobulins. A condition called *combined immunodeficiency* affects animals in early life, after serum levels of maternally derived antibodies have declined. Arabian foals with this disease often die from opportunistic infection due to an absence or deficiency of immunoglobulins.

Lymphoma, a type of tumor characterized by uncontrolled proliferation of lymphocytes, is another abnormality of the immune system. The immune system normally recognizes and destroys cancer cells before they become established in the body, but sometimes the cancer seems to become resistant and escapes the immune defense mechanisms.

PRINCIPLES OF COMMON IMMUNOLOGIC LABORATORY TESTS

Tests of Humoral Immunity

The science of detection and measurement of antibodies or antigens is called *serology.* Detection depends on the binding of antibodies and antigens. Unfortunately, this binding phenomenon is ordinarily invisible. Visualization, and thus detection, of the antigen-antibody reaction depends on secondary events by which the union is easily detected and therefore of diagnostic use in veterinary practice.

Commercial production of monoclonal antibodies to many different antigens has resulted in a variety of test kits for use in the veterinary laboratory. Specific antibodies to many different antigens can be produced and used in the laboratory for rapid identification of disease-producing organisms.

Immunization with viruses, bacteria, or other entities stimulates antibody production in an animal. The antibody-secreting, transformed lymphocytes (plasma cells) can be isolated from the animal and chemically fused with a type of "immortal" cell that propagates indefinitely, such as mouse myeloma cells. The antibodies these hybrid cells produce, called *monoclonal antibodies,* are collected. Because each monoclonal antibody attaches to only one specific part of one type of molecule (antigen), use of these antibodies in diagnostic kits makes the tests very specific and greatly reduces interpretation problems of the result. For example, the feline leukemia virus antigen only reacts with the feline leukemia virus antibody. A specific reaction is diagnostically significant for this complicated disease. In addition to their specificity, these procedures allow rapid identification of the pathogen.

Many serologic tests use monoclonal antibodies. Enzyme immunoassay, latex agglutination, and immunodiffusion are three methodologies used in veterinary laboratories. These are discussed following. Other methods, such as complement fixation, immunofluorescence, immunoelectron microscopy, virus neutraliza- tion, and polymerase chain reaction (PCR) DNA amplification are used in veterinary reference laboratories and research facilities and will not be included in this discussion. Many of the principles are the same, however, and under- standing a few procedures will give you a good basis for understanding others.

Reference laboratories offer myriad serologic tests specifically developed for veterinary samples. Tests for equine infectious anemia, bovine leukemia, toxoplasmosis, feline infectious peritonitis, and rabies are but a few of the diagnostic procedures available (Table 9-1).

ELISA.   ELISA is an acronym for enzyme-linked immunosorbent assay. This enzyme immunoassay has been adapted to many agents commonly tested for in the veterinary laboratory (Figures 9-2 to 9-5 and Table 9-1). Using monoclonal antibodies, the specificity of ELISA is very high; that is, there is little cross-reactivity with other agents. This makes ELISA an accurate way to detect specific antigens, such as viruses, bacteria, parasites, or hormones in serum. ELISA may also be used to test for an antibody in the serum, in which case the test kit contains the specific antigen. Some of the available ELISA kits detect heartworms, feline leukemia virus, feline immunodeficiency virus, canine parvovirus, and progesterone (Procedures 9-1 to 9-3).

For the ELISA antigen detection system, monoclonal antibody is bound to the walls of wells in a test tray, to a membrane, or to a plastic wand. Antigen, if present in the sample, will bind to this antibody, as well as to a second enzyme-labeled antibody that is added to aid in detection of the antigen. When a chromogenic (color-producing) substrate is added to the mixture, it reacts

Text continued on p. 496.

TABLE 9-1. Some commercially available immunologic test kits

DISEASE/CONDITION	PRODUCT NAME	MANUFACTURER	TYPE OF TEST	USE
Allergies	Pet ELISA	Bio-Medical Services	ELISA	For detection of dog and cat allergens (food, inhalants, fleas, *Staphylococcus*)
Borreliosis (Lyme disease)	Lymechek	Synbiotics	ELISA	For detection of *B. burgdorferi* antibodies in dogs
Bovine leukemia virus infection	Leukassay B	Synbiotics	Agar-gel immunodiffusion	For detection of antibodies to bovine leukemia virus in cattle
Bovine mastitis	Rapid Mastitis Test	ImmuCell Corporation	Latex agglutination	For detection of *S. agalactiae* and *S. aureus* in cattle
Brucellosis	CITE *Brucella abortus* Antibody	IDEXX	Enzyme immunoassay	For detection of antibodies to *Brucella abortus* in cattle
Equine endotoxemia	ETOX-DX	Ken Vet	Hemagglutination inhibition	For detection of Gram-negative bacterial endotoxin in equine blood
Equine infectious anemia	D-Tec EIA	Synbiotics	Agar-gel immunodiffusion	For diagnosis of infectious anemia in horses

Equine medication status	Insight Test Kits	ELISA Technologies	ELISA	To determine the medication status of horses
Failure of passive transfer	CITE Foal IgG Test Kit	IDEXX	Enzyme immunoassay	For semiquantitative measurement of IgG levels in equine serum, plasma, or whole blood
Feline infectious peritonitis	SNAP FIP Antibody Test Kit	IDEXX	CELISA	For detection of antibodies to FIP virus in cats
Feline immunodeficiency virus infection	CITE Anti-FIV	IDEXX	Enzyme immunoassay	For detection of antibodies to FIV in cats
Feline leukemia virus infection	Assure/FeLV	Synbiotics	ELISA	For detection of FeLV antigens in cats
	CITE PROBE FeLV Test Kit	IDEXX	ELISA	For detection of FeLV antigens in cats
	Uni-Tec FeLV	Synbiotics	ELISA	For detection of FeLV antigens in cats
	Virachek	Synbiotics	ELISA	For detection of FeLV antigens in cats

Continued.

Table 9-1.—Continued

Disease/condition	Product name	Manufacturer	Type of test	Use
Feline leukemia virus and immunodeficiency virus infection	CITE PROBE Combo FeLV Ag/FIV Ab	IDEXX	ELISA	For detection of FeLV antigens and FIV antibodies in cats
Flea allergy	Allergenic Extract-Flea Ag	Greer Laboratories	Skin test	Aid in diagnosis of flea-bite allergy in dogs and cats
Heartworm infection	Assure/CH	Synbiotics	ELISA	For detection of heartworm antigens in dogs
	Dirochek	Synbiotics	ELISA	For detection of heartworm antigens in dogs
	Vetred	Rhone Merieux	RBC agglutination	For detection of heartworm antigens in dogs
Johne's disease	PROBE *M. paratuberculosis* DNA Test Kit	IDEXX	PCR DNA amplification	For detection of *M. paratuberculosis* in bovine feces
	Rapid Johne's Test	ImmuCell	Agarose gel immunodiffusion	For detection of antibodies to *M. paratuberculosis* in bovine serum

Newcastle disease	Flockchek: Anti-NDV	IDEXX	Enzyme immunoassay	For detection of antibodies to Newcastle disease virus in chicken serum
Parvovirus infection	CITE PROBE Canine Parvovirus Antigen Test Kit	IDEXX	ELISA	For detection of parvovirus antigens in canine feces
Pregnancy	MIP Color-Chek	Synbiotics	Rapid chromatographic immunoassay	For detection of PMSG as an aid in diagnosis of pregnancy in mares
Progesterone	Estruchek	Synbiotics	ELISA	For approximate determination of progesterone levels in the milk of cows and in the blood of dogs and horses
Pseudorabies	ClinEase-PRV	SmithKline Beecham	ELISA	For detection of pseudorabies virus antibodies in the serum of pigs
Rheumatoid arthritis	CRF	Synbiotics	Latex agglutination	For detection of rheumatoid arthritis factor in canine serum

Continued.

Table 9-1.—Continued

Disease/Condition	Product Name	Manufacturer	Type of Test	Use
Salmonellosis	Flockchek *S. enteritidis* Test Kit	IDEXX	Enzyme immunoassay	For detection of antibodies to *S. enteritidis* in chicken serum or egg yolk
T_4	CITE Semiquantitative T_4 Test Kit	IDEXX	ELISA	For semiquantitative determination of total serum T_4 levels in dogs and cats
Tuberculosis	Tuberculin PPD	Synbiotics	Intradermal test	For intradermal testing of cattle for bovine TB
von Willebrand factor deficiency	Botrocetin	American Diagnostica	Macroscopic agglutination test	For detection of *v*WF deficiency in multiple species

American Diagnostica, 222 Railroad Avenue, P.O. Box 1165, Greenwich, CT 06836-1165.
Bio-Medical Services, 3921 Steck Avenue, Suite A-101, Austin, TX 78759.
ELISA Technologies, A Division of Neogen Corporation, 628 East 3RD Street, Lexington, KY 40505.
Greer Laboratories, Box 800, 639 Nuway Circle, Lenoir, NC 28645.
IDEXX Laboratories, One Idexx Drive, Westbrook, ME 04092.
ImmuCell Corporation, 56 Evergreen Drive, Portland, ME 04103.
Ken Vet, 7TH and Orange Streets, Ashland, OH 44805.
Rhone Merieux, 115 Transtech Drive, Athens, GA 30601.
SmithKline Beecham Animal Health, 812 Springdale Drive, Exton, PA 19341.
Synbiotics, 11011 Via Frontera, San Diego, CA 92127.

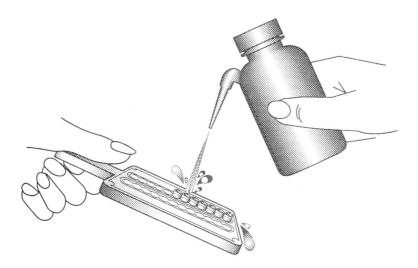

FIGURE 9-2.   A critical step in the microwell enzyme immunoassay is washing away the unbound enzyme-labeled antibodies. (Pet Check Heartworm PF Antigen Test Kit, courtesy IDEXX Laboratories.)

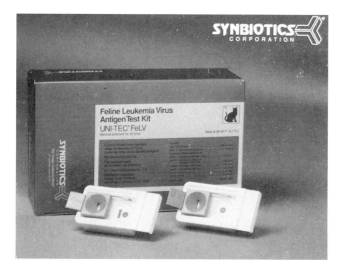

FIGURE 9-3.   Kit to detect FeLV antigens (Uni-Tec FeLV; Synbiotics) based on the ELISA membrane format. The vertical line and dot on the left cassette indicate a positive reaction. The single control dot on the right cassette represents a negative reaction. (Courtesy Synbiotics.)

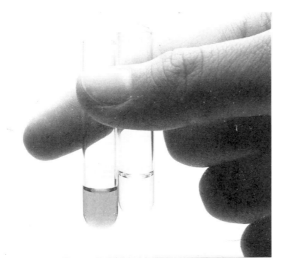

FIGURE 9-4. With the ELISA wand format to test for FeLV (Assure/FeLV; Synbiotics), a positive reaction is indicated by color development in the tube on the left. The wands have been removed from both tubes. (Courtesy Synbiotics.)

with the enzyme to develop a specific color, indicating the presence of antigen in the sample. If the sample contained no antigen, the second antibody would be washed away in a rinsing process and no color reaction would develop.

A similar procedure is used for ELISA antibody detection. In this procedure, antigen is bound to the wells, membrane, or wand, and the patient sample is assayed for the presence of a specific antibody.

CELISA. CELISA is an acronym for competitive enzyme-linked immunosorbent assay. If used to test for patient antigen, this assay uses an enzyme-labeled antigen as well as monoclonal antibodies. Patient antigen, if present, competes with enzyme-labeled antigens for the antibodies coating the test wells. Color developer reacts with the enzyme to produce a color. The intensity of the color produced varies with the concentration of the patient antigen (Procedure 9-4).

LATEX AGGLUTINATION. This test uses small, spherical latex particles coated with antibody (or antigen) and suspended in water. If serum containing the corresponding antigen is added to the mixture, formation of antibody-antigen complexes causes agglutination (clumping). This changes the appearance of the latex suspension from smooth and milky to clumpy because the latex particles have clustered together. If no antigen is present in the sample, the mixture of

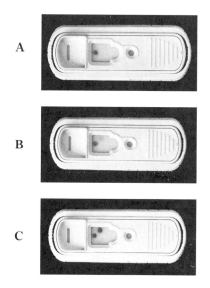

FIGURE 9-5.   Enzyme immunoassay for heartworm antigen (Snap Whole Blood Heartworm Antigen Test; IDEXX). **A,** Negative reaction. **B,** Weak positive reaction. **C,** Strong positive reaction. (Courtesy IDEXX Laboratories.)

latex and serum remains evenly dispersed. Serum for canine rheumatoid factor can be tested using this method (Figure 9-6, Table 9-1, and Procedure 9-5).

IMMUNODIFFUSION.   In this procedure, patient serum samples (possibly containing antibodies) and the antigen to this antibody (supplied in the test kit) are placed into separate wells in an agar gel plate. Both components diffuse into the agar and form a visible band of precipitation when they combine. If no band forms, there is no antibody in the patient's serum sample or the patient's antibody levels are insufficient to cause precipitation in the gel. Diseases that can be detected by immunodiffusion include paratuberculosis, equine infectious anemia, and bovine leukemia virus infection (Figure 9-7, Table 9-1, and Procedure 9-6).

COOMBS' TEST.   The direct Coombs' test is used for diagnosis of autoimmune hemolytic anemia, in which erythrocytes become coated with antibodies and are subsequently removed from circulation by the reticuloendothelial system.

Procedure 9-1. Protocol for microwell ELISA

1. Plastic wells are pre-coated with antibodies specific for the antigen being tested.
2. Samples (that may contain antigen) and a second antibody, labeled with an enzyme, are added to the wells.
3. Antigen, if present, binds to both the solid phase (wells) and enzyme-labeled antibodies.
4. Unbound enzyme-labeled antibodies are washed away.
5. Chromogenic substrate is added that reacts with the enzyme, causing a color to develop.
6. Development of a color indicates the presence of the antigen in the sample.

Procedure 9-2. Protocol for membrane ELISA

1. Sample is added to a membrane, which is precoated with antibodies specific for the antigen being tested.
2. Any antigens in the sample are captured by the antibodies on the membrane.
3. Typically, positive-control spots containing the antigen have also been precoated on the membrane.
4. A second antibody, enzyme-labeled, is then added to the membrane. This also binds to the captured patient antigen and the control antigen. The antigen is now "sandwiched" between two antibodies.
5. Unbound enzyme-labeled antibodies are washed away.
6. Chromogen is added to the membrane and reacts with the enzyme on the second antibody to produce a color.
7. Color appears where the positive control and patient antigens are present on the membrane.

The causative antibodies can be detected on the surface of RBCs by using antiserum that is specific for the antibodies on the RBCs.

Intradermal tests. Skin tests are used to diagnose various allergies to allergens in the environment and in food or water. Allergies are mediated by IgE antibody molecules and can be detected by using allergenic extracts of grasses,

PROCEDURE 9-3. Protocol for wand ELISA

1. The bulbous ends of plastic wands are precoated with antibodies specific for the antigen being tested.
2. Any antigens in the sample are captured by the antibodies on the wand.
3. A second antibody, labeled with an enzyme, is also incubated with the sample and wand. These antibodies will also bind with the antigen.
4. Any unbound enzyme-labeled antibody is washed away and a chromogenic reagent is added.
5. The reagent reacts with the enzyme-labeled antibodies that are bound to the antigens, producing a color reaction.

PROCEDURE 9-4. Protocol for CELISA

1. Test wells are precoated with monoclonal antibodies.
2. Patient samples (that may contain antigen) are added to test wells.
3. Enzyme-labeled antigens are then added to the same test wells.
4. The two antigens compete for antibodies on the test wells. The antigen in higher concentration binds more antibodies.
5. After incubation, the wells are rinsed to wash away excess enzyme-labeled antigens.
6. Color developer is added that reacts with the enzyme on the enzyme-labeled antigen.
7. If the sample contains low levels of patient antigen, most of the antigen bound to the antibodies on the test wells is enzyme-labeled antigen and a deep color develops.
8. If the sample contains high levels of patient antigen, most of the antigen bound to the antibodies on the test wells is antigen from the patient and little color develops.

pollens, ragweed, and other possibly offending antigens. The extracts are injected intradermally, and the injection sites are monitored for allergic reactions. A positive reaction indicates the presence of antibodies, meaning that the animal is allergic to that antigen.

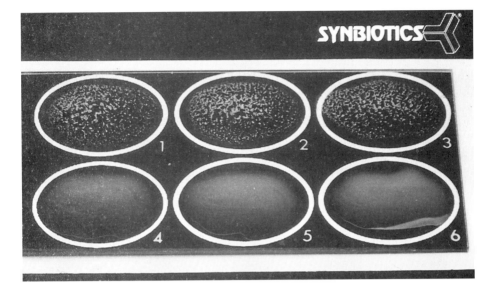

FIGURE 9-6. Clumped latex particles, representing antigen-antibody complexes. Samples 1, 2, and 3 indicate a positive reaction. Samples 4, 5, and 6, showing no clumping, indicate a negative reaction. (Canine RF Test; courtesy Synbiotics.)

PROCEDURE 9-5. Protocol for latex agglutination

1. A dark glass slide is used to read the agglutination reactions.
2. Positive and negative reference sera (positive contains antibodies being tested) and patient sera (with possible antibodies) are separately deposited on the glass slide.
3. A suspension of latex particles that have been coated with antigens that will react with the test antibodies is added to each sample on the slide.
4. The slide is rotated and observed for the appearance of visible agglutination. Agglutination indicates a positive result.

TESTS OF CELL-MEDIATED IMMUNITY

Whereas tests of humoral immunity involve detection of circulating antibodies, evaluation of cell-mediated immunity is much more difficult.

TUBERCULIN SKIN TEST. The tuberculin skin test is one test that correlates with a specific cell-mediated immune reaction. Animals infected with *Mycobacterium*

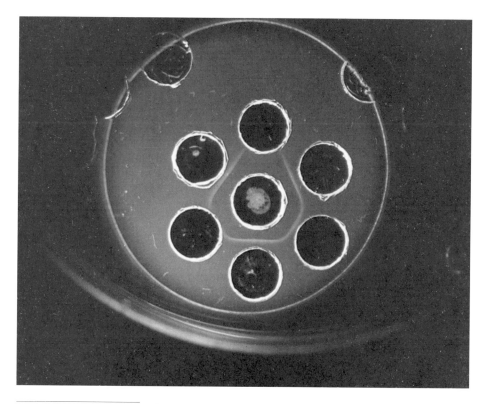

FIGURE 9-7. Agar plate showing lines of precipitation. No lines of precipitation are evident near negative patient wells. (EIA Immunodiffusion, courtesy Synbiotics.)

bacteria develop characteristic delayed hypersensitivity reactions when exposed to purified derivatives of the organism called *tuberculin*.

In the tuberculin skin test, tuberculin is injected intradermally at a site in the cervical region or in a skinfold at the base of the tail in large animals (Table 9-1). A delayed, local inflammatory reaction is observed if the animal has been exposed to mycobacteria. The reaction to injection is delayed because it takes a day or more for the T-lymphocytes to migrate to the foreign antigen injected into the dermis.

COLLECTING SAMPLES FOR SEROLOGIC TESTING

Nearly all serologic tests require serum or plasma as the sample. Whole blood should not be sent to the diagnostic laboratory when serum or plasma is

PROCEDURE 9-6.   Protocol for immunodiffusion

1. An agar plate with one central well and multiple surrounding wells is used.
2. Antigens from the test kit are placed in the center well.
3. Patient serum samples (with possible antibodies) and positive controls (with antibodies) are placed in alternating surrounding wells. Control samples are used for comparison.
4. Antigen from the center well and antibodies from the surrounding wells migrate through the agar toward each other.
5. Where the antigens and antibodies meet, a line of visible precipitation forms. A line of precipitate in front of a patient well indicates antibodies present in the patient serum.

specified. The most practical method of collection is the Vacutainer System (Becton-Dickinson, Rutherford, NJ), commonly available from many veterinary and medical supply companies. A red-top vacuum tube is used when serum is required and a lavender-top tube is used to collect plasma, unless heparinized plasma (green-top tube) is specifically requested.

Reference laboratories have strict requirements concerning specimen type, quality, and handling. For each test, read the requirements carefully and submit exactly what is requested. If a blood sample is to be collected in a syringe, a 5-ml syringe and 20-gauge needle combination causes the least hemolysis.

HANDLING SEROLOGIC SAMPLES

When serum is to be submitted, allow the blood sample to clot for 20 to 30 minutes at room temperature and then centrifuge for 10 minutes at a speed not faster than 1500 rpm. If little serum has separated after centrifuging, "rimming" the tube with a wooden applicator stick to loosen the clot may help; however, this may also cause hemolysis. If plasma is desired, the sample can be centrifuged immediately after collection.

After centrifugation, use a small pipette to aspirate the serum or plasma (upper layer) off the packed erythrocytes. Place the aspirate into a transfer tube or other sealable test tube and label clearly. The serum or plasma can be tested immediately or may be frozen or refrigerated for later use.

Samples for most serologic tests need not be frozen but should be shipped cold, especially during hot weather. The major problem with shipping tubes is breakage. The tubes must be packed firmly in place so they do not move around when the package is jarred. Use paper towels, packing material, or even newspaper but pack the tubes tightly. Be sure to label each sample clearly and correctly and enclose the pertinent paperwork to facilitate proper reporting of the results from the laboratory.

REFERENCES

1. Kuby: *Immunology,* ed 2, New York, 1991, WH Freeman.

2. Lewis and Picut: *Veterinary clinical immunology: from classroom to clinic,* Philadelphia, PA, 1989, Lea & Febiger.

3. McKenzie: *Textbook of hematology,* Philadelphia, PA, 1988, Lea & Febiger.

4. Roitt, et al: *Immunology,* ed 2, Philadelphia, 1989, Lippincott.

5. Tizard: *Veterinary immunology: an introduction,* ed 5, Philadelphia, 1996, WB Saunders.

6. Tortora, et al: *Microbiology: an introduction,* ed 3, Redwood City, CA, 1989, Benjamin/Cummings Publishing.

7. Kanzler: *Veterinary pharmaceuticals and biologicals,* ed 10, Lenexa, KS, 1997, Veterinary Medicine Publishing.

NECROPSY

A.C. Strafuss

This chapter on necropsy (postmortem examination) is written to help veterinary technicians better understand procedures involved in establishing a diagnosis. Information obtained from a properly performed necropsy is correlated with clinical and laboratory findings to establish a diagnosis.

Necropsy is an underused veterinary diagnostic technique. Necropsies should be used to understand disease pathogenesis and to distinguish one disease from another. A skillfully performed necropsy, with proper specimen processing, yields maximal diagnostic information.

Necropsy technique and specimen processing are easy to misuse and difficult to use well. A necropsy carelessly done or attempted by improperly trained people is likely to provide misinformation or no information. Before lesions can be studied, one must have a systematic plan and an orderly necropsy technique. An excellent beginning is to learn how to perform a necropsy on a dog. Then appropriate procedural modifications can be applied to other domestic animals.

The organizational concept of necropsy and supportive laboratory procedures should stress a "collect and do" approach, instead of a "collect and send" philosophy. If isolated from readily accessible reference laboratories, a veterinary practice can easily perform many laboratory procedures using "diagnostic kits" to establish a diagnosis. A common mistake is to omit laboratory procedures or to do difficult tests that are needed infrequently without first perfecting simple tests that are supportive, inexpensive, and more rewarding. The veterinary technician can contribute to the diagnostic process by doing the necropsy, recording the findings, and performing cytologic, clinical chemistry, and microbiologic procedures.

REASONS FOR NECROPSY

Necropsies are performed for a number of reasons. A necropsy is a diagnostic tool and is aided by the history, clinical signs, and laboratory findings. Apart from diagnosis, necropsies play a vital role in understanding diseases and their pathogenesis. In disease surveillance, data from necropsies may provide answers to management problems in herd or flock problems. Necropsy also provides an early warning system to correct a disease trend before it becomes catastrophic. Finally, a necropsy is of legal significance when forensic tests are performed on valuable, insured animals that suddenly die.

NECROPSY PROTOCOL

To gain confidence in doing a necropsy, you should become skilled first in necropsy of dogs and cats. These cadavers are easily manipulated, and their digestive tract is short and simple. The procedural sequence learned on dogs and cats can be applied to other species. Some procedures are common to necropsy of all species. All animals are placed on their left side, except horses, which are placed on their right side. A midline skin incision is made from the lips to the cranial brim of the pelvis, superficial to the linea alba. The lower jaw, tongue, and organs of the neck are removed along with the thoracic organs. Pelvic skeletal cuts, removal of the pelvic organs and urogenital male or female tract, and removal of the brain and spinal cord are all done in the same manner in the various species. The anatomic differences of the gastrointestinal tract of different species necessitate a different sequence in removal of abdominal viscera.

An informative necropsy requires knowledge of general and special pathology of organs and organ systems. More important, developing a standardized necropsy protocol ensures that pathologic conditions are not overlooked. Each organ system is grossly observed in turn. Thoroughness eventually becomes routine and allows for neatness and precision. A standardized necropsy protocol allows for uniform, rapid, systematic, and complete necropsies that are the key to accurate interpretation of lesions. "Shortcuts" lead to an incorrect diagnosis or no diagnosis at all.

Sequential removal of tissues from the cadaver during necropsy allows for proper evaluation of gross lesions and tissues. Visualization of gross lesions at necropsy often is not sufficient for definitive diagnosis; such lesions or tissues must be submitted for diagnostic tests. Therefore the necropsy becomes crucial to selection of appropriate samples for adjunctive histopathologic, microbiologic, toxicologic, virologic, and parasitologic examinations. Careful selection of tissues is necessary to arrive at a pathologic diagnosis.

The history is vital and, when submitted with animals for necropsy, enables the diagnostician to make a more accurate and complete diagnosis. Failure to submit a history may lead to incorrect diagnosis. The history is an integral part of the necropsy procedure, which guides the dissector in proper selection of tests.

SPECIMEN COLLECTION AND SUBMISSION

Test results from the diagnostic laboratory directly reflect the quality and consideration given to selection and handling of specimen samples submitted. If tissues for submission are handled improperly, the time and effort expended in doing the necropsy may be wasted. Careful selection and collection of specimens are among the most important steps in the necropsy procedure. The appropriate specimens must arrive at the laboratory in good condition. In the final analysis, the veterinarian submitting the specimen has the responsibility of properly collecting, packaging, and sending specimens to the laboratory for the requested tests. In many instances, collecting, packaging, and shipping specimens to the laboratory are the responsibility of the technician.

Tissues from autolyzed or frozen birds are usually unrewarding for use in laboratory procedures. Because dry plumage slows the escape of body heat and accelerates autolysis, recently dead birds should immediately be soaked with water and detergent containing a germicide. This decreases the insulating capability of plumage and allows body heat to escape more rapidly. Dead birds should be chilled in a refrigerator before packaging and transport to the laboratory.

The quality of specimens submitted for laboratory tests has more of an influence on the diagnosis than the history or clinical findings. Considering all of the tests that are performed, it follows that appropriately selected and properly handled specimens are more likely to provide an accurate diagnosis than specimens not so treated.

Each tissue in a specimen container is an island of information unto itself, and great care should be given to proper packaging of the specimen. The common practice of submitting intestine (even if tied off) and parenchymatous organs together in the knotted arm of an obstetric sleeve should be avoided. Bacterial contamination rapidly spreads when tissues lack proper refrigeration and tissue fluids are present in the tissue container. Packaging intestines with parenchymatous organs typically prevents the diagnostic laboratory from extracting useful information from all of the commingled specimens.

When an animal is euthanized, tissues can be immediately collected and refrigerated. This allows more tests to be performed on the specimen, especially enzymatic analysis.

Tissues collected from animals found dead are of limited value, as autolysis precludes enzymatic or other chemical analyses. Agonal changes cause breakdown of macrophages and the reticuloendothelial system by enzymatic digestion. The reticuloendothelial system may then release bacteria, leading to contamination of organs. While an animal is alive, bacteria are continually cleared from the bloodstream by the reticuloendothelial system. After the animal dies, these bacteria are then released in many organs.

In ruminants, bacteria are present in the rumen in great numbers and continue to multiply after death. This increases the cadaver temperature and accelerates tissue liquefaction and gas production.

Such factors as humidity and temperature influence the rapidity of cadaver decomposition after death. When animals suddenly die from lightning strike, blackleg, or poisoning, bacteria in the digestive tract continue to generate heat and accelerate tissue autolysis. Stopping the putrefactive processes as soon as possible after death is of high priority.

Cool the tissues immediately for a few hours in a refrigerator before packing them for shipment. Add sufficient fixative to samples submitted for histopathologic examination. Then pack specimens in a package surrounded by cooling packets and insulating material. Choose a courier that can deliver the specimen to the diagnostic laboratory within 24 hours. The quicker the specimens are delivered and processed, the better the results. Poor specimen handling results in hemolyzed blood samples, toxic serum samples, and bacterial infiltration of organs.

SHIPPING SPECIMENS TO THE LABORATORY

It is essential to submit a complete and detailed history along with tissues, including gross lesions observed during the necropsy. Specimens may be delivered to the laboratory by bus, postal service, air, or private courier.

Veterinary medical diagnostic specimens are subject to U.S. Postal Service regulations (Code of Federal Regulations, Title 39, Part III amended). Mailing of clinical specimens is prohibited unless items are properly prepared for mailing and handling in transit. The regulation states that clinical specimens "must be packaged in a securely sealed primary container(s) with sufficient absorbent material to take up the contents in case of leakage, and in an outer shipping container with secondary leakproof material so that, if there should be a leakage of the primary container during shipment, the contents will not escape from the outer shipping container. Shock resistant material shall be used to withstand conditions incident to ordinary handling in transit, including but not limited to shock and pressure changes." It is in the best interest of our profession to comply with these regulations.

Many diagnostic laboratories can supply you with preaddressed mailers for submission of diagnostic specimens, ranging from test tube samples to fresh tissue for microbiologic evaluation. Consult the reference laboratory near your clinic and check with postal authorities to determine which types of containers are acceptable for mailing.

METHODS OF EUTHANASIA

It is best to collect tissues from a cadaver immediately after death. Necropsy done immediately after euthanasia helps ensure more accurate results.

There is no best or single method of euthanasia for all circumstances. Several euthanasia options are available, and you must consider their ethical repercussions before selecting one. Most animals are killed by rapid intravenous injection of euthanasia solution.

A gas chamber can be used on small animals. The size of animals that can be euthanized in a chamber depends on the chamber's size. An overdose of a gaseous anesthetic is administered until the animal is dead. For most small animals, a cylinder of CO_2 can be connected to the chamber. For small birds, a cotton ball can be saturated with ether or chloroform and placed in a container (bell jar) with the bird. A larger chamber may be constructed from a trash can, with a tube entering the lid. Halothane is more expensive but creates less excitement for the animal.

In addition to intravenous injections, large animals may be humanely killed using a captive-bolt gun. The gun is placed against the animal's forehead at the intersection of two imaginary lines drawn from the base of the ear to the opposite medial canthus of the eye. Electrocution with a 110-volt system has been used for euthanasia of animals. Adequate contacts on the animal, along with a shock-proof safety switch, are an absolute necessity. Electrocution is quick and effective on all animals. If the proper switches and contacts are used, it is safe for the operator.

POSTMORTEM CHANGES

Immediately following euthanasia, the jugular vein, axillary vessels (axillary space), or femoral vessels (disarticulating the coxofemoral joint) can be severed to exsanguinate (bleed out) the cadaver. Exsanguination is important because excessive blood in tissues or body cavities tends to obscure lesions. Therefore it is best to allow as much blood as possible to escape from the vascular system.

In cases of natural death, the necropsy should be performed as soon as possible after death. Postmortem destruction of tissues by the body's own enzymes begins immediately after death. Antemortem fever or high ambient temperature hastens decomposition of the carcass by speeding up the rate of enzyme reactions. Obese animals or those with a dense haircoat (wool) decompose more rapidly due to heat entrapment. Ruminants with active rumen fermentation at the time of death generate gas and heat, enhancing postmortem changes.

Postmortem changes (changes occurring after death) have profound effects on normal and diseased tissues. If you do not recognize postmortem changes in tissues, you may mistake such changes for antemortem lesions. An example is hemoglobin staining of intestinal contents, which is frequently mistaken for hemorrhagic enteritis. The diffuse red coloration tends to obscure interpretation of antemortem lesions of hyperemia and hemorrhage. Postmortem changes are found to varying degrees and may be confusing when present concurrently. A detailed description of postmortem changes can be found elsewhere in the literature.

DISPOSAL OF DEAD ANIMALS AND BIRDS

Proper disposal of dead animals is becoming increasingly difficult. Fewer and fewer landfill areas are available, especially near metropolitan areas. Local ordinances may forbid the use of landfills for disposal of dead animals because rodents and insects could carry diseases to residential areas. Although certain chemicals can be applied to carcasses to speed breakdown of body tissue and kill infectious agents in tissues, chemical contamination of underground water supplies may be a problem in certain types of soils. Also, cost may be prohibitive.

Rendering plants can be used for large animal disposal. These plants are designed for carcass disposal and are inspected by government authorities. Disposal of small animal carcasses can often be arranged locally through municipal incineration units or preexcavated burial pits. A crematorium is a prohibitively expensive item for most veterinary hospitals.

COSMETIC NECROPSY

A cosmetic necropsy is restrictive because it limits examination of the animal to the extent that the client will tolerate. However, the internal organs can usually be examined with relative completeness by making a ventral midline incision from the xiphoid cartilage to the cranial brim of the pubis. The thoracic organs can usually be removed after cutting the diaphragm and pulling them caudally, to the exterior. Splitting the sternum allows the thoracic cage to be pulled apart for removal of the lungs and heart. These incisions can be sutured after the examined organs are replaced or the thoracic and abdominal cavities are filled with paper to absorb fluids and maintain the shape of the cavities.

If the brain is to be removed, an incision should be made on the dorsum of the neck, extending rostrally over the calvarium and reflecting the skin laterally to the zygomatic process and eye. The calvarium and then the brain should be removed. The skull should be replaced, suturing the skin over the calvarium, leaving only a suture line. An inverted suture pattern is probably most desirable for this area.

NECROPSY OF RABIES SUSPECTS

Animals with clinical signs of viral encephalitis or those that show abnormal behavior patterns should always be considered as rabies suspects. Proper protective clothing should be worn when handling a dead or live animal with abnormal behavior. Clients should be instructed not to pick up live animals in pain under any circumstances, so possible exposure can be avoided. They should be instructed to call animal control authorities to handle such cases, or call public health officials or the local government veterinarian to help them evaluate the situation. The veterinarian should always instruct the client or persons exposed to possibly rabid animals to call their local physician for proper treatment. The veterinarian should also call the reference laboratory for specific instructions on how to submit specimens for rabies examination.

NECROPSY EQUIPMENT

Elaborate equipment is not required to do a necropsy. Frequently you or the veterinarian are judged on how you conduct a necropsy more than on your knowledge of disease. The client probably will formulate an opinion more from the veterinarian's tools of the trade, rather than from the science of diagnosis. It is therefore logical to assume that the owner and others viewing the necropsy will judge you by your expertise in opening the cadaver and removing organs.

Equipment includes shears for cutting bones, enterotome scissors for incising the gut, and a knife for cutting skin and muscle. A sharp knife is the most important tool for necropsy. A sharp knife is as important to the dissector as a scalpel is to a surgeon. Never attempt to do a necropsy with a dull knife; a sharp knife is imperative. A scalpel, scissors, and forceps are desirable in dissecting small caged birds. A supply of sterile syringes and needles, vials for liquid specimens, and Petri dishes for microbiologic samples should be at hand.

NECROPSY PROCEDURE

A cadaver is examined to determine the pathologic processes in relation to the history and clinical findings regarding the cause of death. The necropsy procedure should be planned, with the various specimens collected according to the diagnosis anticipated.

All animals should be placed in left lateral recumbency, except for horses, which are placed in right lateral recumbency. This accommodates the anatomic differences of the equine gastrointestinal tract, which necessitate a different sequence for removal of abdominal viscera. Maintaining the same position for most animals during necropsy helps familiarize the examiner with the normal relative location of the viscera.

Before starting a necropsy, an external examination should assess: position of the animal at the time of death; general appearance of the carcass (bloat, rigor, postmortem decomposition, dehydration); body condition or nutritional status (obese, cachectic); condition of the haircoat and presence of external parasites; color and appearance of visible mucous membranes; presence or absence of discharges from body openings and the mammary glands; and evidence of swellings, wounds, hernias, and fractures.

There is no single correct way to do a necropsy. The procedure detailed here is an efficient approach.

NECROPSY OF DOGS AND CATS

Dogs and cats are placed on their left side. The dissector faces the ventral abdomen to perform the necropsy.

OPENING THE CADAVER

Start a paramedian ventral skin incision at the sternum and extend it to the symphysis of the mandible. Extend the incision from the sternum caudally to the groin, lateral to the umbilicus, mammary gland, or external male genitalia (Figure 10-1).

Lift the front leg and cut the muscle attachments close to the thorax and reflect the leg dorsolaterally. Reflect the skin dorsolaterally from the midline incision of the neck to the base of the ear. Grasp the proximal rear leg and incise the adductor, gracilis, and quadratus muscles. Disarticulate the coxofemoral joint and reflect the leg dorsolaterally so it lies flat on the table surface. Reflect the abdominal skin dorsolaterally from the paramedian incision to the transverse processes of the spinal column (Figure 10-2).

The legs (front and rear) and integument of the cadaver are reflected dorsolaterally as one unit. Do not remove the legs from the cadaver or from the abdominal skin. Reflect the skin of the left side of the body laterally for about 5 cm (2 inches) along the entire length of the initial incision.

To remove the lower jaw, cut the masseter muscle by inserting the knife at the commissure just lateral to the ramus (Figure 10-3). Extend the cut to the angle of the ramus and sever the masseter muscle from the lateral surface of the angle of the ramus. The mandibular symphysis is cut with pruning shears or a saw. Grasp and pull the right ramus caudally. Cut the muscles caudal to the molar teeth and continue cutting the muscle attachments medial to the ramus and around the caudal border of the angle of the ramus. Pull the right ramus caudally by rotating it laterally in one movement to disarticulate it. Twist the disarticulated ramus and cut the remaining muscle attachments to remove it. Grasp the tongue and cut it loose from the medial surface of the left ramus. Cut

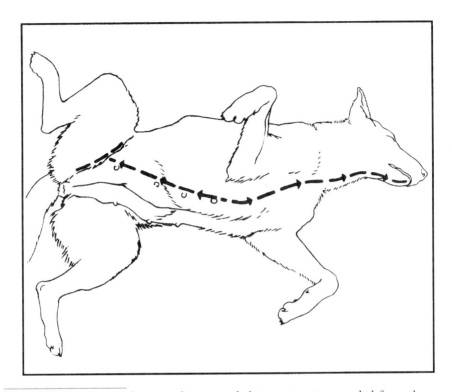

Figure 10-1. An initial paramedian ventral skin incision is extended from the sternum to the mandibular symphysis and to the groin. (Strafuss AC: *Necropsy procedures and basic diagnostic methods for practicing veterinarians,* Springfield, IL, 1988, Charles C Thomas.)

caudal to the hard palate and around the pharynx to the level of the hyoid bones (Figure 10-4). Disarticulate the hyoid bones and continue reflecting the tongue, pharynx, esophagus, and trachea to the thoracic inlet (Figure 10-5).

Open the abdomen by cutting the muscles along the costal arch, from the transverse process of the spinal column to the sternum and caudally along the linea alba to the brim of the pelvis (Figure 10-6). Examine the inguinal canal for evidence of cryptorchidism, incarcerated hernias, infarcted spermatic cord, or hemorrhage from faulty castration.

Remove the ribcage by cutting the ribs with rib shears (or pruning shears, cleaver) along the line of proposed cuts. The cuts are made from the xiphoid cartilage cranially to the thoracic inlet (just ventral to the esophagus, trachea, and tongue, reflected to the thoracic inlet). The next cut begins from the most dorsal aspect of the first rib (dorsal to the reflected neck organs) and extends caudally to the transverse process of the first lumbar vertebra. In heavily

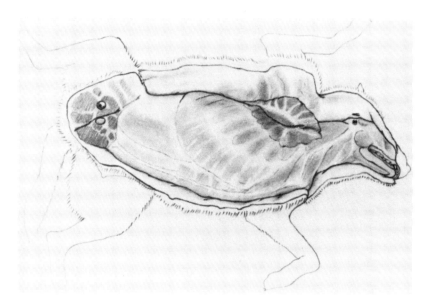

FIGURE 10-2. The rear leg is disarticulated, and the legs and skin are reflected dorsolaterally as a unit. (Strafuss AC: *Necropsy procedures and basic diagnostic methods for practicing veterinarians,* Springfield, IL, 1988, Charles C Thomas.)

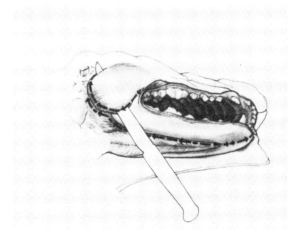

FIGURE 10-3. The knife is inserted just laterally to the ramus of the mandible. (Strafuss AC: *Necropsy procedures and basic diagnostic methods for practicing veterinarians,* Springfield, IL, 1988, Charles C Thomas.)

muscled animals, reflect the muscles of the ribcage along the proposed cuts. After the ribs are detached, note the color of the exposed tissues and organs that may indicate hemorrhage, congestion, postmortem imbibition, or autolysis. Observe the anatomic relationships of organs before removal for signs of volvulus, torsion, intussusception, hernia, or other anomalies. Note the

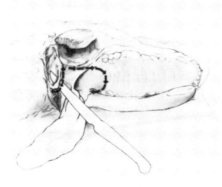

FIGURE 10-4. The tongue is cut loose with an incision around the pharynx to the level of the hyoid bones. (Strafuss AC: *Necropsy procedures and basic diagnostic methods for practicing veterinarians,* Springfield, IL, 1988, Charles C Thomas.)

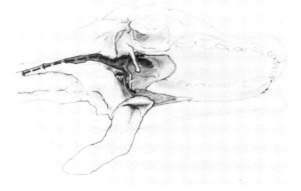

FIGURE 10-5. The hyoid bones are disarticulated, and the tongue, pharynx, esophagus, and trachea are pulled caudally. (Strafuss AC: *Necropsy procedures and basic diagnostic methods for practicing veterinarians,* Springfield, IL, 1988, Charles C Thomas.)

presence of hydropericardium, hydrothorax or hydroperitoneum, and the characteristics of any fluid.

Specimens for microbiologic cultures or direct microscopic examination should be collected at this time, before any organ is contaminated by manipulation or handling of viscera. Pericardial, pleural, or abdominal effusions, fluid from cysts, bile, and urine are best collected before the organs are handled.

Grasp the tongue, esophagus, and trachea, and pull the thoracic organs (heart, lungs, thymus) from the thoracic cavity. Open the esophagus and check for ulcers or parasites. Examine the thyroid and parathyroid glands, which lie adjacent to the trachea and caudal to the larynx. Open the trachea and extend the incision into the bronchi and bronchioles. Palpate and incise each lung lobe to observe for lesions. *Do not detach the heart from the lungs.*

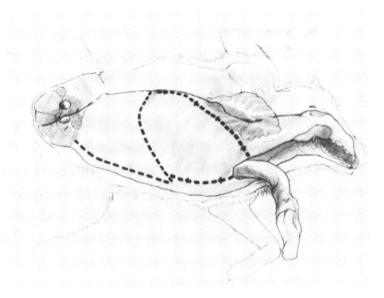

Figure 10-6. The abdomen is opened with an incision caudal to the costal arch and caudally along the linea alba. (Strafuss AC: *Necropsy procedures and basic diagnostic methods for practicing veterinarians,* Springfield, IL, 1988, Charles C Thomas.)

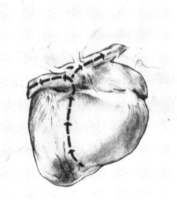

Figure 10-7. The right ventricle is opened near the interventricular septum, and the incision is extended into the caudal vena cava. (Strafuss AC: *Necropsy procedures and basic diagnostic methods for practicing veterinarians,* Springfield, IL, 1988, Charles C Thomas.)

EXAMINING THE HEART

Lay out the thoracic organs so the tongue, esophagus, and trachea are to your right and open the pericardial sac. Hold the heart in your left hand, with the apex toward you. With scissors, make a cut in the right ventricle adjacent to the septum and extend the cut caudodorsally into the caudal vena cava (Figure

10-7). Extend the initial cut in the right ventricle craniodorsally, adjacent to the septum, continuing out to the conus arteriosus and pulmonary artery (Figure 10-8). Examine all valves and openings of the right auricle and ventricle.

Rotate the heart counterclockwise until the left auricle is uppermost. Hold the heart in your left hand, with your thumb over the left auricle. Bisect the left ventricle near the apex and extend the cut dorsally into the pulmonary veins (Figure 10-9). Examine the left atrioventricular (AV) valve.

With your left index finger and thumb, grasp the left half of the left ventricle. With scissors in your right hand, cut through the left ventricle, going beneath the left AV valve (Figure 10-10). Extend the incision distally to the aorta. Examine the origins of the coronary, subclavian, and brachiocephalic arteries (Figure 10-11).

REMOVING THE GASTROINTESTINAL TRACT

Grasp the duodenum and pancreas and reflect them dorsolaterally over the vertebral column. Grasp the omentum and pull it ventrally. The cecum is usually visible as an inflated, comma-shaped structure surrounded by intestine and ventral to the right kidney. Find the ileum at the apex of the cecum, cut the small intestine from its mesenteric attachment to the caudal duodenum, and stop where the duodenum loops under the large intestine (Figures 10-12 and 10-13).

Holding the cecum in your left hand, cut craniodorsally to the cecum and the mesenteric lymph node. Pull the cecum, terminal ileum, colon, and

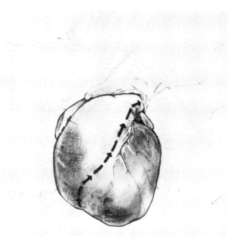

FIGURE 10-8. The right ventricular incision is extended to the conus arteriosus and pulmonary artery. (Strafuss AC: *Necropsy procedures and basic diagnostic methods for practicing veterinarians,* Springfield, IL, 1988, Charles C Thomas.)

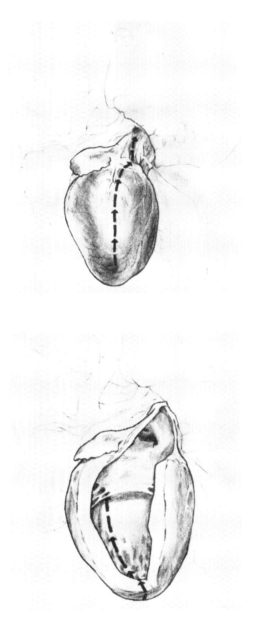

FIGURE 10-9.   The left ventricle is bisected near its apex, and the incision is extended into the pulmonary veins. (Strafuss AC: *Necropsy procedures and basic diagnostic methods for practicing veterinarians,* Springfield, IL, 1988, Charles C Thomas.)

FIGURE 10-10.   Scissors are used to cut through the left ventricle. (Strafuss AC: *Necropsy procedures and basic diagnostic methods for practicing veterinarians,* Springfield, IL, 1988, Charles C Thomas.)

mesenteric lymph node toward you, cutting the mesenteric attachment at the same time (Figure 10-14).

Grasp the caudal duodenum, cut it loose from any remaining attachments, and lay it outside the abdominal cavity. The pancreas can be examined *in situ* (in its natural position) within the abdominal cavity. Cut the duodenum at the tail

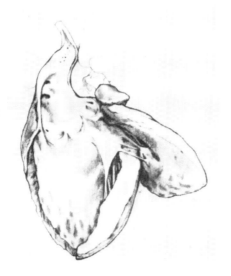

Figure 10-11. The origins of the coronary, subclavian, and brachycephalic arteries are examined. (Strafuss AC: *Necropsy procedures and basic diagnostic methods for practicing veterinarians,* Springfield, IL, 1988, Charles C Thomas.)

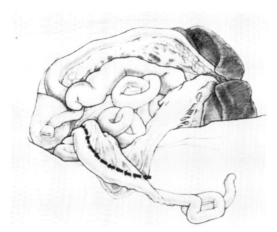

Figure 10-12. The small intestine is cut from its mesenteric attachment to the caudal duodenum. (Strafuss AC: *Necropsy procedures and basic diagnostic methods for practicing veterinarians,* Springfield, IL, 1988, Charles C Thomas.)

of the pancreas and remove the small intestine for examination. Then reflect the cecum, terminal ileum, colon, and mesenteric lymph nodes over the paralumbar region.

Grasp the right kidney and cut craniolateral to the kidney and adrenal gland. Reflect the right kidney, adrenal gland, and ureter caudally to the pelvic inlet and lay them dorsally over the paralumbar region. Repeat for the left kidney, adrenal gland, and ureter (Figure 10-15).

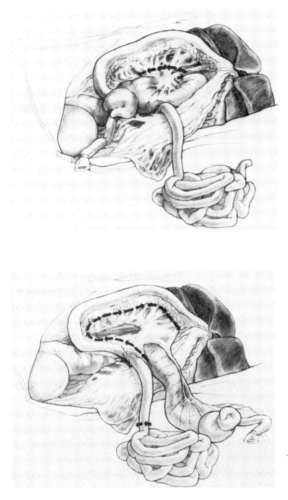

FIGURE **10-13.**   The mesenteric incision is extended to the point where the duodenum loops under the large intestine. (Strafuss AC: *Necropsy procedures and basic diagnostic methods for practicing veterinarians,* Springfield, IL, 1988, Charles C Thomas.)

FIGURE **10-14.**   The mesenteric attachments of the cecum, terminal ileum, colon, and mesenteric lymph nodes are cut, and the duodenum is severed at the tail of the pancreas. (Strafuss AC: *Necropsy procedures and basic diagnostic methods for practicing veterinarians,* Springfield, IL, 1988, Charles C Thomas.)

Check bile duct patency by squeezing the gallbladder and noting whether bile flows into the opened duodenum. Remove the stomach by cutting it from the hilus of the liver. Remove the spleen, duodenum, and pancreas with the stomach (Figure 10-16). Remove the liver and diaphragm together by cutting the diaphragm from its costal attachment.

PELVIC CUTS AND UROGENITAL TRACT REMOVAL

Before the genital tract, urinary system, and caudal alimentary tract are removed, it is necessary to remove the lateral aspects of the pelvis. *Three cuts are required,* and all are made close to the exposed coxofemoral joint (Figure 10-17).

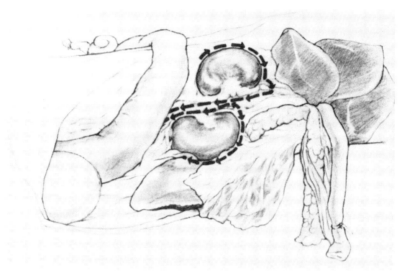

FIGURE 10-15. Incisions are made to free the kidneys, adrenal glands, and ureters. (Strafuss AC: *Necropsy procedures and basic diagnostic methods for practicing veterinarians,* Springfield, IL, 1988, Charles C Thomas.)

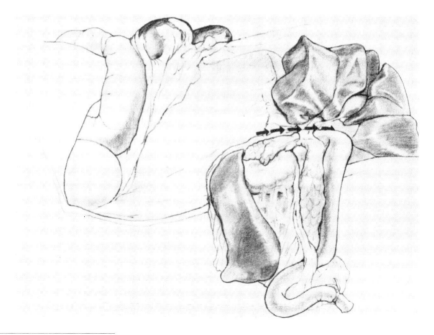

FIGURE 10-16. The spleen, duodenum, and pancreas are removed with the stomach. (Strafuss AC: *Necropsy procedures and basic diagnostic methods for practicing veterinarians,* Springfield, IL, 1988, Charles C Thomas.)

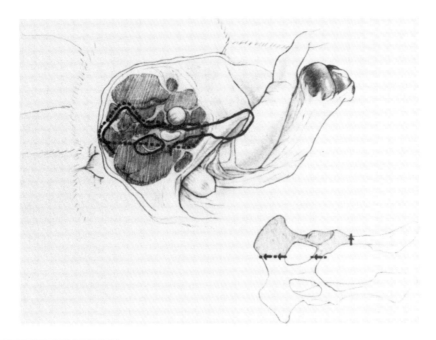

FIGURE 10-17. Three cuts are made to remove the lateral aspects of the pelvis. (Strafuss AC: *Necropsy procedures and basic diagnostic methods for practicing veterinarians,* Springfield, IL, 1988, Charles C Thomas.)

The first cut is made from the cranial brim of the pelvis to the obturator foramen. The second is made from the obturator foramen to the ischial arch, parallel to the long axis of the vertebral column. The third is made across the shaft of the ileum, cranial to the disarticulated coxofemoral joint. Cut the ligaments and muscles surrounding the detached lateral bony pelvis and remove the detached bony pelvis from the cadaver.

In females, grasp the kidneys, attached adrenal glands, ureters, uterus, and large intestine and reflect them caudally to the level of the ischial arch, cutting all attachments close to the abdominal wall and bony pelvis. Cut the fascial attachments from the ventral floor of the pelvis, extending the cut adjacent to the ischial arch to remove the vulva, with the internal reproductive tract intact (Figure 10-18). A gravid uterus with full-term fetuses may be examined *in situ* or cut at the cervix and removed separately.

In males, grasp the kidneys, attached adrenal glands, ureters, and large intestine and cut their pelvic attachments at a point just cranial to the ischial arch. Reflect the external genitalia caudally (scrotum included) to near the caudoventral border of the ischial arch. Grasp the external genitalia and reflected pelvic organs and cut the ligaments and crura close to the caudal

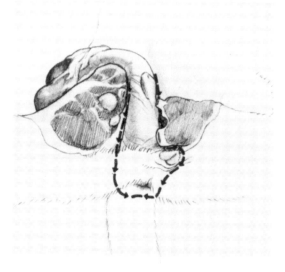

FIGURE 10-18. The reproductive tract of females is removed intact. (Strafuss AC: *Necropsy procedures and basic diagnostic methods for practicing veterinarians,* Springfield, IL, 1988, Charles C Thomas.)

border of the symphysis of the pubis and ischial arch; continue to reflect ventrally around the anus. Remove the urogenital organs and large intestine together (Figure 10-19). This step permits removal of an intact internal and external urethra for examination.

COLLECTING CEREBROSPINAL FLUID

Cut caudal to the angle of the mandible, deep to the caudal border of the occipital condyle, exposing the foramen magnum (Figure 10-20). Cerebrospinal fluid may be removed at this time for microbiologic and clinicopathologic examinations (Figure 10-20, *inset*).

REMOVING THE BRAIN

The brain should be examined in all cases in which the clinical history suggests neurologic disturbances.

Leave the head attached to the spinal column and reflect the skin from the head. An easy way to remove the brain is through a ventral paramedian incision, 1/4 to 1/2 inch to one side of the ventral midline. Saw the head from the ventral side and extend the incision caudally to the level of the occipital

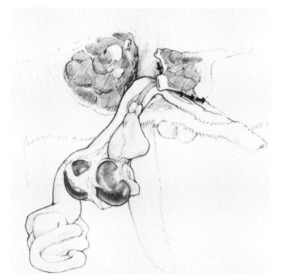

FIGURE 10-19.   In males, the
urogenital organs and large
intestine are removed together.
(Strafuss AC: *Necropsy procedures and
basic diagnostic methods for practicing
veterinarians,* Springfield, IL, 1988,
Charles C Thomas.)

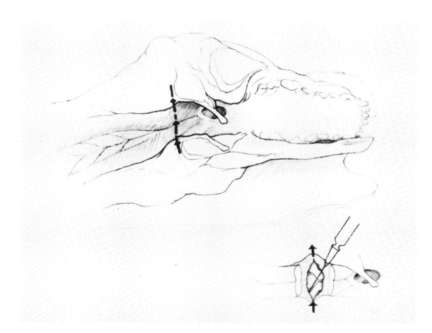

FIGURE 10-20.   The foramen magnum is exposed with an incision deep to the
caudal border of the occipital condyle. Cerebrospinal fluid may then be collected
(*inset*). (Strafuss AC: *Necropsy procedures and basic diagnostic methods for practicing veterinarians,*
Springfield, IL, 1988, Charles C Thomas.)

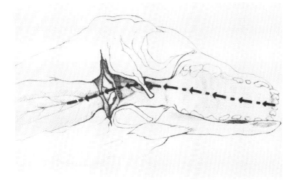

Figure 10-21. The brain can be exposed through a ventral paramedian incision. (Strafuss AC: *Necropsy procedures and basic diagnostic methods for practicing veterinarians,* Springfield, IL, 1988, Charles C Thomas.)

condyle (Figure 10-21). After the calvarium and brain are exposed, each half is removed by gentle traction and passive gravitational force. The brain typically peels out of the calvarium after the cranial nerves and dural attachments are cut with curved pointed scissors. *Do not squeeze or handle the brain roughly,* as it is easily damaged.

Alternatively, the head may be removed from the cadaver and the brain removed through a dorsal approach. Make a dorsal midline cutaneous incision from the frontal prominence to a point caudal to the occiput. Reflect the skin back on either side to expose the temporal muscles to the zygomatic arch. Cut the temporal muscles free from their proximal attachments and from the bone over the dorsolateral surfaces of the skull in the temporal fossa. Remove the head by making a deep transverse cut through the extensor muscles immediately caudal to the occipital protuberance to the atlantooccipital articulation.

After the head is removed, make three cuts through the calvarium to open the cranial cavity. Saw on a line from the dorsolateral periphery of the foramen magnum, cutting the dorsal one third of the occipital condyle and medial to the orbit. Extend the incision rostrally on a line to the medial canthus of the opposite eye. Repeat this cut for the other side.

Cut the frontal bone transversely at the rostral limit of the cranial cavity (line varies with species, age, and breed) on a line caudal to the supraorbital process. Lift or pry the severed calvarium off the cerebral hemispheres and cerebellum. With scissors, cut the meninges and falx cerebri (dura between cerebral hemispheres and cerebellum) and reflect the meninges from the dorsal aspect of the brain. Invert the head so gravity helps ease the brain out of the cranial cavity. By cutting the cranial nerve roots and ventral dural attachments, the brain is easily removed from the cranial cavity. Handle the brain carefully, as it easily becomes an amorphous mass if mishandled.

The brain may be sectioned immediately or placed *in toto* (whole) in 10% buffered neutral formalin and sectioned after preliminary fixation for 12 to 24 hours. The brain may be placed in a container to which concentrated formalin (37% w/v) is added until the brain floats. This rapidly makes the brain firm for sectioning. To section a fresh brain, place the organ on its ventral surface and press the olfactory lobes against a block or the lip of the table. Moisten the knife in physiologic saline or water before each cut so that tissue does not adhere to it. Carefully make a series of transverse cuts (1 cm apart) through both lobes. When diffuse changes or large focal lesions are present, sectioning when the brain is fresh provides better fixation. Small focal lesions are best detected grossly in fixed brains. Lesions in fixed brain tissue are grossly observed as darkened foci and are often easily distinguishable.

REMOVING THE SPINAL CORD

Cut the muscles and tendons from the dorsal, ventral, and transverse processes of the spinal column. A cleaver or ax may be used to chip away the exposed transverse processes along the vertebral column in large animals. Continue chipping parallel to the transverse process until the right side of the vertebral column is removed and the spinal cord is exposed. In small animals, a rongeur may be used to accomplish the same end. An oscillating Stryker saw may be used if one is not adept at handling a cleaver or ax. Starting at the atlantooccipital joint, remove the spinal cord by grasping the meninges with forceps to hold the spinal cord at an obtuse angle. Cut the dorsal and ventral nerve roots to free the cord from the vertebral column. *Do not squeeze, mash, or pull the spinal cord* at acute angles from the spinal column.

After the cord is removed from the spinal column, cut the meninges along the entire length of the spinal cord and examine grossly. Place the cord in 10% buffered neutral formalin to fix for 24 hours before sectioning. Transverse cuts may be made in the fresh cord, using gentle handling and a sharp knife, to examine for lesions.

OPENING LIMB JOINTS

Make a medial skin incision over the joint, reflect the skin, and open the joint to observe the type and amount of fluid and to look for erosions of the articular surfaces.

Any of three approaches is recommended if joint fluid is to be cultured. Saw across the long bone midshaft proximal and distal to the joint and send the joint intact to a diagnostic laboratory for culture. Alternatively, reflect the skin from the joint surface and, with a sterile syringe and needle, aspirate joint fluid or exudate for culture.

Using the last method, reflect the skin from the joint surface, sear the tissue surface, and open the joint with a sterile blade. With a sterile loop, streak a sample of joint contents directly onto a blood agar plate, or take a sample with a sterile swab and send it to the diagnostic laboratory.

NECROPSY OF SWINE

The same procedure described for dogs and cats is used for opening swine cadavers (Figures 10-1 to 10-6) and for examining the heart (Figures 10-7 to 10-11). The entire pharynx must be removed because the tonsil of swine is a flattened structure embedded in the pharynx and is easily overlooked.

REMOVING THE GASTROINTESTINAL TRACT

Grasp the ileum near its entry into the cecum. Cut the small intestine away from its mesenteric attachment to the point where the small intestine courses under the large intestine. At this point, sever the ileum and caudal duodenum and remove the small intestine (Figure 10-22, *bottom*). By cutting the small intestine close to its mesenteric attachment, the attached border is freed so that the intestine is easily opened for examination.

Bluntly dissect the rectum and colon cranially, from the pelvic inlet to the right kidney. Sever the colon and place it over the paralumbar fossa (Figure 10-22, *top*). Examine the pancreas, sever the duodenum caudal to the gallbladder, and bluntly dissect the duodenum from the stomach (Figure 10-22, *top*). Grasp the large intestine (spiral colon) in the left hand and pull it tautly from its mesenteric attachments; sever and remove it from the abdominal cavity.

Reflect the kidneys, adrenal glands, ureters, urinary bladder, and nongravid uterus caudally to the pelvic inlet and place them over the paralumbar region. A gravid uterus with fetuses may be examined *in situ* or removed at the cervix.

Check bile duct patency by squeezing the gallbladder and remove the stomach, spleen, and duodenum together. Sever the costal attachments of the diaphragm and remove the liver and diaphragm.

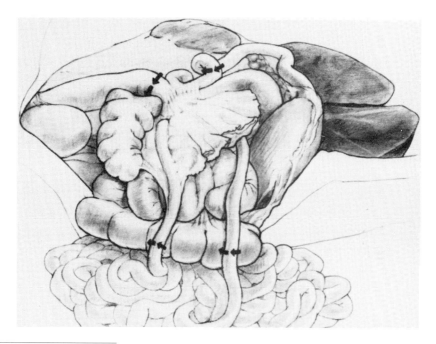

Figure 10-22. Incisions are made at the ileum and caudal duodenum to remove the small intestine (*bottom*). The colon is severed near the right kidney, and the duodenum is severed caudal to the gallbladder (*top*). (Strafuss AC: *Necropsy procedures and basic diagnostic methods for practicing veterinarians,* Springfield, IL, 1988, Charles C Thomas.)

Pelvic cuts and removal of the urogenital organs, caudal gastrointestinal tract, brain, and spinal cord are the same as for dogs and cats (Figures 10-17 to 10-19).

NECROPSY OF CATTLE, SHEEP, AND GOATS

All ruminants are placed on their left side, with the dissector facing the ventral abdomen. The same procedures described for dogs and cats are used for opening ruminant cadavers (Figures 10-1 to 10-6) and for examining the heart (Figures 10-7 to 10-11).

REMOVING THE GASTROINTESTINAL TRACT

Grasp the ileum with the left thumb and index finger near its entry into the cecum and cut the small intestine away from its mesentery attachment to the point where the small intestine disappears beneath the large intestine (duodenojejunal flexure). Cut the small intestine close to its mesenteric attachment, freeing the attached border so that the intestine is easily straightened and opened for examination. Sever and remove the small intestine. Cut the duodenum caudal to the gallbladder, check bile duct patency by squeezing the gallbladder, and bluntly dissect the duodenum to the abomasum (Figure 10-23, *bottom*). Bluntly dissect the rectum cranially, from the pelvic inlet to the right kidney. Sever the rectum and place it over the paralumbar region (Figure 10-23, *top*).

Grasp the large intestine in your left hand, pulling it taut from its mesenteric attachments. Sever and remove it from the abdominal cavity. Reflect the kidneys, adrenal glands, ureters, urinary bladder, and nongravid uterus caudally to the pelvic inlet and place them over the paralumbar fossa. Near-term fetuses in the uterus can be removed and the uterus examined *in situ*. Alternatively, the uterus may be severed at the cervix and removed.

Palpate between the reticulum and diaphragm for lesions associated with foreign bodies before removing the rumen. Sever the dorsal attachments of the rumen from the abdominal wall and pull the rumen counterclockwise. Sever

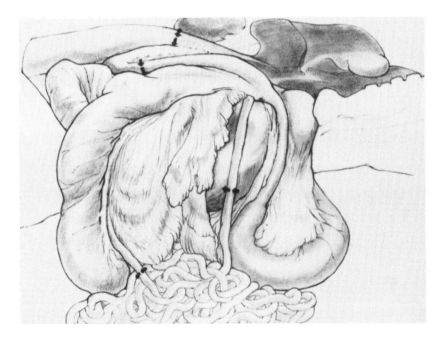

FIGURE **10-23.** The ileum and duodenum are severed to remove the small intestine (*bottom*). The rectum is severed near the right kidney (*top*). (Strafuss AC: *Necropsy procedures and basic diagnostic methods for practicing veterinarians,* Springfield, IL, 1988, Charles C Thomas.)

the attachments between the liver and omasum and ventrally and clockwise pull the omasum and abomasum from the abdominal cavity. Grasp the caudodorsal area of the rumen, sever the remaining dorsal attachments, and pull the rumen counterclockwise out of the abdominal cavity. The spleen lies on top of the rumen and can be examined. Sever the costal attachments of the diaphragm and remove the liver and diaphragm.

Pelvic cuts and removal of the urogenital tract, caudal gastrointestinal tract, brain, and spinal cord are the same as for dogs and cats (Figures 10-17 to 10-19).

NECROPSY OF HORSES

Horses are placed on their right side, with the dissector facing the ventral abdomen. The same procedures described for cats and dogs are used for opening equine cadavers (Figures 10-1 to 10-6) and for removing and examining the thoracic organs (Figures 10-7 to 10-11).

REMOVING THE GASTROINTESTINAL TRACT

Ligate and remove the spleen. (Ligation prevents blood from flowing over abdominal viscera.) Grasp the small colon and lay it over the paralumbar area.

Grasp the pelvic flexure of the great colon and pull it out of the abdominal cavity so that it is at right angles to the long axis of the cadaver. Locate the ileum adjacent to the cecum. Cut the small intestine from the mesenteric attachment cranially, to the point where the duodenum disappears beneath and is attached to the transverse colon. Cut the small intestine close to its mesenteric attachment so that the intestine is easily straightened and opened for examination (Figure 10-24, *bottom*).

Grasp the duodenum (usually ventral to the left kidney) and bluntly tear it loose from its mesenteric attachments and from the large intestine cranial to the stomach. Pull the stomach cranially and cut the esophageal portion loose from the diaphragm. Grasp the duodenum at the pylorus and bluntly dissect it from its mesenteric attachments caudally until it is freed. Sever the duodenum near the right kidney and tie the proximal end in a knot. Grasp the stomach and pull it and the first portion of the duodenum cranially from the abdominal wall. Sever and ligate the small colon 4 cm caudal to the transverse colon and lay it over the paralumbar region (Figure 10 24, *top*).

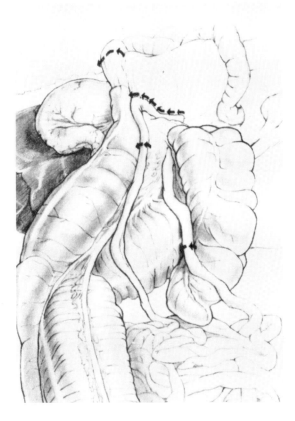

Figure 10-24. The small colon is severed and ligated 4 cm caudal to the transverse colon (*top*). The small intestine is cut near its mesenteric attachment to remove it from the abdomen (*bottom*). (Strafuss AC: *Necropsy procedures and basic diagnostic methods for practicing veterinarians,* Springfield, IL, 1988, Charles C Thomas.)

Cut lateral to the left kidney and reflect the kidney medially. Extend the incision craniomedially to remove the left adrenal gland, left kidney, and left ureter as a unit, pulling them caudally (Figure 10-25). Lay them over the cranial brim of the pelvis or paralumbar region. Check major abdominal blood vessels for thrombi. Start at the most cranial aspect of the abdominal aorta and open it to its termination (internal and external iliacs). Open the celiac, cranial mesenteric, and renal arteries and check the three major branches of the cranial mesenteric artery.

Sever the abdominal aorta caudal to the cranial mesenteric artery and remove this section along with the large colon from the abdominal cavity (Figure 10-26). When reflecting the large colon, *do not remove the right kidney and adrenal gland* with it. The right kidney and adrenal gland lie partially beneath the liver and may be torn loose when removing the large intestine and abdominal aorta.

Cut craniolateral to the right kidney and adjacent adrenal gland (beneath the liver) and reflect them caudally to the cranial brim of the pelvis. Reflect the

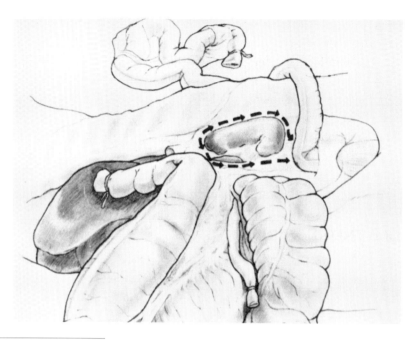

Figure 10-25. The left kidney, adrenal gland, and ureter are removed as a unit. (Strafuss AC: *Necropsy procedures and basic diagnostic methods for practicing veterinarians,* Springfield, IL, 1988, Charles C Thomas.)

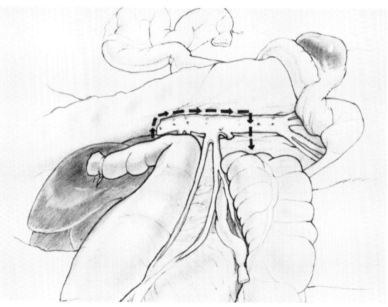

Figure 10-26. A section of the caudal aorta is removed with the large colon. (Strafuss AC: *Necropsy procedures and basic diagnostic methods for practicing veterinarians,* Springfield, IL, 1988, Charles C Thomas.)

left kidney, adrenal gland, ureter, and nongravid uterus caudally to the pelvic inlet and place them over the paralumbar region. A gravid uterus with full-term fetus can be examined *in situ,* or the gravid uterus may be removed at the cervix.

Sever the costal attachments of the diaphragm and remove the liver and diaphragm. Pelvic cuts and removal of urogenital organs, caudal gastrointestinal tract, brain, and spinal cord are the same as for dogs and cats (Figures 10-17 to 10-19).

Recommended Reading

Andrews: Necropsy techniques, *Vet Clin North Am* (Food Animal) 2:1 *et seqq,* 1986.

Brown: Necropsy techniques in small animal medicine, *Vet Tech* 16:409-419, 1995.

Crocker: *Veterinary post-mortem technic,* Philadelphia, 1918, Lippincott.

Feldman: Necropsy, *Proc Ann Mtg AAHA,* pp 542-547, 1973.

Jones and Gleiser: *Veterinary necropsy procedures,* Philadelphia, 1954, Lippincott.

Monlux: Routine necropsy procedure in the bovine, *Southwestern Vet* 5:121-129, 1952.

Rooney: *Autopsy of the horse: technique and interpretation,* 1970, Williams & Wilkins.

Runnells, et al: *Principles of veterinary pathology,* ed 7, Ames, IA, 1965, Iowa State University Press, pp 932-937.

Sheahan: The necropsy in small animal practice, *J Small Anim Pract* 16:569-574, 1975.

Strafuss: *Necropsy procedures and basic diagnostic methods for practicing veterinarians,* Springfield, IL, 1988, Charles C Thomas.

Van Kruiningen: Veterinary autopsy procedure, *Vet Clin North Am* 1:163-169, 1971.

Winter: *Post-mortem examination of ruminants,* St Lucia, Queensland, Australia, 1966, University of Queensland.

CYTOLOGIC EXAMINATION

R.L. Cowell

COLLECTION AND SMEAR PREPARATION

Cytologic samples can be collected by swabbing, scraping, and/or aspirating the lesion. The technique(s) used to collect cytologic samples and prepare slides vary, depending on the anatomic location, characteristics of the tissue being sampled, and characteristics of the patient (e.g., tractability).

When possible, several smears should be prepared, leaving some unstained, so smears are available for special stains if necessary. General considerations for collection and preparation of cytologic samples are discussed following. Cytology texts should be consulted for more information on procedures for cytologic examination of specific tissues.

IMPRINTS

Imprints for cytologic evaluation can be prepared from external lesions on the living animal or from tissues removed during surgery or necropsy. They are easy to collect and require minimal restraint, but they collect fewer cells than scrapings and contain greater contamination (bacterial and cellular) than fine-needle aspiration biopsies (FNABs). As a result, imprints from superficial lesions often only reflect a secondary bacterial infection and/or inflammation-induced tissue dysplasia. This markedly hinders their use in diagnosis of neoplasia.

Ulcers should be imprinted before they are cleaned. The lesion should then be cleaned with a saline-moistened surgical sponge and reimprinted and/or scraped. A fine-needle aspirate of the tissue underlying the surface of the lesion should also be collected. In some conditions, such as *Dermatophilus congolensis* infection (streptothricosis) and *Coccidioides immitis* infection, impressions from the uncleaned lesion often contain far more organisms than impressions from cleaned lesions and samples collected by FNAB. Imprints of the underside of the scabs from *Dermatophilus congolensis* lesions are usually most rewarding. Other conditions may yield more information on the imprints from cleaned lesions than the imprints from uncleaned lesions.

To collect imprints from cleaned cutaneous lesions or tissues collected during surgery or necropsy, blood and tissue fluid should first be removed from the surface of the lesion being imprinted by blotting with a clean absorbent material. Excessive blood and tissue fluids inhibit tissue cells from adhering to the glass slide, producing a poorly cellular preparation. Also, excessive fluid inhibits cells from spreading and assuming the size and shape they usually have in air-dried smears. The middle of a clean glass microscope slide is then touched against the blotted surface of the tissue to be imprinted. Although multiple imprints generally are made on each slide, one imprint per slide usually is sufficient. When possible, several slides are imprinted so slides are available for special stains if necessary.

SCRAPINGS

Smears of scrapings can be prepared from tissues collected during necropsy or surgery or from external lesions on the living animal. Scraping has the advantage of collecting many cells from the tissue and, therefore, is advantageous when the lesion is firm and yields few cells. The major disadvantages of scrapings are that they are more difficult to collect and they collect only superficial samples. As a result, scrapings from superficial lesions often only reflect a secondary bacterial infection and/or inflammation-induced tissue dysplasia. This markedly hinders their use in diagnosis of neoplasia.

Scrapings are prepared by holding a scalpel blade perpendicular to the lesion's cleaned and blotted surface and pulling the blade toward oneself several times. The material collected on the blade is transferred to the middle of a glass microscope slide and spread by one or more of the techniques described following for preparation of smears from aspirates of solid masses.

SWABS

Generally, swabs are collected only when imprints, scrapings, and aspirates cannot be made, as with fistulous tracts and vaginal collections. The lesion is swabbed with a moist, sterile cotton swab. Sterile isotonic fluid, such as 0.9% saline, should be used to moisten the swab. Moistening the swab helps minimize cell damage during sample collection and smear preparation. If the lesion is very moist, the swab need not be moistened. After sample collection, the swab is gently rolled along the flat surface of a clean glass microscope slide. *Do not rub the swab across the slide surface,* as this causes excessive cell damage.

ASPIRATION OF MASSES

Fine-needle aspiration biopsies can be collected from masses, including lymph nodes, nodular lesions, and internal organs. For cutaneous lesions, they avoid superficial contamination (bacterial and cellular) but collect fewer cells than scrapings.

SELECTION OF SYRINGE AND NEEDLE.   Fine-needle aspiration biopsies are collected with a 21- to 25-gauge needle and a 3- to 20-ml syringe. The softer the tissue being aspirated, the smaller the needle and syringe used. It is seldom advantageous, however, to use a needle larger than 21 gauge for aspiration, even for firm tissues, such as fibromas. When needles larger than 21 gauge are used, tissue cores tend to be aspirated, resulting in a poor yield of free cells suitable for cytologic preparation. Also, larger needles tend to cause greater blood contamination.

The size of syringe used is influenced by the consistency of the tissue being aspirated. Softer tissues, such as lymph nodes, often can successfully be aspirated with a 3-ml syringe. Firm tissues, such as fibromas and squamous-cell carcinomas, require a larger syringe to maintain adequate suction for sufficient collection of cells. Because the ideal size of the syringe is not known for many masses before aspiration, a 12-ml syringe is a good all-around size.

PREPARATION OF THE SITE FOR ASPIRATION.   If microbiologic tests are to be performed on a portion of the sample collected or a body cavity (peritoneal and thoracic cavities, joints, etc.) is to be penetrated, the area of aspiration is surgically prepared. Otherwise, skin preparation is essentially that required for a vaccination or venipuncture. An alcohol swab can be used to clean the area.

ASPIRATION PROCEDURE. The mass to be aspirated is held firmly to aid penetration of the skin and mass and to control the direction of the needle. The needle, with syringe attached, is introduced into the center of the mass and strong negative pressure is applied by withdrawing the plunger to about three fourths the volume of the syringe (Figure 11-1). Several areas of the mass should be sampled, but aspiration of the sample into the barrel of the syringe and contamination of the sample by aspiration of tissue surrounding the mass must be avoided. To accomplish this, when the mass is large enough to allow the needle to be redirected and moved to several areas in the mass without danger of the needle's leaving the mass, negative pressure is maintained during redirection and movement of the needle. However, when the mass is not large enough for the needle to be redirected and moved without danger of the needle's leaving the mass, negative pressure is relieved during redirection and

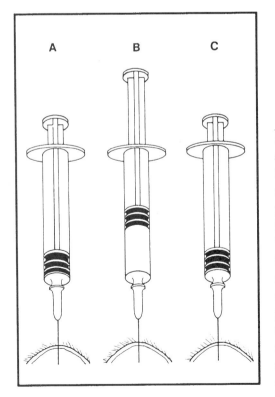

FIGURE 11-1. A, Fine-needle aspiration from a solid mass. **B,** Negative pressure is placed on the syringe by rapidly withdrawing the plunger (usually one half to three fourths the volume of the syringe). The needle is redirected several times while negative pressure is maintained if this can be accomplished without the needle's point leaving the mass. **C,** Before removing the needle from the mass, the plunger is released, relieving negative pressure on the syringe.

movement of the needle. In this situation, negative pressure is applied only when the needle is static. Often, high-quality collections do not have aspirate material visible in the syringe and sometimes not even in the hub of the needle.

After several areas are sampled, the negative pressure is relieved from the syringe and the needle is withdrawn from the mass and skin. Next the needle is removed from the syringe and air is drawn into the syringe. Then the needle is replaced onto the syringe and some of the tissue in the barrel and hub of the needle is expelled onto the middle of a glass microscope slide by rapidly depressing the plunger. When possible, several preparations should be made as described following.

NON-ASPIRATE PROCEDURE (CAPILLARY TECHNIQUE).   The technique described here is a modification of the procedure first described by Drs. Menard and Papageorges.[1] Technically, this technique is easier to perform than aspiration because one does not have to attempt to both direct the syringe and needle and pull the plunger with the same hand. A 22-gauge needle is attached to a 10-ml syringe that has been prefilled with air. The mass to be sampled is held firmly to aid penetration of the skin and mass and to help direct the needle. Grasping at the base of the needle gives one better control. The needle, with syringe attached, is introduced into the mass. The needle is moved rapidly back and forth through the mass five to six times. There is no need to aspirate, as the cells are collected by shearing and capillary action. The needle is removed from the mass, and the material is expelled onto a clean glass microscope slide by rapidly depressing the plunger. The expelled material should be smeared using one of the techniques described following.

Generally, one only collects enough material to make one smear. Therefore the procedure should be repeated two or three times in different sites of the mass so as to have adequate slide numbers and areas of the mass to evaluate.

PREPARATION OF SMEARS
FROM ASPIRATES OF SOLID MASSES

Several methods can be used to prepare smears for cytologic evaluation of solid masses, including lymph nodes. The experience of the person preparing the smears and characteristics of the sample influence the choice of smear preparation technique. We suggest a combination of slide preparation techniques. Some cytologic preparation techniques are described following.

Combination technique. One combination procedure involves spraying the aspirate onto the middle of a clean glass microscope slide (*prep slide*). Keeping the prep slide on a flat, solid, horizontal surface, pull another slide (*spreader slide*) backward at a 45-degree angle to the first slide until it contacts about one third of the aspirate (Figure 11-2). Then slide the spreader slide smoothly and rapidly forward, as if making a blood smear. Next, place the spreader slide horizontally over the back one third of the aspirate at a right angle to the prep slide. Allow the weight of the spreader slide (top slide) to spread the material, resisting the temptation to compress the slides manually. Keeping the spreader slide flat and horizontal, quickly and smoothly slide it across the prep slide.

This makes a squash preparation (see following) of the back third of the aspirate. The middle third of the aspirate is left untouched. This procedure leaves the front third of the aspirate gently spread. If the aspirate is of fragile tissue, this area should contain sufficient unruptured cells to evaluate. The back third of the aspirate has been spread with the shear forces of a squash preparation. If the aspirate contains clumps of cells that are difficult to spread, there should be some clumps sufficiently spread in the back one third of the preparation. If the aspirate is of very low cellularity, the middle third remains more concentrated and is the most efficient area to study.

Squash Preparation. In expert hands, the squash preparation can yield excellent cytologic smears. However, in less experienced hands, it often yields cytologic smears that are unreadable because too many cells are ruptured or the sample is not sufficiently spread. A squash preparation is made by expelling the aspirate onto the middle of one slide and then placing a second slide over the aspirate horizontal with and at right angles to the first slide (Figure 11-3). The second slide is then quickly and smoothly slid across the first slide.

Other spreading techniques. A modification of the squash preparation that has less tendency to rupture cells is to lay the second slide over the aspirate, then rotate the second slide 45 degrees and lift it upward (Figure 11-4).

Another technique for spreading aspirates is to drag the aspirate peripherally in several directions with the point of a syringe needle, producing a starfish shape (Figure 11-5). This technique tends not to damage fragile cells but does allow a thick layer of tissue fluid to remain around the cells. Sometimes the thick layer of fluid prevents the cells from spreading well and interferes with evaluation of cell detail. Usually, however, some acceptable areas are present.

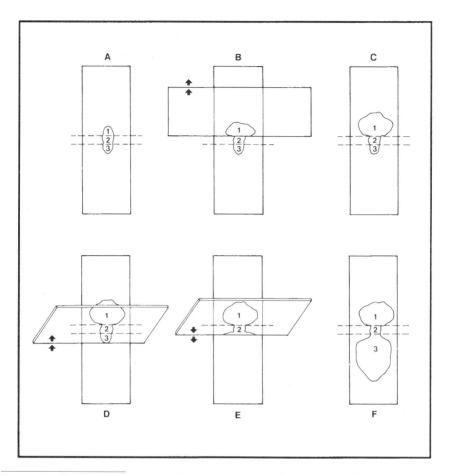

FIGURE 11-2.   Combination cytologic preparation. **A,** A portion of the aspirate is expelled onto a glass microscope slide (prep slide). **B,** Another glass microscope slide is placed over about one third of the preparation. If additional spreading of the aspirate is needed, gentle digital pressure can be used. Excessive pressure should be avoided. **C,** The spreader slide is smoothly slid forward. This makes a squash prep of about one third of the aspirate (*area 1*). The spreader slide also contains a squash prep (*not depicted*). Next, the edge of a tilted glass microscope slide (second spreader slide) is slid backward from the end opposite the squash prep until it contacts about one third the expelled aspirate (**D** and **E**). **F,** Then the second spreader slide is slid rapidly and smoothly forward. This produces an area (*3*) that is spread with mechanical forces like those of a blood smear preparation. The middle area (*2*) is left untouched and contains a high concentration of cells.

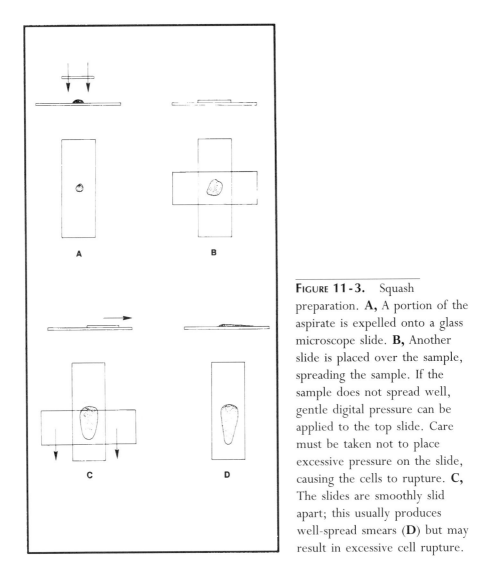

FIGURE 11-3. Squash preparation. **A,** A portion of the aspirate is expelled onto a glass microscope slide. **B,** Another slide is placed over the sample, spreading the sample. If the sample does not spread well, gentle digital pressure can be applied to the top slide. Care must be taken not to place excessive pressure on the slide, causing the cells to rupture. **C,** The slides are smoothly slid apart; this usually produces well-spread smears (**D**) but may result in excessive cell rupture.

PREPARATION OF SMEARS FROM FLUIDS

Cytologic smears should be prepared immediately after fluid collection. When possible, fluid samples for cytologic examination should be collected in ethylenediaminetetraacetic acid (EDTA) tubes. Smears can be prepared directly from fresh, well-mixed fluid or from the sediment of a centrifuged sample by blood smear (Figure 11-6), line smear (Figure 11-7), and squash preparation

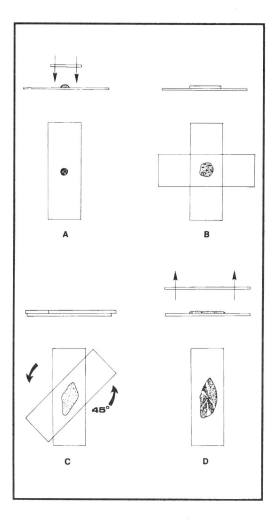

FIGURE 11-4. Modification of the squash preparation. **A,** A portion of the aspirate is expelled onto a glass microscope slide. **B,** Another slide is placed over the sample, causing the sample to spread. If necessary, gentle digital pressure can be applied to the top slide to spread the sample more. Care must be taken not to place excessive pressure on the slide, causing the cells to rupture. **C,** The top slide is rotated about 45 degrees and lifted directly upward, producing a squash preparation with subtle ridges and valleys of cells (**D**).

(Figure 11-3) techniques. The cellularity, viscosity, and homogeneity of the fluid influence the selection of smear technique.

The squash preparation technique often spreads viscous samples and samples with flecks of particulate material better than the blood smear and line smear techniques. The blood smear technique usually produces well-spread smears of sufficient cellularity from homogeneous fluids containing ≥5000 cells/μl but often produces smears of insufficient cellularity from fluids containing <5000 cells/μl. The line smear technique can be used to concentrate fluids of low cellularity but often does not sufficiently spread cells from highly cellular fluids. In general, translucent fluids are of low to moderate cellularity, whereas opaque

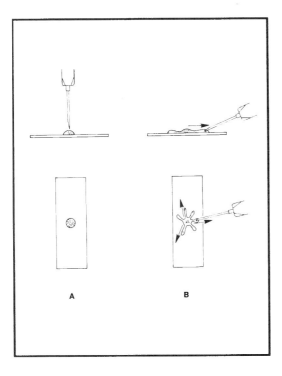

Figure 11-5. Needle spread or "starfish" preparation. **A,** A portion of the aspirate is expelled onto a glass microscope slide. **B,** The tip of a needle is placed in the aspirate and moved peripherally, pulling a trail of the sample with it. This procedure is repeated in several directions, resulting in a preparation with multiple projections.

fluids are usually highly cellular. Therefore, translucent fluids often require concentration, either by centrifugation or by the line smear technique. When possible, concentration by centrifugation is preferred.

To prepare a smear by the blood smear technique, place a small drop of the fluid on a glass slide about 1.0 to 1.5 cm from the end (Figure 11-6). Pull another slide backward at a 30- to 40-degree angle until it contacts the drop. When the fluid flows sideways along the juncture between the slides, quickly and smoothly push the second slide forward until the fluid has all drained away from the second slide. This makes a smear with a feathered edge.

To concentrate fluids by centrifugation, the fluid is centrifuged 5 minutes at 165 to 360 G. This is achieved by operating a centrifuge with a radial arm length of 14.6 cm (the arm length of most urine centrifuges) at 1000 to 1500 rpm. After centrifugation, the supernatant is separated from the sediment and analyzed for total protein concentration. The sediment is resuspended in a few drops of supernatant by gently thumping the side of the tube. A drop of the resuspended sediment is placed on a slide, and a smear is made by the blood smear or squash preparation technique. When possible, several smears should be made by each technique.

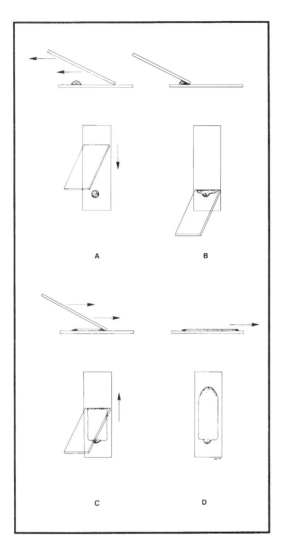

FIGURE 11-6. Blood smear technique. **A,** A drop of fluid sample is placed on a glass microscope slide close to one end, then another slide is slid backward to contact the front of the drop (**B**). When the drop is contacted, it rapidly spreads along the juncture between the two slides. **C** and **D,** The spreader slide is then smoothly and rapidly slid forward the length of the slide, producing a smear with a feathered edge.

When the fluid cannot be concentrated by centrifugation or the centrifuged sample is of low cellularity, the line smear technique (Figure 11-7) can be used to concentrate cells in the smear. A drop of fluid is placed on a clean glass slide and the blood smear technique is used, except the spreading slide is raised directly upward about three fourths of the way through the smear, yielding a line containing a much higher concentration of cells than the rest of the slide. Unfortunately, an excessive amount of fluid may also remain in the "line" and prevent the cells from spreading well.

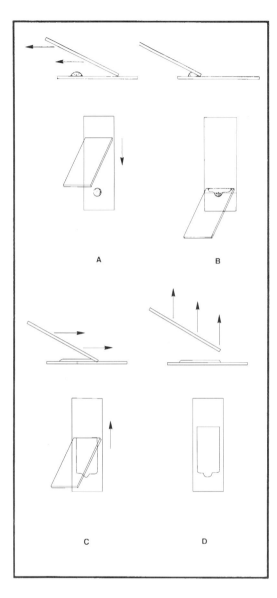

Figure 11-7. Line smear concentration technique. **A,** A drop of fluid sample is placed on a glass microscope slide close to one end, then another slide is slid backward to contact the front of the drop (**B**). When the drop is contacted, it rapidly spreads along the juncture between the two slides. **C,** The spreader slide is then smoothly and rapidly slid forward (**D**). After the spreader slide has been advanced about two thirds to three fourths the distance required to make a smear with a feathered edge, the spreader slide is raised directly upward. This produces a smear with a line of concentrated cells at its end, instead of a feathered edge.

STAINING

Types of stains

Several types of stains have been used for cytologic preparations. The two general types most commonly used are the Romanowsky-type stains (Wright's, Giemsa, Diff-Quik) and Papanicolaou stain and its derivatives, such as Sano's trichrome. The advantages and disadvantages of both types of stains are discussed following. However, because the Romanowsky-type stains are more rewarding, practical, and readily available in practice situations, the remainder of this discussion deals predominantly with Romanowsky-stained preparations.

ROMANOWSKY STAINS.   Romanowsky stains are inexpensive, readily available, and easy to prepare, maintain, and use. They stain organisms and the cytoplasm of cells excellently. Although nuclear and nucleolar detail cannot be perceived as well with Romanowsky stains as with Papanicolaou stains, nuclear and nucleolar detail usually is sufficient for differentiating neoplasia and inflammation and for evaluating neoplastic cells for cytologic evidence of malignant potential (criteria of malignancy).

Smears to be stained with Romanowsky stains are first air dried. Air drying partially preserves ("fixes") the cells and causes them to adhere to the slide so they do not fall off during the staining procedure.

There are many commercially available Romanowsky stains, including Diff-Quik, DipStat, and other quick Wright's stains. Most, if not all, Romanowsky stains are acceptable for staining cytologic preparations. Diff-Quik stain does not undergo the metachromatic reaction. As a result, granules of some mast cells do not stain. When mast-cell granules do not stain, the mast cells may be misclassified as macrophages. This can lead to confusion in examination of some mast-cell tumors. The variations among different Romanowsky stains should not cause a problem once the evaluator has become familiar with the stain he/she uses routinely.

Each stain usually has its own unique recommended staining procedure. These procedures should be followed in general but should be adapted to the type and thickness of smear being stained and to the evaluator's preference. The thinner the smear and the lower the total protein concentration of the fluid, the less time needed in the stain. The thicker the smear and the greater the total protein concentration of the fluid, the more time needed in the stain. As a result, fluid smears with low protein and low cellularity, such as abdominal fluid, may stain better using half or less of the recommended time. Thick smears, such as smears of neoplastic lymph nodes, may need to be stained twice the recommended time or longer. Each person tends to have a different staining technique he/she prefers. By trying variations in the recommended time intervals for stains, the evaluator can establish which times produce the preferred staining characteristics.

NEW METHYLENE BLUE STAIN.   New methylene blue (NMB) stain is a useful adjunct to Romanowsky stains. It stains cytoplasm weakly, if at all, but gives excellent nuclear and nucleolar detail. Because NMB stains cytoplasm weakly, often the nuclear detail of cells in cell clumps can be visualized. Generally, RBCs do not stain with NMB but may develop a pale blue tint. As a result, marked RBC contamination of smears does not obscure nucleated cells.

Papanicolaou stains. The delicate Papanicolaou stains give excellent nuclear detail and delicate cytoplasmic detail. They allow the viewer to see through layers of cells in cell clumps and to evaluate nuclear and nucleolar changes very well. They do not stain cytoplasm as strongly as Romanowsky stains and, therefore, do not demonstrate cytoplasmic changes as well as Romanowsky stains. They also do not demonstrate bacteria and other organisms as well as Romanowsky stains.

Papanicolaou staining requires multiple steps and considerable time. Also the reagents often are difficult to locate, prepare, and maintain in practice. Papanicolaou stains and their derivatives require the specimen to be wet-fixed (i.e., the smear must be fixed before the cells have dried). Usually this is achieved by spraying the smear with a cytologic fixative or placing it in ethanol immediately after preparation. When the smear is to be placed in ethanol, it should be made on a protein-coated slide. This prevents the cells from falling off the slide when it is immersed.

STAINING PROBLEMS

Poor stain quality often perplexes both the novice and experienced cytologist. Most staining problems can be avoided if the following precautions are taken:

- Use new slides, fresh, well-filtered (if periodic filtration is required) stain(s) and fresh buffer solution (if a buffer is required).
- Stain cytologic preparations immediately after air drying.
- Take care not to touch the surface of the slide or smear at any time.

Occasionally a sample may be contaminated with a foreign substance, such as K-Y Jelly, that alters the specimen's staining. Table 11-1 gives some of the problems that can occur with Romanowsky stains and some proposed solutions to these problems.

MICROSCOPIC EVALUATION

A detailed discussion of microscopic evaluation and cytologic interpretation is beyond the scope of this book. Reference sources contain detailed information.[2-7] However, the basic principles are as follows.

TABLE 11-1. Some possible solutions to problems seen with common Romanowsky stains

PROBLEM	SOLUTION
EXCESSIVE BLUE STAINING (RBC MAY BE BLUE-GREEN)	
Prolonged stain contact	Decrease staining time
Inadequate wash	Wash longer
Specimen too thick	Make thinner smears if possible
Stain, diluent, buffer or wash water too alkaline	Check with pH paper and correct pH
Exposure to formalin vapors	Store and ship cytologic preps separate from formalin containers
Wet fixation in ethanol	Air dry smears before fixation
Delayed fixation	Fix smears sooner if possible
Surface of the slide was alkaline	Use new slides
EXCESSIVE PINK STAINING	
Insufficient staining time	Increase staining time
Prolonged washing	Decrease duration of wash
Stain or diluent too acidic	Check with pH paper and correct pH; fresh methanol may be needed
Excessive time in red stain solution	Decrease time in red solution
Inadequate time in blue stain solution	Increase time in blue stain solution
Mounting coverslip before preparation is dry	Allow preparation to dry completely before mounting coverslip
WEAK STAINING	
Insufficient contact with one or more of the stain solutions	Increase staining time
Fatigued (old) stains	Change stains
Another slide covered specimen during staining	Keep slides separate

Continued.

TABLE 11-1. Some possible solutions to problems seen with common Romanowsky stains—*continued*

PROBLEM	SOLUTION
UNEVEN STAINING	
Variation of pH in different areas of slide surface (may be due to slide surface being touched or slide being poorly cleaned)	Use new slides and avoid touching their surface before and after preparation
Water allowed to stand on some areas of the slide after staining and washing	Tilt slides close to vertical to drain water from the surface or dry with a fan
Inadequate mixing of stain and buffer	Mix stain and buffer thoroughly
PRECIPITATE ON PREPARATION	
Inadequate stain filtration	Filter or change the stain(s)
Inadequate washing of slide after staining	Rinse slides well after staining
Dirty slides used	Use clean new slides
Stain solution dries during staining	Use sufficient stain and do not leave it on slide too long
MISCELLANEOUS	
Overstained preparations	Destain with 95% methanol and restain; Diff-Quik-stained smears may have to be destained in the red Diff-Quik stain solution to remove the blue color; however, this damages the red stain solution
Refractile artifact on RBC with Diff-Quik stain (usually due to moisture in fixative)	Change the fixative

After the smear has been stained and dried, it is scanned at low magnification (4X to 10X objective) to determine if all areas of the smear are stained adequately and to detect any localized areas of increased cellularity or areas with unique staining features. If the smear is inadequately stained, it can be restained. However, not all areas of a slide must be adequately stained. For example, even if only the edges of thick smears are stained adequately, they may still be adequately evaluated.

Any areas of increased and/or unique cellularity should be mentally noted for later evaluation. Also, large objects, such as crystals, foreign bodies, parasites, and fungal hyphae, may be seen while scanning the slide at low magnification. When proper staining is ensured and all areas of increased and/or unique cellularity are recognized, magnification is increased to the 10X or 20X objective. An impression of the cellularity and cellular composition (inflammatory cells, epithelial cells, spindle cells, etc.) of the smear and of cell size is usually developed at this magnification. Areas of increased cellularity and/or unique cellularity are evaluated.

Next the smear is viewed with the 40X objective. To improve resolution by decreasing light diffraction, a drop of oil can be placed on the smear; then a coverslip is placed over the drop of oil. At this magnification, individual cells are evaluated and compared to other cells in the smear. Usually, nucleoli and the chromatin pattern can be discerned. With experience, one can see most organisms that are visible microscopically with the 40X objective. However, it may be necessary to use the 100X (oil-immersion) objective to identify some organisms and inclusions and to confirm the identity of organisms seen with the 40X objective. Cell morphology (nuclear chromatin pattern, nucleoli, etc.) is evaluated in detail with the 100X (oil-immersion) objective.

Cell types encountered depend on the origin of the specimen. Familiarity with the appearance of erythrocytes, neutrophils, lymphocytes, plasma cells, eosinophils, mast cells, macrophages, mesothelial cells, squamous (keratinized and nonkeratinized) epithelial cells (Figures 11-8 and 11-9), and neoplastic cells is required. Appreciation of the difference between pyknosis, karolysis, and mechanical disruption of cells (smear artifact) is mandatory for proper interpretation (Figure 11-10). *Pyknosis* represents slow cell death (aging) and refers to a small, condensed, dark nucleus that may fragment (*karyorrhexis*) (Figure 11-11). *Karolysis* represents rapid cell death, as in some septic (bacterial) inflammatory reactions and refers to a swollen, ragged nucleus with reduced staining intensity (Figure 11-12). Macrophages and neutrophils should be noted as nonphagocytic, phagocytic (with a description of the ingested material), nonvacuolated, or vacuolated (Figure 11-11).

Neoplastic cells must be classified as cytologically benign or malignant. As a generalization, a cytologically benign neoplasm has a uniform population of cells, whereas a cytologically malignant neoplasm tends to have a pleomorphic population of cells, with cells, nuclei, and nucleoli tending to be large, usually with a disproportionately large nucleus (referred to as a high nucleus : cytoplasm

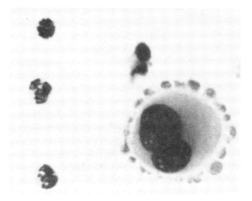

FIGURE 11-8. Large binucleate epithelial cell in equine peritoneal fluid. Cytoplasmic "pseudopods" around the cell are an artifact of slide preparation. (Wright's stain, 1140X)

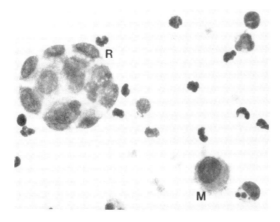

FIGURE 11-9. A raft of mesothelial cells (*R*) in peritoneal fluid from a horse with resolving peritonitis. Several neutrophils and erythrocytes, a phagocytic macrophage, and a mesothelial cell (*M*) are also present. (Wright's stain, 810X)

ratio). Malignant neoplastic cells frequently have multiple, pleomorphic, bizarre (angular) nucleoli and a high mitotic index, with active (basophilic) cytoplasm (Figure 11-13, Table 11-2).

Histopathologic verification of cytologic findings is important for most tumors (whether cytologically benign or malignant). Also it is important to realize that cytologically benign cells may be obtained from malignant tumors. Histopathologic examination offers the advantage of enabling assessment of such factors as local tissue infiltration and vessel or lymphatic invasion by tumor cells. These are characteristics of malignant tumors that are not evident cytologically.

The cytology report should indicate the cell types present, their appearance, and relative proportions. The flow chart in Figure 11-14 on p. 557 shows

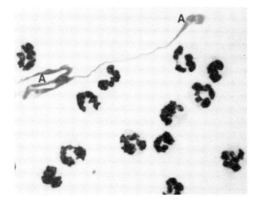

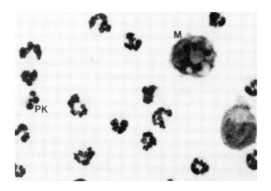

FIGURE **11-10.**   Blood smear artifact. Note that most neutrophils are intact, with normal morphology. However, the nucleus of one cell (*A*) has been mechanically disrupted. (Wright's stain, 780X)

FIGURE **11-11.**   Peritoneal fluid smear from a horse with resolving peritonitis. Numerous neutrophils with normal morphology are present. One neutrophil nucleus (*PK*) is pyknotic (condensed and has increased affinity for stain) and karyorrhectic (fragmented). A macrophage that has phagocytosed cellular debris is also present (*M*). (Wright's stain, 780X)

the steps taken to arrive at a general cytologic diagnosis. Obviously such a diagnosis must be interpreted relative to other findings in that animal.

SUBMISSION OF CYTOLOGIC PREPARATIONS AND SAMPLES FOR INTERPRETATION

When in-house evaluation of a cytologic preparation does not furnish sufficient reliable information for managing a case, the preparation can be submitted to a

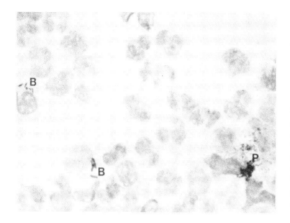

FIGURE 11-12. Peritoneal fluid smear from a dog with acute, septic, suppurative peritonitis, secondary to a ruptured bile duct. Note that all nuclei are karyolytic (swollen, with decreased affinity for stain). Bacteria (*B*) and bile pigment (*P*) are also present. (Wright's stain, 780X)

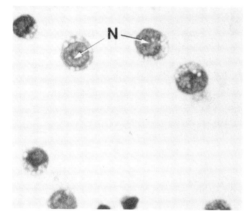

FIGURE 11-13. Smear of feline thoracic effusion due to lymphoblastic lymphosarcoma. Note the large immature lymphocytes with prominent nucleoli (*N*). (Wright's stain, 780X)

veterinary clinical pathologist/cytologist for interpretation, or an alternative procedure, such as biopsy and histopathologic evaluation, can be performed. If possible, the person to whom the cytologic preparation is sent should be contacted, and specifics concerning sample handling should be discussed, such as the number of smears to send, whether to fix or stain the smears before mailing, etc. The following discussion gives some general guidelines for submitting cytologic preparations for interpretation.

When possible, two or three air-dried unstained smears, and two or three air-dried Romanowsky-stained smears should be submitted. The air-dried unstained smears can be stained by the pathologist with the Romanowsky or new methylene blue stains of his/her choice. The Romanowsky-stained smears are a safety factor. Some tissues stain poorly when they are air dried but not

TABLE 11-2. Easily recognized general and nuclear criteria of malignancy

CRITERIA	DESCRIPTION	SCHEMATIC REPRESENTATION
GENERAL CRITERIA		
Anisocytosis and macrocytosis	Variation in cell size, with some cells $\geq$ 1.5 times larger than normal.	
Hypercellularity	Increased cell exfoliation due to decreased cell adherence.	Not depicted
Pleomorphism (except in lymphoid tissue)	Variable size and shape in cells of the same type.	
NUCLEAR CRITERIA		
Macrokaryosis	Increased nuclear size. Cells with nuclei larger than 10 μ in diameter suggest malignancy.	RBC
Increased nucleus: cytoplasm ratio (N:C)	Normal nonlymphoid cells usually have a N:C of 1:3 to 1:8, depending on the tissue. Ratios $\geq$ 1:2 suggest malignancy.	See "Macrokaryosis"
Anisokaryosis	Variation in nuclear size. This is especially important if the nuclei of multinucleated cells vary in size.	
Multinucleation	Multiple nucleation in a cell. This is especially important if the nuclei vary in size.	
Increased mitotic figures	Mitosis is rare in normal tissue.	normal abnormal

Continued.

TABLE 11-2. Easily recognized general and nuclear criteria of malignancy—*continued*

CRITERIA	DESCRIPTION	SCHEMATIC REPRESENTATION
Abnormal mitosis	Improper alignment of chromosomes.	See "Increased mitotic figures"
Coarse chromatin pattern	The chromatin pattern is coarser than normal. It may appear ropy or cord-like.	
Nuclear molding	Deformation of nuclei by other nuclei within the same cell or adjacent cells.	
Macronucleoli	Nucleoli are increased in size. Nucleoli ≥ 5 μ strongly suggest malignancy. For reference RBC are 5 to 6 μ in cats; 7 to 8 μ in dogs.	RBC
Angular nucleoli	Nucleoli are fusiform or have other angular shapes, instead of their normal round to slightly oval shape.	
Anisonucleoliosis	Variation in nucleolar shape or size (especially important if the variation is within the same nucleus).	See "Angular nucleoli"

stained for several days. Also slides occasionally are shattered during transport and cannot be stained upon receipt. Sometimes, microscopic examination of shards from the broken prestained smears allows diagnosis. If only a couple of smears can be prepared from the sample, one should be submitted air dried and unstained and the other submitted air dried and stained. Smears should be well labeled with alcohol-resistant ink or another permanent labeling method.

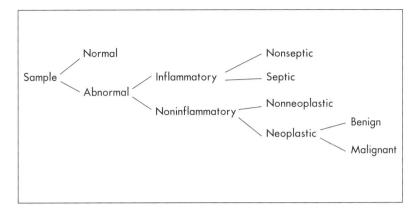

FIGURE 11-14.   Steps involved in making a general cytologic diagnosis.

If a Papanicolaou stain is to be used, several wet-fixed smears should be submitted.

Fluid samples should have smears prepared from them immediately. Both direct smears and concentrated smears should be submitted. Also, an EDTA (lavender top) and sterile serum tube (red top) fluid sample should be submitted. A total nucleated cell count and total protein concentration can be performed on the EDTA tube sample and, if necessary, chemical analyses can be performed on the serum tube sample.

Slides must be protected when mailed. Simple cardboard mailers do not provide sufficient protection to prevent slide breakage if they are mailed in unpadded envelopes. Marking the envelope with such phrases as "Fragile," "Glass," "Breakable," and "Please Hand Cancel" have little success. Placing a pad of bubble-paper or polystyrene on each side of the slide holder usually prevents slide breakage. Also, slides can be mailed in plastic slide holders or innovative holders, such as small pill bottles.

Slides should not be mailed with formalin-containing samples and should be protected against moisture. Formalin fumes alter the staining characteristics of smears and water causes cell lysis.

SUBMISSION OF SAMPLES FOR CULTURE

Culture results are strongly influenced by sample collection, preparation, and transport (see Chapter 4). The following procedures are suggested to optimize success in culturing lesions and fluids:

- Call the laboratory before collecting the sample.
- Collect the sample as aseptically as possible.
- Submit fresh samples for culture.
- Use proper equipment for collection and transport of the sample.
- Use a timely courier service.

CALL THE LAB BEFORE COLLECTING THE SAMPLE

Techniques, media, days when cultures are read or subcultures are performed, etc., often vary from laboratory to laboratory. By contacting the laboratory to which the sample will be submitted, such things as optimum sample type, transport medium, day of the week to submit the sample, etc., can be discussed. Also, some laboratories furnish culture supplies. Expensive and/or quickly outdated supplies, such as blood culture tubes, may be ordered from the laboratory as needed. Early communication with the laboratory also allows the laboratory to prepare for the sample and ensure that any special media required are available.

COLLECT SAMPLES AS ASEPTICALLY AS POSSIBLE

All samples should be collected as aseptically as possible. Even samples collected from lesions that naturally are exposed to secondary contamination, such as cutaneous ulcers, should be protected from further contamination. When samples are collected from more than one lesion, care should be taken not to cross-contaminate the samples. Finding the same organism in several different lesions is strong evidence that the organism is involved in development of the lesions. Therefore, cross-contamination of samples from different lesions can lead to misinterpretation of culture results. When fluids are collected, anticoagulant and serum tubes should not be assumed to be sterile. Also, EDTA, through its effect on bacterial cell walls, can be bacteriostatic or bactericidal.

SUBMIT FRESH SAMPLES

Samples should be submitted as soon after collection as possible. Fluid aspiration, resection of lesions to be cultured, exploratory surgeries during which culture is anticipated, and other procedures that may produce samples to be cultured should be scheduled to allow immediate transport of samples to the laboratory. During transport, samples should be kept cool but not frozen.

Tissue and fluid samples usually are more rewarding than swab samples for isolation of a causative agent. Individual tissue samples submitted for culture should be about 4 cm square or larger. Whirl-Pak (NASCO), Ziploc, or heat-sealed plastic bags are excellent for submitting tissue samples for culture. Such samples as abscesses and skin, known to contain bacteria, must be packaged separately from other tissues. Culturette-type transport systems should be used to prevent small biopsies from drying during transport. Avoid shipping biopsies in sterile saline, as this may cause negative culture results.

Fluid samples (urine, milk, joint fluid, thoracic fluid, abdominal fluid, abscess aspirates) can be submitted in sterile Vacu-Tainer tubes, small Whirl-Pak bags, or sterile disposable syringes. Fluids for anaerobic cultures should be collected in syringes, with air expelled, and then capped and transported immediately to the laboratory for culture. However, for optimal results or if a time delay is anticipated, the fluid should be placed in a transport system that supports both aerobic and anaerobic bacteria. These systems often can be obtained from the laboratory performing the culture. Transport culture tubes, such as Port-A-Cul Tubes (BBL Microbiology Systems, Cockeysville, MD), are commercially available for samples obtained on swabs. Containers, such as Port-A-Cul Vials (BBL), are commercially available for fluid samples. These systems usually support a wide variety of anaerobic and aerobic organisms for up to 72 hours at 20° to 25 C°.

If separate aerobic and anaerobic transport systems are used, a Culturette-like transport system, such as Culture Collection and Transport Tube (Curtis Matheson Scientific, Burbank, CA) containing Amies medium with charcoal, is suggested for aerobic cultures. These seem to be excellent transport and holding media for fastidious bacteria. Anaerobic transport systems, such as B-D Vacu-Tainer Anaerobic Specimen Collector (Becton-Dickinson, Rutherford, NJ), can be used to transport fluid, small tissue specimens, or swabs. However, they are large and cumbersome for mailing and must be packaged well to prevent the glass vial from breaking. Anaerobic transport systems, such as the Anaerobic Culturette (Marion Scientific, Kansas City, MO), have prereduced Cary-Blair transport medium to prevent the swab from drying. These small plastic units are unbreakable and easy to handle and mail. However, they can only be used for swabs.

When biopsies or aspirates are not obtainable or warranted, swabs are useful for sample collection, especially swabs of mucosal surfaces and deep within soft tissue lesions. Culturette-type transport swabs are preferred; those containing Amies medium with charcoal are superior for fastidious organisms. Anaerobic systems, such as mentioned previously, are necessary for transport of swabs for anaerobic culture. Swabs without medium can dry out in transport, resulting in false-negative results, whereas swabs submitted in broth medium often are overgrown by contaminants. Separate swabs should be submitted if additional cultures for fungi and/or viruses are desired.

In general, samples submitted for fungal culture should be collected and transported in the same manner as samples for bacterial culture. Again, tissues and body fluids are preferred to swabs. Swab samples should never be submitted for dermatophyte cultures. Instead, plucked hair and skin scrapings from the periphery of lesions should be transported in clean, dry containers. Communication with the laboratory chosen to perform the cultures is especially important before samples for fungal culture are collected.

References

1. Menard and Papageorges: Technique for ultrasound-guided fine-needle biopsies, *Vet Radiol Ultrasound* 36:137-138, 1995.

2. Cowell and Tyler: *Diagnostic cytology of the dog and cat,* St Louis, 1989, Mosby.

3. Cowell and Tyler: *Hematology and cytology of the horse,* St Louis, 1992, Mosby.

4. DeNicola: Diagnostic cytology, collection techniques, and sample handling, *Proc 4th Ann Mtg ACVIM,* pp 15-25, 1987.

5. Meyer and Franks: Clinical cytology, management of clinical specimens, *Mod Vet Prac* 67:255-259, 1986.

6. O'Rourke: Cytology techniques, *Mod Vet Prac* 64:185-189, 1983.

7. Meyer: Management of cytology specimens, *Compend Cont Ed Pract Vet* 9:10-16, 1987.

MISCELLANEOUS LABORATORY TECHNIQUES

B.W. Parry

The main topics covered in this chapter are cytology, detection of fecal occult blood, toxicology, and skin biopsy. The cytology section begins with a general review of specimen handling, preparation, and evaluation. This is followed by individual sections on routine procedures used to examine samples of cerebrospinal fluid, aqueous humor, peritoneal fluid, pleural fluid, synovial fluid, transtracheal washes, nasal flushes, ear swabs, lymph node and other aspirates, vaginal smears, semen, prostatic fluid, and milk. The toxicology section discusses general aspects of specimen collection, handling, and submission to a toxicology laboratory. Simple procedures for incriminating lead, thallium, antimony, arsenic, mercury, phenols, nitrites, anticoagulant rodenticides, compounds that damage the hemoglobin of red blood cells, and ethylene glycol in clinical poisonings are presented. The section on skin biopsy considers indications, instruments, methods, and specimen handling.

BIOPSY

Tissue biopsy refers to the sampling of a piece of tissue for cytologic and/or histopathologic examination. Many organs or tissues, including kidney, liver, lung, lymph node, prostate, skin, spleen and thyroid, or masses (tumors) can be biopsied. Biopsy techniques include gentle abrasion with a blade, needle aspiration, and excision. The technique used varies with the tissue to be biopsied. Considerations include its location, accessibility, and nature. Methods for making cytologic preparations from biopsy specimens have been described in Chapter 11.

Tissue samples for histopathologic examination often are fixed in 10% formalin. To ensure adequate fixation, slabs of tissue no more than 1 cm wide should be placed in fluid-tight jars containing formalin at about 10 times the specimen's volume.

EXFOLIATIVE CYTOLOGY

Exfoliative cytology refers to the study of cells shed from body surfaces. Thus, in its broadest sense, it refers to examination of cells present in body fluids (such as cerebrospinal, peritoneal, pleural, and synovial fluids), on mucosal surfaces (such as the trachea or vagina), or in secretions (such as semen, prostatic fluid, and milk). Samples typically are collected by imprint, swab, or aspiration. Common laboratory procedures used in conjunction with cytology in evaluation of these samples are presented in the following sections.

Certain gross characteristics of body fluids should be recorded at collection, including ease of sample collection, color, and turbidity. Subsequently, total nucleated cell counts, cell types, and their morphology are determined.

EASE OF COLLECTION

Ease of collection may reflect the volume of fluid present and/or the pressure within that body cavity. It is also influenced by the technical proficiency of the operator and, in the case of conscious animals, the cooperation of the animal.

COLOR, TURBIDITY

Color and turbidity are influenced by protein concentration and cell numbers. Gross discoloration, with increased turbidity, may be due to iatrogenic contamination with peripheral blood, recent or old hemorrhage, inflammation, or a combination thereof.

Perforation of superficial vessels during collection can result in contamination with peripheral blood. Such admixture of blood with the sample may be obvious as a streaking of blood in otherwise clear fluid at some stage during collection. Blood-tinged fluid may also be due to recent or old hemorrhage into the body cavity being sampled. Both peripheral blood contamination and recent hemorrhage result in a clear supernatant and a red (erythrocyte-rich) sediment after centrifugation. Recent hemolysis imparts a reddish discoloration to the supernatant. Hemorrhage that occurred at least 2 days previously generally causes a yellowish supernatant (due to hemoglobin breakdown products), usually with little erythrocytic sediment.

Cytologic examination of the fluid may also assist in determining the time of hemorrhage. Clumps of platelets may be observed in recent, often iatrogenic (operator-induced) hemorrhage (Figure 12-1). Such clumps are not obvious after an hour or so.

Blood must be present in the cavity for several hours before macrophage ingestion of erythrocytes becomes evident (erythrophagocytic macrophages, Figure 12-2). If the hemorrhage occurred a day or so before collection, hemoglobin-breakdown products, such as hemosiderin, may be seen in the macrophages (Figure 12-3).

Inflammation can also discolor body fluids, with the degree of turbidity reflecting leukocyte numbers. Color can vary from an off-white or cream to a red-cream or dirty brown, depending on the number of erythrocytes also involved and the integrity of the cells present.

CEREBROSPINAL FLUID ANALYSIS

Analysis of cerebrospinal fluid (CSF) is useful in evaluation of some neurologic disorders. Fluid is collected aseptically from the anesthetized animal by percutaneous insertion of a spinal needle through either the atlantooccipital or lumbosacral space, into the subarachnoid space of the spinal column. Care must be taken not to advance the needle too far and consequently damage the spinal

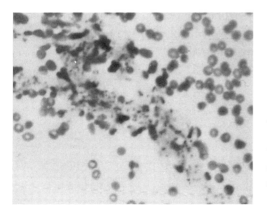

FIGURE 12-1. Synovial fluid from a dog. Recent hemorrhage, probably at collection, is indicated by the clumped platelets. (May Grünwald Giemsa stain, 400X)

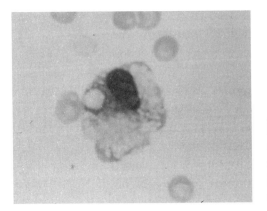

FIGURE 12-2. Synovial fluid from a dog. The erythrophagocytic macrophage indicates hemorrhage before collection. (May Grünwald Giemsa stain, 1000X)

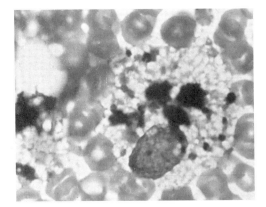

FIGURE 12-3. Prostatic wash fluid from a dog. The hemosiderin-laden macrophages indicate chronic hemorrhage. (May Grünwald Giemsa stain, 1000X)

cord. If the animal is in lateral recumbency, CSF pressure can be measured with a spinal manometer. Fluid is then collected by free flow, not aspiration, into an ethylenediaminetetraacetic acid (EDTA) tube and perhaps a serum (plain) blood tube. The plain tube of CSF should be centrifuged and the supernatant (with normal CSF there is very little sediment) used for biochemical tests, such as protein, glucose, lactate, and creatine kinase determinations.

COLOR, TURBIDITY

Normal CSF is colorless and transparent (it looks grossly like distilled water, and newsprint is easily read through it) because it has a very low protein concentration and very few cells. About 500 cells/μl must be present before turbidity is noticeable. Gross discoloration (with increased turbidity) is most frequently due to iatrogenic contamination with peripheral blood. Interpretation of discolored fluid has been discussed earlier in this chapter. Yellow CSF is referred to as *xanthochromia,* which is generally due to erythrocytic breakdown products (predominantly bilirubin). It may sometimes be due to a markedly elevated serum conjugated bilirubin concentration, with passive diffusion of the water-soluble molecule into the CSF.

CELL COUNTS

Cells in CSF are thought to deteriorate rapidly following collection. It is generally recommended that total and differential nucleated cell counts be performed within 15 minutes (at latest, within 30 minutes) of collection in EDTA. Somewhat longer delays are possible, especially if the sample is kept cool. However, if the sample will not be processed within several hours, the sample may be diluted 1:1 with 40% to 50% ethanol to help preserve cells. This dilution should be taken into account in subsequent calculations.

Nucleated cell counts may be performed using a leukocyte pipette. A suitable diluting fluid is Rosenthal's solution (made by adding 0.1 g of crystal violet to a mixture of 10 ml of glacial acetic acid and 90 ml of distilled water). It should be filtered before use to remove debris that could be confused with cells. The pipette is filled to the 1 mark with diluting fluid and then to the 11 mark with CSF. After thorough mixing, the first few drops are discarded and both sides of a Neubauer hemacytometer chamber are charged with fluid. After 2 minutes (to allow erythrocytes to lyse and nucleated cells to settle), all nucleated cells within the entire boxed area of both sides are counted. The count is multiplied by 0.6 to give the number of cells/μl. (If ethanol-diluted CSF was used, multiply by 1.2.) As a cross-species generalization, normal CSF contains less than 25 nucleated cells/μl (usually 0-10/μl). *Pleocytosis* refers to an elevated CSF nucleated cell count.

Normal CSF contains virtually no erythrocytes. Erythrocytes may be counted by charging a Neubauer hemacytometer with a well-mixed sample of undiluted and unstained CSF. All cells in the entire boxed area of one side are counted. With this method both erythrocytes and nucleated cells are observed. It is usually possible to distinguish between these two groups of cells but not to subcategorize the nucleated cells, as can often be done if Rosenthal's solution is used (see previous discussion). Cell counts for undiluted CSF can be multiplied by 1.1 to give the total number of cells/μl. (If ethanol-diluted CSF is used, multiply by 2.2.)

If difficulty is experienced distinguishing erythrocytes from nucleated cells in unstained CSF, the total number of cells counted using the latter method can be subtracted from the number of nucleated cells counted, using Rosenthal's solution, to calculate the erythrocyte count.

Use of various "correction factors" has been advocated to adjust CSF nucleated cell counts for any peripheral blood leukocytic contamination. As normal CSF contains virtually no erythrocytes, the observed nucleated cell count can be corrected if the number of erythrocytes/μl of CSF is known. The simplest approach is to consider that each 500 to 1000 erythrocytes would be accompanied by one leukocyte. A more complicated method is to use the equation:

$$\text{Corrected Nucleated Cell Count} = \text{Observed Nucleated Cell Count} - \frac{WBC_{blood} \times RBC_{CSF}}{RBC_{blood}}$$

However, this equation requires values for blood leukocyte (WBC_{blood}) and erythrocyte (RBC_{blood}) counts, as well as a CSF erythrocyte count (RBC_{CSF}). Despite its complexity, it is no more accurate than the preceding approximation. Ideally, CSF samples should be free of iatrogenic peripheral blood contamination. Use of the previous "correction factor" is, at best, a rough guide to the uncontaminated CSF nucleated cell count.

CYTOLOGIC EXAMINATION

With experience, especially when total nucleated cell counts are normal, one can perform a preliminary differential cell count on the fluid in the counting chamber, if Rosenthal's solution (or another stain) is used.

When a cytologic smear is to be made of fluid with a cell count below 500/μl, concentration of cells is mandatory. (Such concentration may be helpful even at higher cell counts.) Four methods have been described.

LOW-SPEED CENTRIFUGATION.   Cells may be concentrated by low-speed centrifugation (about 1500 rpm for 5 minutes). The supernatant is carefully removed, and a direct smear is made from the sediment after resuspension in a small quantity of CSF supernatant or cell-free plasma from the same animal. Because CSF normally has a low protein concentration, addition of plasma may help cells adhere to the microscope slide. After air drying, the slide may be stained with Romanowsky stains. Because of the very small numbers of cells in normal CSF, few cells may be present in these smears.

GRAVITATIONAL SEDIMENTATION. This is another method used to concentrate cells. One method uses a glass cylinder (which can be made by cutting the end off a test tube) attached to a microscope slide with paraffin wax. (The smooth tube end is dipped in melted wax and placed on a warm slide.) The cells in about 1 ml of CSF are allowed about 30 minutes to settle. The supernatant is then carefully removed with a pipette and the tube detached. (Excess CSF may be gently removed with absorbent paper.) The slide is air-dried, and residual paraffin carefully scraped off. The slide may be stained with Romanowsky stains.

MEMBRANE FILTRATION. Membrane filtration of alcohol-diluted CSF can also be used to concentrate cells.[1] A membrane pore size of 5 μ is usually satisfactory. Filter holders that attach to a syringe are available. The CSF is permitted to gravity-feed from the syringe barrel, or it is very gently injected through the filter at no more than 1 drop/second. The filter paper must be kept horizontal to evenly distribute the cells. Increased resistance to filtration suggests that the pores are becoming obstructed by cells and/or protein, and no more CSF should be forced through the filter. Filtration of another, smaller volume of CSF through fresh filter paper results in a less crowded preparation.

After removal from the syringe holder, the filter is fixed in 95% ethanol for at least 30 minutes. Holders are available for easy handling of the filter paper during fixation and staining. A trichrome-type stain must be used. Romanowsky stains are unsuitable because they stain the filter paper too intensely. A satisfactory staining procedure is as follows.[1]

Immerse the filter paper for 2 minutes in each of the following (in order): 80%, 70%, 50%, and 30% ethanol and then distilled water, then 4 minutes in hematoxylin, 5 minutes in running tap water, 4 minutes in Pollak's stain, 1 minute in 0.3% acetic acid, 1 minute in 95% ethanol, 2 minutes in n-propyl-alcohol (propanol), 2 minutes in a 1:1 mixture of propanol and xylene, and finally three rinses of 2 minutes each in xylene. At all stages the filter must be treated gently to avoid dislodging cells. Depending on the size of the filter, it may need to be cut to a suitable size before placement on a microscope slide (cell side up). The filter is then flooded with a mounting medium with a refractive index similar to that of filter paper (about 1.5) and a coverslip applied.

Cytologically, the cells trapped by the membrane filter are rounder than those seen following sedimentation (and therefore may be harder to distinguish), and they are in slightly different planes of focus. Further, the filter produces a patterned background that may be distracting. This distraction is minimized by ensuring the sample is not overstained and by using the appropriate mounting medium. The pore size generally used is far too large to trap free bacteria. Quantitatively, more cells are collected by filtration than by the two sedimentation methods.

CYTOCENTRIFUGATION. As with any fluid of low cellularity, a cytocentrifuge (e.g., Shandon cytospin) can be used for preparation of CSF cytologic smears. Such equipment is generally too expensive for a veterinary practice to justify purchasing. However, it is often used in a referral laboratory. This technique allows cells to be concentrated within a small, circular area on the slide.

Normal CSF contains 95% to 100% mononuclear cells, almost all of which are lymphocytes (Figure 12-4).

Bacterial infections involving CSF generally cause marked pleocytosis, mostly due to neutrophils. Inflammation associated with viruses, fungi, neoplasia, or degenerative conditions generally causes less dramatic pleocytosis, with a significant proportion of mononuclear cells (often lymphocytes). Eosinophils are sometimes seen, especially in parasitic inflammatory responses. In general, the causative agent is often not cytologically apparent. Neoplastic cells are seldom observed in CSF.

PROTEIN CONCENTRATION

Normal CSF (from all species) has a very low protein concentration, generally 10 to 50 mg/dl, almost all of which is albumin. Any condition that disrupts the normal blood-brain barrier, such as hemorrhage, inflammation, or neoplasia,

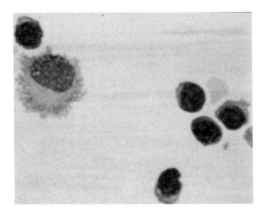

FIGURE 12-4. Cerebrospinal fluid from a dog. Note the several small mononuclear cells (lymphocytes) and a large mononuclear cell (nonphagocytic macrophage). (May Grünwald Giemsa stain, 1000X)

results in an increased CSF protein concentration due to increases in both albumin and globulin. The protein concentration of CSF may be measured qualitatively or quantitatively.

The Pandy test and the Nonne-Apelt test are commonly used as qualitative screening procedures for CSF protein. They detect high-molecular-weight globulins (basically immunoglobulins) but are relatively insensitive tests. The biuret procedure, used to quantitate total serum protein concentration, is not sensitive enough for use with CSF. Two simple quantitative procedures use either sulfosalicylic acid or trichloroacetic acid reactions.

PANDY TEST. For the Pandy test, 1 drop of CSF is added to 1 ml of saturated aqueous phenol. Turbidity is observed before and after the mixture is shaken. Phenol and CSF are immiscible; therefore, after shaking, the CSF disperses as small droplets in the phenol. This should not be confused with a positive reaction (i.e., development of turbidity). If the sample is normal, there is no appreciable immunoglobulin present and the solution remains clear (at most, slightly turbid). This is considered a negative result. If immunoglobulin is present at a concentration of 25 mg/dl or more, the solution becomes cloudy white. The degree of turbidity may be subjectively graded from 1+ to 4+, corresponding to increasing immunoglobulin concentration.

NONNE-APELT TEST. For the Nonne-Apelt test, 1 ml of saturated ammonium sulfate solution is carefully overlaid with 1 ml of CSF and allowed to stand undisturbed for 3 minutes. The junction between the two fluids remains clear with normal CSF. However, if CSF immunoglobulin concentration is increased, a white-gray zone forms at the junction. This reaction may be subjectively graded from 1+ to 4+, reflecting increasing immunoglobulin concentration.

SULFOSALICYLIC ACID TEST. For the sulfosalicylic acid procedure, 0.5 ml of CSF is added to 4.5 ml of 1.5% sulfosalicylic acid, mixed, and allowed to stand for 10 minutes at room temperature. The optical density of the resuspended mixture is read at 420 nm and compared with a protein standard treated in the same manner. (If the protein standard used for blood protein concentration measurement is used, it must be diluted 1:100 with distilled water.)

TRICHLOROACETIC ACID TEST. For the trichloroacetic acid procedure, 0.5 ml of CSF is added to 1.5 ml of 5% trichloroacetic acid, mixed, and allowed to stand for 5 minutes at room temperature. The optical density of the resuspended mixture is read at 420 nm and compared with a standard treated likewise.

OTHER TESTS.   Biochemistry methods used for measurement of urinary protein concentration are often suitable for measurement of CSF protein concentration. These techniques are most likely to be performed by a referral laboratory.

Peripheral blood contamination of a sample may increase its protein concentration. Ideally, an uncontaminated sample should be obtained (possibly by subsequent repeat collection). However, if this is impossible, the amount of protein contributed by peripheral blood may be crudely approximated by considering that every 1000 erythrocytes present will be accompanied by about 1 mg of protein. The equation used to correct the CSF nucleated cell count (see previous discussion) may be modified by replacing observed and corrected nucleated cell counts by protein concentrations and peripheral blood WBC count (WBC_{blood}) by the blood protein concentration. The reservations concerning such "correction factors," expressed earlier, are equally valid for corrections of protein concentration.

PROTEIN ELECTROPHORESIS.   This complex procedure may be performed on CSF; however, it is rarely done in routine clinical cases.

FIBRINOGEN CONCENTRATION

Normal CSF contains no appreciable quantity of fibrinogen and therefore does not clot. Inflammation, hemorrhage, or gross blood contamination increases the CSF fibrinogen concentration. Sample clotting is possible in these circumstances unless the CSF is collected in a tube containing an anticoagulant, such as EDTA.

SPECIFIC GRAVITY

The specific gravity can be measured using a refractometer (see Chapter 5). As a generalization, normal CSF has a specific gravity between 1.004 and 1.008. Its clinical usefulness is not well established.

GLUCOSE CONCENTRATION

Normal CSF glucose concentration varies directly with blood glucose concentration, such that it is generally about 60% to 80% of the blood value. Thus, animals with hyperglycemia and normal CSF usually have higher CSF glucose concentrations than those with normoglycemia, while animals with hypoglycemia and normal CSF usually have lower CSF glucose concentrations than those with normoglycemia. Consequently, for meaningful interpretation, concurrent CSF and blood glucose concentrations should be measured. Methodology is the same as for blood glucose determinations.

Measurement of CSF glucose concentration is most useful as an aid to diagnosis of acute septic suppurative inflammation involving CSF. In this situation, CSF glucose concentration is often much less than 60% of the blood value because of glucose metabolism by bacteria and neutrophils. With successful treatment, the CSF glucose concentration returns to normal.

LACTATE CONCENTRATION

Lactate (lactic acid) is produced by anaerobic cellular metabolism. (For a more detailed consideration of lactate, see the following section on Peritoneal Fluid Analysis.) The value of CSF lactate measurement in animals has not been reported. Increased CSF lactate concentration has been used to assist in diagnosis of septic meningitis in people, although it is not specific for such conditions. Paired blood and CSF lactate values may augment similar glucose measurements.

ELECTROLYTE CONCENTRATIONS

Paired blood and CSF sodium, potassium, chloride, calcium, and magnesium concentrations have been measured but are generally of little practical value. Measurement techniques are the same as for blood samples.

CREATINE KINASE CONCENTRATION

Creatine kinase (CK), previously referred to a creatine phosphokinase (CPK), is probably the enzyme most frequently measured in CSF. Like most other enzymes, CK has a high molecular weight; therefore, its movement between blood and CSF is limited by the normal blood-brain barrier. Normal CSF CK activity is very low and values vary with the measurement technique. Methodology is as for blood CK determination.

Because CK activity in nervous tissue is relatively high, its measurement in CSF has been suggested as an ancillary diagnostic test for nonspecific damage to neural tissue (e.g., neural hypoxia, trauma, inflammation, or compression by a space-occupying lesion, such as a tumor). The CSF CK value may, therefore, be a useful guide to prognosis in canine neurologic cases and in premature foals. Increased values may also be observed following seizures.

AQUEOUS HUMOR ANALYSIS

Samples of fluid may be aspirated from the eye of an anesthetized animal. Such fluid is similar to CSF in that it has very low cellularity, being composed mostly of small mononuclear cells, essentially no erythrocytes, and a very low protein concentration. Interpretation of changes in aqueous humor is similar to that for CSF.

Aqueous (and vitreous) humor may be collected from a dead animal to investigate the concentration of urea and electrolytes before death. The concentration of urea, calcium, and magnesium in these fluids is closely related to that in blood. Consequently, if an animal is thought to have died from renal failure, hypocalcemia ("eclampsia" in dogs, "milk fever" in ruminants) or hypomagnesemia ("grass tetany" in ruminants), collection of aqueous humor may help confirm the diagnosis.

PERITONEAL FLUID ANALYSIS

The normal peritoneal cavity contains only sufficient fluid to ensure lubrication of the surfaces of the intraabdominal organs and the cavity wall. This fluid can be sampled by abdominocentesis. The procedure is well described for many species and is usually performed in the standing animal.

An area at the most dependent point in the ventral midline of the abdomen is aseptically prepared. *Abdominocentesis* (abdominal paracentesis) is performed using a sterile needle or cannula. Peritoneal fluid is collected into an EDTA blood tube for a total nucleated cell count, cytologic examination, and refractometric protein and specific gravity measurement. It may also be collected into a fluoride oxalate blood tube for glucose and lactate measurement and a plain tube for other laboratory tests, including measurement of protein concentration.

Indications for abdominocentesis in all species include investigation of ascites and inflammatory exudation into the peritoneal cavity. In horses, peritoneal fluid is frequently examined in cases of colic and chronic weight loss.

Volume

Subjective estimation of the volume of peritoneal fluid in the abdominal cavity should be attempted at collection. Such an estimate is based on the ease of fluid collection (volume obtained/unit of time) and therefore requires familiarity with the technique of abdominocentesis in a given species. Useful categories are normal, slightly to moderately increased, and plentiful (markedly increased). The small volume of peritoneal fluid in clinically normal animals sometimes makes collection impossible; however, several abdominocenteses should be attempted before the procedure is considered nonproductive.

Color, turbidity

Normal peritoneal fluid is colorless to straw-yellow and transparent to slightly turbid. Gross discoloration and increased turbidity may be due to increased cell numbers and/or protein concentration. Interpretation of such findings have been discussed earlier in this chapter. Discoloration could also be due to free ingesta in the sample. This may be the result of bowel rupture or accidental bowel perforation during abdominocentesis (*enterocentesis*). These conditions may be distinguishable cytologically and by reference to other clinical findings.

Odor

Normal peritoneal fluid has no odor. Collection of malodorous peritoneal fluid at abdominocentesis may indicate a very necrotic segment of bowel within the peritoneal cavity, a ruptured segment of bowel with free gut contents in the cavity, or accidental enterocentesis. These conditions may be distinguishable cytologically and by reference to other clinical findings.

Cell counts

A total nucleated cell count is performed by the same method as for a CBC (see Chapter 2). As a cross-species generalization, normal peritoneal fluid has less than 10,000 nucleated cells/µl, usually 2000 to 6000/µl. Mononuclear cells may be visible as clusters of cells, which can make counting individual cells difficult.

CYTOLOGIC EXAMINATION

Smears of peritoneal fluid are made as outlined earlier. The technique varies with the total nucleated cell count and fluid viscosity. Romanowsky stains are usually used. As previously discussed, the smear should be examined at 40X, 100X, and 1000X magnification.

A differential count of at least 100 nucleated cells should be performed, noting cell type and morphology. Nucleated cells are categorized as neutrophils, large mononuclear cells (a collective grouping of mesothelial cells and macrophages), lymphocytes, eosinophils, and any other nucleated cells. Notes on cell morphology should include comments on nuclear and cytoplasmic appearance. If bacteria are present, their morphology (bacilli, coccobacilli, cocci) and location (free or intracellular, i.e., phagocytosed) must be recorded. In such cases, another smear can be stained with Gram stain and the fluid cultured.

Normal peritoneal fluid contains few erythrocytes. The number present on a smear should be estimated. Suitable categories include rare, few, many, and large numbers. The number present varies with the method of sample preparation. Iatrogenic contamination and acute and chronic hemorrhage are distinguished grossly as outlined earlier (see Exfoliative Cytology). If erythrocytes have been present in the fluid for several hours, they may be phagocytosed by macrophages (*erythrophagocytosis*).

Published normal values for peritoneal fluid cytology of dogs and cats are scanty. Normal horses generally have an average of about 56% neutrophils, 28% large mononuclear cells, 15% lymphocytes, and an occasional eosinophil (1%). Values for cattle are somewhat similar, but normal animals often have comparable numbers of neutrophils and lymphocytes.

Exudates are fluids with increased cellularity and protein concentration because of inflammation. The following cross-species generalization may be made. Acute inflammatory reactions increase the total cell count and the percentage (and absolute numbers) of neutrophils to greater than 95% of the nucleated cells. Subacute to chronic inflammatory reactions usually cause high-normal to elevated total nucleated cell counts, with elevated neutrophil percentages and numerous mesothelial cells and/or macrophages. Many of the latter cells may phagocytize degenerate cells or cellular debris (Figure 12-5). Some mesothelial cells may be present as clusters or rafts of cells (Figure 12-5.) The latter finding confirms that an effusion is present.

Migrating parasite larvae can cause increased neutrophil and eosinophil percentages, with or without an elevated total nucleated cell count.

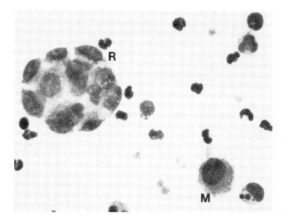

FIGURE 12-5. Raft of mesothelial cells (*R*) in peritoneal fluid from a horse with resolving peritonitis. Several neutrophils and erythrocytes, a phagocytic macrophage, and a mesothelial cell (*M*) are also present. (Wright's stain, 810X)

Septic (bacterial) peritonitis generally causes a marked increase in the total cell count, predominantly due to neutrophils. Cellular morphology depends on the microorganism(s) present and may vary from cytoplasmic vacuolation with few nuclear changes evident to marked cytoplasmic vacuolation, marked karolysis, and general cellular degeneration or fragmentation (see Chapter 2). Cases of simple peritonitis may have a single type of bacterium evident, whereas the bacterial population is frequently mixed in peritonitis due to devitalization or rupture of the bowel. Accidental penetration of the bowel during abdominocentesis may result in a mixed population of bacteria in the smear. However, in the latter case, leukocyte numbers and morphology are usually normal, and the bacteria are frequently not phagocytosed. Large ciliated organisms may also be noted in large-bowel enterocentesis in horses (Figure 12-6).

Transudates (as in ascites due to congestive heart failure) typically have low total nucleated cell counts (less than 500/μl), with fairly normal differential counts or possibly an increase in the percentage of large mononuclear cells and very low protein concentrations. The mononuclear cells are principally mesothelial cells, which may be in clusters or rafts and may be quite reactive in appearance (i.e., multinucleate, with variable nucleus and cell size, prominent nucleoli, and basophilic cytoplasm). Reactive mesothelial cells can be difficult to distinguish from some tumor cells.

Intraabdominal tumors may exfoliate cells into the peritoneal fluid. Cytologic diagnosis of such neoplasia can be quite difficult and is often a task for a specialist cytologist. However, the technician should be able to recognize abnormal lymphocytes (using the hallmarks of malignancy outlined in Chapter

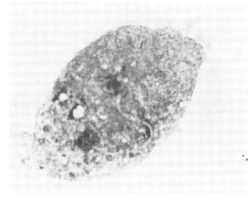

Figure 12-6. This sample collected by accidental enterocentesis in a horse contains a ciliated protozoal organism from the large bowel. A mixed population of bacteria is also usually present, with little evidence of inflammation. (May Grünwald Giemsa stain, 1000X)

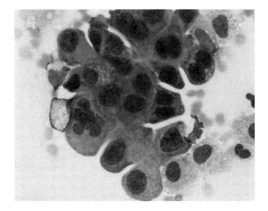

Figure 12-7. Tracheal wash from a dog with a bronchogenic carcinoma. Note the clusters of large mononuclear cells, with moderate variation in cell size, nucleus size, shape, and number, and nucleus-to-cytoplasm ratio. Several cells also have prominent nucleoli of varying size, shape, and number. These findings are typical of malignancy. (May Grünwald Giemsa stain, 1000X)

11) and be suspicious of clusters of pleomorphic, secretory-type cells. Figure 12-7 shows this type of cell.

TOTAL PROTEIN CONCENTRATION

The total protein concentration (of the peritoneal fluid supernatant) can be measured by refractometry or by the biuret procedure (both as for blood samples). Normal peritoneal fluid has a total protein concentration of less than 2.5 g/dl. Because of peritoneal fluid's low protein concentration, refractometric specific gravity (measured as for a urine specimen) may be determined instead of refractometric total protein concentration. Normal peritoneal fluid has a specific gravity of less than 1.018.

The most common causes of increased protein or specific gravity values in peritoneal fluid are inflammation and hemorrhage. Cats with peritoneal effusion due to feline infectious peritonitis (FIP) virus infection frequently have very high peritoneal fluid protein concentrations (up to 8 g/dl) due mainly to gamma globulins. Fluid viscosity is also increased considerably in many cats with FIP.

Fibrinogen concentration

Normal peritoneal fluid has very little fibrinogen (less than 50 mg/dl in horses) and consequently does not clot. Fibrinogen concentration increases with inflammation and/or hemorrhage. Collection into an EDTA tube prevents clotting in such situations. Fibrinogen concentration is not routinely measured, but, if the total protein concentration in peritoneal fluid is greater than 2.5 g/dl, fibrinogen concentration can be determined as outlined for blood fibrinogen measurement, using the EDTA supernatant.

Lactate concentration

Use of paired blood and peritoneal fluid lactate (lactic acid) measurements has been advocated as a diagnostic aid in equine colic cases. The normal resting blood lactate concentration of horses is about 8 to 12 mg/dl. Regardless of the actual values, the blood lactate concentration of normal horses is always greater than that of peritoneal fluid. Horses with GI disorders generally have peritoneal fluid lactate concentrations greater than corresponding blood values. Lactate is produced by anaerobic glycolysis, especially in ischemic tissues. Hypoxia of a section of bowel wall results in increased lactate production, much of which diffuses into the peritoneal cavity before entering the circulation to be removed by the liver. Less severe GI disorders, such as impactions, tend to cause a smaller difference between peritoneal fluid and blood lactate concentrations than do serious ones, such as intestinal torsion (a twisted section of bowel). Peritonitis also increases peritoneal fluid lactate values.

The sample for lactate measurement (blood or peritoneal fluid) should be collected in a fluoride oxalate tube unless it is deproteinized immediately, in which case no preservative/anticoagulant is required. The fluoride stops cellular metabolism of glucose and consequent production of lactate, and the oxalate prevents sample clotting. Whole blood or peritoneal fluid, or their centrifuged supernatants, can be used for lactate measurements. (Fluoride oxalate plasma samples are stable for several days at $4°$ C.) An aliquot of the sample (volume varies with the technique used for lactate measurement) is deproteinized in ice-cold 0.6-N perchloric acid and then centrifuged. The supernatant is used for lactate measurement.

The usefulness of paired blood and peritoneal fluid lactate measurement in other species has not yet been reported.

GLUCOSE CONCENTRATION

The glucose concentration in peritoneal fluid of normal horses is slightly higher (usually 1 to 10 mg/dl higher) than corresponding blood values. Measurement of paired blood and peritoneal fluid glucose concentrations may have diagnostic value in equine colic cases, especially those associated with peritonitis. Leukocyte and (possibly) bacterial metabolism of peritoneal fluid glucose in such cases lowers its concentration, occasionally to undetectable levels. Repeated measurement of peritoneal fluid glucose levels may help monitor the effectiveness of treatment. Successful therapy typically is associated with increasing peritoneal fluid glucose values, possibly before peritoneal fluid leukocyte numbers decrease markedly. The method of peritoneal fluid glucose measurement is as for a blood specimen.

The merit of paired blood and peritoneal fluid glucose determination in other species has not been reported.

UREA NITROGEN CONCENTRATION

The concentration of urea nitrogen in peritoneal fluid can be determined by the same method as blood urea nitrogen measurement. It is normally slightly higher than the blood urea nitrogen level (by 0.5 to 4.0 mg/dl in horses). An animal with a ruptured bladder may have a markedly elevated urea nitrogen concentration in peritoneal fluid. Diagnosis of a ruptured bladder may be confirmed by injecting a dye, such as methylene blue, into the bladder through a urethral catheter and subsequently visualizing its presence in the peritoneal fluid.

PLEURAL FLUID ANALYSIS

As in the peritoneal cavity, the normal pleural (thoracic) cavity contains only enough fluid to adequately lubricate the surfaces of the intrathoracic organs and the cavity wall. Techniques for thoracic fluid collection (*thoracentesis*) are well described for many species. Fluid is collected in EDTA tubes for total nucleated cell counts, cytologic examination, and refractometric protein and specific gravity measurements, and in a plain tube for determination of the total protein concentration. Other clinical chemistry determinations are infrequently performed on pleural fluid.

The main indication for thoracentesis in all species is evaluation of increased thoracic fluid volume (*thoracic effusion*). This may be due to transudation, hemorrhage, ruptured thoracic lymphatic duct (chylothorax), inflammation, or neoplasia.

VOLUME

The volume may be subjectively judged, as when performing abdominocentesis.

COLOR, TURBIDITY

Normal pleural fluid is colorless to straw-yellow and transparent to slightly turbid. It has no odor. Interpretation of most pleural fluid discolorations is as presented earlier (see Exfoliative Cytology). An exception is chylothorax, which, although infrequently seen, is most common in cats and dogs.

Chylothorax usually produces a very "milky" fluid, especially if the animal has recently eaten, because of the chylous effusion's high fat content and large number of lymphocytes. In fasted animals, the fluid may be a tan color. Unlike fluids with high leukocyte counts (which may also have a whitish color), chylous fluid does not have a clear supernatant after centrifugation. The fat in chylous fluid is present as small droplets (*chylomicrons*), which can be stained with Sudan III or IV. The fat in chylous fluid can be dissolved with ether, after the fluid has been alkalinized with sodium hydroxide or sodium bicarbonate. If significant numbers of erythrocytes are present, the fluid may have a reddish color.

Cell counts

A total nucleated cell count is performed by the same technique as for a blood WBC count (see Chapter 2). There are few published normal values for most species. However, as a cross-species generalization, normal pleural fluid has less than 10,000 nucleated cells/μl, usually 2000 to 6000/μl. Many normal animals may have fewer than 1000 cells/μl. Mononuclear cells may be present in clusters, making the counting of individual cells difficult.

Cytologic examination

Most of the comments concerning cytologic evaluation of peritoneal fluid can be extrapolated to pleural fluid. Normal pleural fluid may contain a slightly higher percentage of neutrophils (about 75%).

Chylothorax is characterized cytologically by a predominance of small lymphocytes with normal morphology. Fat droplets may be visible in smears stained with Sudan III or IV.

Total protein and fibrinogen concentrations

Procedures and normal values are the same as for peritoneal fluid. Chylomicron fat increases the pleural fluid refractive index. Consequently, in chylothorax, refractometric "protein" values are usually 2.0 to 6.0 g/dl.

SYNOVIAL FLUID ANALYSIS

Synovial fluid is collected aseptically by *arthrocentesis*, from the unanesthetized or anesthetized animal, generally using a needle and syringe. Arthrocentesis is usually performed as part of a lameness evaluation. Approaches to particular joints vary and have been well described for several species. When in doubt, refer to an anatomy book.

Simple tests on synovial fluid can yield much useful information. The volume of fluid collected influences the tests that can be run. If only 1 or 2 drops can be obtained, as in some normal joints of cats and dogs, gross assessment of fluid color and turbidity and cytologic examination of a direct smear, possibly with concurrent subjective assessment of viscosity, may be all that is practical. If 0.5 to 1 ml is collected, a total nucleated cell count and refractometric protein measurement (on EDTA-preserved fluid) may be added to the list of tests. Collection of larger volumes permits additional tests, such as the mucin clot test.

VOLUME

The volume should be subjectively assessed at collection and compared to the expected (normal) volume. This varies tremendously among joints and species. Experience is the best guide. Generally, the volume of fluid is not increased in normal joints and those with degenerative joint disease, while it is often increased in inflamed joints. The volume of fluid actually collected should also be recorded, with a comment on the ease of collection.

COLOR, TURBIDITY

Normal synovial fluid is clear to straw-yellow and nonturbid. Yellow synovial fluid is very common in large animals, especially horses. Turbidity, when present, is due to cells, protein (or fibrin), or cartilage.

Normal synovial fluid contains very few erythrocytes. Iatrogenic contamination at arthrocentesis is common. Differentiation of contamination and recent or old hemorrhage is as previously described (see Exfoliative Cytology).

VISCOSITY

Viscosity reflects the quality and concentration of hyaluronic acid, which is part of the synovial fluid mucin complex. The function of mucin is joint lubrication. Viscosity may be quantitated with a viscometer; however, subjective assessment is most often used.

Normal synovial fluid is quite sticky. If a drop is placed between thumb and forefinger, as the digits are separated it forms a 1- to 2-inch strand before breaking. Similarly, when gently expressed through a needle on a horizontally held syringe, it hangs in a 1- to 2-inch strand before separating from the needle tip.

In general, viscosity is not decreased in normal joints and those with degenerative problems. It is frequently decreased in joints with bacterial inflammation, due to mucin degradation by bacterial hyaluronidase, and in joints with hydrarthrosis or effusions, due to mucin (and hyaluronic acid) dilution.

Because EDTA may degrade hyaluronic acid, both viscosity and mucin clot formation are usually assessed on fluid to which no anticoagulant has been added. If an anticoagulant is necessary, due to a high fluid fibrinogen concentration, heparin is the preferred anticoagulant.

MUCIN CLOT TEST

Synovial fluid mucin forms a clot when added to acetic acid. The nature of the resultant clot reflects the quality and concentration of hyaluronic acid. One method is as follows:

Initially, 0.1 ml of 7-N glacial acetic acid is diluted with 4 ml of distilled water. Then 1 ml of synovial fluid (not EDTA preserved) is added, without touching the sides of the test tube. For smaller volumes of fluid, use proportionately less dilute acetic acid. The solution is gently mixed and allowed to stand at room temperature for 1 hour. The mucin clot is generally graded as good (large, compact, ropy clot in a clear solution); fair (soft clot in a slightly turbid solution); poor (friable clot in a cloudy solution); or very poor (no actual clot, but some large flecks in a very turbid solution). Clot assessment is enhanced by gently shaking the tube. Good clots remain ropy, whereas poor clots fragment (Figure 12-8).

If only a few drops of synovial fluid are obtained at arthrocentesis, an abbreviated mucin clot test can be performed. If available after preparation of a cytologic smear (and possibly total nucleated cell count), a drop of non-EDTA-preserved fluid is placed on a clean microscope slide. Three drops of diluted acetic acid (see previous discussion) are added and mixed. The resultant clot is graded (as previously mentioned) after about 1 minute. Assessment may be easier against a dark background.

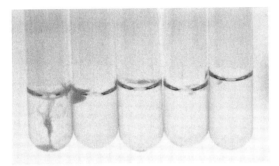

FIGURE 12-8. Mucin clot tests. Reading from *left to right*, these tests are graded as good (normal), good, fair, poor, and poor.

PROTEIN CONCENTRATION

The protein concentration of synovial fluid may be determined by the biuret method or by refractometry (as for a blood sample). In most species, synovial fluid protein concentration is less than 2.5 g/dl. The pig is an exception, with normal values of 3 to 5 g/dl.

Normal synovial fluid contains no appreciable quantity of fibrinogen and consequently does not clot. However, the fluid may gel if left undisturbed for a few hours. This gelling, called *thixotropy,* is reversible; normal fluidity is restored simply by agitating the specimen.

Samples from traumatized or inflamed joints generally contain increased fibrinogen and clot rapidly, possibly even in the syringe at collection. Such samples should be immediately transferred into EDTA for cell counts and cytologic examination and into heparin for the mucin clot test.

CELL COUNTS

Cell counts are performed on EDTA-preserved synovial fluid. Normal synovial fluid contains very few erythrocytes; however, iatrogenic contamination at collection is not uncommon. Erythrocytes may also be present in the synovial fluid of traumatized and inflamed joints. If erythrocytes have been present for several hours, erythrophagocytosis may be evident. Erythrocyte numbers are not usually determined.

Leukocyte numbers vary considerably among joints and species. As a broad generalization, normal joints of all species contain less than 3000 nucleated cells/µl, with horses usually below about 500/µl, cattle usually below about 1000/µl and dogs and cats usually below about 1500/µl. A WBC pipette and

Neubauer hemacytometer are suitable for leukocyte quantitation. The sample is normally used for dilution of blood for leukocyte counts, cannot be used because it causes synovial fluid mucin to clot, invalidating results. The sample is diluted and counted as for a blood WBC count (see Chapter 2). In general, total nucleated cell counts are mildly elevated in traumatic and degenerative joint diseases and moderately or markedly elevated in nonseptic and septic inflammation (Figure 12-9).

Cytologic examination (cell counts)

Slides for cytologic examination may be prepared on EDTA-preserved fluid or fluid without anticoagulant, the latter especially if only a few drops are obtained and the smear is made immediately. Thin smears are made by slowly advancing the spreader slide. Due to the high viscosity of normal synovial fluid, cells do not usually accumulate at the feathered edge of the smear. Margination of cells increases as viscosity of the fluid decreases. At low cell counts, especially below 500/μl, concentration of cells by centrifugational sedimentation and subsequent resuspension of cells in a small volume of supernatant fluid produces a more cellular smear. Slides are usually stained with any Romanowsky stain (Wright's, Giemsa) or with new methylene blue.

Cells in synovial fluid with good viscosity tend to align in a linear fashion in the direction of the smear, giving a "windrow" appearance (Figure 12-10). Mucin precipitation produces an eosinophilic granular background in Romanowsky-stained smears, the density of which reflects smear thickness. Cells in smears from very viscous fluid may not spread out well on the slide,

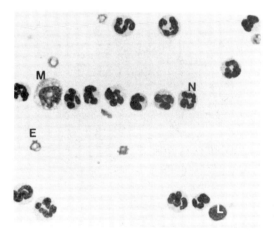

FIGURE 12-9.   Smear of synovial fluid from a dog with acute, suppurative arthritis. Cell types present are neutrophils (N), erythrocytes (E), lymphocytes (L), and a large, slightly vacuolated macrophage (M). Note the normal (eosinophilic), granular, proteinaceous background. (Wright's stain, 780X)

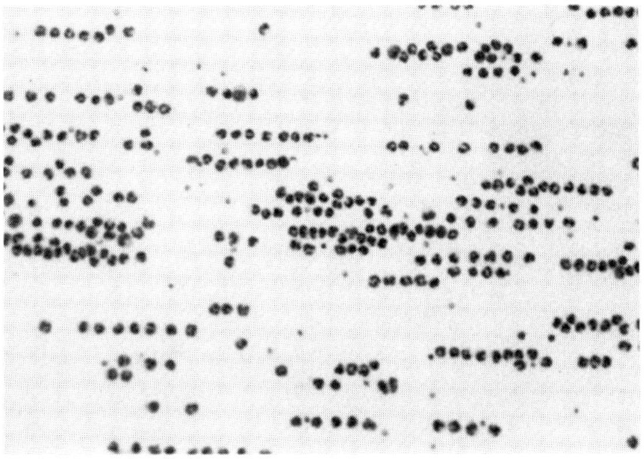

FIGURE 12-10. Smear of synovial fluid from a dog with acute, suppurative arthritis. Note the linear arrangement of cells ("windrowing") suggesting good fluid viscosity. (Wright's stain, 140X)

which can make their identification difficult. Such fluid may be diluted 1:1 with saline-reconstituted hyaluronidase (Sigma Chemical, St. Louis, MO) (150 U/ml). This decreases sample viscosity after a few minutes, allowing more accurate cell morphology when smeared.

Normal synovial fluid generally contains at least 90% mononuclear cells and less than 10% neutrophils. Eosinophils are rarely observed. Mononuclear cells comprise about equal numbers of lymphocytes and monocytic/macrophage-type cells, which are nonvacuolated and nonphagocytic. Large, vacuolated or phagocytic mononuclear cells comprise less than 10% of the differential count of normal synovial fluid (Figure 12-9). Macrophages become vacuolated in normal synovial fluid that is not processed soon after collection.

As a generalization, mononuclear cells predominate in traumatic and degenerative arthropathies, usually with increased numbers of large vacuolated or phagocytic cells. Occasionally when joint erosion has progressed through to subchondral bone, osteoclasts may be observed (Figure 12-11). In contrast, neutrophils predominate in infectious arthropathies (due to bacteria, viruses, mycoplasmas, etc.) and many noninfectious conditions, such as rheumatoid arthritis and systemic lupus erythematosus. When cells are clumped together in a smear, new methylene blue stain usually demonstrates interlocking fibrin strands. Rarely, the causative organism in septic joint fluid may be observed cytologically, especially when phagocytosed. Culture is recommended when an infectious process is suspected. A chronic-active type of arthropathy is suggested when neutrophils and vacuolated/phagocytic macrophages are both increased in number. *Lupus erythematosus cells* (neutrophils containing phagocytosed nuclear chromatin) are occasionally seen in the synovial fluid of animals with systemic lupus erythematosus.

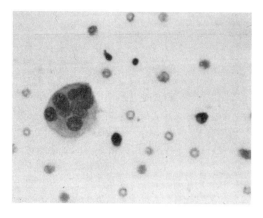

Figure 12-11. Synovial fluid from a dog. The large multinucleated cell is an osteoclast. Its presence suggests erosion of joint cartilage through to underlying subchondral bone. (May Grünwald Giemsa stain, 400X)

Glucose concentration

The glucose concentration of normal synovial fluid is infrequently measured and is about the same as that of blood. Interpretation of findings is similar to that for CSF and peritoneal fluid.

Miscellaneous tests

Particulate analysis may be performed on synovial fluid to assess the degree of cartilage damage. *Synovial fluid aldehyde concentrations* also reflect the degree of cartilage damage. Both tests have been done in horses and require submission of samples to a laboratory specializing in these techniques.

TRACHEAL WASH

Cytologic evaluation of samples obtained from the trachea, bronchi, or bronchioles may assist with diagnosis of pulmonary disease in animals. Tracheal washes can be performed by passage of a catheter through the mouth into an endotracheal tube in an anesthetized animal (orotracheal), via the nasal passages (nasotracheal) or through the skin and trachea (transtracheal) in a conscious, sedated animal. The transtracheal route minimizes pharyngeal contamination of the specimen, but it is an invasive procedure and consequently requires aseptic technique. These procedures are well described for small and large animals.[1,2]

Depending on the placement of the catheter tip, a tracheal, bronchial, or bronchoalveolar wash is obtained. Sterile physiologic saline is used as the wash fluid. Several milliliters are infused (the quantity varies with the animal's size) and immediately withdrawn into the same syringe. The aspirated fluid can be transported to the laboratory in the collection syringe, a plain blood tube, or an EDTA blood tube. The last is preferable if a delay is anticipated before smears are made. However, because cells in tracheal washes are often poorly preserved and delayed sample processing causes artifactual degeneration, delays should be avoided.

Samples with little mucus (generally corresponding to small numbers of cells) should be centrifuged at low speed, and smears prepared from the sediment. Samples containing much mucus (and usually numerous cells) may not need to be centrifuge-concentrated before a smear is made. A gentle squash preparation is usually the best procedure, especially when mucus is present (see Chapter 11). Romanowsky stains are generally satisfactory.

Total nucleated cell counts are not performed on tracheal wash fluids. Cell numbers are subjectively recorded from evaluation of the smear. A tracheal wash smear from a normal animal contains few cells, usually with a small amount of mucus (Figure 12-12). The mucus often appears miroscopically as eosinophilic to purple strands that may enmesh the cells. Epithelial cells are the principal cell type.

If the sample is collected from the level of the trachea, ciliated epithelial cells predominate. These cells are columnar to cuboidal, with a polar nucleus on the border opposite the cilia (Figure 12-12). If the specimen is collected from the bronchi, bronchoalveolar epithelial cells are also fairly common. They are round, nonciliated cells with basophilic cytoplasm and may occur in clumps (Figure 12-13). A few goblet cells (secretory epithelial cells) may also be observed.

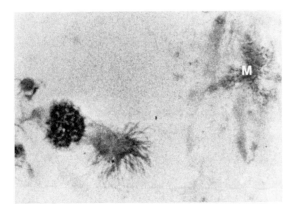

FIGURE 12-12.   Transtracheal wash from a normal horse. Note the ciliated columnar epithelial cell and small amount of mucus (*M*) in the background. (Wright's stain, 1050X)

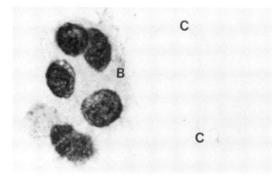

FIGURE 12-13. Transtracheal wash from a normal horse. Note the bronchoalveolar cells (B) and free cilia (C) from ciliated epithelial cells. (Wright's stain, 1050X)

If the sample is a bronchoalveolar wash, alveolar macrophages may predominate. These are large individual cells with a large round to oval nucleus and a moderate amount of basophilic cytoplasm. If they become reactive or activated, the cytoplasm increases in volume and becomes more granular and vacuolated (Figure 12-14). Neutrophils, lymphocytes, eosinophils, plasma cells, mast cells, and erythrocytes are rarely seen in specimens from normal animals. Because cell preservation is often only fair, free eosinophil granules rather than intact eosinophils may be noted.

Abnormal tracheal washes are generally exudates. Such samples contain numerous mucus strands and are very cellular (Figure 12-15). Eosinophilic, spiral casts from small bronchioles (*Curschmann's spirals*) suggest a chronic bronchiolar problem (Figure 12-16). Cell morphology is highly variable among and within samples. Many cells may be unidentifiable. Neutrophils and

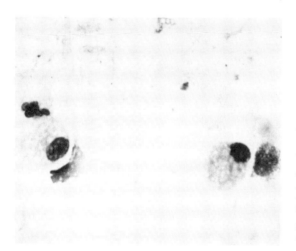

FIGURE 12-14. Transtracheal wash from a horse with a chronic-active inflammatory problem. Note the neutrophil and two vacuolated alveolar macrophages. (Wright's stain, 780X)

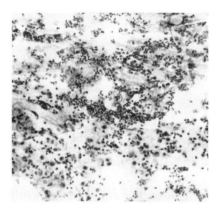

FIGURE 12-15.   Transtracheal wash from a horse with an acute, septic suppurative, inflammatory reaction. Note the marked cellularity and high mucus content. (Wright's stain, 140X)

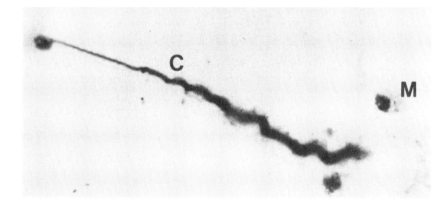

FIGURE 12-16.   Transtracheal wash from a dog with a chronic inflammation. Note the alveolar macrophages (*M*) and Curschmann's spiral (*C*). (Wright's stain, 345X)

macrophages are numerous. In acute inflammation, neutrophils are the predominant cell type and may represent more than 95% of nucleated cells. As the process becomes more chronic, mononuclear macrophages increase in number. The causative agent, possibly bacterial or fungal, may be noted, free and/or phagocytosed, in the smear. Tracheal wash samples can be cultured by routine microbiologic procedures.

The presence of bacteria or fungi in a tracheal wash does not necessarily mean the organism is pathogenic. Plant or fungal spores sometimes contaminate tracheal washes from herbivores (inhaled from feed) and may be phagocytosed by macrophages (Figure 12-17). Oral or pharyngeal contamination of the collection apparatus, or increased inspiratory effort with contamination of the

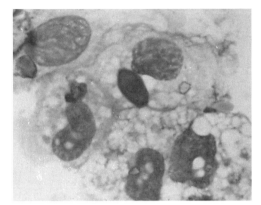

FIGURE 12-17. This tracheal wash from a horse contains reactive, vacuolated macrophages, one of which has ingested pollen (large, dark, elliptic structure). (May Grünwald Giemsa stain, 1000X)

upper tracheal mucosa by pharyngeal microflora, can cause inclusion of bacteria in a tracheal wash specimen. Such bacteria are frequently associated with or adherent to squamous epithelial cells of the pharyngeal mucosa (Figure 12-18).

Eosinophils are prominent (possibly more than 10% of nucleated cells) in inflammatory reactions with an allergic or parasitic component (Figure 12-19). Rarely, parasite eggs or larvae may be noted in the smear.

Erythrocytes are rarely seen in normal tracheal wash specimens. Recent hemorrhage may be evidenced by numerous intact erythrocytes in the smear. In contrast, with old hemorrhage, few erythrocytes may be noted and many of the macrophages may contain hemosiderin granules (dark-blue or red cytoplasmic granules) (see Figure 12-3 for such cells).

Neoplastic cells may be detected in tracheal wash specimens (Figure 12-7). Criteria for malignancy are as outlined earlier (see Chapter 11). Neoplastic

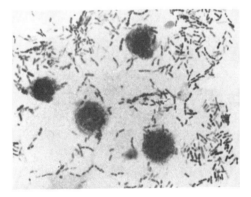

FIGURE 12-18. Bovine tracheal wash containing squamous epithelial cells, with adherent bacteria. These bacteria represent nasopharyngeal contamination of the sample. (Wright's stain, 780X)

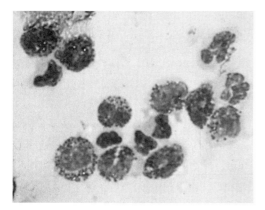

FIGURE 12-19. Tracheal wash from a dog. Large numbers of eosinophils suggest an allergic or hypersensitivity reaction, or possibly parasitism. (May Grünwald Giemsa stain, 1000X)

cells are frequently in clusters, generally epithelial in origin, and frequently "secretory" in appearance (i.e., their cytoplasm is basophilic and vacuolated).

NASAL FLUSH

Cytologic evaluation of samples obtained from the nasal cavity may be useful in investigation of diseases affecting the upper airway. Fluid (normal saline) may be infused into the nasal cavity via the nose, using a syringe and tubing, and then aspirated. This procedure is referred to as a *nasal flush*. Such specimens are processed as for a tracheal wash.

A nasal flush from a normal animal contains cornified and noncornified squamous epithelial cells, often with adherent bacteria, and negligible evidence of hemorrhage or inflammation (Figure 12-20).

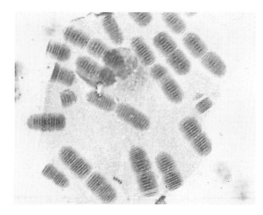

FIGURE 12-20. This nasal flush from a dog shows a cornified squamous epithelial cell with adherent bacteria (*Simonsiella*). These bacteria are part of the normal microflora of the upper airways. (May Grünwald Giemsa stain, 1000X)

Various abnormalities may be demonstrated with this procedure, such as inflammation secondary to sepsis, fungi and yeasts, and neoplasia (Figure 12-21).

EAR SWABS

Cotton-tipped swabs may be used to collect a specimen from the ear canal for cytologic and microbiologic examination. The swab should be gently rolled along a clean glass slide to allow cells and organisms to adhere. The slide is then stained with a Romanowsky stain or Gram's stain. "Normal" specimens contain cornified squamous epithelial cells, with negligible evidence of inflammation and few microorganisms. Common abnormal findings are bacteria and yeasts, with or without inflammation (Figure 12-22).

LYMPH NODE ASPIRATE BIOPSY

Fine-needle aspiration is a useful diagnostic procedure when investigating enlarged lymph nodes. Cytologic evaluation of lymph node aspirates is usually a task for a specialist. However, technicians should know how to prepare good-quality smears. General principles of the technique are described Chapter 11. Causes of lymph node enlargement include:

- *Hyperplasia:* Increased lymphoid cell numbers are associated with inflammation and/or infection in adjacent tissues or surfaces. The

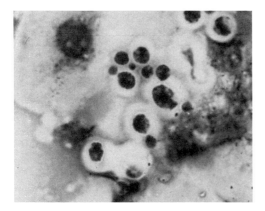

FIGURE 12-21. Nasal flush from a dog. Note the numerous cryptococcal organisms with surrounding (clear) capsule. Some organisms show typical "budding" divisions. (May Grünwald Giemsa stain, 1000X)

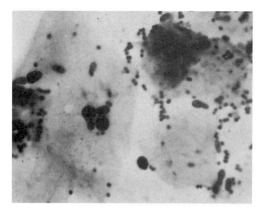

FIGURE 12-22.   This ear swab from a dog shows cornified squamous epithelial cells, with large numbers of bacterial cocci and *Malassezia pachydermatis* organisms. The latter are dark "skittle"-shaped structures (larger than the cocci). (May Grünwald Giemsa stain, 1000X)

numbers of lymphocytes in the node increase, but their morphology and relative proportions appear normal.

- *Inflammation of the lymph node (lymphadenitis):* In this situation, the lymph node is inflamed, and numbers of neutrophils and macrophages are increased. Lymphadenitis usually occurs when bacteria or other microorganisms are present in the node.
- *Lymphoid neoplasia (lymphosarcoma):* This may involve one or more nodes. It may also involve other organs (spleen, kidney, bone marrow) and possibly leukemia (see Chapter 2).
- *Plasma-cell myeloma:* This is a special type of lymphoid tumor involving antibody-producing cells (plasma cells or B-lymphocytes). These cells are usually present in relatively low numbers in normal and hyperplastic nodes. Plasma-cell myeloma is also called multiple myeloma or plasmacytoma.
- *Metastatic neoplasia:* If the lymph node is "draining" an area in which a tumor develops, the tumor may spread to the node, causing it to enlarge (Figure 12-23).

OTHER ASPIRATES AND IMPRESSIONS

Other organs and palpable masses can be aspirated and smears prepared as is done for lymph nodes. Impressions can be prepared from excision biopsies or from swabs of mucosal and cutaneous surfaces. Basic evaluation involves differentiating inflammation from hyperplasia and neoplasia. Differentiation of

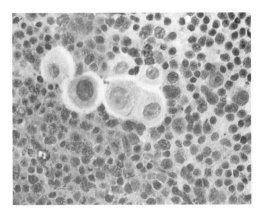

FIGURE 12-23. Lymph node aspirate from a dog. Note the group of large mononuclear cells among the lymphocytes. This is evidence of metastatic squamous-cell carcinoma. (May Grünwald Giemsa stain, 1000X)

the latter possibilities is often done by a specialist; however, as with lymph node aspirates, the technician should be familiar with preparation of smears from these areas, including evaluating the quality of the smear before submission to the laboratory. General principles are described in Chapter 11.

VAGINAL CYTOLOGY

Exfoliative vaginal cytology is a useful adjunct to the history and clinical examination in determining the stage of the estrous cycle in bitches and queens. It assists with optimal timing of mating or artificial insemination in small animals but is not of practical value for these purposes in mares, cows, does, ewes, or sows.

The sample is readily collected with the animal restrained in a standing position and the tail elevated. The vulva is cleansed and rinsed. A lubricated speculum or smooth plastic tube is inserted to a point just cranial to the urethral orifice in the vagina. A sterile swab (which may be moistened with sterile saline) is introduced and gently rotated against the vaginal wall. The swab is removed and carefully rolled along two or three clean microscope slides. After air drying, the smears are stained, generally with a Romanowsky stain. The cells collected are those exfoliated (shed) from the vaginal wall (epithelial cells and neutrophils) and those passing through the vagina from the uterus (especially erythrocytes in proestrus and estrus in the bitch).

Cytologic findings must be interpreted in conjunction with the history and clinical signs. The findings at each stage of the canine estrous cycle are detailed following. These stages are convenient divisions in a continuum of change, brought about by variations in blood estrogen and progesterone concentrations. Because it can be difficult to determine the stage of the estrous cycle based on a single examination, repeat examinations every few days may be necessary.

ANESTRUS

The anestrual bitch has no vulvar swelling and does not attract male dogs. A vaginal smear reveals predominantly noncornified squamous epithelial cells (large cells with a rounded border, abundant basophilic cytoplasm, and a large, round nucleus; Figure 12-24). Based on size, these cells may be categorized as intermediate (larger) or parabasal (smaller) squamous epithelial cells. The smear may also contain some neutrophils but no erythrocytes. Anestrus is variable in length but generally lasts less than 4.5 months.

PROESTRUS

A bitch in proestrus has a swollen vulva, with a reddish vulvar discharge. The bitch attracts but will not accept male dogs attempting to breed. As proestrus progresses toward estrus, the noncornified squamous epithelial cells of anestrus are replaced by cornified squamous epithelial cells. These are cells with angular,

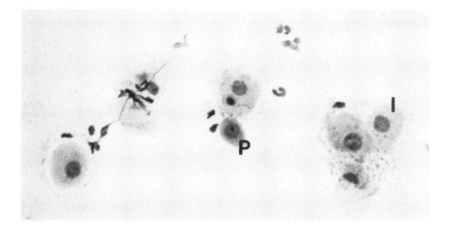

FIGURE 12-24.   Canine anestrual vaginal smear. Note the noncornified squamous epithelial cells, which are predominantly intermediate-type cells (*I*) with a parabasal cell (*P*). Neutrophils and bacteria are also present. (Wright's stain, 345X)

jagged borders, fairly homogeneous, eosinophilic cytoplasm, and a pyknotic nucleus; they are also called "superficial cells." Concurrently, neutrophil numbers in the smear decrease and erythrocyte numbers increase. Proestrus may last 4 to 13 days, with an average of about 9 days.

ESTRUS

The estrual bitch has a history of recent proestrus and a swollen vulva, with possibly a pinkish to straw-colored discharge (becoming whiter as metestrus approaches). Bitches in estrus accept male dogs attempting to mate. A vaginal smear reveals that all squamous epithelial cells are cornified (many appear to have no nucleus), neutrophils are absent, and erythrocytes are present (Figure 12-25). Erythrocyte numbers decrease and neutrophil numbers increase as diestrus approaches. Estrus generally lasts 4 to 13 days, with an average of about 9 days.

METESTRUS

A bitch in metestrus has a history of recent estrus. The vulvar swelling and discharge have decreased, and she no longer attracts or is receptive to male dogs. Cornified squamous epithelial cells are replaced by noncornified squamous epithelial cells and abundant cytologic debris. By about the tenth day after estrus, all epithelial cells are noncornified. Neutrophils increase in number until

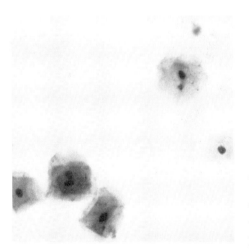

FIGURE 12-25.   Canine estrual vaginal smear. Note the cornified squamous epithelial cells. Bacteria are also present. (Wright's stain, 345X)

about the third day of metestrus and then decrease to very few by about the tenth day. Erythrocytes are generally absent throughout metestrus. Metestrus may last about 2 to 3 months. Cytologically, metestrus and anestrus are often difficult to differentiate.

PREGNANCY

Pregnancy is not cytologically distinguishable from metestrus or anestrus.

VAGINITIS, METRITIS

Inflammation of the vagina or uterus results in a pinkish-white vulvar discharge, usually without vulvar swelling or clinical signs of proestrus or estrus. A vaginal swab reveals noncornified squamous epithelial cells and massive numbers of neutrophils, possibly with free and/or phagocytosed bacteria.

BACTERIA

Bacteria may be present in vaginal smears at any stage of the estrous cycle (but especially during estrus) and usually have no pathologic significance (i.e., they are part of the normal vaginal microflora).

Unlike the bitch, the queen (female cat) ovulates after coital stimulation. Cytologic findings at different stages of the estrous cycle are similar to those of the bitch for epithelial cells and neutrophils; however, erythrocytes are not present at any stage.

SEMEN EVALUATION

The American Society of Theriogenologists has published some guidelines for examination of male animals for breeding soundness. Evaluation of semen is a very important part of such an assessment. Techniques for semen collection in common domestic animals are well described elsewhere.

When handling semen samples, it is important to avoid exposure to marked changes in temperature (especially cold), water, disinfectants, or variations in pH. Consequently, all laboratory equipment used in semen collection and examination should be clean and dry and warmed to about 37° C (98.6° F). This includes microscope slides, coverslips, and pipettes. Stains and diluents should also be warmed to about 37° C. Samples should be processed in a warm room as soon as possible after collection.

The following characteristics are readily determined in the laboratory: volume of ejaculate, gross appearance, wave motion, microscopic motility, spermatozoal concentration, ratio of live:dead spermatozoa, assessment of morphology, and presence of foreign cells or material.

It is important to record the animal's species, breed, age, brief history with salient clinical findings, suspected abnormalities, and the method of semen collection (e.g., artificial vagina, electroejaculation, massage).

VOLUME OF EJACULATE

The volume of ejaculate is easily measured with a volumetric flask, which may be incorporated into the collection receptacle. Marked species variations occur and the method of collection greatly influences the volume obtained, its gross appearance, and spermatozoal concentration. As a generalization, ejaculate volume is larger but spermatozoal concentration lower (and the specimen apparently more dilute) when collected by electroejaculation than when collected by artificial vagina. Further, repeated ejaculation, whether associated with semen collection or sexual activity, decreases the volume and concentration of semen obtained at subsequent collections. Semen volume tends to be greater if collection is preceded by a period of sexual arousal ("teasing").

The ejaculate can be considered to comprise three portions: a sperm-free watery secretion, a sperm-rich fraction, and a sperm-poor fraction. The first and third fractions are derived from accessory sex glands. In bucks, bulls, rams, and toms, all three fractions are collected together. However, with boars, dogs, and stallions, the third fraction may be conveniently collected separately. This is advisable, as the third fraction is voluminous in these three animals and is therefore an unnecessary encumbrance in subsequent evaluation of the semen sample. In these three species, the first two fractions (collected together) are used in the other procedures that follow.

Approximate average total ejaculate volumes (all three fractions) are boar, 250 ml; buck and ram, 1 ml; bull, 5 ml; dog, 10 ml; stallion, 65 ml; and tom, 0.04 ml. Ejaculate volume does not necessarily correlate with fertility. In general, spermatozoal number, motility, and morphology are better guides to fertility. Obviously, however, very small ejaculates may give cause for concern in species with voluminous ejaculates. Knowledge of the ejaculate volume is necessary for determination of total spermatozoal numbers if the sample is to be divided (and possibly diluted) for artificial insemination procedures.

Gross appearance of ejaculate

The opacity and color of the sample should be recorded. Opacity subjectively reflects the concentration of spermatozoa. Categories used include thick, creamy, opaque; milky opaque; opalescent milky; and watery white. This rule of thumb works best for semen from bucks, bulls, and rams, which normally have opaque, creamy-white semen due to high spermatozoal concentration. As the density of spermatozoa decreases, the specimen becomes more translucent and "milkier" in appearance. Semen from boars, dogs, and stallions is normally fairly translucent and white to gray. Contaminants, especially intact or degenerate erythrocytes, cause discoloration of semen.

Sperm motility

Sperm motility (movement) is assessed subjectively and depends on careful handling of the sample for meaningful results. Variations in temperature and exposure to nonisotonic fluids or destructive chemicals (including detergents) must be avoided. Motility is correlated with fertility; however, improper specimen handling adversely affects its assessment. If other tests, especially sperm morphology, suggest the semen is normal but sperm motility is poor, another sample should be examined to ensure that technical errors were not responsible for the poor motility. Motility may be conveniently assessed in two ways.

Wave motion.   Wave motion is a subjective assessment of the gross motility of sperm. Four general classifications are used: very good, good, fair, and poor, based on the amount of "swirling" activity observed in a drop of semen on a microscope slide at low-power (40X) magnification. These categories respectively correspond to distinct vigorous swirling, moderate slow swirling, barely discernible swirling, and lack of actual swirling but with motile sperm present, which may cause the sample to have an irregular oscillating appearance. Wave motion depends on high sperm density and is therefore best in samples from bucks, bulls, and rams, which normally have high sperm concentrations. Wave motion decreases as sperm concentration decreases. Consequently, normal boars, dogs, stallions and toms may have fair or poor wave motion. As a guide, if wave motion is very good or good, the sample should be diluted for evaluation of the percentage of motile sperm and their rate of motility.

MOTILITY.   Progressive motility of individual spermatozoa is determined on a relatively dilute drop of coverslipped semen, examined at 100X magnification. Because the motility of individual spermatozoa is difficult to appreciate in dense samples, such concentrated samples should be diluted before examination. Warm physiologic saline or fresh, buffered 2.9% sodium citrate solutions are suitable diluents.

A drop of semen is placed on a slide and diluted until a satisfactory concentration of spermatozoa is observed. The sample is then coverslipped to produce a monolayer of cells. Excessive dilution of the sample makes evaluation of motility difficult. The rate of motility is generally subjectively classified as very good, good, fair, or poor, corresponding to rapid linear activity, moderate linear activity, slow linear or erratic activity, and very slow erratic activity, respectively. The percentage of motile spermatozoa is broadly categorized as very good, good, fair, or poor, corresponding to about 80% to 100%, 60% to 80%, 40% to 60%, and 20% to 40% motile cells, respectively. As a generalization, to be considered satisfactory, a sample should have at least 60% moderately active spermatozoa. The importance of careful specimen processing cannot be overemphasized.

SPERM CONCENTRATION

Several solutions are satisfactory for semen dilution before counting sperm numbers, including 5 g of sodium bicarbonate or 9 g of sodium chloride with 1 ml of formalin in 1 L of distilled water; 3% chlorazene; or 12.5 g of sodium sulfate with 33.3 ml of glacial acetic acid in 200 ml of distilled water (Gower's solution). The sample is diluted using an erythrocyte dilution pipette. Semen is drawn to the 0.5 mark, then diluent is drawn to the 101 mark, giving a 1:200 dilution. After thorough mixing, several drops are discarded from the pipette and a Neubauer hemacytometer is charged with fluid. The sample is allowed to settle for a few minutes and then checked for homogeneous distribution of spermatozoa. If this is not present, the sample in the pipette should be mixed thoroughly again and the cleaned hemacytometer recharged.

The number of spermatozoa in the central grid area (erythrocyte counting area) of one side of the chamber is counted at 400X magnification. The number of spermatozoa/ml of semen is calculated by multiplying the number observed by 2 million. If spermatozoal concentration is high (e.g., in bucks, bulls, and toms), fewer squares may be counted and the multiplication factor adjusted accordingly. Spermatozoal concentration can also be determined by colorimetric and electronic particle counter techniques.

As outlined earlier, sperm concentration varies with the method of collection. As a generalization, average sperm concentrations (in millions/ml) are about 150 for boars and stallions, 3000 for bucks and rams, 1200 for bulls, 300 for dogs, and 1700 for toms.

LIVE:DEAD SPERM RATIO

Staining with a vital dye permits discrimination between live and dead spermatozoa. An eosin/nigrosin mixture is popular for this purpose and also permits examination of sperm morphology. The stain is prepared by adding 1 g of eosin B and 5 g of nigrosin to a 3% solution of sodium citrate dihydrate. This solution is stable for at least a year.

A small drop of warm stain is mixed gently with a small drop of semen on a warm microscope slide. After several seconds of contact between specimen and dye, the mixture is smeared as when making a blood smear, and then rapidly dried. Once the smear is dried, microscopic examination may be delayed. Live sperm resist staining and appear white (clear) against the blue-black nigrosin background. In contrast, dead sperm passively take up the eosin and are stained a pinkish red. The ratio of live:dead sperm, expressed as a percentage, is determined by examination at 400X or 1000X magnification, preferably by observing 200 cells.

Unfortunately, this procedure is very susceptible to technical problems. Conditions that kill sperm, especially temperature changes, produce misleading results. Findings should always be interpreted with regard to other results, such as sperm concentration, motility, and morphology.

SPERM MORPHOLOGY

Sperm morphology is readily assessed on a nigrosin-and-eosin-stained smear, prepared as outlined previously. Other stains, such as India ink, hematoxylin and eosin, Wright's, Giemsa, and Cavarett's (a mixture of eosin B and phenol), have been used but offer no distinct advantages over nigrosin and eosin.

Species differences exist with respect to the fine points of sperm morphology, but all sperm have the same basic structure (Figure 12-26). The percentage of abnormal spermatozoa and their types are recorded after observing 100 to 500 cells. Counting the lower number of cells (100) is usually adequate once the technician has become proficient. Abnormalities are conveniently divided into head, midpiece, and tail problems. Abnormalities are often categorized as primary or secondary.

Primary defects occur during spermatozoal production and include the following: heads that are double, too large, too small, or oddly shaped (e.g., pear-like, round, twisted, knobby) (Figure 12-27); midpieces that are swollen, kinked, twisted, double, or eccentrically attached to a head (abaxial) (Figure 12-28); and tails that are coiled (Figure 12-28). Primary abnormalities are generally considered more serious than secondary ones. Their percentage is fairly consistent if another semen sample is collected within several days. Slightly abaxial midpiece attachment in boars is probably not as significant as in other species because it may be found in numerous spermatozoa of apparently normal boars.

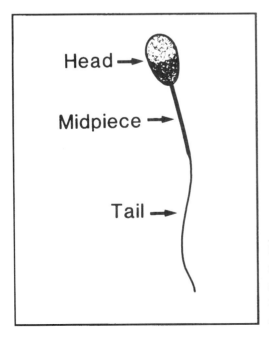

Figure 12-26. Diagrammatic representation of a normal spermatozoon, showing its three main components: head, midpiece, and tail.

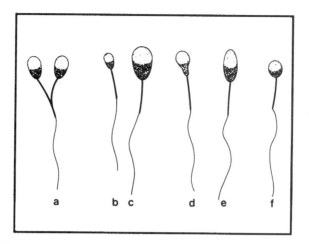

FIGURE 12-27. Diagrammatic representation of primary spermatozoal abnormalities involving the head. Abnormalities depicted are double head (bicephaly) (*a*), small head (microcephaly) (*b*), large head (macrocephaly) (*c*), pear-shaped head (pyriform) (*d*), elongated head (*e*), and round head (*f*).

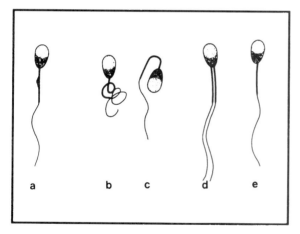

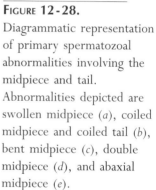

FIGURE 12-28. Diagrammatic representation of primary spermatozoal abnormalities involving the midpiece and tail. Abnormalities depicted are swollen midpiece (*a*), coiled midpiece and coiled tail (*b*), bent midpiece (*c*), double midpiece (*d*), and abaxial midpiece (*e*).

Secondary defects can occur at any time, from storage in the epididymis until the smear is made. Thus, because secondary abnormalities may be artifactual, careful specimen handling, as outlined earlier, is mandatory. Minimization of technique-induced secondary abnormalities permits easier sample interpretation. Secondary defects include tailless heads, protoplasmic droplets on the midpiece, and bent or broken tails (Figure 12-29). Obviously, for every tailless

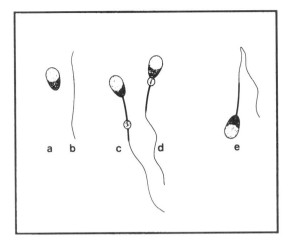

Figure 12-29. Diagrammatic representation of secondary spermatozoal abnormalities involving the midpiece and tail. Abnormalities depicted are tailless head (*a*), headless tail (*b*), distal protoplasmic droplets (*c*), proximal protoplasmic droplets (*d*), and bent tail (*e*).

head there is a headless tail, so the latter need not be counted. Protoplasmic droplets are distinct from swollen midpieces. Protoplasmic droplets are normally present while spermatozoa are in the epididymis. The droplets migrate caudally along the midpiece while the sperm cells mature in the epididymis. The droplets are usually shed before the spermatozoa leave the epididymis.

As a broad generalization, less than 20% of spermatozoa are abnormal in a normal animal and usually less than 10%. Higher percentages of abnormal spermatozoa may compromise fertility. Obviously, however, it is the total number of normal spermatozoa that is important, not the percentage of abnormal sperm.

OTHER CELLS IN SEMEN

Normal semen contains few (if any) leukocytes, erythrocytes or epithelial cells, and no bacteria or fungi. If present, their approximate quantity should be noted. If bacteria or fungi are observed without an inflammatory response, sample contamination by the normal preputial microflora should be suspected. Attention to preputial sanitation before sample collection should remedy the problem. If indicated, a semen sample may be submitted for microbiologic examination.

Cells from the germinal layers of the testis are a very unusual finding in semen and represent severe testicular damage. Such cells would include spermatids, spermatocytes, and large ciliated cells (often called medusa heads).

Precise categorization is unimportant, provided these cells are classified as immature sperm cells.

EVALUATION OF PROSTATIC SECRETIONS

Disorders of the prostate are not uncommon in dogs but they are rare in other domestic animals. Cells of prostatic origin can be collected by urethral catheterization, combined with prostatic massage (or penile massage) performed per rectum to stimulate prostatic secretion. Prostatic tissue can be aspirated by transcutaneous needle biopsy. Cytologic smears are prepared as outlined earlier in this chapter.

An enlarged prostate may be the result of prostatic hypertrophy, hyperplasia, metaplasia, neoplasia, or inflammation. Cytologic characteristics of these conditions are briefly considered following. Prostatic cells may occur singly or in clusters. Spermatozoa may be present in some fluid samples, especially those collected by penile massage.

NORMAL CELLS

Normal prostatic cells have a uniform size and shape, with a fairly high nucleus:cytoplasm ratio, transparent to gray cytoplasm, homogeneous nuclear chromatin, and no obvious nucleoli (Figure 12-30). Normal prostatic fluid or tissue contains few leukocytes.

PROSTATIC HYPERTROPHY

Hypertrophy refers to gland enlargement because of increased size of individual cells, without increased cell numbers. A hypertrophic prostate is not cytologically distinguishable from a normal prostate. The distinction is based on gland size at palpation or radiography.

PROSTATIC HYPERPLASIA

Hyperplasia refers to gland enlargement because of increased numbers of cells. The cells are uniform in size and appearance and have a high nucleus:cytoplasm ratio, basophilic cytoplasm that is often vacuolated, and a nucleus with a

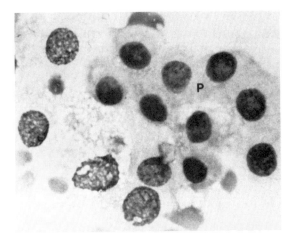

Figure 12-30. Cells in a prostatic biopsy from an old dog with prostatic adenocarcinoma. This field contains some normal prostatic cells (*P*) and some mechanically disrupted cells. (Wright's stain, 1050X)

"roughened" chromatin pattern, and a uniform, small single nucleolus. Few leukocytes are present.

Prostatic metaplasia

Metaplasia refers to a change (from normal) in the population of prostatic cells. Exfoliated or biopsied cells have the appearance of noncornified squamous epithelial cells. Consequently, they have a low nucleus:cytoplasm ratio and a somewhat pyknotic nucleus.

Prostatic neoplasia

Neoplasia is characterized by a pleomorphic population of cells with a high nucleus:cytoplasm ratio and very basophilic cytoplasm (Figure 12-31). Nuclear size varies among cells and they contain variable numbers of large, irregular (angular), and pleomorphic nucleoli.

Prostatic abscessation

A cytologic diagnosis of prostatic *abscessation* is based on finding large numbers of neutrophils in the fluid or tissue sample. Macrophages and lymphocytes may also be present in variable numbers.

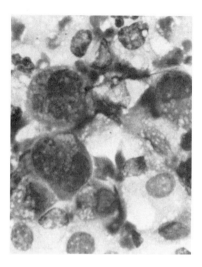

FIGURE 12-31. Needle aspirate from a prostatic adenocarcinoma in an old dog. Note the variation in the sizes of cells and nuclei and the high nucleus:cytoplasm ratio of several cells. Secretory vacuoles overlying the nucleus should not be confused with nucleoli. Some cells have been mechanically disrupted. Erythrocytes are present. (Wright's stain, 780X)

EXAMINATION OF MILK

Subclinical and clinical bovine mastitis (mammary gland infection) is an important economic concern for dairy farmers. Mastitis can be detected by several laboratory procedures. Those most frequently used indirectly or directly reflect milk nucleated cell counts and/or bacterial counts. Tests are performed on milk samples from individual quarters, all four quarters pooled together, or bulk milk (several cows together; usually the whole herd).

When individual animals are being screened, foremilk (sample obtained before milking begins) is generally used. It has more cells than a sample obtained in the middle of milking but fewer cells than one collected at the end of milking. Cell counts also vary with the stage of lactation. Milk samples from normal cows within the first week and at the end of lactation have higher cell counts than throughout the interim.

CALIFORNIA MASTITIS TEST

The California (rapid) mastitis test is a simple, rapid, "cowside" test that detects the amount of cellular nucleoprotein (specifically, DNA) in milk. The reagent comprises an anionic surface-active detergent (e.g., alkyl arylsulfonate) and a pH indicator (bromcresol purple).

The udder is cleaned (and disinfected if a specimen is concurrently collected for bacterial culture) before sample collection. A couple of streams of milk are often discarded because such milk is generally considered to reflect the bacterial and nucleated cell population of the teat canal rather than the mammary gland itself. If the sample cannot be tested immediately or is also being collected for bacteriologic examination and/or direct cell counts, it should be collected in a clean, dry, sterile bottle with an airtight seal.

Care must be exercised to avoid contamination of the bottle by debris and bacteria. As a precaution, the bottle may be held almost horizontally and the lid held with its inside facing down, while the milk is squirted in. About 2 ml are required for the California mastitis test and about 5 ml are often collected for bateriologic examination. It is very important to accurately identify each sample with respect to quarter and cow so that results can be properly recorded. The bottled specimen is refrigerated until used, preferably on the same day, but certainly within 36 hours. Heating, freezing, preservatives that denature protein (e.g., formalin), aging, and bacterial contamination of the sample must be avoided because they decrease the mastitis test reaction by destroying DNA.

Small amounts of milk and reagent are mixed by gentle swirling in the cups of a special plastic paddle (one cup is used for each quarter of the udder). The reaction is graded immediately, as outlined in Table 12-1. The intensity of the reaction is proportional to the number of neutrophils present.

Other "cow-side" mastitis tests, similar to the California mastitis test, include the field Whiteside test, the milk quality test, and the Michigan mastitis test. Laboratory procedures, usually for bulk milk specimens, to evaluate milk viscosity include the Brabant test and the Wisconsin mastitis test. As with the California mastitis test, all of these tests indirectly measure the concentration of "inflammatory products" (specifically, DNA), which do not necessarily correspond to the sample's bacterial content.

Microbiologic examination

Sample collection has been outlined previously, and microbiologic principles are detailed elsewhere (see Chapter 4). Numerous bacterial species have been implicated as causes of mastitis in cattle, including *Staphylococcus aureus, Escherichia coli,* and various species of *Streptococcus, Corynebacterium, Klebsiella, Mycobacterium,* and *Nocardia.*

Bacteria may be seen on direct smears of milk samples. Nucleated cell counts (indirect or direct) do not necessarily parallel bacterial numbers. For example, if nucleated cells are numerous and fairly effectively combating the infection, bacterial numbers may be low. In contrast, early in the course of an

TABLE 12-1. Recording and interpretation of California mastitis test results

SYMBOL	MEANING	DESCRIPTION OF VISIBLE REACTION	GENERAL INTERPRETATION
−	Negative	The mixture remains liquid, with no precipitation.	Less than 200,000 cells/ml, with about 0-25% neutrophils.
T	Trace	A slight precipitate forms. Seen most readily as the paddle is gently rocked back and forth. Continued rocking of the fluid may cause a trace reaction to disappear.	150,000-500,000 cells/ml, with about 30-40% neutrophils.
1	Weakly positive	A distinct precipitate, with no tendency to form a gel. Continued movement may dissipate the precipitate.	400,000-1,500,000 cells/ml, with about 40-60% neutrophils.
2	Distinctly positive	A thick precipitate, with gel formation. Continued swirling causes the mixture to move as a mass, exposing the bottom of the cup. Once halted, the precipitated mixture levels out to cover the bottom of the cup.	800,000-5,000,000 cells/ml, with about 60-70% neutrophils.
3	Strongly positive	A viscous gel, with convex (peaked) surface that usually remains after swirling is stopped. Tends to adhere to the bottom of the cup.	Generally more than 5,000,000 cells/ml and 70-80% neutrophils.
+	Alkaline	Deep-purple mixture.	Secretory activity of the udder is decreased, as in inflammation or drying-off.
y	Acidic	Yellow mixture.	Rare. Suggests fermentation of lactose by bacteria.

infection, bacterial numbers may be high while the neutrophil count is low (but increasing).

MISCELLANEOUS TESTS

Other procedures for detection of bovine mastitis in general veterinary practice have been largely superceded by such tests as the California mastitis test because of the latter's simplicity and reliability. Such procedures include the following:

pH.   Normal milk has a pH of 6.4 to 6.8. Abnormal milk may be more acidic, more alkaline, or normal in pH. Refrigerated or, preferably, freshly collected samples are added to a pH-sensitive dye, such as bromthymol blue or bromcresol purple. Measurement of pH is incorporated into the California mastitis test.

CATALASE TEST.   The catalase activity of normal milk is low. It increases in proportion to the elevation in cell numbers of the sample. It is not a "cow-side" test.

NUCLEATED (SOMATIC) CELL COUNT.   Nucleated cell counts (also called somatic cell counts) can be performed on fresh, well-mixed milk samples. A simple technique is to evenly spread 0.01 ml of milk over exactly 1 cm^2 of a clean microscope slide. (A card with 1 cm^2 borders marked on it can be placed under the slide.) The slide is air-dried, placed into modified Newman-Lampert stain for 2 minutes, drained, and air-dried, then gently washed in warm water to remove excess stain. The modified Newman-Lampert stain is made by adding 0.6 g of methylene blue chloride to a mixture of 52 ml of 95% ethanol and 44 ml of tetrachloroethane. This is stored at 4° to 7° C for 12 to 24 hours, then mixed with 4 ml of glacial acetic acid, filtered, and stored. This stain fixes and removes lipids from the smear, while staining nucleated cells and bacteria. Cells and bacteria tend to be more numerous at the center of the smear.

Such manual counts are really estimates of cell numbers. However, rigid standardization of procedures and use of an optical lens micrometer to measure microscopic field size increase accuracy. Such considerations are well reviewed elsewhere. Microscopic field area may vary among technicians, due to differences in interpupillary distance and eyepiece focal adjustment. Consequently, the field area at 1000X magnification can be measured with an ocular eyepiece micrometer. The equation to calculate microscopic field area at 1000X is area $= \pi d^2/4$. At 1000X magnification, field diameter (d) is often about 0.16 mm. Therefore, field area is about 2×10^{-4} cm^2 (1/5000 cm^2). The number of cells/ml of milk equals the average number of cells per 1000X magnification field multiplied by the microscope factor. The microscope factor is calculated as Microscope Factor $= 1$/field area $\times$ sample volume. In this example, the microscope factor is 500,000. Random examination of 20 to 50 fields is recommended to determine the average cell number per field.

Automated techniques are available for nucleated cell counts, including an electronic particle counter method (Coulter Milk Cell Counter: Coulter Electronics, Hialeah, FL) and a fluorescent dye technique (Fossomatic: Foss Electric, Hillerod, Denmark). However, equipment cost precludes their use in general veterinary practice.

Nucleated cell counts of normal milk are generally less than 300,000 to 500,000 cells/ml. Counts above 500,000 cells/ml indicate mastitis.

Differential cell counts are sometimes performed. Nucleated cells are categorized as neutrophils or mononuclear cells. Normal milk in mid-lactation generally has less than 10% neutrophils, whereas in severe acute mastitis, the milk may have up to 95% neutrophils.

EXAMINATION OF FECES FOR OCCULT BLOOD

A direct fecal smear, stained with Wright's stain, can be microscopically examined to look for intact erythrocytes in feces. However, unless the hemorrhage occurs in the terminal segments of the intestinal tract, erythrocytes are destroyed before passage in the feces. Reagent tablet tests (e.g., Hematest: Ames, Elkhart, IN) are available for detection of erythrocytes and/or hemoglobin in feces. The procedure relies on the peroxidase-like activity of hemoglobin to enhance the oxidation of a chromagen in the tablet to orthotoluidine, which has a blue color.

TECHNIQUE

A small quantity of fresh feces is smeared onto a filter paper square (provided with the kit) and placed on a clean, impermeable surface. A reagent tablet is placed on top of the center of the fecal smear and a drop of water is placed on top of the tablet. After 5 to 10 seconds, another drop of water is added and allowed to run down the side of the tablet. Blue discoloration of the filter paper at 2 minutes constitutes a positive reaction. Because blood or hemoglobin may not be evenly distributed in the feces, testing of more than one portion of a sample may be advisable. Obviously, hands and equipment must be free of blood contamination to avoid a false-positive result. A quality control can be run by using a 1:20,000 dilution of blood, instead of feces, in the test.

Because the test reagent cross-reacts with myoglobin of muscle, the animal should be fed a diet free of raw meat beginning at least 3 days before testing. Any meat in the diet must be well cooked to minimize the likelihood of a false-positive result. False positives can also be obtained if the diet is supplemented with iron or if compounds with peroxidase activity are present in the diet or are produced by intestinal bacteria.

Similar tests are available to examine vomitus (or gastric contents) for blood. These procedures are best used on specimens with a low pH.

TOXICOLOGY

The clinical signs and treatments of common poisonings of dogs, cats, horses, and food animals have been well reviewed in reference texts. Numerous agents may be involved, including herbicides, fungicides, insecticides, rodenticides, heavy metals (especially lead), household products (including phenols), automotive products (especially ethylene glycol), drugs (including medication), and various poisonous plants and animals. Often a presumptive diagnosis can be attained from an accurate history, including environmental factors, and a thorough clinical examination, followed by response to therapy or by necropsy. However, establishing a specific etiologic diagnosis can be quite difficult in some cases.

A few simple tests can be performed in the veterinary practice laboratory. In such situations, personnel must be familiar and competent with the test procedure, reagents must not be outdated, and special equipment may be required. These requirements, together with a sporadic demand for such tests, frequently dictate that practitioners send all toxicologic specimens to a specially equipped laboratory for analysis.

TOXICOLOGIC SPECIMENS

Suggestions on appropriate specimens and preferred methods of handling, packaging, and transport can be obtained by consultation with the toxicology laboratory. Such contact also ensures that the laboratory offers the procedures requested.

Submitted specimens should be free from contamination by extraneous environmental compounds or debris. Specimens should not be washed, as this may remove toxic residues. Samples of different fluids, tissues, feeds, etc., must be submitted in separate leakproof (airtight), clean, plastic, or glass containers. All containers should be individually identified by the owner's and veterinarian's names, animal's name or identification number, and the nature of the specimen before packaging into a large container for submission to the laboratory.

Samples of whole blood (at least 10 ml, usually heparinized), serum (at least 10 ml), vomitus, gastric lavage fluid, feces, and urine (about 50 ml) may be submitted from live animals. Samples of feed (portions of at least 200 g), water, suspected baits, etc., may also be helpful in some cases. In fatal poisoning, samples collected during a thorough necropsy should include whole blood or serum, urine, gut (especially stomach) contents (at least 200 g, noting site of collection), and organ or tissue samples, especially liver and kidney, but sometimes brain, bone, spleen, or fat (generally, where practical, at least 100 g of each tissue). Chapter 10 contains a detailed description of necropsy procedures. It is always better to send too large a sample, as excess can be discarded.

In general, serum or blood samples are best submitted refrigerated, whereas gut contents and tissues are best frozen. Preservatives are usually not required. An exception would be tissue samples submitted for histopathologic examination, which require fixation in 10% formalin and must not be frozen. If a preservative is used on a specimen submitted for chemical analysis, it is probably worthwhile to also submit an aliquot of preservative for reference analysis. Frozen samples should be insulated from other specimens and should arrive at the laboratory while still frozen. Dispatch to the laboratory by courier is recommended.

As litigation may result from poisoning cases, accurate and detailed records should be kept from the outset of the case. Establishment of a good working relationship with the toxicology laboratory, including provision of a good case history (and necropsy findings in fatal poisonings) when samples are submitted, helps ensure the best results.

The main advantages of the following tests are that they can be performed reasonably quickly in the practice laboratory. Results are therefore available more rapidly than if the sample were sent to a toxicology laboratory. However, they are best viewed as screening procedures, suggesting appropriate avenues of investigation and treatment. Verification of findings (especially positive ones) by a reputable toxicology laboratory is advisable, especially if subsequent legal action by the client is a possibility.

Lead poisoning

Lead is a fairly common environmental pollutant, not only in the air of cities, but also in old lead-based paints, lead shot (ammunition), linoleum, car batteries, solder, roofing materials, and petroleum products. Lead poisoning (plumbism) can occur in all species. Clinical signs vary with the species and are related chiefly to the GI tract and nervous system. Hematologic examination of blood from an animal with lead poisoning may reveal basophilic stippling of some erythrocytes and increased numbers of circulating nucleated red blood cells (metarubricytosis) (see also Chapter 2). Such findings in an animal that is not anemic and has clinical signs consistent with lead poisoning strongly suggest plumbism.

There are no simple, reliable tests to detect lead in blood, feces, urine, milk, or tissues. Blood lead levels can be readily determined (by atomic absorption spectrophotometry) at a toxicology laboratory on whole blood, collected in EDTA, heparin, or citrate blood tubes. Tissue samples (especially liver and kidney), feces, etc., can also be tested. Histopathologic examination of liver, kidney, or bone, stained by the Ziehl-Neelsen technique, may reveal characteristic eosinophilic, acid-fast intranuclear inclusion bodies in hepato-cytes, renal tubular cells, and osteoclasts, respectively.

One of the many toxic effects of lead involves inhibition of hemoglobin synthesis, with a consequent increase in delta-aminolevulinic acid (δ-ALA), a compound in the hemoglobin synthesis pathway. As a result, the blood δ-ALA concentration increases and, as enzyme is excreted by the kidney, the urinary δ-ALA concentration also increases. The latter can be easily measured by a commercially available kit (Davis Urinary ALA Test: Bio-Rad Labs, Richmond, CA). Only 0.5 ml of urine is required for the test.

Specimens should be refrigerated at 4° C until tested. As δ-ALA is unstable in alkaline urine, the sample should be acidified to a pH of 4 to 6 and refrigerated if analysis is to be delayed more than 4 hours. About 0.1 ml of glacial acetic acid usually acidifies 10 ml of urine to a pH of 4 to 6. At pH 5 and 4° C, δ-ALA is stable for at least 3 weeks.

Urine δ-ALA concentration can be quantitated by spectrophotometry at 535 nm. Alternatively, the reaction endpoint can be visually appraised. For example, normal dogs have a urinary δ-ALA concentration of less than 0.6

mg/dl, whereas dogs with lead poisoning have values above 1.0 mg/dl. On visual inspection, the former test solutions are yellowish, whereas the latter are obviously pink to red. The test is quite reliable as a screening procedure for diagnosis of clinical lead toxicity in the dog. However, it is not satisfactory for diagnosis of subclinical lead poisoning. The latter requires measurement of blood lead concentration or measurement of urine lead concentration changes after treatment for lead poisoning. The clinical usefulness of urinary δ-ALA measurement in other species of domestic animals is not well reported.

THALLIUM POISONING

Thallium is a potent, heavy-metal rodenticide that persists for long periods in the environment and is slowly metabolized in the body. It may be detected in the urine of poisoned animals within hours and up to 10 days after the onset of clinical signs. A qualitative test procedure follows.

A blank (distilled water), a standard (0.1 g of thallium sulfate in 100 ml of distilled water), and the urine specimen are tested concurrently. Three drops each of water, standard, and urine are added to each of three appropriately labeled 10-ml tubes. Three drops of bromine water are added to each and the tubes are agitated. (A saturated bromine water solution is made by dissolving bromine in distilled water. The solution should be prepared at least 12 hours in advance and stored in a glass-stoppered bottle.) If the resultant slight yellow color persists, no more bromine water is added. Otherwise, bromine water is added, by drops, with mixing, until the color remains. A 10% sulfosalicylic acid solution is added, by drops, with mixing, until the yellow color is just removed. At this stage, the urine mixture tube should be filtered to remove protein, which might otherwise cause a false-positive reading. Next, 1 drop of concentrated hydrochloric acid is added, followed by 1 to 2 drops of rhodamine B solution. (The latter is prepared by adding 0.05 g of rhodamine B to 100 ml of concentrated hydrochloric acid.) After mixing, 1 ml of benzene is added and the tubes are again agitated. Finally, the samples are centrifuged to separate the benzene and aqueous phases.

Purple or bluish discoloration of the benzene (upper) phase indicates a positive reaction. Reddish discoloration of the aqueous phase may occur in all tubes (because of rhodamine B). Color reactions are more easily evaluated against a white background. A positive reaction fluoresces yellow-green under ultraviolet light.

POISONING WITH OTHER HEAVY METALS

REINSCH TEST. The Reinsch test may be used to detect toxic quantities of antimony, arsenic, and mercury, as well as other metals, especially bismuth and silver.

A mixture of 10 ml of concentrated hydrochloric acid and 90 ml of distilled water is added to about 25 g of finely diced gut contents or tissue (usually kidney or liver) in a Pyrex beaker. A length of pure copper wire or foil, previously brightened with nitric acid or steel wool, is then placed into the beaker. A flask of cold water is placed over the mouth of the beaker and the beaker's contents gently boiled for about 45 minutes. The piece of copper is then removed, rinsed well in distilled water, and allowed to air dry. A positive reaction causes discoloration or coating of the copper.

Antimony produces a purple to blue-violet coating. Arsenic and bismuth cause a gray to black coating. If due to arsenic, this coating can be removed by placing the copper strip in 2 ml of 10% potassium cyanide. Bismuth (and antimony) deposits cannot be thus removed. Mercury produces a silvery deposit on the copper strip. Silver, and some other metals in high concentrations, can also cause discoloration or coating of the copper strip.

Positive tests should be confirmed by a toxicology laboratory.

POISONING BY PHENOLS

Phenolic compounds are present in numerous products, including some fungicides, herbicides, household disinfectants, photographic developers, and wood preservatives. They are rapidly absorbed through the skin or gut mucosa and can produce serious poisoning, especially in cats. Presumptive evidence of their presence can be obtained by testing urine samples.

The simplest test requires 10 ml of urine, to which is added 1 ml of a 20% ferric chloride solution (20 g in 100 ml of distilled water). Phenols are present if the mixture turns purple. Another test requires boiling a mixture of 10 ml of urine and 1 to 2 ml of Millon's reagent. Phenolic compounds produce a red color. The drawback of this procedure lies in the preparation of Millon's reagent, made by dissolving 10 g of mercury in 20 ml of nitric acid, diluting this 1:1 with distilled water and then allowing the mixture to stand for 2 hours before decanting the excess water.

NITRATE/NITRITE POISONING

Nitrate/nitrite poisoning may occur in ruminants, pigs, and horses ingesting feeds with high concentrations of these compounds. Such may be the case in cereals, grasses, and root crops heavily fertilized with nitrogenous compounds. Water, especially from deep wells filled with seepage from heavily fertilized ground, may contain large quantities of nitrate. Nitrates are converted to nitrites in the feed or within the intestinal tract. Nitrites, absorbed from the gut, decrease the oxygen-carrying capacity of the blood by degrading hemoglobin to methemoglobin in erythrocytes. Consequently, the animal's blood becomes dark-red to brown. The severity of clinical signs is related to the quantity ingested. Death can be acute and many animals can be affected.

A rapid, fairly specific, semiqualitative test uses diphenylamine, which is converted to quinodial compounds with an intensely blue color, by nitrates and nitrites. Diphenylamine (0.5 g) is dissolved in 20 ml of distilled water and the solution made up to 100 ml with concentrated sulfuric acid. This stock solution may be used undiluted or diluted 1:1 with 80% sulfuric acid. The solution is applied to the inner portion of the plant's stem. An intense blue color within 10 seconds of application of the undiluted solution suggests greater than 1% nitrate is present (and the feed is potentially toxic). False positives may occur with numerous substances, the most significant of which is iron. Such iron is generally on the outside of the stalk; thus, careful application circumvents this problem.

A more dilute diphenylamine solution (the previous stock solution diluted 1:7 with concentrated sulfuric acid) can be used to test for nitrates/nitrites in serum or plasma, other body fluids, and urine. Three drops of the diluted diphenylamine are added to 1 drop of the sample on a glass slide over a white background. Nitrate/nitrite produces an intense blue color immediately. Hemolysis may mask the color change.

ANTICOAGULANT RODENTICIDES

Anticoagulant rodenticides (e.g., warfarin, diphacinone, pindone) act by inhibiting metabolism of vitamin K in the body. The latter is required for production of factors II, VII, IX, and X in the liver. Anticoagulant rodenticide poisoning initially prolongs the prothrombin time (PT) because factor VII is the first to be depleted. Subsequently, the partial thromboplastin time (PTT) and activated coagulation time (ACT) are prolonged as the other factors also become depleted. When an animal is bleeding as a result of such poisoning, both the PT and PTT (or ACT) are usually prolonged. Diagnosis of anticoagulant rodenticide poisoning is commonly based on these "screening tests" and the response to treatment with vitamin K.

CHEMICALS THAT DENATURE HEMOGLOBIN

A variety of compounds, when ingested, may result in damage to (oxidative denaturation of) hemoglobin in erythrocytes, with the formation of Heinz bodies (see also Chapter 2). Such substances include paracetamol and methylene blue (cats), onions (dogs), red maple leaves (horses), and onions and brassicas (ruminants). Demonstration of Heinz bodies on a blood film is diagnostic of such poisoning.

Selenium-deficient animals are more prone to such oxidative injury because of a deficiency of glutathione peroxidase (an enzyme in erythrocytes that helps protect them against such damage).

ETHYLENE GLYCOL

Ethylene glycol is the major constituent of most antifreeze solutions. Accidental ingestion can cause serious or fatal toxicosis, usually in dogs and cats.

Ethylene glycol and its metabolites can be detected in whole blood or serum samples by a toxicology laboratory. Its presence is strongly suggested when urine sediments from poisoned dogs or cats contain masses of hippurate-like crystals and/or calcium oxalate crystals (Figure 12-32). The latter crystals may be oxalate monohydrate (morphology very similar to the hippurate-like crystals in Figure 12-32) or oxalate dihydrate (see Chapter 5). Histopathologic examination of the kidney of fatally affected animals reveals renal tubular nephrosis and numerous oxalate crystals. The latter are most readily seen under polarizing light.

SKIN BIOPSY

P.J. Ihrke

Skin biopsy is a valuable tool in diagnosis of skin diseases. In addition, skin biopsy may have benefits other than offering a diagnosis. Ruling out such

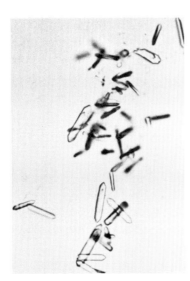

FIGURE 12-32. Crystals (presumably hippurate-like) in the urine sediment of a dog with ethylene glycol (antifreeze) poisoning. (Unstained, 345X) (Courtesy Dr. R.L. Cowell, Oklahoma State University.)

serious diseases as neoplasia may be of equal or greater importance. Skin biopsy also may be valuable in evaluating the prognosis and response to therapy.

In general, skin biopsies are not performed as often as they should be in veterinary practice. The potential usefulness of a skin biopsy, unfortunately, is often reduced by poor timing, poor selection of biopsy sites, and poor biopsy technique. If basic guidelines are followed as to when, what, and how to biopsy, the chances of deriving beneficial information from a skin biopsy are greatly increased.

INDICATIONS FOR SKIN BIOPSY

The most important reason for performing a skin biopsy is to establish a definitive diagnosis. A biopsy may be useful if a disease is not visually identifiable, other laboratory tests have not been diagnostic, or a disease has not responded to apparently rational therapy. Diseases that are clinically subtle or unusual also warrant biopsy. Most suspected or obviously neoplastic lesions should be biopsied. In addition, any severe or persistently ulcerated or eroded skin lesion should be sampled. In difficult cases, a biopsy may help rule out other diseases even though the suspected disease may not have definitive histopathologic characteristics.

Skin biopsy may also be used to formulate a prognosis. Biopsy may be helpful in assessing the degree of chronicity, determining the permanency of changes, or determining response to therapy.

Once an animal becomes a possible candidate for skin biopsy, the biopsy should be performed as soon as possible because chronicity, self-trauma, and topical or systemic therapy can potentially obscure a diagnosis. Lesions biopsied within 2 to 3 weeks after their development are much more likely to yield diagnostic results than those sampled long after they first appeared.

What to biopsy

If multiple lesions are present, those most representative should be sampled. Fully developed lesions are usually preferred to either very early or chronic lesions. An exception would be if a bullous autoimmune disease is suspected, as early lesions are more likely to be useful. Because the stage of the lesion may be very important in biopsy site selection, both the animal's owner and the veterinarian should be consulted when a site is selected. Traumatized lesions, acute ulcerations or chronic lesions often do not yield worthwhile results.

Smaller lesions should be resected in their entirety, or the advancing edge of a larger lesion should be biopsied.

Biopsy of ulcers or progressive ulcerative skin disease represents a special circumstance. Focal or indolent ulceration commonly reflects extensive preceding dermal changes (infectious, neoplastic, or collagenolytic diseases) underlying the ulcer. Consequently, diagnosis is accomplished by biopsy of the ulcer. Areas immediately adjacent to ulcers, as well as the ulcerated area, should be sampled in progressive ulcerative skin disease. The diagnostic lesion usually is present at the junction of the epidermis and dermis. The area at the margin of the ulcer with intact epithelium is critical to establishing a diagnosis, as sampling the ulcer provides the pathologist with a specimen of the dermis lacking the overlying epidermis.

If different stages of a disease are present, it may be beneficial to obtain multiple biopsy specimens. Often two or three tissue samples provide an answer, while a single sample may not. Most laboratories charge no more for processing and evaluating two or three samples than for a single sample. Consequently, multiple biopsies usually are indicated.

Ordinarily, the biopsy site should include abnormal skin only, particularly when the punch technique is used (see following). Identification of histopathologic lesions usually does not require comparison with normal skin. If hair loss is the primary clinical sign, the area of most complete hair loss should be selected. In addition, a separate specimen of normal skin should be sampled and identified for the pathologist. In this way, changes that might not be obvious in an isolated abnormal specimen may be clarified by comparison with a normal specimen.

Specimen selection for direct immunofluorescent testing or immunohistochemical testing is slightly different in that areas *directly adjacent* to well-developed new lesions (bullae or vesicles) should be sampled. The erythematous zone adjacent to a bulla or ulcer should be obtained for direct immunofluorescent tetsing if a bullous autoimmune disease is suspected. Lesional skin may yield false-negative immunofluorescent results because deposited immunoglobulins and complement may be swept away by inflammation.

Necessary instruments

A separate cold-sterilization tray containing the necessary instruments for performing a skin biopsy should be dedicated to this procedure. Because delicate handling of fragile biopsy specimens is imperative, the tray should include a small pair of curved iris scissors and several pairs of very fine eye forceps of various types. Small curved hemostats, a small needleholder, and suture scissors should also be available. The only necessary specialized instruments are Keyes cutaneous biopsy punches (4-, 6- and 8-mm disposable skin biopsy punches: Accuderm, Fort Lauderdale, FL). Used punches may be placed in the sterilization tray and reused until dull. Most disposable punches may be reused at least three or four times.

Methods of skin biopsy

Wedge Biopsy. Elliptic wedge biopsy specimens are commonly obtained with a scalpel. The wedge biopsy offers the advantages of a large, variably sized specimen that is easily oriented by the pathology technician. Solitary lesions are often best removed using this technique.

When a wedge biopsy specimen is taken, a sharp scalpel blade is used to totally excise the entire lesion, or the wedge is taken from an area of the lesion, through a transition zone, to normal tissue (Figure 12-33). The pathology technician then can trim the specimen on its long axis to provide the pathologist with a slide showing abnormal tissue, a transition zone, and normal tissue.

Excisional skin biopsy by the wedge method is indicated for solitary lesions. In addition, wedge biopsy is the method of choice if bullae or vesicles are

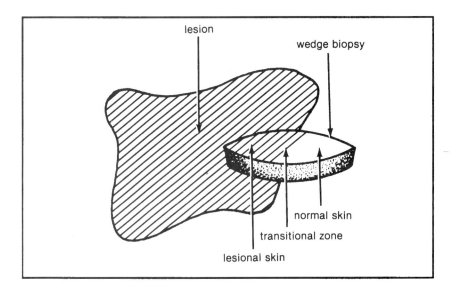

FIGURE 12-33. A wedge biopsy should include areas of the lesion, the transitional zone, and some normal skin.

present because it is potentially less traumatic to fragile tissues. A wedge biopsy is also recommended if diseases of the subcutaneous fat are suspected, as the subcutaneous fat is often lost when punch biopsy specimens are obtained.

The major disadvantage of the wedge biopsy technique is the time required to obtain the specimen. Because wedge biopsy procedures require substantially more time, may require general anesthesia, and require more sutures, wedge biopsy specimens are taken less frequently than warranted in many veterinary hospitals.

PUNCH BIOPSY. The punch biopsy technique has a number of advantages over wedge biopsy. Of greatest importance, the ease and speed of the procedure encourage more frequent use of skin biopsy. Using the biopsy punch, 4-mm specimens require no sutures and 6- or 8-mm biopsy specimens require only one or two sutures.

Sample selection is different for performing a punch biopsy than for obtaining wedge biopsy specimens. Only abnormal tissue is sampled by punch biopsy. If a significant portion of normal skin is obtained, rotation of the sample in the wrong direction during processing could result in histopathologic examination of only normal skin. Consequently, the plug of tissue is taken entirely within the boundary of the lesion. Ideally, two or three punch biopsy specimens of various lesions should be submitted.

SIZE OF THE SPECIMEN

Large specimens may not be adequately fixed in formalin. Therefore individual wedge biopsy specimens should never be more than 2 cm wide or long, regardless of the size of the lesion removed.

Disposable skin biopsy punches of 4 mm, 6 mm, and 8 mm diameter are used most commonly (Figure 12-34). The 4-mm biopsy punches usually are reserved for difficult sites, such as the planum nasale and the skin surrounding the eye. The 6-mm punch specimens generally are the minimal acceptable size, as specimens obtained from larger punches have more tissue to examine and less procurement artifact and thus are more likely to yield diagnostic lesions.

Michel's fixative and transport medium, used for direct immunofluorescence testing, does not penetrate tissue as readily as formalin. Consequently, specimens should not be thicker than 4 mm in diameter. A 4-mm punch biopsy specimen or tissue trimmed from a larger specimen may be used.

TECHNIQUE

Most biopsies are accomplished with local anesthesia and restraint. Occasionally, anesthesia or tranquilization is necessary for a fractious animal or cases involving biopsy of difficult body regions, such as the planum nasale, periorbital region, or footpads, where total restraint is crucial. General or dissociative anesthesia is required more often for feline skin biopsy.

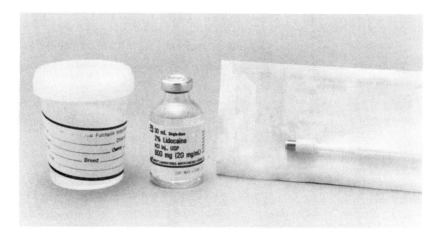

FIGURE 12-34.   Materials needed for punch biopsy include a disposable biopsy punch, lidocaine, and a container of fixative.

Haired prospective skin biopsy sites are carefully clipped to avoid skin irritation so as not to induce an inflammatory artifact. Cleansing of the site is neither recommended nor necessary. It is extremely important not to scrub the lesion or otherwise disturb any scales, crusts, or surface debris, as they may offer valuable diagnostic clues.

After clipping, the site is marked with an indelible marker (Sharpie: Sanford) and undermined with 1 to 2 ml of 2% lidocaine deposited subcutaneously using a 25- or 26-gauge needle. Rinsing the syringe barrel with epinephrine before filling it with lidocaine restricts spread of the anesthetic and aids hemostasis. One ml of lidocaine generally is sufficient for each skin biopsy site. Proper anesthesia is enhanced by gently repositioning the needle several times and depositing the anesthetic in a fan-like pattern. Because sensory nerves radiate peripherally from the spine, the recommended site of injection is the side of the biopsy site that is closest to the spinal column so that needle repositioning will not cause additional discomfort to the patient.

Local anesthesia with subcutaneous lidocaine should not be used if a disease of the subcutaneous fat (panniculitis) is suspected, as subcutaneous injection will damage the tissue to be evaluated. "Ring block" regional anesthesia or general anesthesia is recommended to obtain subcutaneous tissue without artifacts.

The biopsy specimen can be obtained about 5 minutes after injection of the local anesthetic. The indelible marker dots prevent inadvertent sampling of unanesthetized regions, as the bleb of local anesthetic may no longer be visible.

If a disposable biopsy punch is used, the punch is gently rotated in one direction until the punch blade has entered the subcutaneous tissue. The punch is rotated only in one direction because back-and-forth rotation increases the likelihood of specimen damage from shearing forces. With practice, a sudden easing of pressure will be noted when the punch has successfully entered the subcutaneous tissue.

Once the specimen has been cut free from the surrounding skin, either by the wedge or punch method, the specimen should be removed gently by grasping the margin or the underlying subcutaneous fat with a pair of fine forceps. If necessary, iris scissors can be used to detach the subcutis. Remember that fresh unfixed tissue is extremely fragile. The specimen is then blotted gently on a paper towel to remove excess blood and placed with the subcutaneous side down on a small piece of wooden tongue depressor or cardboard. Gently pressing the biopsy specimen flat facilitates adherence and allows proper anatomic orientation of the specimen in the laboratory.

Specimens with the attached "splint" are then immersed or floated specimen-side down in the fixative. Timely placement of the specimen in the fixative is critical, as artifactual changes may occur within 1 minute after the biopsy specimen is obtained. After these steps are accomplished, the biopsy site may be sutured. Postbiopsy complications, such as infection or dehiscence, are rare.

SPECIMEN HANDLING

Under most circumstances, 10% neutral phosphate-buffered formalin is the fixative of choice. When in doubt, consult the pathology laboratory. The volume of fixative should always be at least 10 times that of the specimen. Adequate specimen fixation requires at least 24 hours before processing. Formalin freezes at $-11°$ C $(-24°$ F), and this freezing can cause substantial artifactual damage in unfixed specimens. Therefore, to ensure proper fixation without freezing artifact, specimens should remain at room temperature for at least 6 hours before exposure to possible extreme cold.

Michel's transport medium and fixative is required for specimens to be processed for immunofluorescence studies. Specimens fixed in Michel's medium cannot be used for routine histopathologic examination. Properly buffered Michel's medium maintains its preservative properties over long periods in airtight containers.

Specimen mailers frequently are provided by pathology laboratories. Formalin-filled specimen containers should be sealed tightly and wrapped with tape to prevent leakage during transport. Because formalin can dissolve water-soluble ink, an indelible ballpoint pen should be used to write the history. Shipment of skin biopsy specimens in the same container with samples stored on ice is not recommended because freezing artifact can result.

Skin biopsy specimens for immunofluorescence or immunoperoxidase testing should be submitted concurrently with specimens for routine histopathologic examination. The pathologist can be requested to hold the specimen and to process it only if necessary for the diagnosis. In this way, time is saved in cases where immunologic studies are indicated, and money is saved in circumstances where these tests are not required to establish a diagnosis.

SUBMITTING THE SPECIMEN

The final step in the skin biopsy procedure is as important as the intermediate steps. The specimen should be sent to a laboratory most likely to arrive at the appropriate diagnosis. The first choice should be a laboratory with a veterinary pathologist with special expertise and an interest in dermatohistopathology. Because of the major differences between species, submission to a human medical pathologist is not recommended.

All biopsy specimens should be accompanied by the animal's breed, age and sex, clinical history, a physical description of the lesions, and clinical observations to aid the pathologist in histopathologic interpretation. Clinical findings, in fact, constitute the gross pathologic observations of the case and hence are critical. The more useful, legible information provided the more likely the pathologist will be able to provide useful diagnostic information.

References

1. Cowell and Tyler: *Diagnostic cytology of the dog and cat,* St Louis, 1989, Mosby.

2. Cowell and Tyler: *Hematology and cytology of the horse,* St Louis, 1992, Mosby.

3. DeNicola: Diagnostic cytology, collection techniques and sample handling, *Proc 4th Ann Mtg ACVIM,* 1987, pp 15-25.

4. Meyer: Management of cytology specimens, *Compend Cont Educ Pract Vet* 9:10-16, 1987.

5. Gross, et al: *Veterinary dermatopathology,* St Louis, 1992, Mosby, pp 3-7.

6. Littlewood: In Harvey and Mason: *Manual of small animal dermatology,* Shurdington, United Kingdom, 1993, BSAVA Publications, pp 33-44.

7. Moriello and Galbreath: In Moriello and Mason: *Handbook of small animal dermatology,* Oxford, United Kingdom, 1995, Pergamon Press, pp 45-48.

INDEX

A

Abdomen, opening, in necropsies, 514, *517*
Abdominal cavities, endoparasites of
  in horses, 345
  in ruminants/cattle, 341
Abdominal lymphocytes, in peritoneal fluid, 575-76
Abdominal worms
  of cattle/ruminants, 341
  of horses, 345
Abdominocentesis, for peritoneal fluid analysis, 572
Abortion specimens, 122-23
Abortions
  bacterial causes of, 129t, 132t, 133t, 140t, 141t,
    146t, 148t, 149t
  from *Campylobacter*, 189
    cultures for, 209
    staining for, 179t
  enzootic, 132t
  epizootic, bovine, 134t
  foothill, 132t
  Petriellidium boydii (Allescheria boydii) and, 231t
Abscessation, prostatic, 606
Abscesses
  bacterial causes of, 129t, 145t, 148t
  Gram stains and, 176, 177t
  jowl, bacterial causes of, 149t
  specimens from, 125-26
Acanthocephalans, 312
  in swine, 347
Acarina; *see* Mites; Ticks
Accuracy, 21, 23
Acetest Reagent Tablets (Ames), for urinary ketone
    analysis, 281
Acetoacetic acid, in urine, 280-81
Acetone, in urine, 280-81
Acetonemia, urine odor and, 271
Acid-fast granulomas, staining for, 181t, 183
Acid-fast stains
  for *Cryptosporidium* in feces, 366, 369
  diagnostic uses of, 181t-182t
  DMSO; *see* DMSO acid-fast stains
  fluorescent; *see* Fluorescent acid-fast stains
  Kinyoun; *see* Kinyoun acid-fast stains
  modified; *see* Modified acid-fast stains
  preparation of, 169
  procedure for, 173-74
  supplies for, 168
Acidity, of urine, 276-77
Acinebacter, primary identification of, 188t
Acquired immune system, 484
  cell-mediated, 486-87
  humoral, 484-86
ACT, 63
ACTH; *see* Adrenocorticotrophic hormone (ACTH)
Actinobacillosis, staining for, 178t, 183
Actinobacillus

differentiation between species of, 208, 208t
  primary identification of, 188t
  specimens for, 129t
  TSI slant/lysine decarboxylase and, 199t
Actinobacillus lignieresii, Gram staining for, 178t, 183
Actinobacillus seminis, vs. Brucella ovis, 208
Actinomyces
  primary identification of, 187t
  specimens for, 130t
  staining for, 177t
Actinomyces bovis, staining for, 178t, 183
Actinomyces (Corynebacterium) pyogenes
  cultures for, 209
  milk cultures for, 203
  tests for, 206
Actinomyces (H) pleuropneumoniae (parahemolyticus),
    cultures for, 211-12, 213t
Actinomyces viscosus
  staining for, 178t, 183, 190-91
  vs. nocardiosis, 208
Actinomycosis
  Gram staining for, 178t, 183
  vs. nocardiosis, 183
Activated clotting time (ACT), 63
Activated partial thromboplastin time (APTT), 64
Acute gastroenteritis, bacterial causes of, 149t
Acute nephritis
  proteinuria and, 279
  urinary casts and, 297, 298
Acute pharyngitis, bacterial causes of, 131t
Acute renal disease, urine specific gravity and, 274
Addison's disease, 466-67
  ACTH response test for, 467-68
Adenoviruses
  in cattle, 244t
  in dogs, 247t-248t
ADH, testing of, 461-63
Adnexa, endoparasites of
  in cats/dogs, 334
  in horses, 345
  in ruminants/cattle, 340
Adrenal axis, 466-68
Adrenal hyperplasia, bilateral, from tumors, 466
Adrenocortical function tests, 466-71
Adrenocorticotrophic hormone (ACTH)
  dexamethasone and, 470, 471
  endogenous concentrations of, 470-71
  testing response of, 466, 467-68
Adria Labs
  Bentiromide from, 446
  BT-PABA test from, 446
Adult stage, of anoplurans/mallophagans, 391
Aedes, 395-96
Aelurostrongylus abstrusus, in cats, 330-31, *332*
Aeromonas
  oxidation-fermentation test for, 193-94, 194t

627